Modelling Survival Data in Medical Research

Third Edition

CHAPMAN & HALL/CRC
Texts in Statistical Science Series

Statistical Theory: A Concise Introduction
F. Abramovich and Y. Ritov

Practical Multivariate Analysis, Fifth Edition
A. Afifi, S. May, and V.A. Clark

Practical Statistics for Medical Research
D.G. Altman

Interpreting Data: A First Course in Statistics
A.J.B. Anderson

Introduction to Probability with R
K. Baclawski

Linear Algebra and Matrix Analysis for Statistics
S. Banerjee and A. Roy

Analysis of Categorical Data with R
C. R. Bilder and T. M. Loughin

Statistical Methods for SPC and TQM
D. Bissell

Introduction to Probability
J. K. Blitzstein and J. Hwang

Bayesian Methods for Data Analysis, Third Edition
B.P. Carlin and T.A. Louis

Second Edition
R. Caulcutt

The Analysis of Time Series: An Introduction, Sixth Edition
C. Chatfield

Introduction to Multivariate Analysis
C. Chatfield and A.J. Collins

Problem Solving: A Statistician's Guide, Second Edition
C. Chatfield

Statistics for Technology: A Course in Applied Statistics, Third Edition
C. Chatfield

Bayesian Ideas and Data Analysis: An Introduction for Scientists and Statisticians
R. Christensen, W. Johnson, A. Branscum, and T.E. Hanson

Modelling Binary Data, Second Edition
D. Collett

Modelling Survival Data in Medical Research, Third Edition
D. Collett

Introduction to Statistical Methods for Clinical Trials
T.D. Cook and D.L. DeMets

Applied Statistics: Principles and Examples
D.R. Cox and E.J. Snell

Multivariate Survival Analysis and Competing Risks
M. Crowder

Statistical Analysis of Reliability Data
M.J. Crowder, A.C. Kimber, T.J. Sweeting, and R.L. Smith

An Introduction to Generalized Linear Models, Third Edition
A.J. Dobson and A.G. Barnett

Nonlinear Time Series: Theory, Methods, and Applications with R Examples
R. Douc, E. Moulines, and D.S. Stoffer

Introduction to Optimization Methods and Their Applications in Statistics
B.S. Everitt

Extending the Linear Model with R: Generalized Linear, Mixed Effects and Nonparametric Regression Models
J.J. Faraway

Linear Models with R, Second Edition
J.J. Faraway

A Course in Large Sample Theory
T.S. Ferguson

Multivariate Statistics: A Practical Approach
B. Flury and H. Riedwyl

Readings in Decision Analysis
S. French

Markov Chain Monte Carlo: Stochastic Simulation for Bayesian Inference, Second Edition
D. Gamerman and H.F. Lopes

Bayesian Data Analysis, Third Edition
A. Gelman, J.B. Carlin, H.S. Stern, D.B. Dunson, A. Vehtari, and D.B. Rubin

Multivariate Analysis of Variance and Repeated Measures: A Practical Approach for Behavioural Scientists
D.J. Hand and C.C. Taylor

Practical Longitudinal Data Analysis
D.J. Hand and M. Crowder

Logistic Regression Models
J.M. Hilbe

Richly Parameterized Linear Models: Additive, Time Series, and Spatial Models Using Random Effects
J.S. Hodges

Statistics for Epidemiology
N.P. Jewell

Stochastic Processes: An Introduction, Second Edition
P.W. Jones and P. Smith

The Theory of Linear Models
B. Jørgensen

Principles of Uncertainty
J.B. Kadane

Graphics for Statistics and Data Analysis with R
K.J. Keen

Mathematical Statistics
K. Knight

Introduction to Multivariate Analysis: Linear and Nonlinear Modeling
S. Konishi

Nonparametric Methods in Statistics with SAS Applications
O. Korosteleva

Modeling and Analysis of Stochastic Systems, Second Edition
V.G. Kulkarni

Exercises and Solutions in Biostatistical Theory
L.L. Kupper, B.H. Neelon, and S.M. O'Brien

Exercises and Solutions in Statistical Theory
L.L. Kupper, B.H. Neelon, and S.M. O'Brien

Design and Analysis of Experiments with R
J. Lawson

Design and Analysis of Experiments with SAS
J. Lawson

A Course in Categorical Data Analysis
T. Leonard

Statistics for Accountants
S. Letchford

Introduction to the Theory of Statistical Inference
H. Liero and S. Zwanzig

Statistical Theory, Fourth Edition
B.W. Lindgren

Stationary Stochastic Processes: Theory and Applications
G. Lindgren

The BUGS Book: A Practical Introduction to Bayesian Analysis
D. Lunn, C. Jackson, N. Best, A. Thomas, and D. Spiegelhalter

Introduction to General and Generalized Linear Models
H. Madsen and P. Thyregod

Time Series Analysis
H. Madsen

Pólya Urn Models
H. Mahmoud

Randomization, Bootstrap and Monte Carlo Methods in Biology, Third Edition
B.F.J. Manly

Introduction to Randomized Controlled Clinical Trials, Second Edition
J.N.S. Matthews

Statistical Methods in Agriculture and Experimental Biology, Second Edition
R. Mead, R.N. Curnow, and A.M. Hasted

Statistics in Engineering: A Practical Approach
A.V. Metcalfe

Statistical Inference: An Integrated Approach, Second Edition
H. S. Migon, D. Gamerman, and F. Louzada

Beyond ANOVA: Basics of Applied Statistics
R.G. Miller, Jr.

A Primer on Linear Models
J.F. Monahan

Applied Stochastic Modelling, Second Edition
B.J.T. Morgan

Elements of Simulation
B.J.T. Morgan

Probability: Methods and Measurement
A. O'Hagan

Introduction to Statistical Limit Theory
A.M. Polansky

Applied Bayesian Forecasting and Time Series Analysis
A. Pole, M. West, and J. Harrison

Statistics in Research and Development, Time Series: Modeling, Computation, and Inference
R. Prado and M. West

Introduction to Statistical Process Control
P. Qiu

Sampling Methodologies with Applications
P.S.R.S. Rao

A First Course in Linear Model Theory
N. Ravishanker and D.K. Dey

Essential Statistics, Fourth Edition
D.A.G. Rees

Stochastic Modeling and Mathematical Statistics: A Text for Statisticians and Quantitative Scientists
F.J. Samaniego

Statistical Methods for Spatial Data Analysis
O. Schabenberger and C.A. Gotway

Bayesian Networks: With Examples in R
M. Scutari and J.-B. Denis

Large Sample Methods in Statistics
P.K. Sen and J. da Motta Singer

Decision Analysis: A Bayesian Approach
J.Q. Smith

Analysis of Failure and Survival Data
P. J. Smith

Applied Statistics: Handbook of GENSTAT Analyses
E.J. Snell and H. Simpson

Applied Nonparametric Statistical Methods, Fourth Edition
P. Sprent and N.C. Smeeton

Data Driven Statistical Methods
P. Sprent

Generalized Linear Mixed Models: Modern Concepts, Methods and Applications
W. W. Stroup

Survival Analysis Using S: Analysis of Time-to-Event Data
M. Tableman and J.S. Kim

Applied Categorical and Count Data Analysis
W. Tang, H. He, and X.M. Tu

Elementary Applications of Probability Theory, Second Edition
H.C. Tuckwell

Introduction to Statistical Inference and Its Applications with R
M.W. Trosset

Understanding Advanced Statistical Methods
P.H. Westfall and K.S.S. Henning

Statistical Process Control: Theory and Practice, Third Edition
G.B. Wetherill and D.W. Brown

Generalized Additive Models: An Introduction with R
S. Wood

Epidemiology: Study Design and Data Analysis, Third Edition
M. Woodward

Practical Data Analysis for Designed Experiments
B.S. Yandell

Texts in Statistical Science

Modelling Survival Data in Medical Research

Third Edition

David Collett
NHS Blood and Transplant
Bristol, UK

CRC Press
Taylor & Francis Group
Boca Raton London New York

CRC Press is an imprint of the
Taylor & Francis Group, an **informa** business
A CHAPMAN & HALL BOOK

First edition published in 1994 by Chapman and Hall.

Second edition published in 2003 by Chapman and Hall/CRC.

Reprint 2019

CRC Press
Taylor & Francis Group
6000 Broken Sound Parkway NW, Suite 300
Boca Raton, FL 33487-2742

ISBN: 978-0-367-24100-1 (hbk)

Digitally Printed at Replika Press Pvt. Ltd.

Library of Congress Cataloging-in-Publication Data

Collett, D., 1952-
Modelling survival data in medical research / David Collett. -- Third edition.
pages cm. -- (Chapman & Hall/CRC texts in statistical science series)
"A Chapman & Hall book."
Includes bibliographical references and index.
ISBN 978-1-4398-5678-9
1. Survival analysis (Biometry) 2. Clinical trials--Statistical methods. I. Title.

R853.S7C65 2015
610.72'7--dc23

2014028554

Visit the Taylor & Francis Web site at
http://www.taylorandfrancis.com

and the CRC Press Web site at
http://www.crcpress.com

For sale in India, Pakistan, Nepal, Bhutan, Bangladesh and Sri Lanka only.

Contents

Preface

This book describes and illustrates the modelling approach to the analysis of survival data, using a wide range of examples from biomedical research. My experience in presenting many lectures and courses on this subject, at both introductory and advanced levels, as well as in providing advice on the analysis of survival data, has had a big influence on its content. The result is a comprehensive practical account of survival analysis at an intermediate level, which I hope will continue to meet the needs of statisticians in the pharmaceutical industry or medical research institutes, scientists and clinicians who are analysing their own data, and students following undergraduate or postgraduate courses in survival analysis.

In preparing this new edition, my aim has been to incorporate extensions to the basic models that dramatically increase their scope, while updating the text to take account of the wider availability of computer software for implementing these techniques. This edition therefore contains new chapters covering frailty models, non-proportional hazards, competing risks, multiple events, event history analysis and dependent censoring. Additional material on variable selection, non-linear models, measures of explained variation and flexible parametric models has also been included in earlier chapters.

The main part of the book is formed by Chapters 1 to 7. After an introduction to survival analysis in Chapter 1, Chapter 2 describes methods for summarising survival data, and for comparing two or more groups of survival times. The modelling approach is introduced in Chapter 3, where the Cox regression model is presented in detail. This is followed by a chapter that describes methods for checking the adequacy of a fitted model. Parametric proportional hazards models are covered in Chapter 5, with an emphasis on the Weibull model for survival data. Chapter 6 describes parametric accelerated failure time models, including a detailed account of their log-linear representation that is used in most computer software packages. Flexible parametric models are also described and illustrated in this chapter, while model-checking diagnostics for parametric models are presented in Chapter 7.

The remaining chapters describe a number of extensions to the basic models. The use of time-dependent variables is covered in Chapter 8, and the analysis of interval-censored data is considered in Chapter 9. Frailty models that allow differences between individuals, or groups of individuals, to be modelled using random effects, are described in Chapter 10. Chapter 11 summarises techniques that can be used when the assumption of proportional hazards cannot be made, and shows how these models can be used in comparing survival outcomes across a number of institutions. Competing risk models that accommodate different causes of death are presented in Chapter 12, while extensions of the Cox regression model to cope with multiple events of the same or different types, including event history analysis, are described in Chapter 13. Chapter 14 summarises methods for analysing data when there is dependent censoring, and Chapter 15 shows how to determine the sample size requirements of a study where the outcome variable is a survival time.

All of the techniques that have been described can be implemented in many software packages for survival analysis, including the freeware package R. However, sufficient methodological details have been included to convey a sound understanding of the techniques and the assumptions on which they are based, and to help in adapting the methodology to deal with non-standard problems. Some examples in the earlier chapters are based on fewer observations than would normally be encountered in medical research programmes. This enables the methods of analysis to be illustrated more easily, as well as allowing tabular presentations of the results to be compared with output obtained from computer software. Some additional data sets that may be used to obtain a fuller appreciation of the methodology, or as student exercises, are given in an Appendix. All of the data sets used in this book are available in electronic form from the publisher's web site at `http://www.crcpress.com/`.

In writing this book, I have assumed that the reader has a basic knowledge of statistical methods, and has some familiarity with linear regression analysis. Matrix algebra is used on occasions, but an understanding of linear algebra is not an essential requirement. Bibliographic notes and suggestions for further reading are given at the end of each chapter, but so as not to interrupt the flow, references in the text itself have been kept to a minimum. Some sections contain more mathematical details than others, and these have been denoted with an asterisk. These sections can be omitted without loss of continuity.

I am indebted to Doug Altman, Alan Kimber, Mike Patefield, Anne Whitehead and John Whitehead for their help in the preparation of the current and earlier editions of the book, and to NHS Blood and Transplant for permission to use data from the UK Transplant Registry in a number of the examples. I also thank James Gallagher and staff of the Statistical Services Centre, University of Reading, and my colleagues in the Statistics and Clinical Studies section of NHS Blood and Transplant, for giving me the opportunity to rehearse the new material through courses and seminars. I am particularly grateful to all those who took the trouble to let me know about errors in earlier editions. Although these have been corrected, I would be very pleased to be informed (`d.collett@btinternet.com`) of any further errors, ambiguities and omissions in this edition. Finally, I would like to thank my wife Janet for her support and encouragement over the period that this book was written.

David Collett
September, 2014

Chapter 1

Survival analysis

Survival analysis is the phrase used to describe the analysis of data in the form of times from a well-defined *time origin* until the occurrence of some particular event or *end-point*. In medical research, the time origin will often correspond to the recruitment of an individual into an experimental study, such as a clinical trial to compare two or more treatments. This in turn may coincide with the diagnosis of a particular condition, the commencement of a treatment regimen or the occurrence of some adverse event. If the end-point is the death of a patient, the resulting data are literally survival times. However, data of a similar form can be obtained when the end-point is not fatal, such as the relief of pain, or the recurrence of symptoms. In this case, the observations are often referred to as *time to event* data, and the methods for analysing survival data that are presented in this book apply equally to data on the time to these end-points. The methods can also be used in the analysis of data from other application areas, such as the survival times of animals in an experimental study, the time taken by an individual to complete a task in a psychological experiment, the storage times of seeds held in a seed bank or the lifetimes of industrial or electronic components. The focus of this book is on the application of survival analysis to data arising from medical research, and for this reason much of the general discussion will be phrased in terms of the survival time of an individual patient from entry to a study until death.

1.1 Special features of survival data

We must first consider the reasons why survival data are not amenable to standard statistical procedures used in data analysis. One reason is that survival data are generally not symmetrically distributed. Typically, a histogram constructed from the survival times of a group of similar individuals will tend to be *positively skewed*, that is, the histogram will have a longer 'tail' to the right of the interval that contains the largest number of observations. As a consequence, it will not be reasonable to assume that data of this type have a normal distribution. This difficulty could be resolved by first transforming the data to give a more symmetric distribution, for example by taking logarithms. However, a more satisfactory approach is to adopt an alternative distributional model for the original data.

The main feature of survival data that renders standard methods inappropriate is that survival times are frequently *censored.* Censoring is described in the next section.

1.1.1 Censoring

The survival time of an individual is said to be censored when the end-point of interest has not been observed for that individual. This may be because the data from a study are to be analysed at a point in time when some individuals are still alive. Alternatively, the survival status of an individual at the time of the analysis might not be known because that individual has been *lost to follow-up.* As an example, suppose that after being recruited to a clinical trial, a patient moves to another part of the country, or to a different country, and can no longer be traced. The only information available on the survival experience of that patient is the last date on which he or she was known to be alive. This date may well be the last time that the patient reported to a clinic for a regular check-up.

An actual survival time can also be regarded as censored when death is from a cause that is known to be unrelated to the treatment. However, it can be difficult to be sure that the death is not related to a particular treatment that the patient is receiving. For example, consider a patient in a clinical trial to compare alternative therapies for prostatic cancer who experiences a fatal road traffic accident. The accident could have resulted from an attack of dizziness, which might be a side effect of the treatment to which that patient has been assigned. If so, the death is not unrelated to the treatment. In circumstances such as these, the survival time until death from all causes, or the time to death from causes other than the primary condition for which the patient is being treated, might also be subjected to a survival analysis.

In each of these situations, a patient who entered a study at time t_0 dies at time $t_0 + t$. However, t is unknown, either because the individual is still alive or because he or she has been lost to follow-up. If the individual was last known to be alive at time $t_0 + c$, the time c is called a censored survival time. This censoring occurs after the individual has been entered into a study, that is, to the right of the last known survival time, and is therefore known as *right censoring.* The right-censored survival time is then less than the actual, but unknown, survival time. Right censoring that occurs when the observation period of a study ends is often termed *administrative censoring.*

Another form of censoring is *left censoring,* which is encountered when the actual survival time of an individual is less than that observed. To illustrate this form of censoring, consider a study in which interest centres on the time to recurrence of a particular cancer following surgical removal of the primary tumour. Three months after their operation, the patients are examined to determine if the cancer has recurred. At this time, some of the patients may be found to have a recurrence. For such patients, the actual time to recurrence is less than three months, and the recurrence times of these patients is left-censored. Left censoring occurs far less commonly than right censoring, and so the emphasis of this book will be on the analysis of right-censored survival data.

Yet another type of censoring is *interval censoring*. Here, individuals are known to have experienced an event within an interval of time. Consider again the example concerning the time to recurrence of a tumour used in the above discussion of left censoring. If a patient is observed to be free of the disease at three months, but is found to have had a recurrence when examined six months after surgery, the actual recurrence time of that patient is known to be between three months and six months. The observed recurrence time is then said to be interval-censored. We will return to interval censoring later, in Chapter 9.

1.1.2 Independent censoring

An important assumption that will be made in the analysis of censored survival data is that the actual survival time of an individual, t, does not depend on any mechanism that causes that individual's survival time to be censored at time c, where $c < t$. Such censoring is termed *independent* or *non-informative censoring*. This means that if we consider a group of individuals who all have the same values of relevant prognostic variables, an individual whose survival time is censored at time c must be representative of all other individuals in that group who have survived to that time. A patient whose survival time is censored will be representative of those at risk at the censoring time if the censoring process operates randomly. Similarly, when survival data are to be analysed at a predetermined point in calendar time, or at a fixed interval of time after the time origin for each patient, the prognosis for individuals who are still alive can be taken to be independent of the censoring, so long as the time of analysis is specified before the data are examined. However, this assumption cannot be made if, for example, the survival time of an individual is censored through treatment being withdrawn as a result of a deterioration in their physical condition. This type of censoring is known as *dependent* or *informative censoring*. The methods of survival analysis presented in most chapters of this book are only valid under the assumption of independent censoring, but techniques that enable account to be taken of dependent censoring will be described in Chapter 14.

1.1.3 Study time and patient time

In a typical study, patients are not all recruited at exactly the same time, but accrue over a period of months or even years. After recruitment, patients are followed up until they die, or until a point in calendar time that marks the end of the study, when the data are analysed. Although the actual survival times will be observed for a number of patients, after recruitment some patients may be lost to follow-up, while others will still be alive at the end of the study.

The calendar time period in which an individual is in the study is known as the *study time*.

The study time for eight individuals in a clinical trial is illustrated diagrammatically in Figure 1.1, in which the time of entry to the study is represented by a '•'.

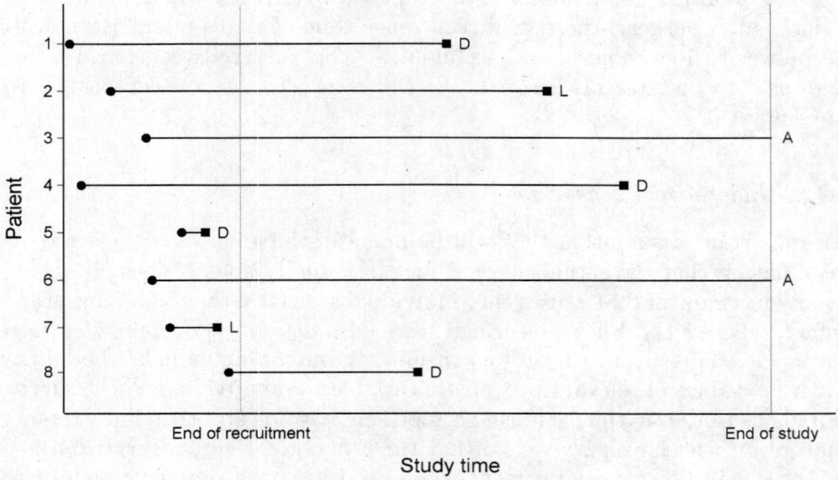

Figure 1.1 *Study time for eight patients in a survival study.*

This figure shows that individuals 1, 4, 5 and 8 die (D) during the course of the study, individuals 2 and 7 are lost to follow-up (L), and individuals 3 and 6 are still alive (A) at the end of the observation period.

As far as each patient is concerned, the trial begins at some time t_0. The corresponding survival times for the eight individuals depicted in Figure 1.1 are shown in order in Figure 1.2. The period of time that a patient spends in the study, measured from that patient's time origin, is often referred to as *patient time*. The period of time from the time origin to the death of a patient (D) is then the survival time, and this is recorded for individuals 1, 4, 5 and 8. The survival times of the remaining individuals are right-censored (C).

In practice, the actual data recorded will be the date on which each individual enters the study, and the date on which each individual dies or was last known to be alive. The survival time in days, weeks or months, whichever is the most appropriate, can then be calculated. Most computer software packages for survival analysis have facilities for performing this calculation from input data in the form of dates.

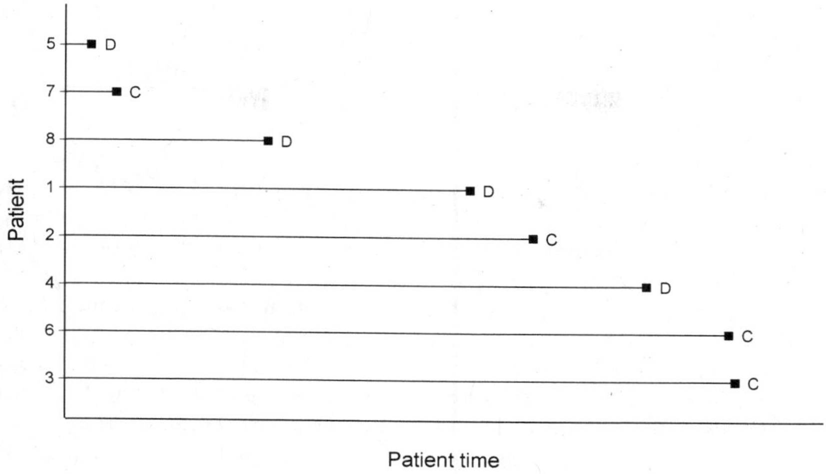

Figure 1.2 *Patient time for eight patients in a survival study.*

1.2 Some examples

In this section, the essential features of survival data are illustrated through a number of examples. Data from these examples will then be used to illustrate some of the statistical techniques presented in subsequent chapters.

Example 1.1 Time to discontinuation of the use of an IUD
In trials involving contraceptives, prevention of pregnancy is an obvious criterion for acceptability. However, modern contraceptives have very low failure rates, and so the occurrence of bleeding disturbances, such as amenorrhoea (the prolonged absence of bleeding), irregular or prolonged bleeding, become important in the evaluation of a particular method of contraception. To promote research into methods for analysing menstrual bleeding data from women in contraceptive trials, the World Health Organisation made available data from clinical trials involving a number of different types of contraceptive (WHO, 1987). Part of this data set relates to the time from which a woman commences use of a particular method until discontinuation, with the discontinuation reason being recorded when known. The data in Table 1.1 refer to the number of weeks from the commencement of use of a particular type of intrauterine device (IUD), known as the Multiload 250, until discontinuation because of menstrual bleeding problems. Data are given for 18 women, all of whom were aged between 18 and 35 years and who had experienced two previous pregnancies. Discontinuation times that are censored are labelled with an asterisk.

In this example, the time origin corresponds to the first day in which a woman uses the IUD, and the end-point is discontinuation because of bleed-

Table 1.1 *Time in weeks to discontinuation of the use of an IUD.*

10	13*	18*	19	23*	30	36	38*	54*
56*	59	75	93	97	104*	107	107*	107*

* Censored discontinuation times.

ing problems. Some women in the study ceased using the IUD because of the desire for pregnancy, or because they had no further need for a contraceptive, while others were simply lost to follow-up. These reasons account for the censored discontinuation times of 13, 18, 23, 38, 54 and 56 weeks. The study protocol called for the menstrual bleeding experience of each woman to be documented for a period of two years from the time origin. For practical reasons, each woman could not be examined exactly two years after recruitment to determine if they were still using the IUD, and this is why there are three discontinuation times greater than 104 weeks that are right-censored.

One objective in an analysis of these data would be to summarise the distribution of discontinuation times. We might then wish to estimate the median time to discontinuation of the IUD, or the probability that a woman will stop using the device after a given period of time. Indeed, a graph of this estimated probability, as a function of time, will provide a useful summary of the observed data.

Example 1.2 Prognosis for women with breast cancer

Breast cancer is one of the most common forms of cancer occurring in women living in the Western world. However, the biological behaviour of the tumour is often unpredictable, and a number of studies have focussed on whether the tumour is likely to have metastasised, or spread, to other organs in the body. Around 80% of women presenting with primary breast cancer are likely to have tumours that have already metastasised to other sites. If these patients could be identified, adjunctive treatment could be focussed on them, while the remaining 20% could be reassured that their disease is surgically curable.

The aim of an investigation carried out at the Middlesex Hospital, documented in Leathem and Brooks (1987), was to evaluate a histochemical marker that discriminates between primary breast cancer that has metastasised and that which has not. The marker under study was a lectin from the albumin gland of the Roman snail, *Helix pomatia*, known as *Helix pomatia* agglutinin, or HPA. The marker binds to those breast cancer cells associated with metastasis to local lymph nodes, and the HPA stained cells can be identified by microscopic examination. In order to investigate whether HPA staining can be used to predict the survival experience of women who present with breast cancer, a retrospective study was carried out, based on the records of women who had received surgical treatment for breast cancer. Sections of the tumours of these women were treated with HPA and each tumour was subsequently classified as being positively or negatively stained, positive staining corresponding to a tumour with the potential for metastasis. The study was concluded in July

1987, when the survival times of those women who had died of breast cancer were calculated. For those women whose survival status in July 1987 was unknown, the time from surgery to the date on which they were last known to be alive is regarded as a censored survival time. The survival times of women who had died from causes other than breast cancer are also regarded as right-censored. The data given in Table 1.2 refer to the survival times in months of women who had received a simple or radical mastectomy to treat a tumour of Grade II, III or IV, between January 1969 and December 1971. In the table, the survival times of each woman are classified according to whether their tumour was positively or negatively stained.

Table 1.2 *Survival times of women with tumours that were negatively or positively stained with HPA.*

Negative staining	Positive staining	
23	5	68
47	8	71
69	10	76*
70*	13	105*
71*	18	107*
100*	24	109*
101*	26	113
148	26	116*
181	31	118
198*	35	143
208*	40	154*
212*	41	162*
224*	48	188*
	50	212*
	59	217*
	61	225*

* Censored survival times.

In the analysis of the data from this study, we will be particularly interested in whether or not there is a difference in the survival experience of the two groups of women. If there were evidence that those women with negative HPA staining tended to live longer after surgery than those with positive staining, we would conclude that the prognosis for a breast cancer patient was dependent on the result of the staining procedure.

Example 1.3 Survival of multiple myeloma patients

Multiple myeloma is a malignant disease characterised by the accumulation of abnormal plasma cells, a type of white blood cell, in the bone marrow. The proliferation of the abnormal plasma cells within the bone causes pain and the destruction of bone tissue. Patients with multiple myeloma also experience anaemia, haemorrhages, recurrent infections and weakness. Unless treated, the condition is invariably fatal. The aim of a study carried out at the Medical Center of the University of West Virginia, USA, was to examine the association between the values of certain *explanatory variables* or *covariates* and the survival time of patients. In the study, the primary response variable was the time, in months, from diagnosis until death from multiple myeloma.

The data in Table 1.3, which were obtained from Krall, Uthoff and Harley (1975), relate to 48 patients, all of whom were aged between 50 and 80 years. Some of these patients had not died by the time that the study was completed, and so these individuals contribute right-censored survival times. The coding of the survival status of an individual in the table is such that zero denotes a censored observation and unity death from multiple myeloma.

At the time of diagnosis, the values of a number of explanatory variables were recorded for each patient. These included the age of the patient in years, their sex (1 = male, 2 = female), the levels of blood urea nitrogen (*Bun*), serum calcium (*Ca*) and haemoglobin (*Hb*), the percentage of plasma cells in the bone marrow (*Pcells*) and an indicator variable (*Protein*) that denotes whether or not the Bence-Jones protein was present in the urine (0 = absent, 1 = present).

The main aim of an analysis of these data would be to investigate the effect of the risk factors *Bun*, *Ca*, *Hb*, *Pcells* and *Protein* on the survival time of the multiple myeloma patients. The effects of these risk factors may be modified by the age or sex of a patient, and so the extent to which the relationship between survival and the important risk factors is consistent for each sex and for each of a number of age groups will also need to be studied.

Example 1.4 Comparison of two treatments for prostatic cancer

A randomised controlled clinical trial to compare treatments for prostatic cancer was begun in 1967 by the Veteran's Administration Cooperative Urological Research Group. The trial was double-blind and two of the treatments used in the study were a placebo and 1.0 mg of diethylstilbestrol (DES). The treatments were administered daily by mouth. The time origin of the study is the date on which a patient was randomised to a treatment, and the end-point is the death of the patient from prostatic cancer.

The full data set is given in Andrews and Herzberg (1985), but the data used in this example are from patients presenting with Stage III cancer, that is, patients for whom there was evidence of a local extension of the tumour beyond the prostatic capsule, but without elevated serum prostatic acid phosphatase. Furthermore, the patients were those who had no history of cardiovascular disease, had a normal ECG result at trial entry, and who were not confined to bed during the daytime. In addition to recording the survival time of each patient in the study, information was recorded on a number of other prognostic factors. These included the age of the patient at trial entry, their serum haemoglobin level in gm/100 ml, the size of their primary tumour in cm^2 and the value of a combined index of tumour stage and grade. This index is known as the Gleason index; the more advanced the tumour, the greater the value of the index.

Table 1.3 *Survival times of patients in a study on multiple myeloma.*

Patient number	Survival time	Status	Age	Sex	*Bun*	*Ca*	*Hb*	*Pcells*	*Protein*
1	13	1	66	1	25	10	14.6	18	1
2	52	0	66	1	13	11	12.0	100	0
3	6	1	53	2	15	13	11.4	33	1
4	40	1	69	1	10	10	10.2	30	1
5	10	1	65	1	20	10	13.2	66	0
6	7	0	57	2	12	8	9.9	45	0
7	66	1	52	1	21	10	12.8	11	1
8	10	0	60	1	41	9	14.0	70	1
9	10	1	70	1	37	12	7.5	47	0
10	14	1	70	1	40	11	10.6	27	0
11	16	1	68	1	39	10	11.2	41	0
12	4	1	50	2	172	9	10.1	46	1
13	65	1	59	1	28	9	6.6	66	0
14	5	1	60	1	13	10	9.7	25	0
15	11	0	66	2	25	9	8.8	23	0
16	10	1	51	2	12	9	9.6	80	0
17	15	0	55	1	14	9	13.0	8	0
18	5	1	67	2	26	8	10.4	49	0
19	76	0	60	1	12	12	14.0	9	0
20	56	0	66	1	18	11	12.5	90	0
21	88	1	63	1	21	9	14.0	42	1
22	24	1	67	1	10	10	12.4	44	0
23	51	1	60	2	10	10	10.1	45	1
24	4	1	74	1	48	9	6.5	54	0
25	40	0	72	1	57	9	12.8	28	1
26	8	1	55	1	53	12	8.2	55	0
27	18	1	51	1	12	15	14.4	100	0
28	5	1	70	2	130	8	10.2	23	0
29	16	1	53	1	17	9	10.0	28	0
30	50	1	74	1	37	13	7.7	11	1
31	40	1	70	2	14	9	5.0	22	0
32	1	1	67	1	165	10	9.4	90	0
33	36	1	63	1	40	9	11.0	16	1
34	5	1	77	1	23	8	9.0	29	0
35	10	1	61	1	13	10	14.0	19	0
36	91	1	58	2	27	11	11.0	26	1
37	18	0	69	2	21	10	10.8	33	0
38	1	1	57	1	20	9	5.1	100	1
39	18	0	59	2	21	10	13.0	100	0
40	6	1	61	2	11	10	5.1	100	0
41	1	1	75	1	56	12	11.3	18	0
42	23	1	56	2	20	9	14.6	3	0
43	15	1	62	2	21	10	8.8	5	0
44	18	1	60	2	18	9	7.5	85	1
45	12	0	71	2	46	9	4.9	62	0
46	12	1	60	2	6	10	5.5	25	0
47	17	1	65	2	28	8	7.5	8	0
48	3	0	59	1	90	10	10.2	6	1

Table 1.4 gives the data recorded for 38 patients, where the survival times are given in months. The survival times of patients who died from other causes, or who were lost during the follow-up process, are regarded as censored. A variable associated with the status of an individual at the end of the study takes the value unity if the patient has died from prostatic cancer, and zero if the survival time is right-censored. The variable associated with the treatment group takes the value 2 when an individual is treated with DES and unity if an individual is on the placebo treatment.

The main aim of this study is to determine the extent of any evidence that patients treated with DES survive longer than those treated with the placebo. Since the data on which this example is based are from a randomised trial, one might expect that the distributions of the prognostic factors, that is the age of patient, serum haemoglobin level, size of tumour and Gleason index, will be similar over the patients in each of the two treatment groups. However, it would not be wise to rely on this assumption. For example, it could turn out that patients in the placebo group had larger tumours on average than those in the group treated with DES. If patients with large tumours have a poorer prognosis than those with small tumours, the size of the treatment effect would be overestimated, unless proper account was taken of the size of the tumour in the analysis. Consequently, it will first be necessary to determine if any of the covariates are related to survival time. If so, the effect of these variables will need to be allowed for when comparing the survival experiences of the patients in the two treatment groups.

1.3 Survivor, hazard and cumulative hazard functions

In summarising survival data, there are three functions of central interest, namely the *survivor function*, the *hazard function*, and the *cumulative hazard function*. These functions are therefore defined in this first chapter.

1.3.1 The survivor function

The actual survival time of an individual, t, can be regarded as the observed value of a variable, T, that can take any non-negative value. The different values that T can take have a *probability distribution*, and we call T the *random variable* associated with the survival time. Now suppose that this random variable has a probability distribution with underlying *probability density function* $f(t)$. The *distribution function* of T is then given by

$$F(t) = \mathrm{P}(T < t) = \int_0^t f(u)\,\mathrm{d}u, \tag{1.1}$$

and represents the probability that the survival time is less than some value t. This function is also called the *cumulative incidence function*, since it summarises the cumulative probability of death occurring before time t.

Table 1.4 *Survival times of prostatic cancer patients in a clinical trial to compare two treatments.*

Patient number	Treatment	Survival time	Status	Age	Serum haem.	Size of tumour	Gleason index
1	1	65	0	67	13.4	34	8
2	2	61	0	60	14.6	4	10
3	2	60	0	77	15.6	3	8
4	1	58	0	64	16.2	6	9
5	2	51	0	65	14.1	21	9
6	1	51	0	61	13.5	8	8
7	1	14	1	73	12.4	18	11
8	1	43	0	60	13.6	7	9
9	2	16	0	73	13.8	8	9
10	1	52	0	73	11.7	5	9
11	1	59	0	77	12.0	7	10
12	2	55	0	74	14.3	7	10
13	2	68	0	71	14.5	19	9
14	2	51	0	65	14.4	10	9
15	1	2	0	76	10.7	8	9
16	1	67	0	70	14.7	7	9
17	2	66	0	70	16.0	8	9
18	2	66	0	70	14.5	15	11
19	2	28	0	75	13.7	19	10
20	2	50	1	68	12.0	20	11
21	1	69	1	60	16.1	26	9
22	1	67	0	71	15.6	8	8
23	2	65	0	51	11.8	2	6
24	1	24	0	71	13.7	10	9
25	2	45	0	72	11.0	4	8
26	2	64	0	74	14.2	4	6
27	1	61	0	75	13.7	10	12
28	1	26	1	72	15.3	37	11
29	1	42	1	57	13.9	24	12
30	2	57	0	72	14.6	8	10
31	2	70	0	72	13.8	3	9
32	2	5	0	74	15.1	3	9
33	2	54	0	51	15.8	7	8
34	1	36	1	72	16.4	4	9
35	2	70	0	71	13.6	2	10
36	2	67	0	73	13.8	7	8
37	1	23	0	68	12.5	2	8
38	1	62	0	63	13.2	3	8

The survivor function, $S(t)$, is defined to be the probability that the survival time is greater than or equal to t, and so from Equation (1.1),

$$S(t) = \mathrm{P}(T \geqslant t) = 1 - F(t). \tag{1.2}$$

The survivor function can therefore be used to represent the probability that an individual survives beyond any given time.

1.3.2 The hazard function

The *hazard function* is widely used to express the risk or hazard of an event such as death occurring at some time t. This function is obtained from the probability that an individual dies at time t, conditional on he or she having survived to that time. For a formal definition of the hazard function, consider the probability that the random variable associated with an individual's survival time, T, lies between t and $t + \delta t$, conditional on T being greater than or equal to t, written $\mathrm{P}(t \leqslant T < t + \delta t \mid T \geqslant t)$. This conditional probability is then expressed as a probability per unit time by dividing by the time interval, δt, to give a *rate*. The hazard function, $h(t)$, is then the limiting value of this quantity, as δt tends to zero, so that

$$h(t) = \lim_{\delta t \to 0} \left\{ \frac{\mathrm{P}(t \leqslant T < t + \delta t \mid T \geqslant t)}{\delta t} \right\}. \tag{1.3}$$

The function $h(t)$ is also referred to as the *hazard rate*, the *instantaneous death rate*, the *intensity rate* or the *force of mortality*.

From the definition of the hazard function in Equation (1.3), $h(t)$ is the event rate at time t, conditional on the event not having occurred before t. Specifically, if the survival time is measured in days, $h(t)$ is the approximate probability that an individual, who is at risk of the event occurring at the start of day t, experiences the event during that day. The hazard function at time t can also be regarded as the expected number of events experienced by an individual in unit time, given that the event has not occurred before then, and assuming that the hazard is constant over that time period.

The definition of the hazard function in Equation (1.3) leads to some useful relationships between the survivor and hazard functions. According to a standard result from probability theory, the probability of an event A, conditional on the occurrence of an event B, is given by $\mathrm{P}(A \mid B) = \mathrm{P}(AB)/\mathrm{P}(B)$, where $\mathrm{P}(AB)$ is the probability of the joint occurrence of A and B. Using this result, the conditional probability in the definition of the hazard function in Equation (1.3) is

$$\frac{\mathrm{P}(t \leqslant T < t + \delta t)}{\mathrm{P}(T \geqslant t)},$$

which is equal to

$$\frac{F(t + \delta t) - F(t)}{S(t)},$$

where $F(t)$ is the distribution function of T. Then,

$$h(t) = \lim_{\delta t \to 0} \left\{ \frac{F(t + \delta t) - F(t)}{\delta t} \right\} \frac{1}{S(t)}.$$

Now,

$$\lim_{\delta t \to 0} \left\{ \frac{F(t + \delta t) - F(t)}{\delta t} \right\}$$

is the definition of the derivative of $F(t)$ with respect to t, which is $f(t)$, and so

$$h(t) = \frac{f(t)}{S(t)}. \tag{1.4}$$

Taken together, Equations (1.1), (1.2) and (1.4) show that from any one of the three functions, $f(t)$, $S(t)$, and $h(t)$, the other two can be determined.

1.3.3 *The cumulative hazard function*

From Equation (1.4), it follows that

$$h(t) = -\frac{\mathrm{d}}{\mathrm{d}t}\{\log S(t)\}, \tag{1.5}$$

and so

$$S(t) = \exp\{-H(t)\}, \tag{1.6}$$

where

$$H(t) = \int_0^t h(u)\,\mathrm{d}u. \tag{1.7}$$

The function $H(t)$ features widely in survival analysis, and is called the *integrated* or *cumulative hazard function*. From Equation (1.6), the cumulative hazard function can also be obtained from the survivor function, since

$$H(t) = -\log S(t). \tag{1.8}$$

The cumulative hazard function, $H(t)$, is the cumulative risk of an event occurring by time t. If the event is death, then $H(t)$ summarises the risk of death up to time t, given that death has not occurred before t. The cumulative hazard function at time t can also be interpreted as the expected number of events that occur in the interval from the time origin to t.

It is possible for the cumulative hazard function to exceed unity. Using Equation (1.8), $H(t) \geqslant 1$, when $-\log S(t) \geqslant 1$, that is when $S(t) \leqslant e^{-1} = 0.37$. The cumulative hazard is then greater than unity when the probability of an event occurring after time t is less than 0.37, and means that more than one event is expected in the time interval $(0, t)$. The survivor function, $S(t)$, is then more correctly defined as the probability that one *or more* events occur after time t. The interpretation of a cumulative hazard function in terms of the expected number of events is only reasonable when repetitions of an event are possible, such as when the event is the occurrence of an infection, migraine or seizure. When the event of interest is death, this interpretation relies on individuals being immediately resurrected after death has occurred! Methods for analysing times to multiple occurrences of an event are considered later in Chapter 13, and a more mathematical interpretation of the hazard and cumulative hazard functions when multiple events are possible is included in Section 13.1 of that chapter.

In the analysis of survival data, the survivor function, hazard function and cumulative hazard function are estimated from the observed survival times. Methods of estimation that do not require the form of the probability density function of T to be specified are described in Chapters 2 and 3, while methods based on the assumption of a particular survival time distribution are presented in Chapters 5 and 6.

1.4 Computer software for survival analysis

Most of the techniques for analysing survival data that will be presented in this book require suitable computer software for their implementation. Many computer packages for survival analysis are now available, but of the commercially available software packages, SAS (SAS Institute Inc.), S-PLUS (TIBCO Software Inc.) and Stata (StataCorp) have the most extensive range of facilities. In addition, the R statistical computing environment (R Core Team, 2013) is free software, distributed under the terms of the GNU General Public License. Both S-PLUS and R are modern implementations of the S statistical programming language, and include a comprehensive range of modules for survival analysis. Any of these four packages can be used to carry out the analyses described in subsequent chapters of this book.

In this book, the data sets used to illustrate the different methods of survival analysis have been analysed using SAS 9.4 (SAS Institute, Cary NC), mainly using the procedures `lifetest`, `lifereg` and `phreg`. Where published SAS macros have been used for more specialised analyses, these are documented in the 'Further reading' section of each chapter.

In some circumstances, numerical results in the output produced by software packages may differ. This is often due to different default methods of calculation being used. A particularly important example of this occurs when a data set includes two or more individuals with the same survival times. In this case, the SAS `phreg` procedure and the R package `survival` (Therneau, 2014) default to different methods of handling these tied observations, leading to differences in the output. The default settings can of course be changed, and the treatment of tied survival times is described in Section 3.3.2 of Chapter 3. Differences in numerical values may also result from different settings being used for parameters that control the convergence of certain iterative procedures, and different methods being used for numerical optimisation.

1.5 Further reading

An introduction to the techniques used in the analysis of survival data is included in a number of general books on statistics in medical research, such as those of Altman (1991) and Armitage, Berry and Matthews (2002). Machin, Cheung and Parmar (2006) provide a practical guide to the analysis of survival data from clinical trials, using non-technical language.

There a number of textbooks that provide an introduction to the methods of survival analysis, illustrated with practical examples. Lee and Wang (2013) provides a broad coverage of topics with illustrations drawn from biology and medicine, and Marubini and Valsecchi (1995) describe the analysis of survival data from clinical trials and observational studies. Hosmer, Lemeshow and May (2008) give a balanced account of survival analysis, with excellent chapters on model development and the interpretation of the parameter estimates in a fitted model. Klein and Moeschberger (2005) include many example data sets and exercises in their comprehensive textbook, and Kleinbaum and Klein (2012) provide a self-learning text on survival analysis. Applications of survival analysis in the analysis of epidemiological data are described by Breslow and Day (1987) and Woodward (2014). Introductory texts that describe the application of survival analysis in other areas include those of Crowder et al. (1991) who focus on the analysis of reliability data, and Box-Steffensmeier and Jones (2004) who give a non-mathematical account of time to event analysis in the social sciences.

Comprehensive accounts of the subject are given by Kalbfleisch and Prentice (2002) and Lawless (2002). These books have been written for the postgraduate statistician or research worker, and are usually regarded as reference books rather than introductory texts. A concise review of survival analysis is given in the research monograph of Cox and Oakes (1984), and in the chapter devoted to this subject in Hinkley, Reid and Snell (1991). The book by Hougaard (2000) on multivariate survival data incorporates more advanced topics, after introductory chapters that cover the basic features of survival analysis. Therneau and Grambsch (2000) base their presentation of survival analysis on the counting process approach, leading to a more mathematical development of the material. Harrell (2001) gives details on many issues that arise in the development of a statistical model not found in other texts, and includes an extensive discussion of two case studies.

There are many general books on the use of particular software packages for data analysis, and some that give a detailed account of how they are used in the analysis of survival data. Allison (2010) provides a comprehensive guide to the SAS software for survival analysis. Der and Everitt (2013) also include material on survival analysis in their text on the use of SAS for analysing medical data. Therneau and Grambsch (2000) give a detailed account of how SAS and S-PLUS are used to fit the Cox regression model, and extensions to it. This book includes a description of a number of SAS macros and S-PLUS functions that supplement the standard facilities available in these packages.

The use of S-PLUS in survival analysis is also described in Everitt and Rabe-Hesketh (2001) and Tableman and Kim (2004), while Broström (2012) shows how R is used in the analysis of survival data. Venables and Ripley (2002) describe how graphical and numerical data analyses can be carried out in the S environment that is implemented in both R and S-PLUS; note that S code generally runs under R. A similarly comprehensive account of the R system is given by Crawley (2013), while Dalgaard (2008) gives a more elementary introduction to R. The short introduction to R of Venables and Smith (2009) is also available from R Core Team (2013). The use of Stata in survival analysis is presented by Cleves et al. (2010), and Rabe-Hesketh and Everitt (2007) give a more general introduction to the use of Stata in data analysis.

Chapter 2

Some non-parametric procedures

An initial step in the analysis of a set of survival data is to present numerical or graphical summaries of the survival times for individuals in a particular group. Such summaries may be of interest in their own right, or as a precursor to a more detailed analysis of the data. Survival data are conveniently summarised through estimates of the survivor function and hazard function. Methods for estimating these functions from a single sample of survival data are described in Sections 2.1 and 2.3. These methods are said to be *non-parametric* or *distribution-free*, since they do not require specific assumptions to be made about the underlying distribution of the survival times.

Once the estimated survivor function has been found, the median and other percentiles of the distribution of survival times can be estimated, as shown in Section 2.4. Numerical summaries of the data, derived on the basis of assumptions about the probability distribution from which the data have been drawn, will be considered later in Chapters 5 and 6.

When the survival times of two groups of patients are being compared, an informal comparison of the survival experience of each group of individuals can be made using the estimated survivor functions. However, there are more formal procedures that enable two groups of survival data to be compared. Two non-parametric procedures for comparing two or more groups of survival times, namely the *log-rank test* and the *Wilcoxon test*, are described in Section 2.6.

2.1 Estimating the survivor function

Suppose first that we have a single sample of survival times, where none of the observations are censored. The survivor function $S(t)$, defined in Equation (1.2), is the probability that an individual survives for a time greater than or equal to t. This function can be estimated by the *empirical survivor function*, given by

$$\hat{S}(t) = \frac{\text{Number of individuals with survival times} \geqslant t}{\text{Number of individuals in the data set}}. \tag{2.1}$$

Equivalently, $\hat{S}(t) = 1 - \hat{F}(t)$, where $\hat{F}(t)$ is the *empirical distribution function*, that is, the ratio of the total number of individuals alive at time t to the total number of individuals in the study. Notice that the empirical survivor function is equal to unity for values of t before the first death time, and zero after the final death time.

The estimated survivor function $\hat{S}(t)$ is assumed to be constant between two adjacent death times, and so a plot of $\hat{S}(t)$ against t is a step-function. The function decreases immediately after each observed survival time.

Example 2.1 Pulmonary metastasis

One complication in the management of patients with a malignant bone tumour, or osteosarcoma, is that the tumour often spreads to the lungs. This pulmonary metastasis is life-threatening. In a study concerned with the treatment of pulmonary metastasis arising from osteosarcoma, Burdette and Gehan (1970) give the following survival times, in months, of eleven male patients.

11 13 13 13 13 13 14 14 15 15 17

Using Equation (2.1), the estimated values of the survivor function at times 11, 13, 14, 15 and 17 months are 1.000, 0.909, 0.455, 0.273 and 0.091. The estimated value of the survivor function is unity from the time origin until 11 months, and zero after 17 months. A graph of the estimated survivor function is given in Figure 2.1.

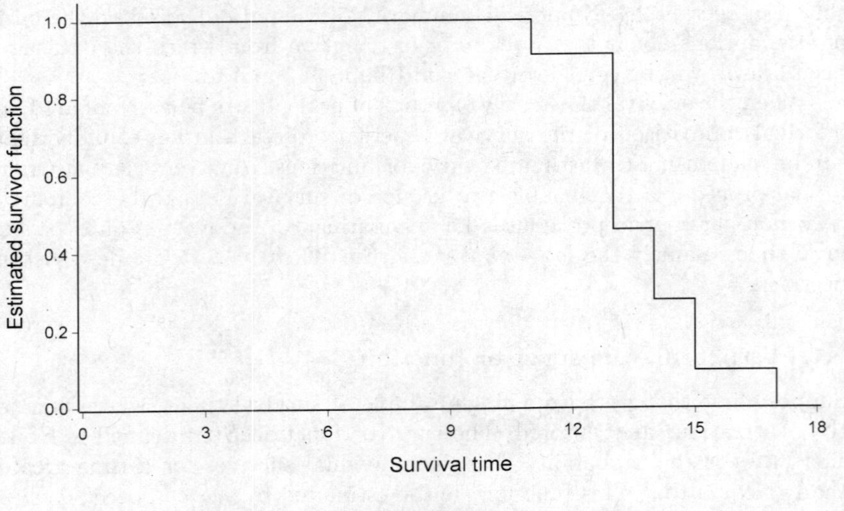

Figure 2.1 *Estimated survivor function for the data from Example 2.1.*

The method of estimating the survivor function illustrated in the above example cannot be used when there are censored observations. The reason for this is that the method does not allow information provided by an individual whose survival time is censored before time t to be used in computing the estimated survivor function at t. Non-parametric methods for estimating $S(t)$, which can be used in the presence of censored survival times, are described in the following sections.

2.1.1 Life-table estimate of the survivor function

The *life-table estimate* of the survivor function, also known as the *actuarial estimate of survivor function*, is obtained by first dividing the period of observation into a series of time intervals. These intervals need not necessarily be of equal length, although they usually are. The number of intervals used will depend on the number of individuals in the study, but would usually be somewhere between 5 and 15.

Suppose that the jth of m such intervals, $j = 1, 2, \ldots, m$, extends from time t'_{j-1} to immediately before time t'_j, where we take $t_0 = 0$ and $t_m = \infty$. Also, let d_j and c_j denote the number of deaths and the number of censored survival times, respectively, in this interval, and let n_j be the number of individuals who are alive, and therefore at risk of death, at the start of the jth interval. We now make the assumption that the censoring process is such that the censored survival times occur uniformly throughout the jth interval, so that the average number of individuals who are at risk during this interval is

$$n'_j = n_j - c_j/2. \tag{2.2}$$

This assumption is sometimes known as the *actuarial assumption*.

In the jth interval, the probability of death can be estimated by d_j/n'_j, so that the corresponding survival probability is $(n'_j - d_j)/n'_j$. Now consider the probability that an individual survives beyond time t'_{j-1}, $j = 2, 3, \ldots, m$, that is, until some time after the start of the jth interval. This will be the product of the probabilities that an individual survives through each of the $j-1$ preceding intervals, and so the life-table estimate of the survivor function is given by

$$S^*(t) = \prod_{i=1}^{j-1} \left(\frac{n'_i - d_i}{n'_i} \right), \tag{2.3}$$

for $t'_{j-1} \leqslant t < t'_j$, $j = 2, 3, \ldots, m$. The estimated probability of surviving beyond the start of the first interval, t'_0, is of course unity, while the estimated probability of surviving beyond t'_m is zero. A graphical estimate of the survivor function will then be a step-function with constant values of the function in each time interval.

Example 2.2 Survival of multiple myeloma patients
To illustrate the computation of the life-table estimate, consider the data on the survival times of the 48 multiple myeloma patients given in Table 1.3. In this illustration, the information collected on other explanatory variables for each individual will be ignored.

The survival times are first grouped to give the number of patients who die, d_j, and the number who are censored, c_j, in each of the first five years of the study, and in the subsequent three-year period. The number at risk of death at the start of each of these intervals, n_j, is then computed, together with the adjusted number at risk, n'_j. Finally, the probability of survival through each interval is estimated, from which the estimated survivor function is obtained using Equation (2.3). The calculations are shown in Table 2.1, in which the time period is given in months, and the jth interval that begins at time t'_{j-1} and ends just before time t'_j, for $j = 1, 2, \ldots, m$, is denoted $t'_{j-1}-$.

Table 2.1 *Life-table estimate of the survivor function for the data from Example 1.3.*

Interval	Time period	d_j	c_j	n_j	n'_j	$(n'_j - d_j)/n'_j$	$S^*(t)$
1	0–	16	4	48	46.0	0.6522	1.0000
2	12–	10	4	28	26.0	0.6154	0.6522
3	24–	1	0	14	14.0	0.9286	0.4013
4	36–	3	1	13	12.5	0.7600	0.3727
5	48–	2	2	9	8.0	0.7500	0.2832
6	60–	4	1	5	4.5	0.1111	0.2124

A graph of the life-table estimate of the survivor function is shown in Figure 2.2.

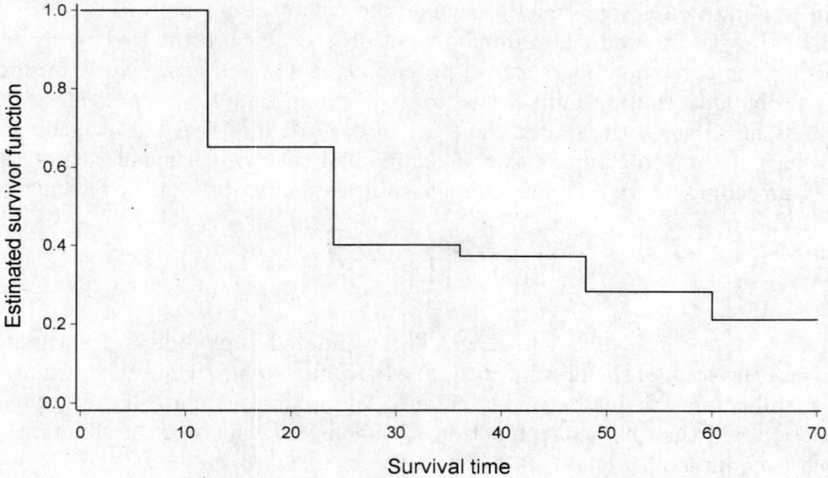

Figure 2.2 *Life-table estimate of the survivor function.*

The form of the estimated survivor function obtained using this method is sensitive to the choice of the intervals used in its construction, just as the shape of a histogram depends on the choice of the class intervals. On the other hand, the life-table estimate is particularly well suited to situations in which the actual death times are unknown, and the only available information is the number of deaths and the number of censored observations that occur in a series of consecutive time intervals. In practice, such interval-censored survival data occur quite frequently.

When the actual survival times are known, the life-table estimate can still be used, as in Example 2.2, but the grouping of the survival times does result in some loss of information. Alternative methods for estimating the survivor function are then more appropriate, such as that leading to the Kaplan-Meier estimate.

2.1.2 *Kaplan-Meier estimate of the survivor function*

The first step in the analysis of ungrouped censored survival data is normally to obtain the *Kaplan-Meier estimate* of the survivor function. This estimate is therefore considered in some detail. To obtain the Kaplan-Meier estimate, a series of time intervals is constructed, as for the life-table estimate. However, each of these intervals is designed to be such that one death time is contained in the interval, and this death time is taken to occur at the start of the interval.

As an illustration, suppose that $t_{(1)}$, $t_{(2)}$ and $t_{(3)}$ are three observed survival times arranged in rank order, so that $t_{(1)} < t_{(2)} < t_{(3)}$, and that c is a censored survival time that falls between $t_{(2)}$ and $t_{(3)}$. The constructed intervals then begin at times $t_{(1)}$, $t_{(2)}$ and $t_{(3)}$, and each interval includes the one death time, although there could be more than one individual who dies at any particular death time. Notice that no interval begins at the censored time of c. Now suppose that two individuals die at $t_{(1)}$, one dies at $t_{(2)}$ and three die at $t_{(3)}$. The situation is illustrated diagrammatically in Figure 2.3, in which D represents a death and C a censored survival time.

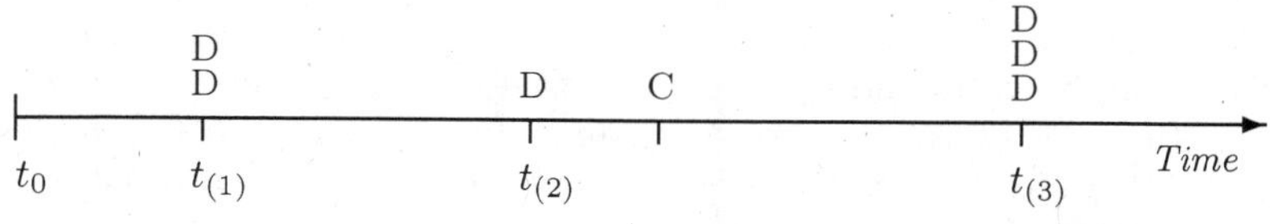

Figure 2.3 *Construction of intervals used in the derivation of the Kaplan-Meier estimate.*

The time origin is denoted by t_0, and so there is an initial period commencing at t_0, which ends just before $t_{(1)}$, the time of the first death. This means that the interval from t_0 to $t_{(1)}$ will not include a death time. The first constructed interval extends from $t_{(1)}$ to just before $t_{(2)}$, and since the second death time is at $t_{(2)}$, this interval includes the single death time at $t_{(1)}$. The second interval begins at time $t_{(2)}$ and ends just before $t_{(3)}$, and includes the death time at $t_{(2)}$ and the censored time c. There is also a third interval beginning at $t_{(3)}$, which contains the longest survival time, $t_{(3)}$.

In general, suppose that there are n individuals with observed survival times $t_1, t_2, \ldots, t_n$. Some of these observations may be right-censored, and there may also be more than one individual with the same observed survival time. We therefore suppose that there are r death times amongst the individuals, where $r \leqslant n$. After arranging these death times in ascending order, the jth is denoted $t_{(j)}$, for $j = 1, 2, \ldots, r$, and so the r ordered death times are $t_{(1)} < t_{(2)} < \cdots < t_{(r)}$. The number of individuals who are alive just before time $t_{(j)}$, including those who are about to die at this time, will be denoted n_j, for $j = 1, 2, \ldots, r$, and d_j will denote the number who die at this time. The time interval from $t_{(j)} - \delta$ to $t_{(j)}$, where δ is an infinitesimal time interval, then includes one death time. Since there are n_j individuals who are alive just before $t_{(j)}$ and d_j deaths at $t_{(j)}$, the probability that an individual dies during the interval from $t_{(j)} - \delta$ to $t_{(j)}$ is estimated by d_j/n_j. The corresponding estimated probability of survival through that interval is then $(n_j - d_j)/n_j$.

It sometimes happens that there are censored survival times that occur at the same time as one or more deaths, so that a death time and a censored survival time appear to occur simultaneously. In this situation, the censored survival time is taken to occur immediately after the death time when computing the values of the n_j.

From the manner in which the time intervals are constructed, the interval from $t_{(j)}$ to $t_{(j+1)} - \delta$, the time immediately before the next death time, contains no deaths. The probability of surviving from $t_{(j)}$ to $t_{(j+1)} - \delta$ is therefore unity, and the joint probability of surviving from $t_{(j)} - \delta$ to $t_{(j)}$ and from $t_{(j)}$ to $t_{(j+1)} - \delta$ can be estimated by $(n_j - d_j)/n_j$. In the limit, as δ tends to zero, $(n_j - d_j)/n_j$ becomes an estimate of the probability of surviving the interval from $t_{(j)}$ to $t_{(j+1)}$.

We now make the assumption that the deaths of the individuals in the sample occur independently of one another. Then, the estimated survivor function at any time, t, in the kth constructed time interval from $t_{(k)}$ to $t_{(k+1)}$, $k = 1, 2, \ldots, r$, where $t_{(r+1)}$ is defined to be ∞, will be the estimated probability of surviving beyond $t_{(k)}$. This is actually the probability of surviving through the interval from $t_{(k)}$ to $t_{(k+1)}$, and all preceding intervals, and leads to the Kaplan-Meier estimate of the survivor function, which is given by

$$\hat{S}(t) = \prod_{j=1}^{k} \left(\frac{n_j - d_j}{n_j} \right), \tag{2.4}$$

for $t_{(k)} \leqslant t < t_{(k+1)}$, $k = 1, 2, \ldots, r$, with $\hat{S}(t) = 1$ for $t < t_{(1)}$, and where $t_{(r+1)}$ is taken to be ∞. If the largest observation is a censored survival time, t^*, say, $\hat{S}(t)$ is undefined for $t > t^*$. On the other hand, if the largest observed survival time, $t_{(r)}$, is an uncensored observation, $n_r = d_r$, and so $\hat{S}(t)$ is zero for $t \geqslant t_{(r)}$. A plot of the Kaplan-Meier estimate of the survivor function is a step-function, in which the estimated survival probabilities are constant between adjacent death times and decrease at each death time.

Equation (2.4) shows that, as for the life-table estimate of the survivor function in Equation (2.3), the Kaplan-Meier estimate is formed as a product of a series of estimated probabilities. In fact, the Kaplan-Meier estimate is the limiting value of the life-table estimate in Equation (2.3) as the number of intervals tends to infinity and their width tends to zero. For this reason, the Kaplan-Meier estimate is also known as the *product-limit estimate* of the survivor function.

Note that if there are no censored survival times in the data set, $n_j - d_j = n_{j+1}$, $j = 1, 2, \ldots, k$, in Equation (2.4), and on expanding the product we get

$$\hat{S}(t) = \frac{n_2}{n_1} \times \frac{n_3}{n_2} \times \cdots \times \frac{n_{k+1}}{n_k}.$$

This reduces to n_{k+1}/n_1, for $k = 1, 2, \ldots, r-1$, with $\hat{S}(t) = 1$ for $t < t_{(1)}$ and $\hat{S}(t) = 0$ for $t \geqslant t_{(r)}$. Now, n_1 is the number of individuals at risk just before the first death time, which is the number of individuals in the sample, and n_{k+1} is the number of individuals with survival times greater than or equal to $t_{(k+1)}$. Consequently, in the absence of censoring, $\hat{S}(t)$ is simply the empirical survivor function defined in Equation (2.1). The Kaplan-Meier estimate is therefore a generalisation of the empirical survivor function that accommodates censored observations.

Example 2.3 Time to discontinuation of the use of an IUD
Data from 18 women on the time to discontinuation of the use of an intra-uterine device (IUD) were given in Table 1.1. For these data, the survivor function, $S(t)$, represents the probability that a woman discontinues the use of the contraceptive device after any time t. The Kaplan-Meier estimate of the survivor function is readily obtained using Equation (2.4), and the required calculations are set out in Table 2.2.

Table 2.2 *Kaplan-Meier estimate of the survivor function for the data from Example 1.1.*

Time interval	n_j	d_j	$(n_j - d_j)/n_j$	$\hat{S}(t)$
0–	18	0	1.0000	1.0000
10–	18	1	0.9444	0.9444
19–	15	1	0.9333	0.8815
30–	13	1	0.9231	0.8137
36–	12	1	0.9167	0.7459
59–	8	1	0.8750	0.6526
75–	7	1	0.8571	0.5594
93–	6	1	0.8333	0.4662
97–	5	1	0.8000	0.3729
107	3	1	0.6667	0.2486

The estimated survivor function, $\hat{S}(t)$, is plotted in Figure 2.4. Note that since the largest discontinuation time of 107 days is censored, $\hat{S}(t)$ is not defined beyond $t = 107$.

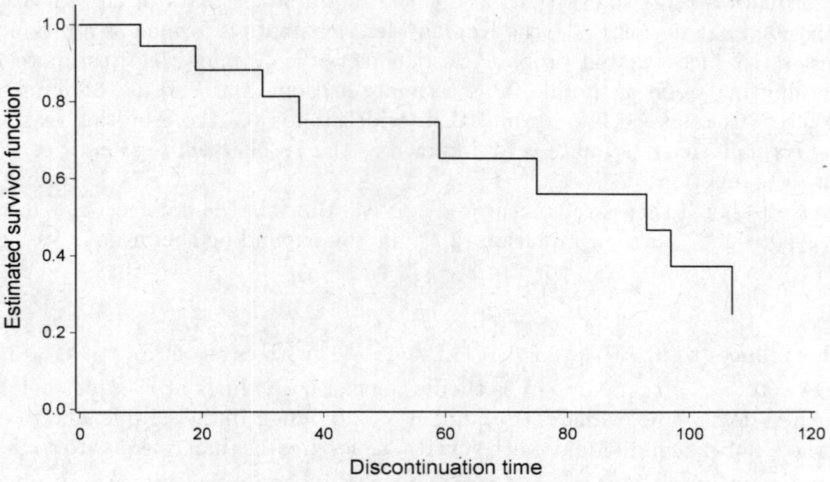

Figure 2.4 *Kaplan-Meier estimate of the survivor function for the data from Example 1.1.*

2.1.3 Nelson-Aalen estimate of the survivor function

An alternative estimate of the survivor function, which is based on the individual event times, is the *Nelson-Aalen estimate*, given by

$$\tilde{S}(t) = \prod_{j=1}^{k} \exp(-d_j/n_j). \tag{2.5}$$

This estimate can be obtained from an estimate of the cumulative hazard function, as shown in Section 2.3.3. Moreover, the Kaplan-Meier estimate of the survivor function can be regarded as an approximation to the Nelson-Aalen estimate. To show this, we use the result that

$$e^{-x} = 1 - x + \frac{x^2}{2} - \frac{x^3}{6} + \cdots,$$

which is approximately equal to $1 - x$ when x is small. It then follows that $\exp(-d_j/n_j) \approx 1 - (d_j/n_j) = (n_j - d_j)/n_j$, so long as d_j is small relative to n_j, which it will be except at the longest survival times. Consequently, the Kaplan-Meier estimate, $\hat{S}(t)$, in Equation (2.4), approximates the Nelson-Aalen estimate, $\tilde{S}(t)$, in Equation (2.5).

The Nelson-Aalen estimate of the survivor function, also known as *Altshuler's estimate*, will always be greater than the Kaplan-Meier estimate at any given time, since $e^{-x} \geqslant 1 - x$, for all values of x. Although the Nelson-Aalen estimate has been shown to perform better than the Kaplan-Meier estimate in small samples, in many circumstances, the estimates will be very similar, particularly at the earlier survival times. Since the Kaplan-Meier estimate is a generalisation of the empirical survivor function, the latter estimate has much to commend it.

Example 2.4 Time to discontinuation of the use of an IUD
The values shown in Table 2.2, which gives the Kaplan-Meier estimate of the survivor function for the data on the time to discontinuation of the use of an intrauterine device, can be used to calculate the Nelson-Aalen estimate. This estimate is shown in Table 2.3.

Table 2.3 *Nelson-Aalen estimate of the survivor function for the data from Example 1.1.*

Time interval	$\exp(-d_j/n_j)$	$\tilde{S}(t)$
0–	1.0000	1.0000
10–	0.9460	0.9460
19–	0.9355	0.8850
30–	0.9260	0.8194
36–	0.9200	0.7539
59–	0.8825	0.6653
75–	0.8669	0.5768
93–	0.8465	0.4882
97–	0.8187	0.3997
107	0.7165	0.2864

From this table we see that the Kaplan-Meier and Nelson-Aalen estimates of the survivor function differ by less than 0.04. However, when we consider the precision of these estimates, which we do in Section 2.2, we see that a difference of 0.04 is of no practical importance.

2.2 Standard error of the estimated survivor function

An essential aid to the interpretation of an estimate of any quantity is the precision of the estimate, which is reflected in the *standard error* of the estimate. This is defined to be the square root of the estimated variance of the estimate, and is used in the construction of an interval estimate for a quantity of interest. In this section, the standard error of estimates of the survivor function are given.

Because the Kaplan-Meier estimate is the most important and widely used estimate of the survivor function, the derivation of the standard error of $\hat{S}(t)$ will be presented in detail in this section. The details of this derivation can be omitted on a first reading.

2.2.1 Standard error of the Kaplan-Meier estimate*

The Kaplan-Meier estimate of the survivor function for any value of t in the interval from $t_{(k)}$ to $t_{(k+1)}$ can be written as

$$\hat{S}(t) = \prod_{j=1}^{k} \hat{p}_j,$$

for $k = 1, 2, \ldots, r$, where $\hat{p}_j = (n_j - d_j)/n_j$ is the estimated probability that an individual survives through the time interval that begins at $t_{(j)}$, $j = 1, 2, \ldots, r$. Taking logarithms,

$$\log \hat{S}(t) = \sum_{j=1}^{k} \log \hat{p}_j,$$

and so the variance of $\log \hat{S}(t)$ is given by

$$\text{var}\left\{\log \hat{S}(t)\right\} = \sum_{j=1}^{k} \text{var}\left\{\log \hat{p}_j\right\}. \tag{2.6}$$

Now, the number of individuals who survive through the interval beginning at $t_{(j)}$ can be assumed to have a *binomial distribution* with parameters n_j and p_j, where p_j is the true probability of survival through that interval. The observed number who survive is $n_j - d_j$, and using the result that the variance of a binomial random variable with parameters n, p is $np(1-p)$, the variance of $n_j - d_j$ is given by

$$\text{var}\,(n_j - d_j) = n_j p_j (1 - p_j).$$

Since $\hat{p}_j = (n_j - d_j)/n_j$, the variance of $\hat{p}_j$ is $\text{var}\,(n_j - d_j)/n_j^2$, that is, $p_j(1 - p_j)/n_j$. The variance of $\hat{p}_j$ may then be estimated by

$$\hat{p}_j(1 - \hat{p}_j)/n_j. \tag{2.7}$$

In order to obtain the variance of $\log \hat{p}_j$, we make use of a general result for the approximate variance of a function of a random variable. According to this result, the variance of a function $g(X)$ of the random variable X is given by

$$\text{var}\,\{g(X)\} \approx \left\{\frac{\mathrm{d}g(X)}{\mathrm{d}X}\right\}^2 \text{var}\,(X). \tag{2.8}$$

This is known as the *Taylor series approximation* to the variance of a function of a random variable. Using Equation (2.8), the approximate variance of $\log \hat{p}_j$ is $\text{var}\,(\hat{p}_j)/\hat{p}_j^2$, and using Expression (2.7), the approximate estimated variance of $\log \hat{p}_j$ is $(1 - \hat{p}_j)/(n_j \hat{p}_j)$, which on substitution for $\hat{p}_j$, reduces to

$$\frac{d_j}{n_j(n_j - d_j)}. \tag{2.9}$$

* Sections marked with an asterisk may be omitted without loss of continuity.

Then, from Equation (2.6),

$$\text{var}\left\{\log \hat{S}(t)\right\} \approx \sum_{j=1}^{k} \frac{d_j}{n_j(n_j - d_j)}, \tag{2.10}$$

and a further application of the result in Equation (2.8) gives

$$\text{var}\left\{\log \hat{S}(t)\right\} \approx \frac{1}{[\hat{S}(t)]^2} \text{var}\left\{\hat{S}(t)\right\},$$

so that

$$\text{var}\left\{\hat{S}(t)\right\} \approx [\hat{S}(t)]^2 \sum_{j=1}^{k} \frac{d_j}{n_j(n_j - d_j)}. \tag{2.11}$$

Finally, the standard error of the Kaplan-Meier estimate of the survivor function, defined to be the square root of the estimated variance of the estimate, is given by

$$\text{se}\left\{\hat{S}(t)\right\} \approx \hat{S}(t) \left\{\sum_{j=1}^{k} \frac{d_j}{n_j(n_j - d_j)}\right\}^{\frac{1}{2}}, \tag{2.12}$$

for $t_{(k)} \leqslant t < t_{(k+1)}$. This result is known as *Greenwood's formula.*

If there are no censored survival times, $n_j - d_j = n_{j+1}$, and Expression (2.9) becomes $(n_j - n_{j+1})/n_j n_{j+1}$. Now,

$$\sum_{j=1}^{k} \frac{n_j - n_{j+1}}{n_j n_{j+1}} = \sum_{j=1}^{k} \left(\frac{1}{n_{j+1}} - \frac{1}{n_j}\right) = \frac{n_1 - n_{k+1}}{n_1 n_{k+1}},$$

which can be written as

$$\frac{1 - \hat{S}(t)}{n_1 \hat{S}(t)},$$

since $\hat{S}(t) = n_{k+1}/n_1$ for $t_{(k)} \leqslant t < t_{(k+1)}$, $k = 1, 2, \ldots, r - 1$, in the absence of censoring. Hence, from Equation (2.11), the estimated variance of $\hat{S}(t)$ is $\hat{S}(t)[1 - \hat{S}(t)]/n_1$. This is an estimate of the variance of the empirical survivor function, given in Equation (2.1), on the assumption that the number of individuals at risk at time t has a binomial distribution with parameters $n_1, S(t)$.

2.2.2 Standard error of other estimates*

The life-table estimate of the survivor function is similar in form to the Kaplan-Meier estimate, and so the standard error of this estimator is obtained in a similar manner. In the notation of Section 2.1.1, the standard error of the life-table estimate is given by

$$\text{se}\,\{S^*(t)\} \approx S^*(t)\left\{\sum_{j=1}^{k}\frac{d_j}{n'_j(n'_j - d_j)}\right\}^{\frac{1}{2}}.$$

The standard error of the Nelson-Aalen estimator is

$$\text{se}\,\left\{\tilde{S}(t)\right\} \approx \tilde{S}(t)\left\{\sum_{j=1}^{k}\frac{d_j}{n_j^2}\right\}^{\frac{1}{2}},$$

although other expressions have been proposed.

2.2.3 *Confidence intervals for values of the survivor function*

Once the standard error of an estimate of the survivor function has been calculated, a *confidence interval* for the corresponding value of the survivor function, at a given time t, can be found. A confidence interval is an interval estimate of the survivor function, and is the interval which is such that there is a prescribed probability that the value of the true survivor function is included within it. The intervals constructed in this manner are sometimes referred to as *pointwise confidence intervals*, since they apply to a specific survival time.

A confidence interval for the true value of the survivor function at a given time t is obtained by assuming that the estimated value of the survivor function at t is normally distributed with mean $S(t)$ and estimated variance given by Equation (2.11). The interval is computed from *percentage points* of the standard normal distribution. Thus, if Z is a random variable that has a standard normal distribution, the upper (one-sided) $\alpha/2$-point, or the two-sided α-point, of this distribution is that value $z_{\alpha/2}$ which is such that $\text{P}(Z > z_{\alpha/2}) = \alpha/2$. This probability is the area under the standard normal curve to the right of $z_{\alpha/2}$, as illustrated in Figure 2.5. For example, the two-sided 5% and 1% points of the standard normal distribution, $z_{0.025}$ and $z_{0.005}$, are 1.96 and 2.58, respectively.

A $100(1-\alpha)\%$ confidence interval for $S(t)$, for a given value of t, is the interval from $\hat{S}(t) - z_{\alpha/2}\,\text{se}\,\{\hat{S}(t)\}$ to $\hat{S}(t) + z_{\alpha/2}\,\text{se}\,\{\hat{S}(t)\}$, where $\text{se}\,\{\hat{S}(t)\}$ is found from Equation (2.12). These intervals for $S(t)$ can be superimposed on a graph of the estimated survivor function, as shown in Example 2.5.

One difficulty with this procedure arises from the fact that the confidence intervals are symmetric. When the estimated survivor function is close to zero or unity, symmetric intervals are inappropriate, since they can lead to confidence limits for the survivor function that lie outside the interval (0,1). A pragmatic solution to this problem is to replace any limit that is greater than unity by 1.0, and any limit that is less than zero by 0.0.

An alternative procedure is to transform $\hat{S}(t)$ to a value in the range $(-\infty, \infty)$, and obtain a confidence interval for the transformed value. The

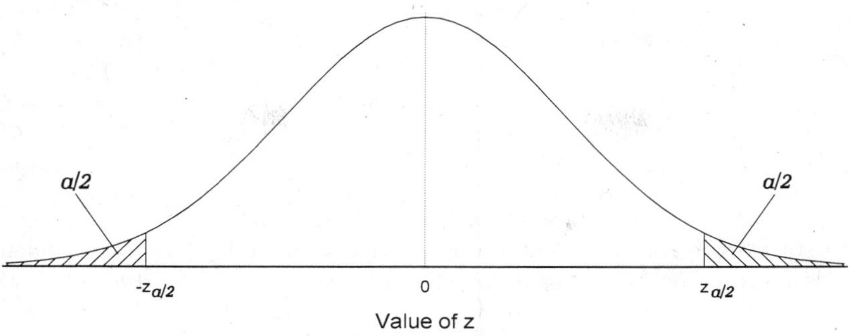

Figure 2.5 *Upper and lower $\alpha/2$-points of the standard normal distribution.*

resulting confidence limits are then back-transformed to give a confidence interval for $S(t)$ itself. Possible transformations are the logistic transformation, $\log[S(t)/\{1 - S(t)\}]$, and the complementary log-log transformation, $\log\{-\log S(t)\}$. Note that from Equation (1.8), the latter quantity is the logarithm of the cumulative hazard function. In either case, the standard error of the transformed value of $\hat{S}(t)$ can be found using the approximation in Equation (2.8).

For example, the variance of $\log\{-\log \hat{S}(t)\}$ is obtained from the expression for $\text{var}\,\{\log \hat{S}(t)\}$ in Equation (2.10). Using the general result in Equation (2.8),

$$\text{var}\,\{\log(-X)\} \approx \frac{1}{X^2}\,\text{var}\,(X),$$

and setting $X = \log \hat{S}(t)$ gives

$$\text{var}\,\left[\log\{-\log \hat{S}(t)\}\right] \approx \frac{1}{\{\log \hat{S}(t)\}^2} \sum_{j=1}^{k} \frac{d_j}{n_j(n_j - d_j)}.$$

The standard error of $\log\{-\log \hat{S}(t)\}$ is the square root of this quantity. This leads to $100(1-\alpha)\%$ limits of the form

$$\hat{S}(t)^{\exp[\pm z_{\alpha/2}\,\text{se}\{\log[-\log \hat{S}(t)]\}]},$$

where $z_{\alpha/2}$ is the upper $\alpha/2$-point of the standard normal distribution.

A further problem is that in the tails of the distribution of the survival times, that is, when $\hat{S}(t)$ is close to zero or unity, the variance of $\hat{S}(t)$ obtained using Greenwood's formula can underestimate the actual variance. In these circumstances, an alternative expression for the standard error of $\hat{S}(t)$ may be used. Peto et al. (1977) propose that the standard error of $\hat{S}(t)$ should be obtained from the equation

$$\text{se}\,\{\hat{S}(t)\} = \frac{\hat{S}(t)\sqrt{\{1 - \hat{S}(t)\}}}{\sqrt{(n_k)}},$$

for $t_{(k)} \leqslant t < t_{(k+1)}$, $k = 1, 2, \ldots, r$, where $\hat{S}(t)$ is the Kaplan-Meier estimate of $S(t)$ and n_k is the number of individuals at risk at $t_{(k)}$, the start of the kth constructed time interval.

This expression for the standard error of $\hat{S}(t)$ is conservative, in the sense that the standard errors obtained will tend to be larger than they ought to be. For this reason, the Greenwood estimate is recommended for general use.

Example 2.5 Time to discontinuation of the use of an IUD
The standard error of the estimated survivor function, and 95% confidence limits for the corresponding true value of the function, for the data from Example 1.1 on the times to discontinuation of use of an IUD, are given in Table 2.4. In this table, confidence limits outside the range $(0, 1)$ have been replaced by zero or unity.

Table 2.4 *Standard error of* $\hat{S}(t)$ *and confidence intervals for* $S(t)$ *for the data from Example 1.1.*

Time interval	$\hat{S}(t)$	se $\{\hat{S}(t)\}$	95% confidence interval
0–	1.0000	0.0000	
10–	0.9444	0.0540	(0.839, 1.000)
19–	0.8815	0.0790	(0.727, 1.000)
30–	0.8137	0.0978	(0.622, 1.000)
36–	0.7459	0.1107	(0.529, 0.963)
59–	0.6526	0.1303	(0.397, 0.908)
75–	0.5594	0.1412	(0.283, 0.836)
93–	0.4662	0.1452	(0.182, 0.751)
97–	0.3729	0.1430	(0.093, 0.653)
107	0.2486	0.1392	(0.000, 0.522)

From this table we see that, in general, the standard error of the estimated survivor function increases with the discontinuation time. The reason for this is that estimates of the survivor function at later times are based on fewer individuals. A graph of the estimated survivor function, with the 95% confidence limits shown as dashed lines, is given in Figure 2.6.

It is important to observe that the confidence limits for a survivor function, illustrated in Figure 2.6, are only valid for any given time. Different methods are needed to produce confidence bands that are such that there is a given probability, 0.95 for example, that the survivor function is contained in the band for all values of t. These bands will tend to be wider than the band formed from the pointwise confidence limits. Details will not be included, but references to these methods are given in the final section of this chapter. Notice also that the width of these intervals is very much greater than the difference between the Kaplan-Meier and Nelson-Aalen estimates of the survivor function, shown in Tables 2.2 and 2.3. Similar calculations lead to confidence limits based on life-table and Nelson-Aalen estimates of the survivor function.

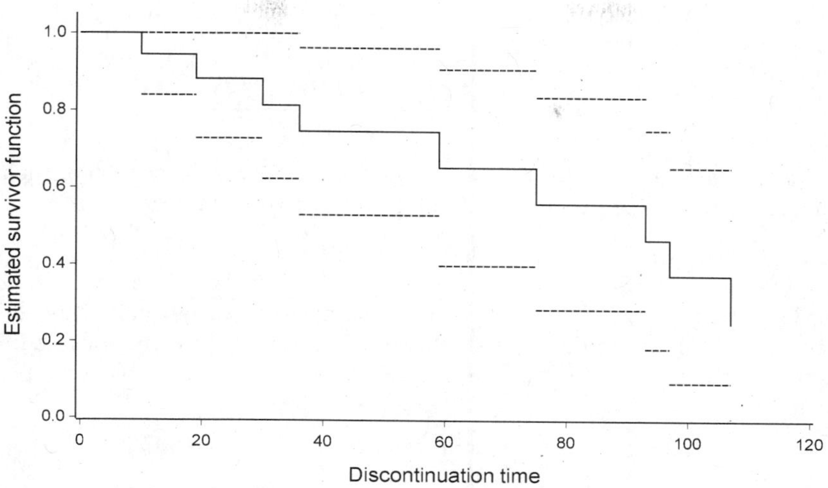

Figure 2.6 *Estimated survivor function and 95% confidence limits for* $S(t)$.

2.3 Estimating the hazard function

A single sample of survival data may also be summarised through the hazard function, which shows the dependence of the instantaneous risk of death on time. There are a number of ways of estimating this function, two of which are described in this section.

2.3.1 Life-table estimate of the hazard function

Suppose that the observed survival times have been grouped into a series of m intervals, as in the construction of the life-table estimate of the survivor function. An appropriate estimate of the average hazard of death per unit time over each interval is the observed number of deaths in that interval, divided by the average time survived in that interval. This latter quantity is the average number of persons at risk in the interval, multiplied by the length of the interval. Let the number of deaths in the jth time interval be d_j, $j = 1, 2, \ldots, m$, and suppose that n'_j is the average number of individuals at risk of death in that interval, where n'_j is given by Equation (2.2). Assuming that the death rate is constant during the jth interval, the average time survived in that interval is $(n'_j - d_j/2)\tau_j$, where τ_j is the length of the jth time interval. The life-table estimate of the hazard function in the jth time interval is then given by

$$h^*(t) = \frac{d_j}{(n'_j - d_j/2)\tau_j},$$

for $t'_{j-1} \leqslant t < t'_j$, $j = 1, 2, \ldots, m$, so that $h^*(t)$ is a step-function.

The asymptotic standard error of this estimate has been shown by Gehan (1969) to be given by

$$\text{se}\,\{h^*(t)\} = \frac{h^*(t)\sqrt{\{1 - [h^*(t)\tau_j/2]^2\}}}{\sqrt{(d_j)}},$$

and confidence intervals for the corresponding true hazard over each of the m time intervals can be obtained in the manner described in Section 2.2.3.

Example 2.6 Survival of multiple myeloma patients
The life-table estimate of the survivor function for the data from Example 1.3 on the survival times of 48 multiple myeloma patients was given in Table 2.1. Using the same time intervals as were used in Example 2.2, calculations leading to the life-table estimate of the hazard function are given in Table 2.5.

Table 2.5 *Life-table estimate of the hazard function for the data from Example 1.3.*

Time period	τ_j	d_j	n'_j	$h^*(t)$
0–	12	16	46.0	0.0351
12–	12	10	26.0	0.0397
24–	12	1	14.0	0.0062
36–	12	3	12.5	0.0227
48–	12	2	8.0	0.0238
60–	36	4	4.5	0.0444

The estimated hazard function is plotted as a step-function in Figure 2.7. The general pattern is for the hazard to remain roughly constant over the first two years from diagnosis, after which time it declines and then increases gradually. However, some caution is needed in interpreting this estimate, as there are few deaths two years after diagnosis.

2.3.2 Kaplan-Meier type estimate

A natural way of estimating the hazard function for ungrouped survival data is to take the ratio of the number of deaths at a given death time to the number of individuals at risk at that time. If the hazard function is assumed to be constant between successive death times, the hazard per unit time can be found by further dividing by the time interval. Thus, if there are d_j deaths at the jth death time, $t_{(j)}$, $j = 1, 2, \ldots, r$, and n_j at risk at time $t_{(j)}$, the hazard function in the interval from $t_{(j)}$ to $t_{(j+1)}$ can be estimated by

$$\hat{h}(t) = \frac{d_j}{n_j\tau_j}, \tag{2.13}$$

for $t_{(j)} \leqslant t < t_{(j+1)}$, where $\tau_j = t_{(j+1)} - t_{(j)}$. Notice that it is not possible to use Equation (2.13) to estimate the hazard in the interval that begins at the final death time, since this interval is open-ended.

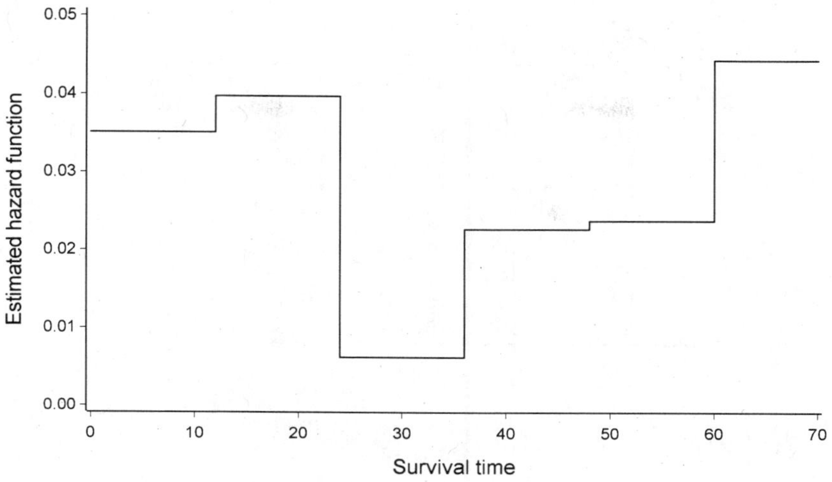

Figure 2.7 *Life-table estimate of the hazard function for the data from Example 1.3.*

The estimate in Equation (2.13) is referred to as a *Kaplan-Meier type estimate*, because the estimated survivor function derived from it is the Kaplan-Meier estimate. To show this, note that since $\hat{h}(t)$, $t_{(j)} \leqslant t < t_{(j+1)}$, is an estimate of the risk of death per unit time in the jth interval, the probability of death in that interval is $\hat{h}(t)\tau_j$, that is, d_j/n_j. Hence an estimate of the corresponding survival probability in that interval is $1 - (d_j/n_j)$, and the estimated survivor function is as given by Equation (2.4).

The approximate standard error of $\hat{h}(t)$ can be found from the variance of d_j, which, following Section 2.2.1, may be assumed to have a binomial distribution with parameters n_j and p_j, where p_j is the probability of death in the interval of length τ. Consequently, $\text{var}\,(d_j) = n_j p_j (1 - p_j)$, and estimating p_j by d_j/n_j gives

$$\text{se}\,\{\hat{h}(t)\} = \hat{h}(t)\sqrt{\frac{n_j - d_j}{n_j d_j}}.$$

However, when d_j is small, confidence intervals constructed using this standard error will be too wide to be of practical use.

Example 2.7 Time to discontinuation of the use of an IUD
Consider again the data on the time to discontinuation of the use of an IUD for 18 women, given in Example 1.1. The Kaplan-Meier estimate of the survivor function for these data was given in Table 2.2, and Table 2.6 gives the corresponding Kaplan-Meier type estimate of the hazard function, computed from Equation (2.13). The approximate standard errors of $\hat{h}(t)$ are also given.

Table 2.6 *Kaplan-Meier type estimate of the hazard function for the data from Example 1.1.*

Time interval	τ_j	n_j	d_j	$\hat{h}(t)$	se $\{\hat{h}(t)\}$
0–	10	18	0	0.0000	–
10–	9	18	1	0.0062	0.0060
19–	11	15	1	0.0061	0.0059
30–	6	13	1	0.0128	0.0123
36–	23	12	1	0.0036	0.0035
59–	16	8	1	0.0078	0.0073
75–	18	7	1	0.0079	0.0073
93–	4	6	1	0.0417	0.0380
97–	10	5	1	0.0200	0.0179

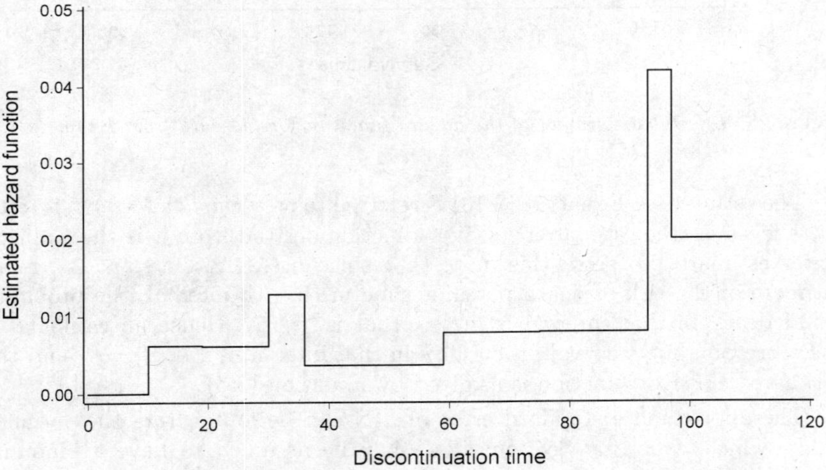

Figure 2.8 *Kaplan-Meier type estimate of the hazard function for the data from Example 1.1.*

Figure 2.8 shows a plot of the estimated hazard function. From this figure, there is some evidence that the longer the IUD is used, the greater is the risk of discontinuation, but the picture is not very clear. The approximate standard errors of the estimated hazard function at different times are of little help in interpreting this plot.

In practice, estimates of the hazard function obtained in this way will often tend to be rather irregular. For this reason, plots of the hazard function may be 'smoothed', so that any pattern can be seen more clearly. There are a number of ways of smoothing the hazard function, that lead to a weighted average of values of the estimated hazard $\hat{h}(t)$ at death times in the neighbourhood of t.

For example, a *kernel smoothed* estimate of the hazard function, based on the r ordered death times, $t_{(1)}, t_{(2)}, \ldots, t_{(r)}$, with d_j deaths and n_j at risk at time $t_{(j)}$, can be found from

$$h^{\dagger}(t) = b^{-1} \sum_{j=1}^{r} 0.75 \left\{ 1 - \left(\frac{t - t_{(j)}}{b} \right)^2 \right\} \frac{d_j}{n_j},$$

where the value of b needs to be chosen. The function $h^{\dagger}(t)$ is defined for all values of t in the interval from b to $t_{(r)} - b$, where $t_{(r)}$ is the greatest death time. For any value of t in this interval, the death times in the interval $(t - b, t + b)$ will contribute to the weighted average. The parameter b is known as the *bandwidth* and its value controls the shape of the plot; the larger the value of b, the greater the degree of smoothing. There are formulae that lead to 'optimal' values of b, but these tend to be rather cumbersome. Fuller details can be found in the references provided in the final section of this chapter. In this book, the use of a modelling approach to the analysis of survival data is advocated, and so model-based estimates of the hazard function will be considered in subsequent chapters.

2.3.3 Estimating the cumulative hazard function

The interpretation of the cumulative hazard function in terms of the expected number of events that occur up to a given time, given in Section 1.3.3 of Chapter 1, means that this function is important in the identification of models for survival data, as will be seen later in Sections 4.4 and 5.2. In addition, since the derivative of the cumulative hazard function is the hazard function itself, the slope of the cumulative hazard function provides information about the shape of the underlying hazard function. For example, a linear cumulative hazard function over some time interval suggests that the hazard is constant over this interval. Methods that can be used to estimate this function will now be described.

The cumulative hazard at time t, $H(t)$, was defined in Equation (1.7) to be the integral of the hazard function, but is more conveniently found using Equation (1.8). According to this result, $H(t) = -\log S(t)$, and so if $\hat{S}(t)$ is the Kaplan-Meier estimate of the survivor function, $\hat{H}(t) = -\log \hat{S}(t)$ is an appropriate estimate of the cumulative hazard function to time t.

Now, using Equation (2.4),

$$\hat{H}(t) = -\sum_{j=1}^{k} \log \left(\frac{n_j - d_j}{n_j} \right),$$

for $t_{(k)} \leqslant t < t_{(k+1)}$, $k = 1, 2, \ldots, r$, and $t_{(1)}, t_{(2)}, \ldots, t_{(r)}$ are the r ordered death times, with $t_{(r+1)} = \infty$.

If the Nelson-Aalen estimate of the survivor function is used, the estimated cumulative hazard function, $\tilde{H}(t) = -\log \tilde{S}(t)$, is given by

$$\tilde{H}(t) = \sum_{j=1}^{k} \frac{d_j}{n_j}.$$

This is the cumulative sum of the estimated probabilities of death from the first to the kth time interval, $k = 1, 2, \ldots, r$, and so this quantity has immediate intuitive appeal as an estimate of the cumulative hazard.

An estimate of the cumulative hazard function also leads to an estimate of the corresponding hazard function, since the differences between adjacent values of the estimated cumulative hazard function provide estimates of the underlying hazard, after dividing by the time interval. In particular, differences in adjacent values of the Nelson-Aalen estimate of the cumulative hazard lead directly to the hazard function estimate in Section 2.3.2.

2.4 Estimating the median and percentiles of survival times

Since the distribution of survival times tends to be positively skewed, the median is the preferred summary measure of the location of the distribution. Once the survivor function has been estimated, it is straightforward to obtain an estimate of the *median survival time*. This is the time beyond which 50% of the individuals in the population under study are expected to survive, and is given by that value $t(50)$ which is such that $S\{t(50)\} = 0.5$.

Because the non-parametric estimates of $S(t)$ are step-functions, it will not usually be possible to realise an estimated survival time that makes the survivor function exactly equal to 0.5. Instead, the estimated median survival time, $\hat{t}(50)$, is defined to be the smallest observed survival time for which the value of the estimated survivor function is less than 0.5.

In mathematical terms,

$$\hat{t}(50) = \min\{t_i \mid \hat{S}(t_i) < 0.5\},$$

where t_i is the observed survival time for the ith individual, $i = 1, 2, \ldots, n$. Since the estimated survivor function only changes at a death time, this is equivalent to the definition

$$\hat{t}(50) = \min\{t_{(j)} \mid \hat{S}(t_{(j)}) < 0.5\},$$

where $t_{(j)}$ is the jth ordered death time, $j = 1, 2, \ldots, r$.

In the particular case where the estimated survivor function is exactly equal to 0.5 for values of t in the interval from $t_{(j)}$ to $t_{(j+1)}$, the median is taken to be the half-way point in this interval, that is $(t_{(j)} + t_{(j+1)})/2$. When there are no censored survival times, the estimated median survival time will be the smallest time beyond which 50% of the individuals in the sample survive.

Example 2.8 Time to discontinuation of the use of an IUD

The Kaplan-Meier estimate of the survivor function for the data from Example 1.1 on the time to discontinuation of the use of an IUD was given in Table 2.2. The estimated survivor function, $\hat{S}(t)$, for these data was shown in Figure 2.4. From the estimated survivor function, the smallest discontinuation time beyond which the estimated probability of discontinuation is less than 0.5 is 93 weeks. This is therefore the estimated median time to discontinuation of the IUD for this group of women.

A similar procedure to that described above can be used to estimate other *percentiles* of the distribution of survival times. The pth percentile of the distribution of survival times is defined to be the value $t(p)$ which is such that $F\{t(p)\} = p/100$, for any value of p from 0 to 100. In terms of the survivor function, $t(p)$ is such that $S\{t(p)\} = 1 - (p/100)$, so that for example the 10th and 90th percentiles are given by

$$S\{t(10)\} = 0.9, \quad S\{t(90)\} = 0.1,$$

respectively. Using the estimated survivor function, the estimated pth percentile is the smallest observed survival time, $\hat{t}(p)$, for which $\hat{S}\{\hat{t}(p)\} < 1 - (p/100)$.

It sometimes happens that the estimated survivor function is greater than 0.5 for all values of t. In such cases, the median survival time cannot be estimated. It would then be natural to summarise the data in terms of other percentiles of the distribution of survival times, or the estimated survival probabilities at particular time points.

Estimates of the dispersion of a sample of survival data are not widely used, but should such an estimate be required, the *semi-interquartile range* (*SIQR*) can be calculated. This is defined to be half the difference between the 75th and 25th percentiles of the distribution of survival times. Hence,

$$SIQR = \frac{1}{2}\left\{t(75) - t(25)\right\},$$

where $t(25)$ and $t(75)$ are the 25th and 75th percentiles of the survival time distribution. These two percentiles are also known as the *first* and *third quartiles*, respectively. The corresponding sample-based estimate of the *SIQR* is $\{\hat{t}(75) - \hat{t}(25)\}/2$. Like the variance, the larger the value of the *SIQR*, the more dispersed is the survival time distribution.

Example 2.9 Time to discontinuation of the use of an IUD

From the Kaplan-Meier estimate of the survivor function for the data from Example 1.1, given in Table 2.2, the 25th and 75th percentiles of the distribution of discontinuation times are 36 and 107 weeks, respectively. Hence, the *SIQR* of the distribution is estimated to be 35.5 weeks.

2.5* Confidence intervals for the median and percentiles

Approximate confidence intervals for the median and other percentiles of a distribution of survival times can be found once the variance of the estimated percentile has been obtained. An expression for the approximate variance of a percentile can be derived from a direct application of the general result for the variance of a function of a random variable in Equation (2.8). Using this result,

$$\text{var}\,[\hat{S}\{t(p)\}] = \left(\frac{\text{d}\hat{S}\{t(p)\}}{\text{d}t(p)}\right)^2 \text{var}\,\{t(p)\}, \tag{2.14}$$

where $t(p)$ is the pth percentile of the distribution and $\hat{S}\{t(p)\}$ is the Kaplan-Meier estimate of the survivor function at $t(p)$. Now,

$$-\frac{\text{d}\hat{S}\{t(p)\}}{\text{d}t(p)} = \hat{f}\{t(p)\},$$

an estimate of the probability density function of the survival times at $t(p)$, and on rearranging Equation (2.14), we get

$$\text{var}\,\{t(p)\} = \left(\frac{1}{\hat{f}\{t(p)\}}\right)^2 \text{var}\,[\hat{S}\{t(p)\}].$$

The standard error of $\hat{t}(p)$, the estimated pth percentile, is therefore given by

$$\text{se}\,\{\hat{t}(p)\} = \frac{1}{\hat{f}\{\hat{t}(p)\}}\,\text{se}\,[\hat{S}\{\hat{t}(p)\}]. \tag{2.15}$$

The standard error of $\hat{S}\{\hat{t}(p)\}$ is found using Greenwood's formula for the standard error of the Kaplan-Meier estimate of the survivor function, given in Equation (2.12), while an estimate of the probability density function at $\hat{t}(p)$ is

$$\hat{f}\{\hat{t}(p)\} = \frac{\hat{S}\{\hat{u}(p)\} - \hat{S}\{\hat{l}(p)\}}{\hat{l}(p) - \hat{u}(p)},$$

where

$$\hat{u}(p) = \max\left\{t_{(j)} \mid \hat{S}(t_{(j)}) \geqslant 1 - \frac{p}{100} + \epsilon\right\},$$

and

$$\hat{l}(p) = \min\left\{t_{(j)} \mid \hat{S}(t_{(j)}) \leqslant 1 - \frac{p}{100} - \epsilon\right\},$$

for $j = 1, 2, \ldots, r$, and small values of ϵ. In many cases, taking $\epsilon = 0.05$ will be satisfactory, but a larger value of ϵ will be needed if $\hat{u}(p)$ and $\hat{l}(p)$ turn out to be equal. In particular, from Equation (2.15), the standard error of the median survival time is given by

$$\text{se}\,\{\hat{t}(50)\} = \frac{1}{\hat{f}\{\hat{t}(50)\}}\,\text{se}\,[\hat{S}\{\hat{t}(50)\}], \tag{2.16}$$

where $\hat{f}\{\hat{t}(50)\}$ can be found from

$$\hat{f}\{\hat{t}(50)\} = \frac{\hat{S}\{\hat{u}(50)\} - \hat{S}\{\hat{l}(50)\}}{\hat{l}(50) - \hat{u}(50)}. \tag{2.17}$$

In this expression, $\hat{u}(50)$ is the largest survival time for which the Kaplan-Meier estimate of the survivor function exceeds 0.55, and $\hat{l}(50)$ is the smallest survival time for which the survivor function is less than or equal to 0.45.

Once the standard error of the estimated pth percentile has been found, a $100(1-\alpha)\%$ confidence interval for $t(p)$ has limits of

$$\hat{t}(p) \pm z_{\alpha/2}\,\text{se}\,\{\hat{t}(p)\},$$

where $z_{\alpha/2}$ is the upper (one-sided) $\alpha/2$-point of the standard normal distribution.

This interval estimate is only approximate, in the sense that the probability that the interval includes the true percentile will not be exactly $1-\alpha$. A number of methods have been proposed for constructing confidence intervals for the median with superior properties, although these alternatives are more difficult to compute than the interval estimate derived in this section.

Example 2.10 Time to discontinuation of the use of an IUD

The data on the discontinuation times for users of an IUD, given in Example 1.1, are now used to illustrate the calculation of a confidence interval for the median discontinuation time. From Example 2.8, the estimated median discontinuation time for this group of women is given by $\hat{t}(50) = 93$ weeks. Also, from Table 2.4, the standard error of the Kaplan-Meier estimate of the survivor function at this time is given by $\text{se}\,[\hat{S}\{\hat{t}(50)\}] = 0.1452$.

To obtain the standard error of $\hat{t}(50)$ using Equation (2.16), we need an estimate of the density function at the estimated median discontinuation time. This is obtained from Equation (2.17). The quantities $\hat{u}(50)$ and $\hat{l}(50)$ needed in this equation are such that

$$\hat{u}(50) = \max\{t_{(j)} \mid \hat{S}(t_{(j)}) \geqslant 0.55\},$$

and

$$\hat{l}(50) = \min\{t_{(j)} \mid \hat{S}(t_{(j)}) \leqslant 0.45\},$$

where $t_{(j)}$ is the jth ordered discontinuation time, $j = 1, 2, \ldots, 9$. Using Table 2.4, $\hat{u}(50) = 75$ and $\hat{l}(50) = 97$, and so

$$\hat{f}\{\hat{t}(50)\} = \frac{\hat{S}(75) - \hat{S}(97)}{97 - 75} = \frac{0.5594 - 0.3729}{22} = 0.0085.$$

Then, the standard error of the median is given by

$$\text{se}\,\{\hat{t}(50)\} = \frac{1}{0.0085} \times 0.1452 = 17.13.$$

A 95% confidence interval for the median discontinuation time has limits of

$$93 \pm 1.96 \times 17.13,$$

and so the required interval estimate for the median ranges from 59 to 127 days.

2.6 Comparison of two groups of survival data

The simplest way of comparing the survival times obtained from two groups of individuals is to plot the corresponding estimates of the two survivor functions on the same axes. The resulting plot can be quite informative, as the following example illustrates.

Example 2.11 Prognosis for women with breast cancer
Data on the survival times of women with breast cancer, grouped according to whether or not sections of a tumour were positively stained with *Helix pomatia* agglutinin (HPA), were given in Example 1.2. The Kaplan-Meier estimate of the survivor function, for each of the two groups of survival times, is plotted in Figure 2.9. Notice that in this figure, the Kaplan-Meier estimates extend to the time of the largest censored observation in each group.

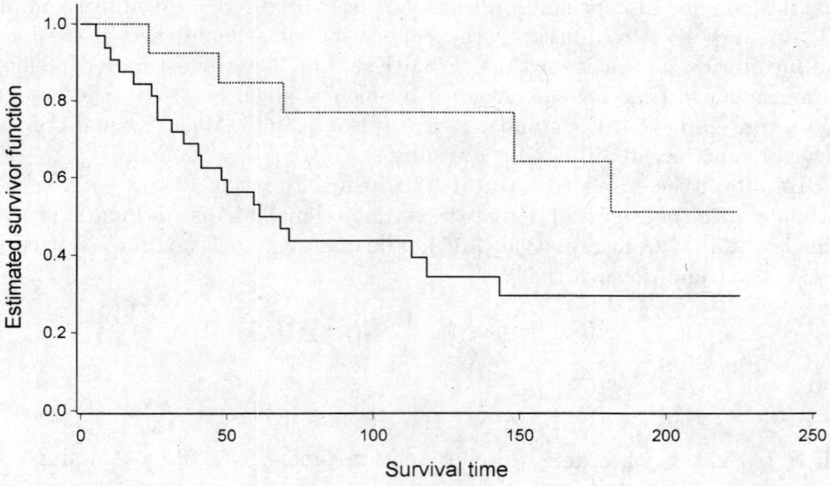

Figure 2.9 *Kaplan-Meier estimate of the survivor functions for women with tumours that were positively stained (—) and negatively stained (······).*

This figure shows that the estimated survivor function for those women with negatively stained tumours is always greater than that for women with positively stained tumours. This means that at any time t, the estimated probability of survival beyond t is greater for women with negative staining, suggesting that the result of the HPA staining procedure might be a useful prognostic indicator. In particular, those women whose tumours are positively stained appear to have a poorer prognosis than those with negatively stained tumours.

There are two possible explanations for an observed difference between two estimated survivor functions, such as those in Example 2.11. One explanation is that there is a real difference between the survival times of the two groups of individuals, so that those in one group have a different survival experience from those in the other. An alternative explanation is that there are no real differences between the survival times in each group, and that the difference that has been observed is merely the result of chance variation. To help distinguish between these two possible explanations, we use a procedure known as the *hypothesis test*. Because the concept of the hypothesis test has a central role in the analysis of survival data, the underlying basis for this procedure is described in detail in the following section.

2.6.1 Hypothesis testing

The hypothesis test is a procedure that enables us to assess the extent to which an observed set of data are consistent with a particular hypothesis, known as the *working* or *null hypothesis*. A null hypothesis generally represents a simplified view of the data-generating process, and is typified by hypotheses that specify that there is no difference between two groups of survival data, or that there is no relationship between survival time and explanatory variables such as age or serum cholesterol level. The null hypothesis is then the hypothesis that will be adopted, and subsequently acted upon, unless the data indicate that it is untenable.

The next step is to formulate a *test statistic* that measures the extent to which the observed data depart from the null hypothesis. In general, the test statistic is so constructed that the larger the value of the statistic, the greater the departure from the null hypothesis. Hence, if the null hypothesis is that there is no difference between two groups, relatively large values of the test statistic will be interpreted as evidence against this null hypothesis.

Once the value of the test statistic has been obtained from the observed data, we calculate the probability of obtaining a value as extreme or more extreme than the observed value, when the null hypothesis is true. This quantity summarises the strength of the evidence in the sample data against the null hypothesis, and is known as the *probability value*, or *P-value* for short. If the P-value is large, we would conclude that it is quite likely that the observed data would have been obtained when the null hypothesis was true, and that there is no evidence to reject the null hypothesis. On the other hand, if the P-value is small, this would be interpreted as evidence against the null hypothesis; the smaller the P-value, the stronger the evidence.

In order to obtain the P-value for a hypothesis test, the test statistic must have a probability distribution that is known, or at least approximately known, when the null hypothesis is true. This probability distribution is referred to as the *null distribution* of the test statistic. More specifically, consider a test statistic, W, which is such that the larger the observed value of the test statistic, w, the greater the deviation of the observed data from that expected under the null hypothesis. If W has a continuous probability distribution, the P-value is then $\text{P}(W \geqslant w) = 1 - F(w)$, where $F(w)$ is the distribution function of W, under the null hypothesis, evaluated at w.

In some applications, the most natural test statistic is one for which large positive values correspond to departures from the null hypothesis in one direction, while large negative values correspond to departures in the opposite direction. For example, suppose that patients suffering from a particular illness have been randomised to receive either a standard treatment or a new treatment, and their survival times are recorded. In this situation, a null hypothesis of interest will be that there is no difference in the survival experience of the patients in the two treatment groups. The extent to which the data are consistent with this null hypothesis might then be summarised by a test statistic for which positive values indicate that the new treatment is superior to the standard, while negative values indicate that the standard treatment is superior. When departures from the null hypothesis in either direction are equally important, the null hypothesis is said to have a *two-sided alternative*, and the hypothesis test itself is referred to as a two-sided test.

If W is a test statistic for which large positive or large negative observed values lead to rejection of the null hypothesis, a new test statistic, such as $|W|$ or W^2, can be defined, so that only large positive values of the new statistic indicate that there is evidence against the null hypothesis. For example, suppose that W is a test statistic that under the null hypothesis has a standard normal distribution. If w is the observed value of W, the appropriate P-value is $\text{P}(W \leqslant -|w|) + \text{P}(W \geqslant |w|)$, which in view of the symmetry of the standard normal distribution, is $2\,\text{P}(W \geqslant |w|)$. Alternatively, we can make use of the result that if W has a standard normal distribution, W^2 has a chi-squared distribution on one degree of freedom, written χ_1^2. Thus, a P-value for the two-sided hypothesis test based on the statistic W is the probability that a χ_1^2 random variable exceeds w^2. The required P-value can therefore be found from the standard normal or chi-squared distribution functions.

When interest centres on departures in a particular direction, the hypothesis test is said to be *one-sided*. For example, in comparing the survival times of two groups of patients where one group receives a standard treatment and the other group a new treatment, it might be argued that the new treatment cannot possibly be inferior to the standard. Then, the only relevant alternative to the null hypothesis of no treatment difference is that the new treatment is superior. If positive values of the test statistic W reflect the superiority of the new treatment, the P-value is then $\text{P}(W \geqslant w)$. If W has a standard normal distribution, this P-value is half of that which would have been obtained for the corresponding two-sided alternative hypothesis.

A one-sided hypothesis test can only be appropriate when there is no interest whatsoever in departures from the null hypothesis in the opposite direction to that specified in the one-sided alternative. For example, consider again the comparison of a new treatment with a standard treatment, and suppose that the observed value of the test statistic is either positive or negative, depending on whether the new treatment is superior or inferior to the standard. If the alternative to the null hypothesis of no treatment difference is that the new treatment is superior, a large negative value of the test statistic would not be regarded as evidence against the null hypothesis. Instead, it would be assumed that this large negative value is simply the result of chance variation. Generally speaking, the use of one-sided tests can rarely be justified in medical research, and so two-sided tests will be used throughout this book.

If a P-value is smaller than some value α, we say that the hypothesis is rejected at the $100\alpha\%$ *level of significance*. The observed value of the test statistic is then said to be significant at this level. But how do we decide on the basis of the P-value whether or not a null hypothesis should actually be rejected? Traditionally, P-values of 0.05 or 0.01 have been used in reaching a decision about whether or not a null hypothesis should be rejected, so that if $P < 0.05$, for example, the null hypothesis is rejected at the 5% significance level. Guidelines such as these are not hard-and-fast rules and should not be interpreted rigidly. For example, there is no practical difference between a P-value of 0.046 and 0.056, even though only the former indicates that the observed value of the test statistic is significant at the 5% level.

Instead of reporting that a null hypothesis is rejected or not rejected at some specified significance level, a more satisfactory policy is to report the actual P-value. This P-value can then be interpreted as a measure of the strength of evidence against the null hypothesis, using a vocabulary that depends on the range within which the P-value lies. Thus, if $P > 0.1$, there is said to be no evidence to reject the null hypothesis; if $0.05 < P \leqslant 0.1$, there is slight evidence against the null hypothesis; if $0.01 < P \leqslant 0.05$, there is moderate evidence against the null hypothesis; if $0.001 < P \leqslant 0.01$, there is strong evidence against the null hypothesis, and if $P \leqslant 0.001$, the evidence against the null hypothesis is overwhelming.

An alternative to quoting the exact P-value associated with a hypothesis test is to compare the observed value of the test statistic with those values that would correspond to particular P-values, when the null hypothesis is true. Values of the test statistic that lead to rejection of the null hypothesis at particular levels of significance can be found from percentage points of the null distribution of that statistic. In particular, if W is a test statistic that has a standard normal distribution, for a two-sided test, the upper $\alpha/2$-point of the distribution, depicted in Figure 2.5, is the value of the test statistic for which the P-value is α. For example, values of the test statistic of 1.96, 2.58 and 3.29 correspond to P-values of 0.05, 0.01 and 0.001. Thus, if the observed value of

W were between 1.96 and 2.58, we would declare that $0.01 < P < 0.05$. On the other hand, if the null distribution of W is chi-squared on one degree of freedom, the upper α-point of the distribution is the value of the test statistic which would give a P-value of α. Then, values of the test statistic of 3.84, 6.64 and 10.83 correspond to P-values of 0.05, 0.01 and 0.001, respectively. Notice that these values are simply the squares of those for the standard normal distribution, which they must be in view of the fact that the square of a standard normal random variable has a chi-squared distribution on one degree of freedom.

For commonly encountered probability distributions, such as the normal and chi-squared, percentage points are tabulated in many introductory text books on statistics, or in statistical tables such as those of Lindley and Scott (1984). Statistical software packages used in computer-based statistical analyses of survival data usually provide the exact P-values associated with hypothesis tests as a matter of course. Note that when these are rounded off to, say, three decimal places, a P-value of 0.000 should be interpreted as $P < 0.001$.

In deciding on a course of action, such as whether or not to reject the hypothesis that there is no difference between two treatments, the statistical evidence summarised in the P-value for the hypothesis test will be just one ingredient of the decision-making process. In addition to the statistical evidence, there will also be scientific evidence to consider. This may, for example, concern whether the size of the treatment effect is clinically important. In particular, in a large trial, a difference between two treatments that is significant at, say, the 5% level may be found when the magnitude of the treatment effect is so small that it does not indicate a major scientific breakthrough. On the other hand, a new formulation of a treatment may prolong life by a factor of two, and yet, because of small sample sizes used in the study, may not appear to be significantly different from the standard.

Rather than report findings in terms of the results of a hypothesis testing procedure, it is more informative to provide an estimate of the size of any treatment difference, supported by a confidence interval for this difference. Unfortunately, the non-parametric approaches to the analysis of survival data being considered in this chapter do not lend themselves to this approach. We will therefore return to this theme in subsequent chapters when we consider models for survival data.

In the comparison of two groups of survival data, there are a number of methods that can be used to quantify the extent of between-group differences. Two non-parametric procedures will now be considered, namely the log-rank test and the Wilcoxon test.

2.6.2 The log-rank test

In order to construct the log-rank test, we begin by considering separately each death time in two groups of survival data. These groups will be labelled Group I and Group II. Suppose that there are r distinct death times, denoted

$t_{(1)} < t_{(2)} < \cdots < t_{(r)}$, across the two groups, and that at time $t_{(j)}$, d_{1j} individuals in Group I and d_{2j} individuals in Group II die, for $j = 1, 2, \ldots, r$. Unless two or more individuals in a group have the same recorded death time, the values of d_{1j} and d_{2j} will either be zero or unity. Suppose further that there are n_{1j} individuals at risk of death in the first group just before time $t_{(j)}$, and that there are n_{2j} at risk in the second group. Consequently, at time $t_{(j)}$, there are $d_j = d_{1j} + d_{2j}$ deaths in total out of $n_j = n_{1j} + n_{2j}$ individuals at risk. The situation is summarised in Table 2.7.

Table 2.7 *Number of deaths at the jth death time in each of two groups of individuals.*

Group	Number of deaths at $t_{(j)}$	Number surviving beyond $t_{(j)}$	Number at risk just before $t_{(j)}$
I	d_{1j}	$n_{1j} - d_{1j}$	n_{1j}
II	d_{2j}	$n_{2j} - d_{2j}$	n_{2j}
Total	d_j	$n_j - d_j$	n_j

Now consider the null hypothesis that there is no difference in the survival experience of the individuals in the two groups. One way of assessing the validity of this hypothesis is to consider the extent of the difference between the observed number of individuals in the two groups who die at each of the death times, and the numbers expected under the null hypothesis. Information about the extent of these differences can then be combined over each of the death times.

If the marginal totals in Table 2.7 are regarded as fixed, and the null hypothesis that survival is independent of group is true, the four entries in this table are solely determined by the value of d_{1j}, the number of deaths at $t_{(j)}$ in Group I. We can therefore regard d_{1j} as a random variable, which can take any value in the range from 0 to the minimum of d_j and n_{1j}. In fact, d_{1j} has a distribution known as the *hypergeometric distribution*, according to which the probability that the random variable associated with the number of deaths in the first group takes the value d_{1j} is

$$\frac{\binom{d_j}{d_{1j}}\binom{n_j - d_j}{n_{1j} - d_{1j}}}{\binom{n_j}{n_{1j}}}. \tag{2.18}$$

In this formula, the expression

$$\binom{d_j}{d_{1j}}$$

represents the number of different ways in which d_{1j} times can be chosen from d_j times and is read as '$d_j\ C\ d_{1j}$'. It is given by

$$\binom{d_j}{d_{1j}} = \frac{d_j!}{d_{1j}!(d_j - d_{1j})!},$$

where $d_j!$, read as 'd_j *factorial*', is such that

$$d_j! = d_j \times (d_j - 1) \times \cdots \times 2 \times 1.$$

The other two terms in Expression (2.18) are interpreted in a similar manner.

The mean of the hypergeometric random variable d_{1j} is given by

$$e_{1j} = n_{1j} d_j / n_j, \tag{2.19}$$

so that e_{1j} is the expected number of individuals who die at time $t_{(j)}$ in Group I. This value is intuitively appealing, since under the null hypothesis that the probability of death at time $t_{(j)}$ does not depend on the group that an individual is in, the probability of death at $t_{(j)}$ is d_j/n_j. Multiplying this by n_{1j}, gives e_{1j} as the expected number of deaths in Group I at $t_{(j)}$.

The next step is to combine the information from the individual 2×2 tables for each death time to give an overall measure of the deviation of the observed values of d_{1j} from their expected values. The most straightforward way of doing this is to sum the differences $d_{1j} - e_{1j}$ over the total number of death times, r, in the two groups. The resulting statistic is given by

$$U_L = \sum_{j=1}^{r} (d_{1j} - e_{1j}). \tag{2.20}$$

Notice that this is $\sum d_{1j} - \sum e_{1j}$, which is the difference between the total observed and expected numbers of deaths in Group I. This statistic will have zero mean, since $\operatorname{E}(d_{1j}) = e_{1j}$. Moreover, since the death times are independent of one another, the variance of U_L is simply the sum of the variances of the d_{1j}. Now, since d_{1j} has a hypergeometric distribution, the variance of d_{1j} is given by

$$v_{1j} = \frac{n_{1j} n_{2j} d_j (n_j - d_j)}{n_j^2 (n_j - 1)}, \tag{2.21}$$

so that the variance of U_L is

$$\operatorname{var}(U_L) = \sum_{j=1}^{r} v_{1j} = V_L, \tag{2.22}$$

say. Furthermore, it can be shown that U_L has an approximate normal distribution, when the number of death times is not too small. It then follows that $U_L/\sqrt{V_L}$ has a normal distribution with zero mean and unit variance, denoted $N(0, 1)$. We therefore write

$$\frac{U_L}{\sqrt{V_L}} \sim N(0, 1),$$

where the symbol '$\sim$' is read as '*is distributed as*'. The square of a standard normal random variable has a chi-squared distribution on one degree of freedom, denoted χ_1^2, and so we have that

$$\frac{U_L^2}{V_L} \sim \chi_1^2. \tag{2.23}$$

This method of combining information over a number of 2×2 tables was proposed by Mantel and Haenszel (1959), and is known as the Mantel-Haenszel procedure. In fact, the test based on this statistic has various names, including *Mantel-Cox* and *Peto-Mantel-Haenszel*, but it is probably best known as the log-rank test. The reason for this name is that the test statistic can be derived from the ranks of the survival times in the two groups, and the resulting rank test statistic is based on the logarithm of the Nelson-Aalen estimate of the survivor function.

The statistic $W_L = U_L^2/V_L$ summarises the extent to which the observed survival times in the two groups of data deviate from those expected under the null hypothesis of no group differences. The larger the value of this statistic, the greater the evidence against the null hypothesis. Because the null distribution of W is approximately chi-squared with one degree of freedom, the P-value associated with the test statistic can be obtained from the distribution function of a chi-squared random variable. Alternatively, percentage points of the chi-squared distribution can be used to identify a range within which the P-value lies. An illustration of the log-rank test is presented below in Example 2.12.

Example 2.12 Prognosis for women with breast cancer

In this example, we return to the data on the survival times of women with breast cancer, grouped according to whether a section of the tumour was positively or negatively stained. In particular, the null hypothesis that there is no difference in the survival experience of the two groups will be examined using the log-rank test. The required calculations are laid out in Table 2.8.

We begin by ordering the observed death times across the two groups of women; these times are given in column 1 of Table 2.8. The numbers of women in each group who die at each death time and the numbers who are at risk at each time are then calculated. These values are d_{1j}, n_{1j}, d_{2j} and n_{2j} given in columns 2 to 5 of the table. Columns 6 and 7 contain the total numbers of deaths and the total numbers of women at risk over the two groups, at each death time. The final two columns give the values of e_{1j} and v_{1j}, computed from Equations (2.19) and (2.21), respectively. Summing the entries in columns 2 and 8 gives $\sum d_{1j}$ and $\sum e_{1j}$, from which the log-rank statistic can be calculated from $U_L = \sum d_{1j} - \sum e_{1j}$. The value of $V_L = \sum v_{1j}$ can be obtained by summing the entries in the final column. We find that $U_L = 5 - 9.565 = -4.565$ and $V_L = 5.929$, and so the value of the log-rank test statistic is $W_L = (-4.565)^2/5.929 = 3.515$.

The corresponding P-value is calculated from the probability that a chi-squared variate on one degree of freedom is greater than or equal to 3.515,

Table 2.8 *Calculation of the log-rank statistic for the data from Example 1.2.*

Death time	d_{1j}	n_{1j}	d_{2j}	n_{2j}	d_j	n_j	e_{1j}	v_{1j}
5	0	13	1	32	1	45	0.2889	0.2054
8	0	13	1	31	1	44	0.2955	0.2082
10	0	13	1	30	1	43	0.3023	0.2109
13	0	13	1	29	1	42	0.3095	0.2137
18	0	13	1	28	1	41	0.3171	0.2165
23	1	13	0	27	1	40	0.3250	0.2194
24	0	12	1	27	1	39	0.3077	0.2130
26	0	12	2	26	2	38	0.6316	0.4205
31	0	12	1	24	1	36	0.3333	0.2222
35	0	12	1	23	1	35	0.3429	0.2253
40	0	12	1	22	1	34	0.3529	0.2284
41	0	12	1	21	1	33	0.3636	0.2314
47	1	12	0	20	1	32	0.3750	0.2344
48	0	11	1	20	1	31	0.3548	0.2289
50	0	11	1	19	1	30	0.3667	0.2322
59	0	11	1	18	1	29	0.3793	0.2354
61	0	11	1	17	1	28	0.3929	0.2385
68	0	11	1	16	1	27	0.4074	0.2414
69	1	11	0	15	1	26	0.4231	0.2441
71	0	9	1	15	1	24	0.3750	0.2344
113	0	6	1	10	1	16	0.3750	0.2344
118	0	6	1	8	1	14	0.4286	0.2449
143	0	6	1	7	1	13	0.4615	0.2485
148	1	6	0	6	1	12	0.5000	0.2500
181	1	5	0	4	1	9	0.5556	0.2469
Total	5						9.5652	5.9289

and is 0.061, written $P = 0.061$. This P-value is sufficiently small to cast doubt on the null hypothesis that there is no difference between the survivor functions for the two groups of women. In fact, the evidence against the null hypothesis is nearly significant at the 6% level. We therefore conclude that the data do provide some evidence that the prognosis of a breast cancer patient is dependent on the result of the staining procedure.

2.6.3 The Wilcoxon test

The Wilcoxon test, sometimes known as the *Breslow test*, is also used to test the null hypothesis that there is no difference in the survivor functions for two groups of survival data. The Wilcoxon test is based on the statistic

$$U_W = \sum_{j=1}^{r} n_j(d_{1j} - e_{1j}),$$

where, as in the previous section, d_{1j} is the number of deaths at time $t_{(j)}$ in the first group and e_{1j} is as defined in Equation (2.19). The difference between U_W and U_L is that in the Wilcoxon test, each difference $d_{1j} - e_{1j}$ is weighted by n_j, the total number of individuals at risk at time $t_{(j)}$. The effect of this is to give less weight to differences between d_{1j} and e_{1j} at those times when the total number of individuals who are still alive is small, that is, at the longest survival times. This statistic is therefore less sensitive than the log-rank statistic to deviations of d_{1j} from e_{1j} in the tail of the distribution of survival times.

The variance of the Wilcoxon statistic U_W is given by

$$V_W = \sum_{j=1}^{r} n_j^2 v_{1j},$$

where v_{1j} is given in Equation (2.21), and so the Wilcoxon test statistic is

$$W_W = U_W^2 / V_W,$$

which has a chi-squared distribution on one degree of freedom when the null hypothesis is true. The Wilcoxon test is therefore conducted in the same manner as the log-rank test.

Example 2.13 Prognosis for women with breast cancer
For the data on the survival times of women with tumours that were positively or negatively stained, the value of the Wilcoxon statistic is $U_W = -159$, and the variance of the statistic is $V_W = 6048.136$. The value of the chi-squared statistic, U_W^2/V_W, is 4.180, and the corresponding P-value is 0.041. This is slightly smaller than the P-value for the log-rank test, and on the basis of this result, we would declare that the difference between the two groups is significant at the 5% level.

2.6.4 Comparison of the log-rank and Wilcoxon tests

Of the two tests, the log-rank test is the more suitable when the alternative to the null hypothesis of no difference between two groups of survival times is that the hazard of death at any given time for an individual in one group is proportional to the hazard at that time for a similar individual in the other group. This is the assumption of *proportional hazards*, which underlies a number of methods for analysing survival data. For other types of departure from the null hypothesis, the Wilcoxon test is more appropriate than the log-rank test for comparing the two survivor functions.

In order to help decide which test is the more suitable in any given situation, we make use of the result that if the hazard functions are proportional, the survivor functions for the two groups of survival data do not cross one another. To show this, suppose that $h_1(t)$ is the hazard of death at time t for an individual in Group I, and $h_2(t)$ is the hazard at that same time for an individual in Group II. If these two hazards are proportional, then we can write

$h_1(t) = \psi h_2(t)$, where ψ is a constant that does not depend on the time t. Integrating both sides of this expression, multiplying by -1 and exponentiating gives

$$\exp\left\{-\int_0^t h_1(u)\,\mathrm{d}u\right\} = \exp\left\{-\int_0^t \psi h_2(u)\,\mathrm{d}u\right\}. \tag{2.24}$$

Now, from Equation (1.6),

$$S(t) = \exp\left\{-\int_0^t h(u)\,\mathrm{d}u\right\},$$

and so if $S_1(t)$ and $S_2(t)$ are the survivor functions for the two groups of survival data, from Equation (2.24),

$$S_1(t) = \{S_2(t)\}^{\psi}.$$

Since the survivor function takes values between zero and unity, this result shows that $S_1(t)$ is greater than or less than $S_2(t)$, according to whether ψ is less than or greater than unity, at any time t. This means that if two hazard functions are proportional, the true survivor functions do not cross. This is a necessary, but not a sufficient condition for proportional hazards.

An informal assessment of the likely validity of the proportional hazards assumption can be made from a plot of the estimated survivor functions for two groups of survival data, such as that shown in Figure 2.9. If the two estimated survivor functions do not cross, the assumption of proportional hazards may be justified, and the log-rank test is appropriate. Of course, sample-based estimates of survivor functions may cross even though the corresponding true hazard functions are proportional, and so some care is needed in the interpretation of such graphs. A more satisfactory graphical method for assessing the validity of the proportional hazards assumption is described in Section 4.4.1 of Chapter 4.

In summary, unless a plot of the estimated survival functions, or previous data, indicate that there is good reason to doubt the proportional hazards assumption, the log-rank test should be used to test the hypothesis of equality of two survivor functions.

Example 2.14 Prognosis for women with breast cancer

From the graph of the two estimated survivor functions in Figure 2.9, we see that the survivor function for the negatively stained women always lies above that for the positively stained women. This suggests that the proportional hazards assumption is appropriate, and that the log-rank test is more appropriate than the Wilcoxon test. However, in this example, there is very little difference between the results of the two hypothesis tests.

2.7* Comparison of three or more groups of survival data

Both the log-rank and the Wilcoxon tests can be extended to enable three or more groups of survival data to be compared. Suppose that the survival distributions of g groups of survival data are to be compared, for $g \geqslant 2$. We then define analogues of the U-statistics for comparing the observed numbers of deaths in groups $1, 2, \ldots, g-1$ with their expected values. In an obvious extension of the notation used in Section 2.6, we obtain

$$U_{Lk} = \sum_{j=1}^{r} \left(d_{kj} - \frac{n_{kj} d_j}{n_j} \right),$$

$$U_{Wk} = \sum_{j=1}^{r} n_j \left(d_{kj} - \frac{n_{kj} d_j}{n_j} \right),$$

for $k = 1, 2, \ldots, g-1$. These quantities are then expressed in the form of a vector with $(g-1)$ components, which we denote by $\boldsymbol{U}_L$ and $\boldsymbol{U}_W$.

We also need expressions for the variances of the U_{Lk} and U_{Wk}, and for the covariance between pairs of values. In particular, the covariance between U_{Lk} and $U_{Lk'}$ is given by

$$V_{Lkk'} = \sum_{j=1}^{r} \frac{n_{kj} d_j (n_j - d_j)}{n_j (n_j - 1)} \left(\delta_{kk'} - \frac{n_{k'j}}{n_j} \right),$$

for $k, k' = 1, 2, \ldots, g-1$, where $\delta_{kk'}$ is such that

$$\delta_{kk'} = \begin{cases} 1 & \text{if } k = k', \\ 0 & \text{otherwise.} \end{cases}$$

These terms are then assembled in the form of a *variance-covariance matrix*, $\boldsymbol{V}_L$, which is a symmetric matrix that has the variances of the U_{Lk} down the diagonal, and covariance terms in the off-diagonals. For example, in the comparison of three groups of survival data, this matrix would be given by

$$\boldsymbol{V}_L = \begin{pmatrix} V_{L11} & V_{L12} \\ V_{L12} & V_{L22} \end{pmatrix},$$

where V_{L11} and V_{L22} are the variances of U_{L1} and U_{L2}, respectively, and V_{L12} is their covariance.

Similarly, the variance-covariance matrix for the Wilcoxon statistic is the matrix $\boldsymbol{V}_W$, whose (k, k')th element is

$$V_{Wkk'} = \sum_{j=1}^{r} n_j^2 \frac{n_{kj} d_j (n_j - d_j)}{n_j (n_j - 1)} \left(\delta_{kk'} - \frac{n_{k'j}}{n_j} \right),$$

for $k, k' = 1, 2, \ldots, g-1$.

Finally, in order to test the null hypothesis of no group differences, we make use of the result that the test statistic $\boldsymbol{U}_L' \boldsymbol{V}_L^{-1} \boldsymbol{U}_L$, or $\boldsymbol{U}_W' \boldsymbol{V}_W^{-1} \boldsymbol{U}_W$, has a chi-squared distribution on $(g-1)$ degrees of freedom, when the null hypothesis is true.

Statistical software for the analysis of survival data usually incorporates this methodology, and because the interpretation of the resulting chi-squared statistic is straightforward, an example will not be given here.

2.8 Stratified tests

In many circumstances, there is a need to compare two or more sets of survival data, after taking account of additional variables recorded on each individual. As an illustration, consider a multicentre clinical trial in which two forms of chemotherapy are to be compared in terms of their effect on the survival times of lung cancer patients. Information on the survival times of patients in each treatment group will be available from each centre. The resulting data are then said to be *stratified* by centre.

Individual log-rank or Wilcoxon tests based on the data from each centre will be informative, but a test that combines information about the treatment difference in each centre provides a more precise summary of the treatment effect. A similar situation would arise in attempting to test for treatment differences when patients are stratified according to variables such as age group, sex, performance status and other potential risk factors for the disease under study.

In situations such as those described above, a stratified version of the log-rank or Wilcoxon test may be employed. Essentially, this involves calculating the values of the U- and V-statistics for each *stratum*, and then combining these values over the strata. In this section, the *stratified log-rank test* will be described, but a stratified version of the Wilcoxon test can be obtained in a similar manner. An equivalent analysis, based on a model for the survival times, is described in Section 11.2 of Chapter 11.

Let U_{Lk} be the value of the log-rank statistic for comparing two treatment groups, computed from the kth of s strata using Equation (2.20). Also, denote the variance of the statistic for the kth stratum by V_{Lk}, where V_{Lk} would be computed for each stratum using Equation (2.21). The stratified log-rank test is then based on the statistic

$$W_S = \frac{\left(\sum_{k=1}^{s} U_{Lk}\right)^2}{\sum_{k=1}^{s} V_{Lk}}, \tag{2.25}$$

which has a chi-squared distribution on one degree of freedom (1 d.f.) under the null hypothesis that there is no treatment difference. Comparing the observed value of this statistic with percentage points of the chi-squared distribution enables the hypothesis of no overall treatment difference to be tested.

Example 2.15 Survival times of patients with melanoma

The aim of a study carried out by the University of Oklahoma Health Sciences Center was to compare two immunotherapy treatments for their ability to prolong the life of patients suffering from melanoma, a highly malignant tumour occurring in the skin. For each patient, the tumour was surgically removed before allocation to *Bacillus Calmette-Guérin* (BCG) vaccine or to a vaccine based on the bacterium *Corynebacterium parvum* (*C. parvum*).

The survival times of the patients in each treatment group were further classified according to the age group of the patient. The data, which were given in Lee and Wang (2013), are shown in Table 2.9.

Table 2.9 *Survival times of melanoma patients in two treatment groups, stratified by age group.*

21–40		41–60		61–	
BCG	*C. parvum*	BCG	*C. parvum*	BCG	*C. parvum*
19	27*	34*	8	10	25*
24*	21*	4	11*	5	8
8	18*	17*	23*		11*
17*	16*		12*		
17*	7		15*		
34*	12*		8*		
	24		8*		
	8				
	8*				

* Censored survival times.

These data are analysed by first computing the log-rank statistics for comparing the survival times of patients in the two treatment groups, separately for each age group. The resulting values of the U-, V- and W-statistics, found using Equations (2.20), (2.22) and (2.23), are summarised in Table 2.10.

Table 2.10 *Values of the log-rank statistic for each age group.*

Age group	U_L	V_L	W_L
21–40	−0.2571	1.1921	0.055
41–60	0.4778	0.3828	0.596
61–	1.0167	0.6497	1.591
Total	1.2374	2.2246	

The values of the W_L-statistic are quite similar for the three age groups, suggesting that the treatment effect is consistent over these groups. Moreover, none of them are significantly large at the 10% level.

To carry out a stratified log-rank test on these data, we calculate the W_S-statistic defined in Equation (2.25). Using the results in Table 2.10,

$$W_S = \frac{1.2374^2}{2.2246} = 0.688.$$

The observed value of W_S is not significant when compared with percentage points of the chi-squared distribution on 1 d.f. We therefore conclude that after allowing for the different age groups, there is no significant difference between the survival times of patients treated with the BCG vaccine and those treated with *C. parvum*.

For comparison, when the division of the patients into the different age groups is ignored, the log-rank test for comparing the two groups of patients leads to $W_L = 0.756$. The fact that this is so similar to the value that allows for age group differences suggests that it is not necessary to stratify the patients by age.

The stratified log-rank test can be extended to compare more than two treatment groups. The resulting formulae render it unsuitable for hand calculation, but the methodology can be implemented using computer software for survival analysis. However, this method of taking account of additional variables is not as flexible as that based on a modelling approach, introduced in the next chapter, and so further details are not given here.

2.9 Log-rank test for trend

In many applications where three or more groups of survival data are to be compared, these groups are ordered in some way. For example, the groups may correspond to increasing doses of a treatment, the stage of a disease, or the age group of an individual. In comparing these groups using the log-rank test described in previous sections, it can happen that the analysis does not lead to a significant difference between the groups, even though the hazard of death increases or decreases across the groups. A test procedure that uses information about the ordering of the groups is more likely to lead to a trend being identified as significant than a standard log-rank test.

The log-rank test for trend across g ordered groups is based on the statistic

$$U_T = \sum_{k=1}^{g} w_k (d_{k.} - e_{k.}), \tag{2.26}$$

where w_k is a *code* assigned to the kth group, $k = 1, 2, \ldots, g$, and

$$d_{k.} = \sum_{j=1}^{r_k} d_{kj}, \qquad e_{k.} = \sum_{j=1}^{r_k} e_{kj},$$

are the observed and expected numbers of deaths in the kth group, where the summation is over the r_k death times in that group. Note that the dot subscript in the notation $d_{k.}$ and $e_{k.}$ stands for summation over the subscript that the dot replaces. The codes are often taken to be equally spaced to correspond to a linear trend across the groups. For example, if there are three groups, the codes might be taken to be 1, 2 and 3, although the equivalent choice of -1, 0 and 1 does simplify the calculations somewhat. The variance of U_T is given by

$$V_T = \sum_{k=1}^{g} (w_k - \bar{w})^2 e_{k.}, \tag{2.27}$$

where $\bar{w}$ is a weighted sum of the quantities w_k, in which the expected numbers of deaths, $e_{k.}$, are the weights, that is,

$$\bar{w} = \frac{\sum_{k=1}^{g} w_k e_{k.}}{\sum_{k=1}^{g} e_{k.}}.$$

The statistic $W_T = U_T^2/V_T$ then has a chi-squared distribution on 1 d.f. under the hypothesis of no trend across the g groups.

Example 2.16 Survival times of patients with melanoma

The log-rank test for trend will be illustrated using the data from Example 2.15 on the survival times of patients suffering from melanoma. For the purpose of this illustration, only the data from those patients allocated to the BCG vaccine will be used. The log-rank statistic for comparing the survival times of the patients in the three age groups turns out to be 3.739. When compared to percentage points of the chi-squared distribution on 2 d.f., this is not significant ($P = 0.154$).

We now use the log-rank test for trend to examine whether there is a linear trend over age. For this, we will take the codes, w_k, to be equally spaced, with values -1, 0 and 1. Some of the calculations required for the log-rank test for trend are summarised in Table 2.11.

Table 2.11 *Values of w_k and the observed and expected numbers of deaths in the three age groups.*

Age group	w_k	$d_{k.}$	$e_{k.}$
21–40	-1	2	3.1871
41–60	0	1	1.1949
61–	1	2	0.6179

The log-rank test for trend is based on the statistic in Equation (2.26), the value of which is

$$U_T = (d_{3.} - e_{3.}) - (d_{1.} - e_{1.}) = 2.5692.$$

Using the values of the expected numbers of deaths in each group, given in Table 2.11, the weighted mean of the w_k's is given by

$$\bar{w} = \frac{e_{3.} - e_{1.}}{e_{1.} + e_{3.}} = 0.5138.$$

The three values of $(w_k - \bar{w})^2$ are 0.2364, 0.2640 and 2.2917, and, from Equation (2.27), $V_T = 2.4849$. Finally, the test statistic is

$$W_T = \frac{U_T^2}{V_T} = 2.656,$$

which is just about significant at the 10% level ($P = 0.103$) when judged against a chi-squared distribution on 1 d.f. We therefore conclude that there is slight evidence of a linear trend across the age groups.

An alternative method of examining whether there is a trend across the levels of an ordered categorical variable, based on a modelling approach to the analysis of survival data, is described and illustrated in Section 3.8.1 of the next chapter.

2.10 Further reading

The life-table, which underpins the calculation of the life-table estimate of the survivor function, is widely used in the analysis of data from epidemiological studies. Fuller details of this application can be found in Armitage, Berry and Matthews (2002), and books on statistical methods in demography and epidemiology, such as Pollard, Yusuf and Pollard (1990) and Woodward (2014).

The product-limit estimate of the survivor function has been in use since the early 1900s. Kaplan and Meier (1958) derived the estimate using the method of maximum likelihood, which is why the estimate now bears their name. The properties of the Kaplan-Meier estimate of the survivor function have been further explored by Breslow and Crowley (1974) and Meier (1975). The Nelson-Aalen estimate is due to Altshuler (1970), Nelson (1972) and Aalen (1978b).

The expression for the standard error of the Kaplan-Meier estimate was first given by Greenwood (1926), but an alternative result is given by Aalen and Johansen (1978). Expressions for the variance of the Nelson-Aalen estimate of the cumulative hazard function are compared by Klein (1991). Although Section 2.2.3 shows how a confidence interval for the value of the survivor function at particular times can be found using Greenwood's formula, alternative procedures are needed for the construction of confidence bands for the complete survivor function. Hall and Wellner (1980) and Efron (1981) have shown how such bands can be computed, and these procedures are also described by Harris and Albert (1991).

Methods for constructing confidence intervals for the median survival time are described by Brookmeyer and Crowley (1982), Emerson (1982), Nair (1984), Simon and Lee (1982) and Slud, Byar and Green (1984). Simon (1986) emphasises the importance of confidence intervals in reporting the results of clinical trials, and includes an illustration of a method described in Slud, Byar and Green (1984). Klein and Moeschberger (2005) include a comprehensive review of kernel-smoothed estimates of the hazard function.

The formulation of the hypothesis testing procedure in the frequentist approach to inference is covered in many statistical texts. See, for example, Altman (1991) and Armitage, Berry and Matthews (2002) for non-technical presentations of the ideas in a medical context.

The log-rank test results from the work of Mantel and Haenszel (1959), Mantel (1966) and Peto and Peto (1972). See Lawless (2002) for details of the rank test formulation. A thorough review of the hypergeometric distribution, used in the derivation of the log-rank test in Section 2.6.2, is included in Johnson, Kemp and Kotz (2005). The log-rank test for trend is derived from the test for trend in a $2 \times k$ contingency table, given in Armitage, Berry and Matthews (2002).

Chapter 3

The Cox regression model

The non-parametric methods described in Chapter 2 can be useful in the analysis of a single sample of survival data, or in the comparison of two or more groups of survival times. However, in most medical studies that give rise to survival data, supplementary information will also be recorded on each individual. A typical example would be a clinical trial to compare the survival times of patients who receive one or other of two treatments. In such a study, demographic variables such as the age and sex of the patient, the values of physiological variables such as serum haemoglobin level and heart rate, and factors that are associated with the lifestyle of the patient, such as smoking history and dietary habits, may all have an impact on the time that the patient survives. Accordingly, the values of these variables, which are referred to as *explanatory variables*, would be recorded at the outset of the study. The resulting data set would then be more complex than those considered in Chapter 2, and the methods described in that chapter would generally be unsuitable.

In order to explore the relationship between the survival experience of a patient and explanatory variables, an approach based on statistical modelling can be used. The particular model that is developed in this chapter, known as the *Cox regression model*, both unifies and extends the non-parametric procedures of Chapter 2.

3.1 Modelling the hazard function

Through a modelling approach to the analysis of survival data, we can explore how the survival experience of a group of patients depends on the values of one or more explanatory variables, whose values have been recorded for each patient at the time origin. For example, in the study on multiple myeloma, given as Example 1.3, the aim is to determine which of seven explanatory variables have an impact on the survival time of the patients. In Example 1.4 on the survival times of patients in a clinical trial involving two treatments for prostatic cancer, the primary aim is to identify whether patients in the two treatment groups have a different survival experience. In this example, variables such as the age of the patient and the size of their tumour are likely to influence survival time, and so it will be important to take account of these variables when assessing the extent of any treatment difference.

In the analysis of survival data, interest centres on the risk or hazard of death at any time after the time origin of the study. As a consequence, the hazard function, defined in Section 1.3.2 of Chapter 1, is modelled directly in survival analysis. The resulting models are somewhat different in form from linear models encountered in regression analysis and in the analysis of data from designed experiments, where the dependence of the mean response, or some function of it, on certain explanatory variables is modelled. However, many of the principles and procedures used in linear modelling carry over to the modelling of survival data.

There are two broad reasons for modelling survival data. One objective of the modelling process is to determine which combination of potential explanatory variables affect the form of the hazard function. In particular, the effect that the treatment has on the hazard of death can be studied, as can the extent to which other explanatory variables affect the hazard function. Another reason for modelling the hazard function is to obtain an estimate of the hazard function itself for an individual. This may be of interest in its own right, but in addition, from the relationship between the survivor function and hazard function described by Equation (1.6), an estimate of the survivor function can be found. This will in turn lead to an estimate of quantities such as the median survival time, which will be a function of the explanatory variables in the model. The median survival time could then be estimated for current or future patients with particular values of these explanatory variables. The resulting estimate could be particularly useful in devising a treatment regimen, or in counselling the patient about their prognosis.

The model for survival data to be described in this chapter is based on the assumption of proportional hazards, introduced in Section 2.6.4 of Chapter 2, and is called a *proportional hazards model.* We first develop the model for the comparison of the hazard functions for individuals in two groups.

3.1.1 A model for the comparison of two groups

Suppose that two groups of patients receive either a standard treatment or a new treatment, and let $h_S(t)$ and $h_N(t)$ be the hazards of death at time t for patients on the standard treatment and new treatment, respectively. According to a simple model for the survival times of the two groups of patients, the hazard at time t for a patient on the new treatment is proportional to the hazard at that same time for a patient on the standard treatment. This proportional hazards model can be expressed in the form

$$h_N(t) = \psi h_S(t), \tag{3.1}$$

for any non-negative value of t, where ψ is a constant. An implication of this assumption is that the corresponding true survivor functions for individuals on the new and standard treatments do not cross, as previously shown in Section 2.6.4.

The value of ψ is the ratio of the hazard of death at any time for an individual on the new treatment relative to an individual on the standard treatment, and so ψ is known as the *relative hazard* or *hazard ratio.* If $\psi < 1$, the hazard of death at t is smaller for an individual on the new drug, relative to an individual on the standard. The new treatment is then an improvement on the standard. On the other hand, if $\psi > 1$, the hazard of death at t is greater for an individual on the new drug, and the standard treatment is superior.

An alternative way of expressing the model in Equation (3.1) leads to a model that can more easily be generalised. Suppose that survival data are available on n individuals and denote the hazard function for the ith of these by $h_i(t)$, $i = 1, 2, \ldots, n$. Also, write $h_0(t)$ for the hazard function for an individual on the standard treatment. The hazard function for an individual on the new treatment is then $\psi h_0(t)$. The relative hazard ψ cannot be negative, and so it is convenient to set $\psi = \exp(\beta)$. The parameter β is then the logarithm of the hazard ratio, that is, $\beta = \log \psi$, and any value of β in the range $(-\infty, \infty)$ will lead to a positive value of ψ. Note that positive values of β are obtained when the hazard ratio, ψ, is greater than unity, that is, when the new treatment is inferior to the standard.

Now let X be an *indicator variable*, which takes the value zero if an individual is on the standard drug, and unity if an individual is on the new drug. If x_i is the value of X for the ith individual in the study, $i = 1, 2, \ldots, n$, the hazard function for this individual can be written as

$$h_i(t) = e^{\beta x_i} h_0(t), \tag{3.2}$$

where $x_i = 1$ if the ith individual is on the new treatment and $x_i = 0$ otherwise. This is the proportional hazards model for the comparison of two treatment groups.

3.1.2 *The general proportional hazards model*

The model of the previous section is now generalised to the situation where the hazard of death at a particular time depends on the values $x_1, x_2, \ldots, x_p$ of p explanatory variables, $X_1, X_2, \ldots, X_p$. The values of these variables will be assumed to have been recorded at the time origin of the study. An extension of the model to cover the situation where the values of one or more of the explanatory variables change over time will be considered in Chapter 8.

The set of values of the explanatory variables in the proportional hazards model will be represented by the vector $\boldsymbol{x}$, so that $\boldsymbol{x} = (x_1, x_2, \ldots, x_p)'$. Let $h_0(t)$ be the hazard function for an individual for whom the values of all the explanatory variables that make up the vector $\boldsymbol{x}$ are zero. The function $h_0(t)$ is called the *baseline hazard function.* The hazard function for the ith individual can then be written as

$$h_i(t) = \psi(\boldsymbol{x}_i) h_0(t),$$

where $\psi(\boldsymbol{x}_i)$ is a function of $\boldsymbol{x}_i$, the vector of values of the explanatory variables for the ith individual, whose components are $x_{1i}, x_{2i}, \ldots, x_{pi}$. The function $\psi(\cdot)$ can be interpreted as the hazard at time t for an individual whose vector of explanatory variables is $\boldsymbol{x}_i$, relative to the hazard for an individual for whom $\boldsymbol{x} = \mathbf{0}$.

Again, since the relative hazard, $\psi(\boldsymbol{x}_i)$, cannot be negative, it is convenient to write this as $\exp(\eta_i)$, where η_i is a linear combination of the values of the p explanatory variables in $\boldsymbol{x}_i$. Therefore,

$$\eta_i = \beta_1 x_{1i} + \beta_2 x_{2i} + \cdots + \beta_p x_{pi},$$

so that $\eta_i = \sum_{j=1}^{p} \beta_j x_{ji}$. In matrix notation, $\eta_i = \boldsymbol{\beta}' \boldsymbol{x}_i$, where $\boldsymbol{\beta} = (\beta_1, \beta_2, \ldots, \beta_p)'$ is the vector of coefficients of the p explanatory variables in the model. The quantity η_i is called the *linear component* of the model, but it is also known as the *risk score* or *prognostic index* for the ith individual. There are other possible forms for the function $\psi(\boldsymbol{x}_i)$, but the choice $\psi(\boldsymbol{x}_i) = \exp(\boldsymbol{\beta}' \boldsymbol{x}_i)$ leads to the most commonly used model for survival data. The general proportional hazards model then becomes

$$h_i(t) = \exp(\beta_1 x_{1i} + \beta_2 x_{2i} + \cdots + \beta_p x_{pi}) h_0(t). \tag{3.3}$$

Notice that there is no constant term in the linear component of this proportional hazards model. If a constant term β_0, say, were included, the baseline hazard function could simply be rescaled by dividing $h_0(t)$ by $\exp(\beta_0)$, and the constant term would cancel out. The model in Equation (3.3) can also be re-expressed in the form

$$\log \left\{ \frac{h_i(t)}{h_0(t)} \right\} = \beta_1 x_{1i} + \beta_2 x_{2i} + \cdots + \beta_p x_{pi},$$

to give a linear model for the logarithm of the hazard ratio.

The model in Equation (3.3), in which no assumptions are made about the actual form of the baseline hazard function $h_0(t)$, was introduced by Cox (1972) and has come to be known as the *Cox regression model* or the *Cox proportional hazards model*. Since no particular form of probability distribution is assumed for the survival times, the Cox regression model is a *semi-parametric model*, and Section 3.3 will show how the β-coefficients in this model can be estimated. Of course, we will often need to estimate $h_0(t)$ itself, and we will see how this can be done in Section 3.10. Models in which specific assumptions are made about the form of the baseline hazard function, $h_0(t)$, will be described in Chapters 5 and 6.

3.2 The linear component of the model

There are two types of variable on which a hazard function may depend, namely *variates* and *factors*. A variate is a variable that takes numerical values that are often on a continuous scale of measurement, such as age or systolic blood pressure. A factor is a variable that takes a limited set of values, which are known as the *levels* of the factor. For example, sex is a factor with two levels, and type of tumour might be a factor whose levels correspond to different histologies, such as squamous, adeno or small cell.

We now consider how variates, factors and terms that combine factors and variates, can be incorporated in the linear component of a Cox regression model.

3.2.1 *Including a variate*

Variates, either alone or in combination, are readily incorporated in a Cox regression model. Each variate appears in the model with a corresponding β-coefficient. As an illustration, consider a situation in which the hazard function depends on two variates X_1 and X_2. The value of these variates for the ith individual will be x_{1i} and x_{2i}, respectively, and the Cox regression model for the ith of n individuals is written as

$$h_i(t) = \exp(\beta_1 x_{1i} + \beta_2 x_{2i}) h_0(t).$$

In models such as this, the baseline hazard function, $h_0(t)$, is the hazard function for an individual for whom all the variates included in the model take the value zero.

3.2.2 *Including a factor*

Suppose that the dependence of the hazard function on a single factor, A, is to be modelled, where A has a levels. The model for an individual for whom the level of A is j will then need to incorporate the term α_j, which represents the effect due to the jth level of the factor. The terms $\alpha_1, \alpha_2, \ldots, \alpha_a$ are known as the *main effects* of the factor A. According to the Cox regression model, the hazard function for an individual with factor A at level j is $\exp(\alpha_j)h_0(t)$. Now, the baseline hazard function $h_0(t)$ has been defined to be the hazard for an individual with values of all explanatory variables equal to zero. To be consistent with this definition, one of the α_j must be taken to be zero. One possibility is to adopt the constraint $\alpha_1 = 0$, which corresponds to taking the baseline hazard to be the hazard for an individual for whom A is at the first level. This is the constraint that will be used in the sequel.

Models that contain terms corresponding to factors can be expressed as linear combinations of explanatory variables by defining *indicator* or *dummy variables* for each factor. This procedure will be required when using computer software for survival analysis that does not allow factors to be fitted directly.

If the first level of the factor A is set to zero, so that this is the *baseline level* of the factor, the term α_j can be included in the model by defining $a - 1$ indicator variables, $X_2, X_3, \ldots, X_a$. These take the values shown in Table 3.1.

Table 3.1 *Indicator variables for a factor with a levels.*

Level of A	X_2	X_3	$\dots$	X_a
1	0	0	$\dots$	0
2	1	0	$\dots$	0
3	0	1	$\dots$	0
$\dots$	$\dots$	$\dots$	$\dots$	$\dots$
a	0	0	$\dots$	1

The term α_j can be incorporated in the linear part of the Cox regression model by including the $a - 1$ explanatory variables $X_2, X_3, \dots, X_a$ with coefficients $\alpha_2, \alpha_3, \dots, \alpha_a$. In other words, the term α_j in the model is replaced by $\alpha_2 x_2 + \alpha_3 x_3 + \cdots + \alpha_a x_a$, where x_j is the value of X_j for an individual for whom A is at level j, $j = 2, 3, \dots, a$. There are then $a - 1$ parameters associated with the main effect of the factor A, and A is said to have $a - 1$ *degrees of freedom.*

3.2.3 Including an interaction

When terms corresponding to more than one factor are to be included in the model, sets of indicator variables can be defined for each factor in a manner similar to that shown above. In this situation, it may also be appropriate to include a term in the model that corresponds to individual effects for each combination of levels of two or more factors. Such effects are known as *interactions.*

For example, suppose that the two factors are the sex of a patient and grade of tumour. If the effect of grade of tumour on the hazard of death is different in patients of each sex, we would say that there is an interaction between these two factors. The hazard function would then depend on the combination of levels of these two factors.

In general, if A and B are two factors, and the hazard of death depends on the combination of levels of A and B, then A and B are said to *interact.* If A and B have a and b levels, respectively, the term that represents an interaction between these two factors is denoted by $(\alpha\beta)_{jk}$, for $j = 1, 2, \dots, a$ and $k = 1, 2, \dots, b$.

In statistical modelling, the effect of an interaction can only be investigated by adding the interaction term to a model that already contains the corresponding main effects. If either α_j or β_k are excluded from the model, the term $(\alpha\beta)_{jk}$ represents the effect of one factor *nested* within the other. For example, if α_j is included in the model, but not β_k, then $(\alpha\beta)_{jk}$ is the effect of B nested within A. If both α_j and β_k are excluded, the term $(\alpha\beta)_{jk}$ represents the effect of the combination of level i of A and level j of B on the response variable. This means that $(\alpha\beta)_{jk}$ can only be interpreted as an interaction effect when included in a model that contains both α_j and β_k, which correspond to the main effects of A and B. We will return to this point when we consider model-building strategy in Section 3.6.

In order to include the term $(\alpha\beta)_{jk}$ in the model, products of indicator variables associated with the main effects are calculated. For example, if A and B have 2 and 3 levels respectively, indicator variables U_2 and V_2, V_3 are defined as in Table 3.2.

Table 3.2 *Indicator variables for two factors with two and three levels, respectively.*

Level of A	U_2	Level of B	V_2	V_3
1	0	1	0	0
2	1	2	1	0
		3	0	1

Let u_j and v_k be the values of U_j and V_k for a given individual, for $j = 2$, $k = 2, 3$. The term $(\alpha\beta)_{jk}$ is then fitted by including variates formed from the products of U_j and V_k in the model. The corresponding value of the product for a given individual is $u_j v_k$. The coefficient of this product is denoted $(\alpha\beta)_{jk}$, and so the term $(\alpha\beta)_{jk}$ is fitted as

$$(\alpha\beta)_{22}u_2v_2 + (\alpha\beta)_{23}u_2v_3.$$

There are therefore two parameters associated with the interaction between A and B. In general, if A and B have a and b levels, respectively, the two-factor interaction AB has $(a-1)(b-1)$ parameters associated with it, in other words AB has $(a-1)(b-1)$ degrees of freedom. Furthermore, the term $(\alpha\beta)_{jk}$ is equal to zero whenever either A or B are at the first level, that is, when either $j = 1$ or $k = 1$.

3.2.4 Including a mixed term

Another type of term that might be needed in a model is a mixed term formed from a factor and a variate. Terms of this type would be used when the coefficient of a variate in a model was likely to be different for each level of a factor. For example, consider a contraceptive trial in which the time to the onset of a period of amenorrhoea, the prolonged absence of menstrual bleeding, is being modelled. The hazard of an amenorrhoea may be related to the weight of a woman, but the coefficient of this variate may differ according to the level of a factor associated with the number of previous pregnancies that the woman has experienced.

The dependence of the coefficient of a variate, X, on the level of a factor, A, would be depicted by including the term $\alpha_j x$ in the linear component of the Cox regression model, where x is the value of X for a given individual for whom the factor A is at the jth level, $j = 1, 2, \ldots, a$. To include such a term, indicator variables U_j, say, are defined for the factor A, and each of these is multiplied by the value of X for each individual. The resulting values of the products U_jX are u_jx, and the coefficient of u_jx in the model is α_j, where j indexes the level of the factor A.

If the same definition of indicator variables in the previous discussion were used, α_1, the coefficient of X for individuals at the first level of A, would be zero. It is then essential to include the variate X in the model as well as the products, for otherwise the dependence on X for individuals at the first level of A would not be modelled. An illustration should make this clearer.

Suppose that there are nine individuals in a study, on each of whom the value of a variate, X, and the level of a factor, A, have been recorded. We will take A to have three levels, where A is at the first level for the first three individuals, at the second level for the next three, and at the third level for the final three. In order to model the dependence of the coefficient of the variate X on the level of A, two indicator variables, U_2 and U_3 are defined as in Table 3.3. Explanatory variables formed as the products U_2X and U_3X, given in the last two columns of Table 3.3, would then be included in the linear component of the model, together with the variate X.

Table 3.3 *Indicator variables for the combination of a factor with three levels and a variate.*

Individual	Level of A	X	U_2	U_3	U_2X	U_3X
1	1	x_1	0	0	0	0
2	1	x_2	0	0	0	0
3	1	x_3	0	0	0	0
4	2	x_4	1	0	x_4	0
5	2	x_5	1	0	x_5	0
6	2	x_6	1	0	x_6	0
7	3	x_7	0	1	0	x_7
8	3	x_8	0	1	0	x_8
9	3	x_9	0	1	0	x_9

Let the coefficients of the values of the products U_2X and U_3X be α_2' and α_3', respectively, and let the coefficient of the value of the variate X in the model be β. Then, the model contains the terms $\beta x + \alpha_2'(u_2x) + \alpha_3'(u_3x)$. From Table 3.3, $u_2 = 0$ and $u_3 = 0$ for individuals at level 1 of A, and so the coefficient of x for these individuals is just β. For those at level 2 of A, $u_2 = 1$ and $u_3 = 0$, and the coefficient of x is $\beta + \alpha_2'$. Similarly, at level 3 of A, $u_2 = 0$ and $u_3 = 1$, and the coefficient of x is $\beta + \alpha_3'$.

Notice that if the term βx is omitted from the model, the coefficient of x for individuals $1, 2$ and 3 would be zero. There would then be no information about the relationship between the hazard function and the variate X for individuals at the first level of the factor A.

The manipulation described in the preceding paragraphs can be avoided by defining the indicator variables in a different way. If a factor A has a levels, and it is desired to include the term α_jx in a model, without necessarily including the term βx, a indicator variables $Z_1, Z_2, \ldots, Z_a$ can be defined for A, where $Z_j = 1$ at level j of A and zero otherwise. The corresponding values of these products for an individual, $z_1x, z_2x, \ldots, z_ax$, are then included in the model with coefficients $\alpha_1, \alpha_2, \ldots, \alpha_a$. These are the coefficients of x for each level of A.

Now, if the variate X is included in the model, along with the a products of the form Z_jX, there will be $a + 1$ terms corresponding to the a coefficients. It will not then be possible to obtain unique estimates of each of these α-coefficients, and the model is said to be *overparameterised.* This overparameterisation can be dealt with by forcing one of the $a + 1$ coefficients to be zero. In particular, taking $\alpha_1 = 0$ would be equivalent to a redefinition of the indicator variables, in which Z_1 is taken to be zero. This then leads to the same formulation of the model that has already been discussed.

The application of these ideas in the analysis of actual data sets will be illustrated in Section 3.4, after we have seen how the Cox regression model can be fitted.

3.3 Fitting the Cox regression model

Fitting the Cox regression model given in Equation (3.3) to an observed set of survival data entails estimating the unknown coefficients of the explanatory variables, $X_1, X_2, \ldots, X_p$, in the linear component of the model, $\beta_1, \beta_2, \ldots, \beta_p$. The baseline hazard function, $h_0(t)$, may also need to be estimated. It turns out that these two components of the model can be estimated separately. The βs are estimated first and these estimates are then used to construct an estimate of the baseline hazard function. This is an important result, since it means that in order to make inferences about the effects of p explanatory variables, $X_1, X_2, \ldots, X_p$, on the relative hazard, $h_i(t)/h_0(t)$, we do not need an estimate of $h_0(t)$. Methods for estimating $h_0(t)$ will therefore be deferred until Section 3.10.

The β-coefficients in the Cox regression model, which are the unknown parameters in the model, can be estimated using the *method of maximum likelihood.* To operate this method, we first obtain the *likelihood* of the sample data. This is the joint probability of the observed data, regarded as a function of the unknown parameters in the assumed model. For the Cox regression model, this is a function of the observed survival times and the unknown β-parameters in the linear component of the model. Estimates of the βs are then those values that are the most likely on the basis of the observed data. These *maximum likelihood estimates* are therefore the values that maximise the likelihood function. From a computational viewpoint, it is more convenient to maximise the logarithm of the likelihood function. Furthermore, approximations to the variance of maximum likelihood estimates can be obtained from the second derivatives of the log-likelihood function. Details will not be given here, but Appendix A contains a summary of relevant results from the theory of maximum likelihood estimation.

Suppose that data are available for n individuals, among whom there are r distinct death times and $n-r$ right-censored survival times. We will for the moment assume that only one individual dies at each death time, so that there are no *ties* in the data. The treatment of ties will be discussed in Section 3.3.2. The r ordered death times will be denoted by $t_{(1)} < t_{(2)} < \cdots < t_{(r)}$, so that $t_{(j)}$ is the jth ordered death time. The set of individuals who are at risk at time $t_{(j)}$ will be denoted by $R(t_{(j)})$, so that $R(t_{(j)})$ is the group of individuals who are alive and uncensored at a time just prior to $t_{(j)}$. The quantity $R(t_{(j)})$ is called the *risk set*.

Cox (1972) showed that the relevant likelihood function for the model in Equation (3.3) is given by

$$L(\boldsymbol{\beta}) = \prod_{j=1}^{r} \frac{\exp(\boldsymbol{\beta}'\boldsymbol{x}_{(j)})}{\sum_{l \in R(t_{(j)})} \exp(\boldsymbol{\beta}'\boldsymbol{x}_l)}, \tag{3.4}$$

in which $\boldsymbol{x}_{(j)}$ is the vector of covariates for the individual who dies at the jth ordered death time, $t_{(j)}$. The summation in the denominator of this likelihood function is the sum of the values of $\exp(\boldsymbol{\beta}'\boldsymbol{x})$ over all individuals who are at risk at time $t_{(j)}$. Notice that the product is taken over the individuals for whom death times have been recorded. Individuals for whom the survival times are censored do not contribute to the numerator of the log-likelihood function, but they do enter into the summation over the risk sets at death times that occur before a censored time.

The likelihood function that has been obtained is not a true likelihood, since it does not make direct use of the actual censored and uncensored survival times. For this reason it is referred to as a *partial likelihood function*. The likelihood function in Equation (3.4) depends only on the ranking of the death times, since this determines the risk set at each death time. Consequently, inferences about the effect of explanatory variables on the hazard function depend only on the rank order of the survival times.

Now suppose that the data consist of n observed survival times, denoted by $t_1, t_2, \ldots, t_n$, and that δ_i is an event indicator, which is zero if the ith survival time t_i, $i = 1, 2, \ldots, n$, is right-censored, and unity otherwise. The partial likelihood function in Equation (3.4) can then be expressed in the form

$$\prod_{i=1}^{n} \left\{ \frac{\exp(\boldsymbol{\beta}'\boldsymbol{x}_i)}{\sum_{l \in R(t_i)} \exp(\boldsymbol{\beta}'\boldsymbol{x}_l)} \right\}^{\delta_i}, \tag{3.5}$$

where $R(t_i)$ is the risk set at time t_i. From Equation (3.5), the corresponding partial log-likelihood function is given by

$$\log L(\boldsymbol{\beta}) = \sum_{i=1}^{n} \delta_i \left\{ \boldsymbol{\beta}'\boldsymbol{x}_i - \log \sum_{l \in R(t_i)} \exp(\boldsymbol{\beta}'\boldsymbol{x}_l) \right\}. \tag{3.6}$$

The maximum likelihood estimates of the β-parameters in the Cox regression model can be found by maximising this log-likelihood function using numerical methods. This maximisation is generally accomplished using the *Newton-Raphson procedure* described below in Section 3.3.3.

Fortunately, most statistical software for survival analysis enables the Cox regression model to be fitted. Such software also gives the standard errors of the parameter estimates in the fitted model.

The justification for using Equation (3.4) as a likelihood function, and further details on the structure of the likelihood function, are given in Section 3.3.1. The treatment of tied survival times is then discussed in Section 3.3.2 and the Newton-Raphson procedure is outlined in Section 3.3.3. These three sections can be omitted without loss of continuity.

3.3.1 Likelihood function for the model*

In the Cox regression model, the hazard of death at time t for the ith individual, $i = 1, 2, \ldots, n$ is given by

$$h_i(t) = \exp(\boldsymbol{\beta}'\boldsymbol{x}_i)h_0(t)$$

where $\boldsymbol{\beta}$ is the vector of coefficients of p explanatory variables whose values are $x_{1i}, x_{2i}, \ldots, x_{pi}$ for the ith individual, and $h_0(t)$ is the baseline hazard function of unspecified form. The basis of the argument used in the construction of a likelihood function for this model is that intervals between successive death times convey no information about the effect of explanatory variables on the hazard of death. This is because the baseline hazard function has an arbitrary form, and so it is conceivable that $h_0(t)$, and hence $h_i(t)$, is zero in those time intervals in which there are no deaths. This in turn means that these intervals give no information about the values of the β-parameters. We therefore consider the probability that the ith individual dies at some time $t_{(j)}$, conditional on $t_{(j)}$ being one of the observed set of r death times $t_{(1)}, t_{(2)}, \ldots, t_{(r)}$. If the vector of values of the explanatory variables for the individual who dies at $t_{(j)}$ is denoted by $\boldsymbol{x}_{(j)}$, this probability is

$$\text{P(individual with variables } \boldsymbol{x}_{(j)} \text{ dies at } t_{(j)} \mid \text{one death at } t_{(j)}). \tag{3.7}$$

Next, from the result that the probability of an event A, given that an event B has occurred, is given by

$$\text{P}(A \mid B) = \text{P}(A \text{ and } B)/\text{P}(B),$$

the probability in Expression (3.7) becomes

$$\frac{\text{P(individual with variables } \boldsymbol{x}_{(j)} \text{ dies at } t_{(j)})}{\text{P(one death at } t_{(j)})}. \tag{3.8}$$

Since the death times are assumed to be independent of one another, the denominator of this expression is the sum of the probabilities of death at time $t_{(j)}$ over all individuals who are at risk of death at that time. If these individuals are indexed by l, with $R(t_{(j)})$ denoting the set of individuals who are at risk at time $t_{(j)}$, Expression (3.8) becomes

$$\frac{\text{P(individual with variables } \boldsymbol{x}_{(j)} \text{ dies at } t_{(j)})}{\sum_{l \in R(t_{(j)})} \text{P(individual } l \text{ dies at } t_{(j)})}. \tag{3.9}$$

The probabilities of death at time $t_{(j)}$, in Expression (3.9), are now replaced by probabilities of death in the interval $(t_{(j)}, t_{(j)} + \delta t)$, and dividing both the numerator and denominator of Expression (3.9) by δt, we get

$$\frac{\text{P\{individual with variables } \boldsymbol{x}_{(j)} \text{ dies in } (t_{(j)}, t_{(j)} + \delta t)\}/\delta t}{\sum_{l \in R(t_{(j)})} \text{P\{individual } l \text{ dies in } (t_{(j)}, t_{(j)} + \delta t)\}/\delta t}.$$

The limiting value of this expression as $\delta t \to 0$ is then the ratio of the probabilities in Expression (3.9). But from Equation (1.3), this limit is also the ratio of the corresponding hazards of death at time $t_{(j)}$, that is,

$$\frac{\text{Hazard of death at time } t_{(j)} \text{ for individual with variables } \boldsymbol{x}_{(j)}}{\sum_{l \in R(t_{(j)})}\{\text{Hazard of death at time } t_{(j)} \text{ for individual } l\}}.$$

If it is the ith individual who dies at $t_{(j)}$, the hazard function in the numerator of this expression can be written $h_i(t_{(j)})$. Similarly, the denominator is the sum of the hazards of death at time $t_{(j)}$ over all individuals who are at risk of death at this time. This is the sum of the values $h_l(t_{(j)})$ over those individuals in the risk set at time $t_{(j)}$, $R(t_{(j)})$. Consequently, the conditional probability in Expression (3.7) becomes

$$\frac{h_i(t_{(j)})}{\sum_{l \in R(t_{(j)})} h_l(t_{(j)})}.$$

On using Equation (3.3), the baseline hazard function in the numerator and denominator cancels out, and we are left with

$$\frac{\exp(\boldsymbol{\beta}' \boldsymbol{x}_{(j)})}{\sum_{l \in R(t_{(j)})} \exp(\boldsymbol{\beta}' \boldsymbol{x}_l)}.$$

Finally, taking the product of these conditional probabilities over the r death times gives the partial likelihood function in Equation (3.4).

In order to throw more light on the structure of the partial likelihood, consider a sample of survival data from five individuals, numbered from 1 to 5. The survival data are illustrated in Figure 3.1. The observed survival times of individuals 2 and 5 will be taken to be right-censored, and the three ordered death times are denoted $t_{(1)} < t_{(2)} < t_{(3)}$. Then, $t_{(1)}$ is the death time of individual 3, $t_{(2)}$ is that of individual 1, and $t_{(3)}$ that of individual 4.

The risk set at each of the three ordered death times consists of the individuals who are alive and uncensored just prior to each death time. Hence,

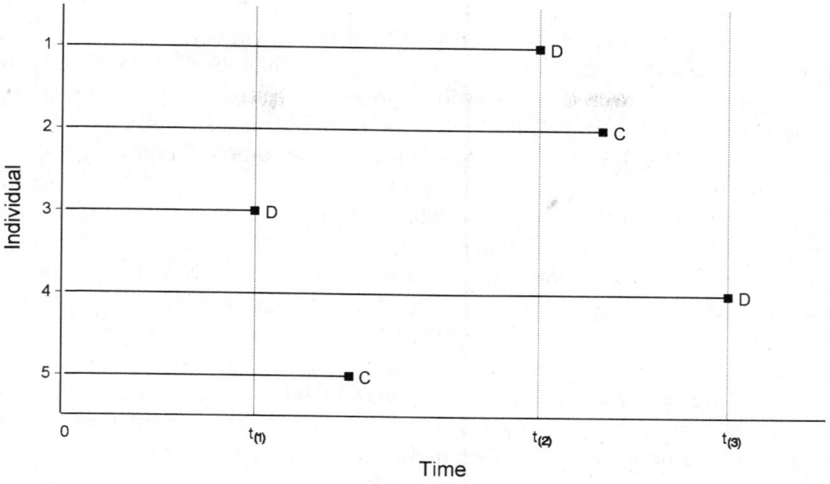

Figure 3.1 *Survival times of five individuals.*

the risk set $R(t_{(1)})$ consists of all five individuals, risk set $R(t_{(2)})$ consists of individuals 1, 2 and 4, while risk set $R(t_{(3)})$ only includes individual 4. Now write $\psi(i) = \exp(\boldsymbol{\beta}'\boldsymbol{x}_i)$, $i = 1, 2, \ldots, 5$, where $\boldsymbol{x}_i$ is the vector of explanatory variables for the ith individual. The numerators of the partial likelihood function for times $t_{(1)}$, $t_{(2)}$ and $t_{(3)}$, respectively, are $\psi(3)$, $\psi(1)$ and $\psi(4)$, since individuals 3, 1 and 4, respectively, die at the three ordered death times. The partial likelihood function over the three death times is then

$$\frac{\psi(3)}{\psi(1)+\psi(2)+\psi(3)+\psi(4)+\psi(5)} \times \frac{\psi(1)}{\psi(1)+\psi(2)+\psi(4)} \times \frac{\psi(4)}{\psi(4)}.$$

It turns out that standard results used in maximum likelihood estimation carry over without modification to maximum partial likelihood estimation. In particular, the results given in Appendix A for the variance-covariance matrix of the estimates of the βs can be used, as can distributional results associated with likelihood ratio testing, to be discussed in Section 3.5.

3.3.2 Treatment of ties*

The Cox regression model for survival data assumes that the hazard function is continuous, and under this assumption, tied survival times are not possible. Of course, survival times are usually recorded to the nearest day, month or year, and so tied survival times can arise as a result of this rounding process. Indeed, Examples 1.2, 1.3 and 1.4 in Chapter 1 all contain tied observations.

In addition to the possibility of more than one death at a given time, there might also be one or more censored observations at a death time. When there are both censored survival times and deaths at a given time, the censoring is assumed to occur after all the deaths. Potential ambiguity concerning which individuals should be included in the risk set at that death time is then resolved and tied censored observations present no further difficulties in the computation of the likelihood function using Equation (3.4). Accordingly, we only need consider how tied survival times can be handled in fitting the Cox regression model.

In order to accommodate tied observations, the likelihood function in Equation (3.4) has to be modified in some way. The appropriate likelihood function in the presence of tied observations has been given by Kalbfleisch and Prentice (2002). However, this likelihood has a very complicated form, and will not be reproduced here. In addition, the computation of this likelihood function can be very time consuming, particularly when there are a relatively large number of ties at one or more death times. Fortunately, there are a number of approximations to the likelihood function that have computational advantages over the exact method. But before these are given, some additional notation needs to be developed.

Let $\boldsymbol{s}_j$ be the vector of sums of each of the p covariates for those individuals who die at the jth death time, $t_{(j)}$, $j = 1, 2, \ldots, r$. If there are d_j deaths at $t_{(j)}$, the hth element of $\boldsymbol{s}_j$ is $s_{hj} = \sum_{k=1}^{d_j} x_{hjk}$, where x_{hjk} is the value of the hth explanatory variable, $h = 1, 2, \ldots, p$, for the kth of d_j individuals, $k = 1, 2, \ldots, d_j$, who die at the jth death time, $j = 1, 2, \ldots, r$.

The simplest approximation to the likelihood function is that due to Breslow (1974), who proposed the approximate likelihood

$$\prod_{j=1}^{r} \frac{\exp(\boldsymbol{\beta}'\boldsymbol{s}_j)}{\left\{\sum_{l \in R(t_{(j)})} \exp(\boldsymbol{\beta}'\boldsymbol{x}_l)\right\}^{d_j}}. \tag{3.10}$$

In this approximation, the d_j deaths at time $t_{(j)}$ are considered to be distinct and to occur sequentially. The probabilities of all possible sequences of deaths are then summed to give the likelihood in Equation (3.10). Apart from a constant of proportionality, this is also the approximation suggested by Peto (1972). This likelihood is quite straightforward to compute, and is an adequate approximation when the number of tied observations at any one death time is not too large. For these reasons, this method is usually the default procedure for handling ties in statistical software for survival analysis, and will be used in the examples given in this book.

Efron (1977) proposed

$$\prod_{j=1}^{r} \frac{\exp(\boldsymbol{\beta}'\boldsymbol{s}_j)}{\prod_{k=1}^{d_j}\left[\sum_{l \in R(t_{(j)})} \exp(\boldsymbol{\beta}'\boldsymbol{x}_l) - (k-1)d_j^{-1} \sum_{l \in D(t_{(j)})} \exp(\boldsymbol{\beta}'\boldsymbol{x}_l)\right]} \tag{3.11}$$

as an approximate likelihood function for the Cox regression model, where $D(t_{(j)})$ is the set of all individuals who die at time $t_{(j)}$. This is a closer approximation to the appropriate likelihood function than that due to Breslow, although in practice, both approximations often give similar results.

Cox (1972) suggested the approximation

$$\prod_{j=1}^{r} \frac{\exp(\boldsymbol{\beta}'\boldsymbol{s}_j)}{\sum_{l \in R(t_{(j)};d_j)} \exp(\boldsymbol{\beta}'\boldsymbol{s}_l)}, \tag{3.12}$$

where the notation $R(t_{(j)}; d_j)$ denotes a set of d_j individuals drawn from $R(t_{(j)})$, the risk set at $t_{(j)}$. The summation in the denominator is the sum over all possible sets of d_j individuals, sampled from the risk set without replacement. The approximation in Expression (3.12) is based on a model for the situation where the time-scale is discrete, so that under this model, tied observations are permissible. Now, from Section 1.3.2 of Chapter 1, the hazard function for an individual with vector of explanatory variables $\boldsymbol{x}_i$, $h_i(t)$, is the probability of death in the unit time interval $(t, t+1)$, conditional on survival to time t. A discrete version of the Cox regression model of Equation (3.3) is the model

$$\frac{h_i(t)}{1 - h_i(t)} = \exp(\boldsymbol{\beta}'\boldsymbol{x}_i)\frac{h_0(t)}{1 - h_0(t)},$$

for which the likelihood function is that given in Equation (3.12). In fact, in the limit as the width of the discrete time intervals becomes zero, this model tends to the Cox regression model of Equation (3.3).

When there are no ties, that is, when $d_j = 1$ for each death time, the approximations in Equations (3.10), (3.11) and (3.12) all reduce to the likelihood function in Equation (3.4).

3.3.3 The Newton-Raphson procedure*

Models for censored survival data are usually fitted by using the Newton-Raphson procedure to maximise the partial likelihood function, and so the procedure is outlined in this section.

Let $\boldsymbol{u}(\boldsymbol{\beta})$ be the $p \times 1$ vector of first derivatives of the log-likelihood function in Equation (3.6) with respect to the β-parameters. This quantity is known as the *vector of efficient scores*. Also, let $\boldsymbol{I}(\boldsymbol{\beta})$ be the $p \times p$ matrix of negative second derivatives of the log-likelihood, so that the (j,k)th element of $\boldsymbol{I}(\boldsymbol{\beta})$ is

$$-\frac{\partial^2 \log L(\boldsymbol{\beta})}{\partial \beta_j \partial \beta_k}.$$

The matrix $\boldsymbol{I}(\boldsymbol{\beta})$is known as the *observed information matrix.*

According to the Newton-Raphson procedure, an estimate of the vector of β-parameters at the $(s+1)$th cycle of the iterative procedure, $\hat{\boldsymbol{\beta}}_{s+1}$, is

$$\hat{\boldsymbol{\beta}}_{s+1} = \hat{\boldsymbol{\beta}}_s + \boldsymbol{I}^{-1}(\hat{\boldsymbol{\beta}}_s)\boldsymbol{u}(\hat{\boldsymbol{\beta}}_s),$$

for $s = 0, 1, 2, \ldots$, where $\boldsymbol{u}(\hat{\boldsymbol{\beta}}_s)$ is the vector of efficient scores and $\boldsymbol{I}^{-1}(\hat{\boldsymbol{\beta}}_s)$ is the inverse of the information matrix, both evaluated at $\hat{\boldsymbol{\beta}}_s$. The procedure can be started by taking $\hat{\boldsymbol{\beta}}_0 = \mathbf{0}$. The process is terminated when the change in the log-likelihood function is sufficiently small, or when the largest of the relative changes in the values of the parameter estimates is sufficiently small.

When the iterative procedure has converged, the variance-covariance matrix of the parameter estimates can be approximated by the inverse of the information matrix, evaluated at $\hat{\boldsymbol{\beta}}$, that is, $\boldsymbol{I}^{-1}(\hat{\boldsymbol{\beta}})$. The square root of the diagonal elements of this matrix are then the standard errors of the estimated values of $\beta_1, \beta_2, \ldots, \beta_p$.

3.4 Confidence intervals and hypothesis tests

When statistical software is used to fit a Cox regression model, the parameter estimates that are provided are usually accompanied by their standard errors. These standard errors can be used to obtain approximate confidence intervals for the unknown β-parameters. In particular, a $100(1-\alpha)\%$ confidence interval for a parameter β is the interval with limits $\hat{\beta} \pm z_{\alpha/2}\,\text{se}\,(\hat{\beta})$, where $\hat{\beta}$ is the estimate of β, and $z_{\alpha/2}$ is the upper $\alpha/2$-point of the standard normal distribution.

If a $100(1-\alpha)\%$ confidence interval for β does not include zero, this is evidence that the value of β is non-zero. More specifically, the null hypothesis that $\beta = 0$ can be tested by calculating the value of the statistic $\hat{\beta}/\,\text{se}\,(\hat{\beta})$. The observed value of this statistic is then compared to percentage points of the standard normal distribution in order to obtain the corresponding P-value. Equivalently, the square of this statistic can be compared with percentage points of a chi-squared distribution on one degree of freedom. This procedure is sometimes called a *Wald test*, and the P-values for this test are often given alongside parameter estimates and their standard errors in computer output.

When attempting to interpret the P-value for a given parameter, β_j, say, it is important to recognise that the hypothesis that is being tested is that $\beta_j = 0$ in the presence of all other terms that are in the model. For example, suppose that a model contains the three explanatory variables X_1, X_2, X_3, and that their true coefficients are $\beta_1, \beta_2, \beta_3$. The test statistic $\hat{\beta}_2/\,\text{se}\,(\hat{\beta}_2)$ is then used to test the null hypothesis that $\beta_2 = 0$ in the presence of β_1 and β_3. If there was no evidence to reject this hypothesis, we would conclude that X_2 was not needed in the model in the presence of X_1 and X_3.

In general, the individual estimates of the βs in a Cox regression model are not all independent of one another. This means that the results of testing separate hypotheses about the β-parameters in a model may not be easy to interpret. For example, consider again the situation where there are three explanatory variables, X_1, X_2, X_3. If $\hat{\beta}_1$ and $\hat{\beta}_2$ were not found to be significantly different from zero, when compared with their standard errors, we could not conclude that only X_3 need be included in the model. This is because the coefficient of X_1, for example, could well change when X_2 is excluded from the model, and vice versa. This would certainly happen if X_1 and X_2 were correlated.

Because of the difficulty in interpreting the results of tests concerning the coefficients of the explanatory variables in a model, alternative methods for comparing different Cox regression models are required. It turns out that the methods to be described in Section 3.5 are much more satisfactory than the Wald tests. The results of these tests given in computer-based analyses of survival data should therefore be treated with some caution.

3.4.1 Standard errors and confidence intervals for hazard ratios

We have seen that in situations where there are two groups of survival data, the parameter β in a Cox regression model is the logarithm of the ratio of the hazard of death at time t for individuals in one group relative to those in the other. Hence the hazard ratio itself is $\psi = e^{\beta}$. The corresponding estimate of the hazard ratio is $\hat{\psi} = \exp(\hat{\beta})$, and the standard error of $\hat{\psi}$ can be obtained from the standard error of $\hat{\beta}$ using the result given as Equation (2.8) in Chapter 2. From this result, the approximate variance of $\hat{\psi}$, a function of $\hat{\beta}$, is

$$\left\{\exp(\hat{\beta})\right\}^2 \text{var}\,(\hat{\beta}),$$

that is, $\hat{\psi}^2 \,\text{var}\,(\hat{\beta})$, and so the standard error of $\hat{\psi}$ is given by

$$\text{se}\,(\hat{\psi}) = \hat{\psi}\,\text{se}\,(\hat{\beta}). \tag{3.13}$$

Generally speaking, a confidence interval for the true hazard ratio will be more informative than the standard error of the estimated hazard ratio. A $100(1-\alpha)\%$ confidence interval for the true hazard ratio, ψ, can be found simply by exponentiating the confidence limits for β. An interval estimate obtained in this way is preferable to one found using $\hat{\psi} \pm z_{\alpha/2}\,\text{se}\,(\hat{\psi})$. This is because the distribution of the logarithm of the estimated hazard ratio will be more closely approximated by a normal distribution than that of the hazard ratio itself.

The construction of a confidence interval for a hazard ratio is illustrated in Example 3.1 below. Fuller details on the interpretation of the parameters in the linear component of a Cox regression model are given in Section 3.9.

3.4.2 Two examples

In this section, the results of fitting a Cox regression model to data from two of the examples introduced in Chapter 1 are given.

Example 3.1 Prognosis for women with breast cancer
Data on the survival times of breast cancer patients, classified according to whether or not sections of their tumours were positively stained, were first

given in Example 1.2. The variable that indexes the result of the staining process can be regarded as a factor with two levels. From the arguments given in Section 3.2.2, this factor can be fitted by using an indicator variable X to denote the staining result, where $X = 0$ corresponds to negative staining and $X = 1$ to positive staining. Under the Cox regression model, the hazard of death at time t for the ith woman, for whom the value of the indicator variable is x_i, is

$$h_i(t) = e^{\beta x_i} h_0(t),$$

where x_i is zero or unity. The baseline hazard function $h_0(t)$ is then the hazard function for a women with a negatively stained tumour. This is essentially the model considered in Section 3.1.1, and given in Equation (3.2).

In the group of women whose tumours were positively stained, there are two who die at 26 months. To cope with this tie, the Breslow approximation to the likelihood function will be used. This model is fitted by finding that value of β, $\hat{\beta}$, which maximises the likelihood function in Equation (3.10). The maximum likelihood estimate of β is $\hat{\beta} = 0.908$. The standard error of this estimate is also obtained from statistical packages for fitting the Cox regression model, and turns out to be given by $\text{se}\,(\hat{\beta}) = 0.501$.

The quantity e^{β} is the ratio of the hazard function for a woman with $X = 1$ to that for a woman with $X = 0$, so that β is the logarithm of the ratio of the hazard of death at time t for positively stained relative to negatively stained women. The estimated value of this hazard ratio is $e^{0.908} = 2.48$. Since this is greater than unity, we conclude that a woman who has a positively stained tumour will have a greater risk of death at any given time than a comparable women whose tumour was negatively stained. Positive staining therefore indicates a poorer prognosis for a breast cancer patient.

The standard error of the hazard ratio can be found from the standard error of $\hat{\beta}$, using the result in Equation (3.13). Since the estimated relative hazard is $\hat{\psi} = \exp(\hat{\beta}) = 2.480$, and the standard error of $\hat{\beta}$ is 0.501, the standard error of $\hat{\psi}$ is given by

$$\text{se}\,(\hat{\psi}) = 2.480 \times 0.501 = 1.242.$$

We can go further and construct a confidence interval for this hazard ratio. The first step is to obtain a confidence interval for the logarithm of the hazard ratio, β. For example, a 95% confidence interval for β is the interval from $\hat{\beta} - 1.96\,\text{se}\,(\hat{\beta})$ to $\hat{\beta} + 1.96\,\text{se}\,(\hat{\beta})$, that is, the interval from -0.074 to 1.890. Exponentiating these confidence limits gives $(0.93, 6.62)$ as a 95% confidence interval for the hazard ratio itself. Notice that this interval barely includes unity, suggesting that there is evidence that the two groups of women have a different survival experience.

Example 3.2 Survival of multiple myeloma patients

Data on the survival times of 48 patients suffering from multiple myeloma were given in Example 1.3. The database also contains the values of seven other variables that were recorded for each patient. For convenience, the values of the variable that describes the sex of a patient have been redefined to be zero and unity for males and females, respectively. The sex of the patient and the variable associated with the occurrence of Bence-Jones protein are factors with two levels, and these terms are fitted using the indicator variables *Sex* and *Protein*. The variables to be used in the modelling process are then as follows:

Age:	Age of the patient
Sex:	Sex of the patient (0 = male, 1 = female)
Bun:	Blood urea nitrogen
Ca:	Serum calcium
Hb:	Serum haemoglobin
Pcells:	Percentage of plasma cells
Protein:	Bence-Jones protein (0 = absent, 1 = present)

The Cox regression model for the ith individual is then

$$h_i(t) = \exp(\beta_1 Age_i + \beta_2 Sex_i + \beta_3 Bun_i + \beta_4 Ca_i + \beta_5 Hb_i + \beta_6 Pcells_i + \beta_7 Protein_i)h_0(t),$$

where the subscript i on an explanatory variable denotes the value of that variable for the ith individual. The baseline hazard function is the hazard function for an individual for whom the values of all seven of these variables are zero. This function therefore corresponds to a male aged zero, who has zero values of *Bun*, *Ca*, *Hb* and *Pcells*, and no Bence-Jones protein. In view of the obvious difficulty in interpreting this function, it might be more sensible to redefine the variables *Age*, *Bun*, *Ca*, *Hb* and *Pcells* by subtracting values for an average patient. For example, if we took $Age - 60$ in place of *Age*, the baseline hazard would correspond to a male aged 60 years. This procedure also avoids the introduction of a function that describes the hazard of individuals whose ages are rather different from the age range of patients in the study. Although this leads to a baseline hazard function that has a more natural interpretation, it will not affect inference about the influence of the explanatory variables on the hazard of death. For this reason, the untransformed variables will be used in this example. On fitting the model, the estimates of the coefficients of the explanatory variables and their standard errors are found to be those shown in Table 3.4.

We see from Table 3.4 that some of the estimates are close to zero. Indeed, if individual 95% confidence intervals are calculated for the coefficients of the seven variables, only those for *Bun* and *Hb* exclude zero. This suggests that the hazard function does not depend on all seven explanatory variables.

We cannot deduce from this that *Bun* and *Hb* are the relevant variables, since the estimates of the coefficients of the seven explanatory variables in the fitted model are not independent of one another. This means that if one of the seven explanatory variables were excluded from the model, the coefficients

Table 3.4 *Estimated values of the coefficients of the explanatory variables on fitting a Cox regression model to the data from Example 1.3.*

Variable	$\hat{\beta}$	se $(\hat{\beta})$
Age	−0.019	0.028
Sex	−0.251	0.402
Bun	0.021	0.006
Ca	0.013	0.132
Hb	−0.135	0.069
Pcells	−0.002	0.007
Protein	−0.640	0.427

of the remaining six might be different from those in Table 3.4. For example, if *Bun* is omitted, the estimated coefficients of the six remaining explanatory variables, *Age*, *Sex*, *Ca*, *Hb*, *Pcells* and *Protein*, turn out to be −0.009, −0.301, −0.036, −0.140, −0.001 and −0.420, respectively. Comparison with the values shown in Table 3.4 shows that there are differences in the estimated coefficients of each of these six variables, although in this case the differences are not very great.

In general, to determine on which of the seven explanatory variables the hazard function depends, a number of different models will need to be fitted, and the results compared. Methods for comparing the fit of alternative models, and strategies for model building are considered in subsequent sections of this chapter.

3.5 Comparing alternative models

In a modelling approach to the analysis of survival data, a model is developed for the dependence of the hazard function on one or more explanatory variables. In this development process, Cox regression models with linear components that contain different sets of terms are fitted, and comparisons made between them.

As a specific example, consider the situation where there are two groups of survival times, corresponding to individuals who receive either a new treatment or a standard. The common hazard function under the model for no treatment difference can be taken to be $h_0(t)$. This model is a special case of the general proportional hazards model in Equation (3.3), in which there are no explanatory variables in the linear component of the model. This model is therefore referred to as the *null model*.

Now let X be an indicator variable that takes the value zero for individuals receiving the standard treatment and unity otherwise. Under a proportional hazards model, the hazard function for an individual for whom X takes the value x is $e^{\beta x} h_0(t)$. The hazard functions for individuals on the standard and new treatments are then $h_0(t)$ and $e^{\beta}h_0(t)$, respectively. The difference between this model and the null model is that the linear component of the latter contains the additional term βx. Since $\beta = 0$ corresponds to no treatment effect, the extent of any treatment difference can be investigated by comparing these two Cox regression models for the observed survival data.

More generally, suppose that two models are contemplated for a particular data set, Model (1) and Model (2), say, where Model (1) contains a subset of the terms in Model (2). Model (1) is then said to be *parametrically nested* within Model (2). Specifically, suppose that the p explanatory variables, $X_1, X_2, \ldots, X_p$, are fitted in Model (1), so that the hazard function under this model can be written as

$$\exp\{\beta_1 x_1 + \beta_2 x_2 + \cdots + \beta_p x_p\} h_0(t).$$

Also suppose that the $p + q$ explanatory variables $X_1, X_2, \ldots, X_p, X_{p+1}, \ldots,$ X_{p+q} are fitted in Model (2), so that the hazard function under this model is

$$\exp\{\beta_1 x_1 + \cdots + \beta_p x_p + \beta_{p+1} x_{p+1} + \cdots + \beta_{p+q} x_{p+q}\} h_0(t).$$

Model (2) then contains the q additional explanatory variables $X_{p+1}, X_{p+2},$ $\ldots, X_{p+q}$. Because Model (2) has a larger number of terms than Model (1), Model (2) must be a better fit to the observed data. The statistical problem is then to determine whether the additional q terms in Model (2) significantly improve the explanatory power of the model. If not, they might be omitted, and Model (1) would be deemed to be adequate.

In the discussion of Example 3.2, we saw that when there are a number of explanatory variables of possible relevance, the effect of each term cannot be studied independently of the others. The effect of any given term therefore depends on the other terms currently included in the model. For example, in Model (1), the effect of any of the p explanatory variables on the hazard function depends on the $p - 1$ variables that have already been fitted, and the effect of X_p is said to be *adjusted* for the remaining $p - 1$ variables. In particular, the effect of X_p is adjusted for $X_1, X_2, \ldots, X_{p-1}$, but we also speak of the effect of X_p *eliminating* or *allowing for* $X_1, X_2, \ldots, X_{p-1}$. Similarly, when the q variables $X_{p+1}, X_{p+2}, \ldots, X_{p+q}$ are added to Model (1), the effect of these variables on the hazard function is said to be adjusted for the p variables that have already been fitted, $X_1, X_2, \ldots, X_p$.

3.5.1 The statistic $-2 \log \hat{L}$

In order to compare alternative models fitted to an observed set of survival data, a statistic that measures the extent to which the data are fitted by a particular model is required. Since the likelihood function summarises the information that the data contain about the unknown parameters in a given model, a suitable summary statistic is the value of the likelihood function when the parameters are replaced by their maximum likelihood estimates. This leads to the maximised likelihood, or in the case of the Cox regression model the maximised partial likelihood, under an assumed model. This statistic can be computed from Equation (3.4) by replacing the βs by their maximum likelihood estimates under the model. For a given set of data, the larger the value of the maximised likelihood, the better is the agreement between the model and the observed data.

For reasons given in the sequel, it is more convenient to use minus twice the logarithm of the maximised likelihood in comparing alternative models. If the maximised likelihood for a given model is denoted by $\hat{L}$, the summary measure of agreement between the model and the data is $-2\log\hat{L}$. From Section 3.3.1, $\hat{L}$ is in fact the product of a series of conditional probabilities, and so this statistic will be less than unity. In consequence, $-2\log\hat{L}$ will always be positive, and for a given data set, the smaller the value of $-2\log\hat{L}$, the better the model.

The statistic $-2\log\hat{L}$ cannot be used on its own as a measure of model adequacy. The reason for this is that the value of $\hat{L}$, and hence of $-2\log\hat{L}$, is dependent upon the number of observations in the data set. Thus if, after fitting a model to a set of data, additional data became available to which the fit of the model was the same as that to the original data, the value of $-2\log\hat{L}$ for the enlarged data set would be different from that of the original data. Accordingly the value of $-2\log\hat{L}$ is only useful when making comparisons between models fitted to the same data.

3.5.2 Comparing nested models

Consider again Model (1) and Model (2) defined earlier, where Model (1) contains p explanatory variables and Model (2) contains an additional q explanatory variables. Let the value of the maximised partial likelihood function for each model be denoted by $\hat{L}(1)$ and $\hat{L}(2)$, respectively. The two models can then be compared on the basis of the difference between the values of $-2\log\hat{L}$ for each model. In particular, a large difference between $-2\log\hat{L}(1)$ and $-2\log\hat{L}(2)$ would lead to the conclusion that the q variables in Model (2), that are additional to those in Model (1), do improve the adequacy of the model. Naturally, the amount by which the value of $-2\log\hat{L}$ changes when terms are added to a model will depend on which terms have already been included. In particular, the difference in the values of $-2\log\hat{L}(1)$ and $-2\log\hat{L}(2)$, that is, $-2\log\hat{L}(1)+2\log\hat{L}(2)$, will reflect the combined effect of adding the variables $X_{p+1}, X_{p+2}, \ldots, X_{p+q}$ to a model that already contains $X_1, X_2, \ldots, X_p$. This is said to be the change in the value of $-2\log\hat{L}$ due to fitting $X_{p+1}, X_{p+2}, \ldots, X_{p+q}$, adjusted for $X_1, X_2, \ldots, X_p$.

The statistic $-2\log\hat{L}(1) + 2\log\hat{L}(2)$, can be written as

$$-2\log\{\hat{L}(1)/\hat{L}(2)\},$$

and this is the log-likelihood ratio statistic for testing the null hypothesis that the q parameters $\beta_{p+1}, \beta_{p+2}, \ldots, \beta_{p+q}$ in Model (2) are all zero. From results associated with the theory of likelihood ratio testing (see Appendix A), this statistic has an asymptotic chi-squared distribution, under the null hypothesis that the coefficients of the additional variables are zero. The number of degrees of freedom of this chi-squared distribution is equal to the difference between the number of independent β-parameters being fitted under the two models. Hence, in order to compare the value of $-2\log\hat{L}$ for Model (1) and Model (2), we use the fact that the statistic $-2\log\hat{L}(1) + 2\log\hat{L}(2)$ has a chi-squared distribution on q degrees of freedom, under the null hypothesis that $\beta_{p+1}, \beta_{p+2}, \ldots, \beta_{p+q}$ are all zero. If the observed value of the statistic is not significantly large, the two models will be adjudged to be equally suitable. Then, other things being equal, the more simple model, that is, the one with fewer terms, would be preferred. On the other hand, if the values of $-2\log\hat{L}$ for the two models are significantly different, we would argue that the additional terms are needed and the more complex model would be adopted.

Although the difference in the values of the $-2\log\hat{L}$ for two nested models has an associated number of degrees of freedom, the $-2\log\hat{L}$ statistic itself does not. This is because the value of $-2\log\hat{L}$ for a particular model does not have a chi-squared distribution. Sometimes, $-2\log\hat{L}$ is referred to as a *deviance*. However, this is inappropriate, since unlike the deviance used in the context of generalised linear modelling, $-2\log\hat{L}$ does not measure deviation from a model that is a perfect fit to the data.

Example 3.3 Prognosis for women with breast cancer

Consider again the data from Example 1.2 on the survival times of breast cancer patients. On fitting a Cox regression model that contains no explanatory variables, that is, the null model, the value of $-2\log\hat{L}$ is 173.968. As in Example 3.1, the indicator variable X, will be used to represent the result of the staining procedure, so that X is zero for women whose tumours are negatively stained and unity otherwise. When the variable X is included in the linear component of the model, the value of $-2\log\hat{L}$ decreases to 170.096. The values of $-2\log\hat{L}$ for alternative models are conveniently summarised in tabular form, as illustrated in Table 3.5.

Table 3.5 *Values of $-2\log\hat{L}$ on fitting Cox regression models to the data from Example 1.2.*

Variables in model	$-2\log\hat{L}$
none	173.968
X	170.096

The difference between the values of $-2\log\hat{L}$ for the null model and the model that contains X can be used to assess the significance of the difference between the hazard functions for the two groups of women. Since one model contains one more β-parameter than the other, the difference in the values of $-2\log\hat{L}$ has a chi-squared distribution on one degree of freedom. The difference in the two values of $-2\log\hat{L}$ is $173.968 - 170.096 = 3.872$, which is just significant at the 5% level ($P = 0.049$). We may therefore conclude that there is evidence, significant at the 5% level, that the hazard functions for the two groups of women are different.

In Example 2.12, the extent of the difference between the survival times of the two groups of women was investigated using the log-rank test. The chi-squared value for this test was found to be 3.515 ($P = 0.061$). This value is not very different from the figure of 3.872 ($P = 0.049$) obtained above. The similarity of these two P-values means that essentially the same conclusions are drawn about the extent to which the data provide evidence against the null hypothesis of no group difference. From the practical viewpoint, the fact that one result is just significant at the 5% level, while the other is not quite significant at that level, is immaterial.

Although the model-based approach used in this example is operationally different from the log-rank test, the two procedures are in fact closely related. This relationship will be explored in greater detail in Section 3.13.

Example 3.4 Treatment of hypernephroma

In a study carried out at the University of Oklahoma Health Sciences Center, data were obtained on the survival times of 36 patients with a malignant tumour in the kidney, or hypernephroma. The patients had all been treated with a combination of chemotherapy and immunotherapy, but additionally a nephrectomy, the surgical removal of the kidney, had been carried out on some of the patients. Of particular interest is whether the survival time of the patients depends on their age at the time of diagnosis and on whether or not they had received a nephrectomy. The data obtained in the study were given in Lee and Wang (2013), but in this example, the age of a patient has been classified according to whether the patient is less than 60, between 60 and 70 or greater than 70. Table 3.6 gives the survival times of the patients in months.

In this example, there is a factor, age group, with three levels (< 60, 60–70, > 70), and a factor associated with whether or not a nephrectomy was performed. There are a number of possible models for these data depending on whether the hazard function is related to neither, one or both of these factors, labelled Model (1) to Model (5). Under Model (1), the hazard of death does not depend on either of the two factors and is the same for all 36 individuals in the study. In Models (2) and (3), the hazard depends on either the age group or on whether a nephrectomy was performed, but not on both. In Model (4), the hazard depends on both factors, where the impact of nephrectomy on the hazard is independent of the age group of the patient. Model (5) includes an interaction between age group and nephrectomy, so that under this model the effect of a nephrectomy on the hazard of death depends on the age group of the patient.

Suppose that the effect due to the jth age group is denoted by α_j, $j = 1, 2, 3$, and that due to nephrectomy status is denoted by ν_k, $k = 1, 2$. The

Table 3.6 *Survival times of 36 patients classified according to age group and whether or not they have had a nephrectomy.*

No nephrectomy			Nephrectomy		
<60	60–70	>70	<60	60–70	>70
9	15	12	104*	108*	10
6	8		9	26	9
21	17		56	14	18
			35	115	6
			52	52	
			68	5*	
			77*	18	
			84	36	
			8	9	
			38		
			72		
			36		
			48		
			26		
			108		
			5		

* Censored survival times.

terms α_j and ν_k may then be included in Cox regression models for $h_i(t)$, the hazard function for the ith individual in the study. The five possible models are then as follows:

$$\text{Model (1):} \quad h_i(t) = h_0(t)$$

$$\text{Model (2):} \quad h_i(t) = \exp\{\alpha_j\}h_0(t)$$

$$\text{Model (3):} \quad h_i(t) = \exp\{\nu_k\}h_0(t)$$

$$\text{Model (4):} \quad h_i(t) = \exp\{\alpha_j + \nu_k\}h_0(t)$$

$$\text{Model (5):} \quad h_i(t) = \exp\{\alpha_j + \nu_k + (\alpha\nu)_{jk}\}h_0(t)$$

To fit the term α_j, two indicator variables A_2 and A_3 are defined with values shown in Table 3.7. The term ν_k is fitted by defining a variable N which takes the value zero when no nephrectomy has been performed and unity when it has. With this choice of indicator variables, the baseline hazard function will correspond to an individual in the youngest age group who has not had a nephrectomy.

Models that contain the term α_j are then fitted by including the variables A_2, A_3 in the model, while the term ν_k is fitted by including N. The interaction is fitted by including the products $A_2N = A_2 \times N$ and $A_3N = A_3 \times N$ in

Table 3.7 *Indicator variables for age group.*

Age group	A_2	A_3
<60	0	0
60–70	1	0
>70	0	1

the model. The explanatory variables fitted, and the values of $-2\log\hat{L}$ for each of the five models under consideration, are shown in Table 3.8. When computer software for modelling survival data enables factors to be included in a model without having to define appropriate indicator variables, the values of $-2\log\hat{L}$ in Table 3.8 can be obtained directly.

Table 3.8 *Values of $-2\log\hat{L}$ on fitting five models to the data in Table 3.6.*

Model	Terms in model	Variables in model	$-2\log\hat{L}$
(1)	null model	none	177.667
(2)	α_j	A_2, A_3	172.172
(3)	ν_k	N	170.247
(4)	$\alpha_j + \nu_k$	A_2, A_3, N	165.508
(5)	$\alpha_j + \nu_k + (\alpha\nu)_{jk}$	A_2, A_3, N, A_2N, A_3N	162.479

The first step in comparing these different models is to determine if there is an interaction between nephrectomy status and age group. To do this, Model (4) is compared with Model (5). The reduction in the value of $-2\log\hat{L}$ on including the interaction term in the model that contains the main effects of age group and nephrectomy status is $165.508 - 162.479 = 3.029$ on 2 d.f. This is not significant ($P = 0.220$) and so we conclude that there is no interaction between age group and whether or not a nephrectomy has been performed.

We now determine whether the hazard function is related to neither, one or both of the factors age group and nephrectomy status. The change in the value of $-2\log\hat{L}$ on including the term α_j in the model that contains ν_k is $170.247 - 165.508 = 4.739$ on 2 d.f. This is significant at the 10% level ($P = 0.094$) and so there is some evidence that α_j is needed in a model that contains ν_k. The change in $-2\log\hat{L}$ when ν_k is added to the model that contains α_j is $172.172 - 165.508 = 6.664$ on 1 d.f., which is significant at the 1% level ($P = 0.010$). Putting these two results together, the term α_j may add something to the model that includes ν_k, and ν_k is certainly needed in the model that contains α_j. This means that both terms are required, and that the hazard function depends on both the patient's age group and on whether or not a nephrectomy has been carried out.

Before leaving this example, let us consider other possible results from the comparison of the five models, and how they would affect the conclusion as to which model is the most appropriate. If the term corresponding to age group, α_j, was needed in a model in addition to the term corresponding to nephrectomy status, ν_k, and yet ν_k was not needed in the presence of α_j, the model containing just α_j, Model (2), is probably the most suitable. To make sure that α_j was needed at all, Model (2) would be further compared with Model (1), the null model. Similarly, if the term corresponding to nephrectomy status, ν_k, was needed in addition to the term corresponding to age group, α_j, but α_j was not required in the presence of ν_k, Model (3) would probably be satisfactory. However, the significance of ν_k would be checked by comparing Model (3) with Model (1). If neither of the terms corresponding to age group and nephrectomy status were needed in the presence of the other, a maximum of one variable would be required. To determine which of the two is necessary, Model (2) would be compared with Model (1) and Model (3) with Model (1). If both results were significant, on statistical grounds, the model that leads to the biggest reduction in the value of $-2 \log \hat{L}$ from that for the null model would be adopted. If neither Model (2) nor Model (3) was superior to Model (1), we would conclude that neither age group nor nephrectomy status had an effect on the hazard function.

There are two further steps in the modelling approach to the analysis of survival data. First, we will need to critically examine the fit of a model to the observed data in order to ensure that the fitted Cox regression model is indeed appropriate. Second, we will need to interpret the parameter estimates in the chosen model, in order to quantify the effect that the explanatory variables have on the hazard function. Interpretation of parameters in a fitted model is considered in Section 3.9, while methods for assessing the adequacy of a fitted model will be considered in Chapter 4. But first, possible strategies for model selection are discussed.

3.6 Strategy for model selection

An initial step in the model selection process is to identify a set of explanatory variables that have the potential for being included in the linear component of a Cox regression model. This set will contain those variates and factors that have been recorded for each individual, but additional terms corresponding to interactions between factors or between variates and factors may also be required.

Once a set of potential explanatory variables has been isolated, the combination of variables that are to be used in modelling the hazard function has to be determined. In practice, a hazard function will not depend on a unique combination of variables. Instead, there are likely to be a number of equally good models, rather than a single 'best' model. For this reason, it is desirable to consider a wide range of possible models.

The model selection strategy depends to some extent on the purpose of the study. In some applications, information on a number of variables will have been obtained, and the aim might be to determine which of them has an effect on the hazard function, as in Example 1.3 on multiple myeloma.

In other situations, there may be one or more variables of primary interest, such as terms corresponding to a treatment effect. The aim of the modelling process is then to evaluate the effect of such variables on the hazard function, as in Example 1.4 on prostatic cancer. Since the other variables that have been recorded might also be expected to influence the magnitude of the treatment effect, these variables will need to be taken account of in the modelling process.

An important principle in statistical modelling is that when a term corresponding to the interaction between two factors is to be included in a model, the corresponding lower-order terms should also be included. This rule is known as the *hierarchic principle*, and means, for example, that interactions between two factors should not be fitted unless the corresponding main effects are present. Models that are not hierarchic are difficult to interpret.

3.6.1 Variable selection procedures

We first consider the situation where all explanatory variables are on an equal footing, and the aim is to identify subsets of variables upon which the hazard function depends. When the number of potential explanatory variables, including interactions, non-linear terms and so on, is not too large, it might be feasible to fit all possible combinations of terms, paying due regard to the hierarchic principle. Alternative nested models can be compared by examining the change in the value of $-2\log\hat{L}$ on adding terms into a model or deleting terms from a model.

Comparisons between a number of possible models, which need not necessarily be nested, can also be made on the basis of *Akaike's information criterion*, given by

$$AIC = -2\log\hat{L} + 2q,$$

in which q is the number of unknown β-parameters in the model. The smaller the value of this statistic, the better the model, but unlike the $-2\log\hat{L}$ statistic, the value of AIC will tend to increase when unnecessary terms are added to the model.

An alternative to the AIC statistic is the *Bayesian Information Criterion*, given by

$$BIC = -2\log\hat{L} + q\log d,$$

where q is the number of unknown parameters in the fitted model and d is the number of uncensored observations in the data set. The BIC statistic is also known as the *Schwarz Bayesian Criterion* and denoted SBC. The Bayesian Information Criterion is an adjusted value of the $-2\log\hat{L}$ statistic that takes account of both the number of unknown parameters in the fitted model and the number of observations to which the model has been fitted. As for the AIC statistic, smaller values of BIC are obtained for better models.

Of course, some terms may be identified as alternatives to those in a particular model, leading to subsets that are equally suitable. The decision on which of these subsets is the most appropriate should not then rest on statistical grounds alone. When there are no subject matter grounds for model choice, the model chosen for initial consideration from a set of alternatives might be the one for which the value of $-2 \log \hat{L}$, AIC or BIC is a minimum. It will then be important to confirm that the model does fit the data using the methods for model checking described in Chapter 4.

In some applications, information might be recorded on a number of variables, all of which relate to the same general feature. For example, the variables height, weight, body mass index (weight/height^2), head circumference, arm length and so on, are all concerned with the size of an individual. In view of inter-relationships between these variables, a model for the survival times of these individuals may not need to include each of them. It would then be appropriate to determine which variables from this group should be included in the model, although it may not matter exactly which variables are chosen.

When the number of variables is relatively large, it can be computationally expensive to fit all possible models. In particular, if there is a pool of p potential explanatory variables, there are 2^p possible combinations of terms, so that if $p > 10$, there are more than a thousand possible combinations of explanatory variables. In this situation, automatic routines for variable selection that are available in many software packages might seem an attractive prospect. These routines are based on *forward selection*, *backward elimination* or a combination of the two known as the *stepwise procedure*.

In forward selection, variables are added to the model one at a time. At each stage in the process, the variable added is the one that gives the largest decrease in the value of $-2 \log \hat{L}$ on its inclusion. The process ends when the next candidate for inclusion in the model does not reduce the value of $-2 \log \hat{L}$ by more than a prespecified amount. This is known as the *stopping rule*. This rule is often couched in terms of the significance level of the difference in the values of $-2 \log \hat{L}$ when a variable is added to a model, so that the selection process ends when the next term for inclusion ceases to be significant at a preassigned level.

In backward elimination, a model that contains the largest number of variables under consideration is first fitted. Variables are then excluded one at a time. At each stage, the variable omitted is the one that increases the value of $-2 \log \hat{L}$ by the smallest amount on its exclusion. The process ends when the next candidate for deletion increases the value of $-2 \log \hat{L}$ by more than a prespecified amount.

The stepwise procedure operates in the same way as forward selection. However, a variable that has been included in the model can be considered for exclusion at a later stage. Thus, after adding a variable to the model, the procedure then checks whether any previously included variable can now be deleted. These decisions are again made on the basis of prespecified stopping rules.

These automatic routines have a number of disadvantages. Typically, they lead to the identification of one particular subset, rather than a set of equally good ones. The subsets found by these routines often depend on the variable selection process that has been used, that is, whether it is forward selection, backward elimination or the stepwise procedure, and generally tend not to take any account of the hierarchic principle. They also depend on the stopping rule that is used to determine whether a term should be included in or excluded from a model. For all these reasons, these automatic routines have a limited role in model selection, and should certainly not be used uncritically.

Instead of using automatic variable selection procedures, the following general strategy for model selection is recommended.

1. The first step is to fit models that contain each of the variables one at a time. The values of $-2 \log \hat{L}$ for these models are then compared with that for the null model to determine which variables on their own significantly reduce the value of this statistic.
2. The variables that appear to be important from Step 1 are then fitted together. In the presence of certain variables, others may cease to be important. Consequently, those variables that do not significantly increase the value of $-2 \log \hat{L}$ when they are omitted from the model can now be discarded. We therefore compute the change in the value of $-2 \log \hat{L}$ when each variable on its own is omitted from the set. Only those that lead to a significant increase in the value of $-2 \log \hat{L}$ are retained in the model. Once a variable has been dropped, the effect of omitting each of the remaining variables in turn should be examined.
3. Variables that were not important on their own, and so were not under consideration in Step 2, may become important in the presence of others. These variables are therefore added to the model from Step 2, one at a time, and any that reduce $-2 \log \hat{L}$ significantly are retained in the model. This process may result in terms in the model determined at Step 2 ceasing to be significant.
4. A final check is made to ensure that no term in the model can be omitted without significantly increasing the value of $-2 \log \hat{L}$, and that no term not included significantly reduces $-2 \log \hat{L}$.

When using this selection procedure, rigid application of a particular significance level should be avoided. In order to guide decisions on whether to include or omit a term, the significance level should not be too small, for otherwise too few variables will be selected for inclusion; a level of 15% is recommended for general use.

In some applications, a small number of interactions and other higher-order terms, such as powers of certain variates, may need to be considered for inclusion in a model. Such terms would be added to the model identified in Step 3 above, after ensuring that any terms necessitated by the hierarchic principle have already been included in the model. If any higher-order term leads to a significant reduction in the value of $-2\log\hat{L}$, that term would be included in the model.

This model selection strategy is now illustrated in an example.

Example 3.5 Survival of multiple myeloma patients

The analysis of the data on the survival times of multiple myeloma patients in Example 3.2 suggested that not all of the seven explanatory variables, *Age*, *Sex*, *Bun*, *Ca*, *Hb*, *Pcells* and *Protein*, are needed in a Cox regression model. We now determine the most appropriate subsets of these variables. In this example, transformations of the original variables and interactions between them will not be considered. We will further assume that there are no medical grounds for including particular variables in a model. A summary of the values of $-2\log\hat{L}$ for all models that are to be considered is given in Table 3.9.

Table 3.9 *Values of* $-2\log\hat{L}$ *for models fitted to the data from Example 1.3.*

Variables in model	$-2\log\hat{L}$
none	215.940
Age	215.817
Sex	215.906
Bun	207.453
Ca	215.494
Hb	211.068
Pcells	215.875
Protein	213.890
Hb + *Bun*	202.938
Hb + *Protein*	209.829
Bun + *Protein*	203.641
Bun + *Hb* + *Protein*	200.503
Hb + *Bun* + *Age*	202.669
Hb + *Bun* + *Sex*	202.553
Hb + *Bun* + *Ca*	202.937
Hb + *Bun* + *Pcells*	202.773

The first step is to fit the null model and models that contain each of the seven explanatory variables on their own. Of these variables, *Bun* leads to the largest reduction in $-2\log\hat{L}$, reducing the value of the statistic from 215.940 to 207.453. This reduction of 8.487 is significant at the 1% level ($P = 0.004$) when compared with percentage points of the chi-squared distribution on 1 d.f. The reduction in $-2\log\hat{L}$ on adding *Hb* to the null model is 4.872, which is also significant at the 5% level ($P = 0.027$). The only other variable that on its own has some explanatory power is *Protein*, which leads to a reduction in $-2\log\hat{L}$ that is nearly significant at the 15% level ($P = 0.152$). Although this P-value is relatively high, we will for the moment keep *Protein* under consideration for inclusion in the model.

The next step is to fit the model that contains *Bun*, *Hb* and *Protein*, which leads to a value of $-2\log\hat{L}$ of 200.503. The effect of omitting each of the three variables in turn from this model is shown in Table 3.9. In particular, when *Bun* is omitted, the increase in $-2\log\hat{L}$ is 9.326, when *Hb* is omitted the increase is 3.138, and when *Protein* is omitted it is 2.435. Each of these changes in the value of $-2\log\hat{L}$ can be compared with percentage points of a chi-squared distribution on 1 d.f. Since *Protein* does not appear to be needed in the model, in the presence of *Hb* and *Bun*, this variable will not be further considered for inclusion.

If either *Hb* or *Bun* is excluded from the model that contains both of these variables, the increase in $-2\log\hat{L}$ is 4.515 and 8.130, respectively. Both of these increases are significant at the 5% level, and so neither *Hb* nor *Bun* can be excluded from the model without significantly increasing the value of the $-2\log\hat{L}$ statistic.

Finally, we look to see if any of variables *Age*, *Sex*, *Ca* and *Pcells* should be included in the model that contains *Bun* and *Hb*. Table 3.9 shows that when any of these four variables is added, the reduction in $-2\log\hat{L}$ is less than 0.5, and so none of them need to be included in the model. We therefore conclude that the most satisfactory model is that containing *Bun* and *Hb*.

We now turn to studies where there are variables of primary importance, such as a treatment effect. Here, we proceed in the following manner.

1. The important prognostic variables are first selected, ignoring the treatment effect. Models with all possible combinations of the variables can be fitted when their number is not too large. Alternatively, the variable selection process might follow similar lines to those described previously in Steps 1 to 4.
2. The treatment effect is then included in the model. In this way, any differences between the two groups that arise as a result of differences between the distributions of the prognostic variables in each treatment group, are not attributed to the treatment.
3. If the possibility of interactions between the treatment and other explanatory variables has not been discounted, these must be considered before the treatment effect can be interpreted.

Additionally, it will often be of interest to fit a model that contains the treatment effect alone. This enables the effect that the prognostic variables have on the magnitude of the treatment effect to be evaluated.

In this discussion on strategies for model selection, the use of statistical criteria to guide the selection process has been emphasised. In addition, due account must be taken of the application area. In particular, on subject area grounds, it may be inappropriate to include particular combinations of variables. On the other hand, there might be some variables that it is not sensible to omit from the model, even if they appear not to be needed in modelling a particular data set. Indeed, there is always a need for non-statistical considerations in model building.

Example 3.6 Comparison of two treatments for prostatic cancer
In the data from Example 1.4 on the survival times of 38 prostatic cancer patients, there are four prognostic variables that might have an effect on the survival times. These are the age of the patient (*Age*), serum haemoglobin level (*Shb*), tumour size (*Size*) and Gleason index (*Index*). All possible combinations of these variates are fitted in a Cox regression model and the values of $-2\log\hat{L}$ computed. These are shown in Table 3.10, together with the values of Akaike's information criterion, obtained from $AIC = -2\log\hat{L} + 2q$ and the Bayesian Information Criterion obtained from $BIC = -2\log\hat{L} + q\log(6)$, where q is the number of terms in a model fitted to a data set with 6 death times.

Table 3.10 *Values of* $-2\log\hat{L}$, *AIC and BIC for models fitted to the data from Example 1.4.*

Variables in model	$-2\log\hat{L}$	*AIC*	*BIC*
none	36.349	36.349	36.349
Age	36.269	38.269	38.061
Shb	36.196	38.196	37.988
Size	29.042	31.042	30.834
Index	29.127	31.127	30.919
Age + *Shb*	36.151	40.151	39.735
Age + *Size*	28.854	32.854	32.438
Age + *Index*	28.760	32.760	32.344
Shb + *Size*	29.019	33.019	32.603
Shb + *Index*	27.981	31.981	31.565
Size + *Index*	23.533	27.533	27.117
Age + *Shb* + *Size*	28.852	34.852	34.227
Age + *Shb* + *Index*	27.893	33.893	33.268
Age + *Size* + *Index*	23.269	29.269	28.644
Shb + *Size* + *Index*	23.508	29.508	28.883
Age + *Shb* + *Size* + *Index*	23.231	31.231	30.398

The two most important explanatory variables when considered separately are *Size* and *Index*. From the change in the value of $-2\log\hat{L}$ on omitting either of them from a model that contains both, we deduce that both variables are needed in a Cox regression model. The value of $-2\log\hat{L}$ is only reduced by a very small amount when *Age* and *Shb* are added to the model that contains *Size* and *Index*. We therefore conclude that only *Size* and *Index* are important prognostic variables.

From the values of Akaike's information criterion in Table 3.10, the model with *Size* and *Index* leads to the smallest value of the statistic, confirming that this is the most suitable model of those tried. Notice also that there are no other combinations of explanatory variables that lead to similar values of the *AIC*-statistic, which shows that there are no obvious alternatives to using

Size and *Index* in the model. The same conclusions follow from the values of the Bayesian Information Criterion.

We now consider the treatment effect. Let *Treat* be a variable that takes the value zero for individuals allocated to the placebo, and unity for those allocated to diethylstilbestrol. When *Treat* is added to the model that contains *Size* and *Index*, the value of $-2 \log \hat{L}$ is reduced to 22.572. This reduction of 0.961 on 1 d.f. is not significant ($P = 0.327$). This indicates that there is no treatment effect, but first we ought to examine whether the coefficients of the two explanatory variables in the model depend on treatment. To do this, we form the products *Tsize* = *Treat* × *Size* and *Tindex* = *Treat* × *Index*, and add these to the model that contains *Size*, *Index* and *Treat*. When *Tsize* and *Tindex* are added to the model, $-2 \log \hat{L}$ is reduced to 20.829 and 20.792, respectively. On adding both of these mixed terms, $-2 \log \hat{L}$ becomes 19.705. The reductions in $-2 \log \hat{L}$ on adding these terms to the model are not significant, and so there is no evidence that the treatment effect depends on *Size* and *Index*. This means that our original interpretation of the size of the treatment effect is valid, and that on the basis of these data, treatment with DES does not appear to affect the hazard of death. The estimated size of this treatment effect will be considered later in Example 3.12.

Before leaving this example, we note that when either *Tsize* or *Tindex* is added to the model, their estimated coefficient, and that of *Treat*, become large. The standard errors of these estimates are also very large. In particular, in the model that contains *Size*, *Index*, *Treat* and *Tsize*, the estimated coefficient of *Treat* is −11.28 with a standard error of 18.50. For the model that contains *Size*, *Index*, *Treat* and *Tindex*, the coefficients of *Treat* and *Tindex* are −161.52 and 14.66, respectively, while the standard errors of these estimates are 18476 and 1680, respectively! This is evidence of *overfitting*.

In an overfitted model, the estimated values of some of the β-coefficients will be highly dependent on the actual data. A very slight change to the values of one of these variables could then have a large impact on the estimate of the corresponding coefficient. This is the reason for such estimates having large standard errors. In this example, overfitting occurs because of the small number of events in the data set: there are only 6 of the 38 patients who die.

An overfitted model is one that is more complicated than is justified by the data, and does not provide a useful summary of the data. This is another reason for not including the mixed terms in the model for the hazard of death from prostatic cancer.

3.7* Variable selection using the lasso

A particularly useful aid to variable selection is the *Least Absolute Shrinkage and Selection Operator*, referred to as the *lasso*. The effect of using the lasso is to shrink the coefficients of explanatory variables in a model towards zero and in so doing, some estimates are set automatically to exactly zero. Explanatory variables whose coefficients become zero in the lasso procedure will be those that have little or no explanatory power, or that are highly correlated with others. The variables selected for inclusion in the model are then those with non-zero coefficients. This *shrinkage* also improves the predictive ability of a model, since the shrunken parameter estimates are less susceptible to changes in the sample data, and so are more stable.

3.7.1 The lasso in Cox regression modelling

Consider a Cox regression model that contains p explanatory variables, where the hazard of an event occurring at time t for the ith of n individuals is $h_i(t) = \exp(\boldsymbol{\beta}'\boldsymbol{x}_i)h_0(t)$, where $\boldsymbol{\beta}'\boldsymbol{x}_i = \beta_1 x_{1i} + \beta_2 x_{2i} + \cdots + \beta_p x_{pi}$, and $h_0(t)$ is the baseline hazard function. In the lasso procedure, the β-parameters in this model are estimated by maximising the partial likelihood function in Equation (3.5), while constraining the sum of their absolute values to be less than or equal to some value s. Denote the set of individuals at risk of an event at time t_i, the observed survival time of the ith individual, by $R(t_i)$, and let δ_i be the event indicator that is zero when t_i is a censored survival time and unity otherwise. The partial likelihood function for the model with p explanatory variables is then

$$L(\boldsymbol{\beta}) = \prod_{i=1}^{n} \left\{ \frac{\exp(\boldsymbol{\beta}'\boldsymbol{x}_i)}{\sum_{l \in R(t_i)} \exp(\boldsymbol{\beta}'\boldsymbol{x}_l)} \right\}^{\delta_i}, \tag{3.14}$$

which is maximised subject to the constraint that $\sum_{j=1}^{p} |\beta_j| \leqslant s$. The quantity $\sum_{j=1}^{p} |\beta_j|$ is called the L_1-norm of the vector $\boldsymbol{\beta}$, and is usually denoted $||\boldsymbol{\beta}||_1$. The estimates $\hat{\boldsymbol{\beta}}$ that maximise the constrained partial likelihood function are also the values that maximise

$$L_\lambda(\boldsymbol{\beta}) = L(\boldsymbol{\beta}) - \lambda \sum_{j=1}^{p} |\beta_j|, \tag{3.15}$$

where λ is called the *lasso parameter*. The likelihood function in Equation (3.15) is referred to as a *penalised* likelihood, since a penalty is assigned to the more extreme values of the βs. The resulting estimates will be closer to zero and have greater precision than the standard estimates on fitting a Cox model, at the cost of introducing a degree of bias in the estimates.

To see the effect of this *shrinkage*, estimates of the coefficients of all the explanatory variables that might potentially be included in the final model are obtained for a range of values of the lasso parameter. A plot of these estimates against λ, known as the *lasso trace*, provides an informative summary of the dependence of the estimates on the value of λ. When λ is small, few variables in the model will have zero coefficients, and the number of explanatory variables will not be reduced by much. On the other hand, large values of λ result in too many variables being excluded and an unsatisfactory model.

Although the lasso trace is a useful graphical aid to identifying a suitable value of λ to use in the modelling process, this is usually supplemented by techniques that enable the optimal value of the lasso parameter to be determined. This value could be taken to be that which maximises the penalised likelihood, $L_\lambda(\boldsymbol{\beta})$ in Equation (3.15), or equivalently the value of λ that minimises $-2\log L_\lambda(\boldsymbol{\beta})$. However, other methods for determining the optimum value of λ are generally preferred, such as the cross-validation method. In this approach, the optimal value of λ is that which maximises the cross-validated partial log-likelihood function. To define this, let $\hat{\boldsymbol{\beta}}_{(-i)}(\lambda)$ be the estimated vector of parameters on maximising the penalised partial likelihood function in Equation (3.15) when the data for the ith individual are omitted from the fitting process, $i = 1, 2, \ldots, n$, and for a given value of the lasso parameter λ. Writing $\log L(\boldsymbol{\beta})$ for the logarithm of the partial likelihood function defined in Equation (3.14), let $\log L_{(-i)}(\boldsymbol{\beta})$ be the partial log-likelihood when the data for the ith individual are excluded. The cross-validated partial log-likelihood function is then

$$\log \hat{L}_{CV}(\lambda) = \sum_{i=1}^{n} \left\{ \log L[\hat{\boldsymbol{\beta}}_{(-i)}(\lambda)] - \log L_{(-i)}[\hat{\boldsymbol{\beta}}_{(-i)}(\lambda)] \right\},$$

and the value of λ that maximises this function is chosen as the optimal value for the lasso parameter. The variables selected for inclusion in the model are then those with non-zero coefficients at this value of λ.

Following use of the lasso procedure, standard errors of the parameter estimates, or functions of these estimates such as hazard ratios, are not usually presented. One reason for this is that they are difficult to compute, but the main reason is that the parameter estimates will be biased towards zero. As a result, standard errors are not very meaningful and will tend to underestimate the precision of the estimates. If standard errors are required, the lasso procedure could be used to determine the variables that should be included in a model, that is those with non-zero coefficients at an optimal value of the lasso parameter. A standard Cox regression model that contains these variables is then fitted, but the advantages of shrinkage are then lost.

3.7.2 Data preparation

Before using the lasso procedure, the explanatory variables must be on similar scales of measurement. When this is not the case, each of the explanatory variables is first standardised to have zero mean and unit variance, by subtracting the sample mean and dividing by the standard deviation.

The lasso process can also be applied to categorical variables, after first standardising the indicator variables associated with the factor. This approach means that a factor is not regarded as a single entity, and the lasso procedure may result in a subset of the associated indicator variables being set to zero.

The variables that are identified by the lasso procedure will then depend on how the corresponding indicator variables have been coded. For example, if the $m-1$ indicator variables corresponding to an m-level factor are such that they are all zero for the first level of the factor, as illustrated in Section 3.2, the indicator variables will measure the effect of each factor level relative to the first. This may be helpful as a means of identifying factor levels that do not differ from a baseline level, but is inappropriate when, for example, the factor levels are ordered. In this case, a coding that reflects differences in the levels of the factor, known as *forward difference coding*, would be more useful. Coefficients that are set to zero in the lasso procedure would then correspond to levels that have similar effects to adjacent levels with non-zero coefficients.

To illustrate this coding, suppose that an ordered categorical variable A has four levels. This factor might be represented by three indicator variables A_1, A_2, A_3, defined in Table 3.11.

Table 3.11 *Indicator variables for a factor using forward difference coding.*

Level of A	A_1	A_2	A_3
1	3/4	1/2	1/4
2	−1/4	1/2	1/4
3	−1/4	−1/2	1/4
4	−1/4	−1/2	−3/4

When these three variables are included in a model with coefficients $\alpha_1, \alpha_2, \alpha_3$, the effect of level 1 of A is $(3\alpha_1 + 2\alpha_2 + \alpha_3)/4$, and that of level 2 is $(-\alpha_1 + 2\alpha_2 + \alpha_3)/4$. The coefficient of A_1, α_1, therefore represents the difference between level 1 and level 2 of A. Similarly, the coefficient of A_2 represents the difference between levels 2 and 3 of A and the coefficient of A_3 represents the difference between levels 3 and 4. In the general case of a factor A with m levels, the $m-1$ indicator variables are such that A_1 has values $(m-1)/m, -1/m, -1/m, \ldots, -1/m$, A_2 has values $(m-2)/m, (m-2)/m, -2/m, -2/m, \ldots, -2/m$, A_3 has values $(m-3)/m, (m-3)/m, (m-3)/m, -3/m, \ldots, -3/m$, and so on until A_{m-1} has values $1/m, 1/m, \ldots, 1/m, -(m-1)/m$. Categorical variables can also be accommodated using the *group lasso*, that enables a complete set of variables to be included or excluded, but further details will not be given here.

Example 3.7 Survival of multiple myeloma patients

The use of the lasso procedure in variable selection will be illustrated using data on the survival times of 48 patients with multiple myeloma that were first given in Example 1.3 of Chapter 1. The seven potential explanatory variables include five continuous variables (*Age*, *Bun*, *Ca*, *Hb*, *Pcells*) and two binary variables (*Sex*, *Protein*). All seven variables have very different scales of measurement, and so they are first standardised to have a sample mean of zero and unit standard deviation. For example, the 48 values of *Age* have a mean of 62.90 and a standard deviation of 6.96, and so the standardised values are $(Age - 62.90)/6.96$.

To apply the lasso procedure, estimates of the seven β-coefficients are obtained by maximising the penalised likelihood function in Equation (3.15) for a range of values of λ. The resulting trace of the coefficients of each variable, plotted against λ, is shown in Figure 3.2. In this plot, the coefficients presented are those of the original variables, obtained by dividing the estimated coefficient of the standardised explanatory variable that maximises the constrained likelihood function, by the standard deviation of that variable.

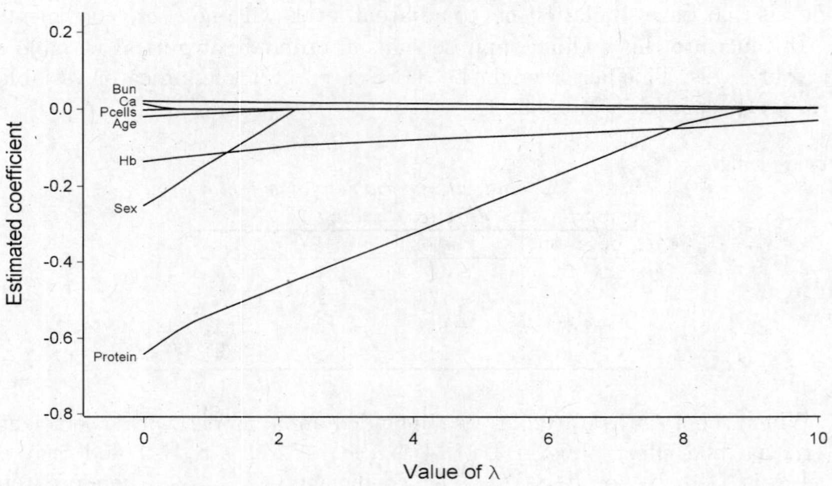

Figure 3.2 *Trace of the estimated coefficients of the explanatory variables as a function of the lasso parameter,* λ.

The estimates when $\lambda = 0$ are the parameter estimates on fitting a Cox regression model that contains all seven explanatory variables. As λ increases, these estimates get closer to zero, but at differing rates. The estimated coefficient of *Ca* has become zero when $\lambda = 0.5$ and that of *Pcells* is zero by $\lambda = 0.75$. The estimated coefficients of *Age* and *Sex* are both zero by $\lambda = 2.5$. This figure also illustrates another property of the lasso, which is that the lasso trace is formed from a number of straight line segments, so that it is *piecewise linear*.

To determine the optimal value of λ, the cross-validated partial log-likelihood, $\log \hat{L}_{CV}(\lambda)$, is evaluated for a range of λ values, and the value that maximises this likelihood function determined. The cross-validated partial log-likelihood is shown as a function of the lasso parameter, λ, in Figure 3.3. This function is a maximum when $\lambda = 3.90$, and at this value of λ, there are three variables with non-zero coefficients, *Hb*, *Bun* and *Protein*. The lasso procedure therefore leads to a model that contains these three variables.

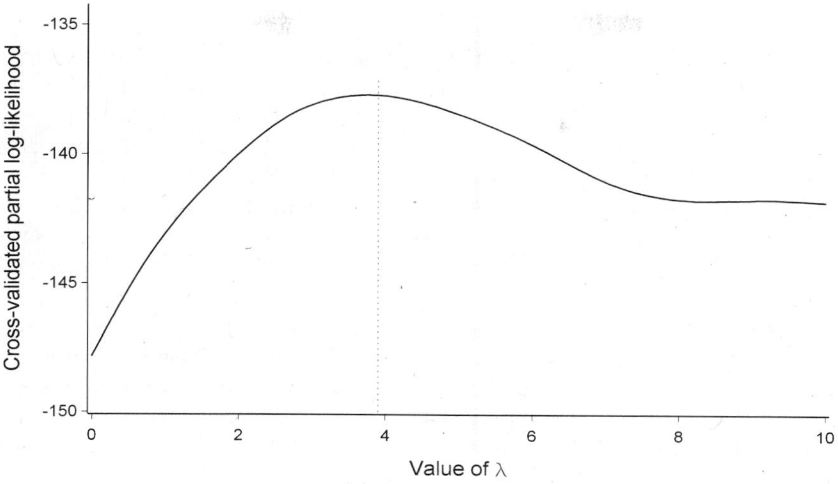

Figure 3.3 *Cross-validated partial log-likelihood as a function of the lasso parameter, showing the optimum value of* λ.

In this example, the cross-validated partial log-likelihood function shown in Figure 3.3 is quite flat around its maximum, and has very similar values for λ between 3 and 5. Also, from Figure 3.2, the same variables would be selected for inclusion in the model for any value of λ between 3 and 5, although the estimated coefficients will differ.

The coefficients of *Hb*, *Bun* and *Protein* in the model with $\lambda = 3.90$ are -0.080, 0.015 and -0.330, respectively. The corresponding estimates from a fitted Cox model with these three variables are -0.110, 0.020, and -0.617. Notice that the estimated coefficients in the model from the lasso procedure are all closer to zero than the corresponding estimates in the Cox model, illustrating the shrinkage effect. In the Cox model, the coefficient of *Protein* is not significantly different from zero ($P = 0.13$), although the lasso procedure suggests that this variable should be retained in the model. Ultimately, one might wish to include *Protein* in the model so as not to miss anything.

3.8 Non-linear terms

When the dependence of the hazard function on an explanatory variable that takes a wide range of values is to be modelled, we should consider whether it is appropriate to include that variable as a linear term in the Cox regression model. If there are reasons for not assuming that a variable is linear, we then need to consider how the non-linearity is modelled.

3.8.1 *Testing for non-linearity*

A straightforward way of examining whether non-linear terms are needed is to add quadratic or cubic terms to the model, and examine the consequent reduction in the value of the $-2 \log \hat{L}$ statistic. If the inclusion of such terms significantly reduces the value of this statistic, we would conclude that there is non-linearity. Polynomial terms might then be included in the model. However, in many situations, non-linearity in an explanatory variable cannot be adequately represented by the inclusion of polynomial terms in a Cox regression model. The following procedure is therefore recommended for general use.

To determine whether a variable exhibits non-linearity, the values of a possibly non-linear variate are first grouped into four or five categories containing approximately equal numbers of observations. A factor is then defined whose levels correspond to this grouping. For example, a variate reflecting the size of a tumour could be fitted as a factor whose levels correspond to very small, small, medium and large.

More specifically, let A be a factor with m levels formed from a continuous variate, and let X be a variate that takes the value j when A is at level j, for $j = 1, 2, \ldots, m$. Linearity in the original variate will then correspond to there being a linear trend across the levels of A. This linear trend can be modelled by fitting X alone. Now, fitting the $m-1$ terms $X, X^2, \ldots, X^{m-1}$ is equivalent to fitting A as a factor in the model, using indicator variables as in Section 3.2.2. Accordingly, the difference between the value of $-2 \log \hat{L}$ for the model that contains X, and that for the model that contains A, is a measure of non-linearity across the levels of A. If this difference is not significant we would conclude that there is no non-linearity and the original variate would be fitted. On the other hand, if there is evidence of non-linearity the actual form of this non-linearity can be further studied from the coefficients of the indicator variables corresponding to A. A plot of these coefficients may help in establishing the nature of any trend across the levels of the factor A.

Example 3.8 Survival of multiple myeloma patients

In Example 3.5, we found that a Cox regression model that contained the explanatory variables *Bun* and *Hb* appeared to be appropriate for the data on the survival times of multiple myeloma patients. We now consider whether there is any evidence of non-linearity in the values of serum haemoglobin level, and examine whether a quadratic term is needed in the model that contains *Bun* and *Hb*. When the term Hb^2 is added to this model, the value of $-2 \log \hat{L}$ is reduced from 202.938 to 202.917. This reduction of 0.021 on 1 d.f. is clearly not significant, which suggests that a linear term in *Hb* is sufficient.

An alternative way of examining the extent of non-linearity is to use a factor to model the effect of serum haemoglobin level on the hazard function. Suppose that a factor with four levels is defined, where level 1 corresponds to values of *Hb* less than or equal to 7, level 2 to values between 7 and 10, level 3 to values between 10 and 13 and level 4 to values greater than 13. This choice of levels corresponds roughly to the quartiles of the distribution of the values of *Hb*. This factor can be fitted by defining three indicator variables, *Hb*2, *Hb*3 and *Hb*4, which take the values shown in Table 3.12.

Table 3.12 *Indicator variables for a factor corresponding to values of the variable Hb.*

Level of factor (X)	Value of *Hb*	*Hb*2	*Hb*3	*Hb*4
1	$Hb \leqslant 7$	0	0	0
2	$7 < Hb \leqslant 10$	1	0	0
3	$10 < Hb \leqslant 13$	0	1	0
4	$Hb > 13$	0	0	1

When a model containing *Bun*, *Hb*2, *Hb*3 and *Hb*4 is fitted, the value of $-2 \log \hat{L}$ is 200.417. The change in the value of this statistic on adding the indicator variables *Hb*2, *Hb*3 and *Hb*4 to the model that contains *Bun* alone is 7.036 on 3 d.f., which is significant at the 10% level ($P = 0.071$). However, it is difficult to identify any pattern across the factor levels.

A linear trend across the levels of the factor corresponding to haemoglobin level can be modelled by fitting the variate X, which takes values 1, 2, 3, 4, according to the factor level. When the model containing *Bun* and X is fitted, $-2 \log \hat{L}$ is 203.891, and the change in the value of $-2 \log \hat{L}$ due to any non-linearity is $203.891 - 200.417 = 3.474$ on 2 d.f. This is not significant when compared with percentage points of the chi-squared distribution on 2 d.f. ($P = 0.176$). We therefore conclude that the effect of haemoglobin level on the hazard of death in this group of patients is adequately modelled by using the linear term *Hb*.

3.8.2 Modelling non-linearity

If non-linearity is detected using the procedure described in Section 3.8.1, it may be tempting to use the factor corresponding to the variable in the modelling process. However, this means that a continuous variable is being replaced by a step-function. Such a representation of an inherently continuous variable is not usually plausible from a subject matter viewpoint. In addition, this procedure requires category boundaries to be chosen, and the process of categorisation leads to a loss in information. The use of polynomial terms to represent non-linear behaviour in an explanatory variable is also not generally recommended. This is because low order polynomials, such as a quadratic or cubic expression, may not be a good fit to the data, and higher-order polynomials do not usually fit well in the extremes of the range of values of an explanatory variable. In addition, variables that have limiting values, or asymptotes, cannot be adequately modelled using polynomial expressions. A straightforward yet flexible solution is to use a model that contains different powers of the same variable, which may be fractional, referred to as *fractional polynomials*.

3.8.3 *Fractional polynomials*

A fractional polynomial in a variable X of order m contains m different powers of X. The expression $\beta_1 X^{p_1} + \beta_2 X^{p_2} + \cdots + \beta_m X^{p_m}$ is then included in the model, where each power p_j, $j = 1, 2, \ldots, m$, is taken to be one of the values in the set $\{-2, -1, -0.5, 0, 0.5, 1, 2, 3\}$, with X^0 taken to be $\log X$. The representation of X to the power of 0 by $\log X$ is called the *Box-Tidwell transformation* of X. Considerable flexibility in modelling the impact of an explanatory variable on the hazard of death can be achieved by using just two different powers of the variable, and so m is generally taken to be either 1 or 2. When $m = 2$, we can without any loss of generality take $p_1 < p_2$, since a model with powers p_1, p_2 is the same as one with powers p_2, p_1, and models with $p_1 = p_2$ are equivalent to the corresponding model with $m = 1$.

With $m = 1$, models with the 8 possible powers would be fitted, and that with the smallest value of $-2 \log \hat{L}$, in the presence of other variables under consideration, is the best fitting model. When $m = 2$, there are 28 possible combinations of the 8 powers in the set, excluding the 8 cases where the variable appears twice with the same power, and again the most appropriate combination would be the one for which $-2 \log \hat{L}$ is minimised. When comparing non-nested models of different orders, for example a model with two powers rather than one, where no power is common to both models, the *AIC* or *BIC* statistics can be used.

Example 3.9 Survival of multiple myeloma patients

In this example, we investigate whether there is evidence of non-linearity in serum haemoglobin level in the data set on the survival times of multiple myeloma patients. Fractional polynomials in *Hb* of order 1 and 2 are fitted, in addition to the variable *Bun*. Thus, *Hb* is included in the model as a single term with powers p_1 and as two terms with powers $p_1 < p_2$, where p_1 and p_2 are drawn from the set of values $\{-2, -1, -0.5, 0, 0.5, 1, 2, 3\}$ and where *Hb* raised to the power of zero is taken to mean log *Hb*. The values of $-2 \log \hat{L}$ for Cox regression models with

$$h_i(t) = \exp(\beta_1 Hb_i^{p_1} + \beta_2 Bun_i) h_0(t),$$

and

$$h_i(t) = \exp(\beta_1 Hb_i^{p_1} + \beta_2 Hb_i^{p_2} + \beta_3 Bun_i) h_0(t),$$

are shown in Table 3.13.

From this table, the best models with just one power of *Hb*, that is for $m = 1$, are those with a linear or a quadratic term, and of these, the model with *Hb* alone is the simplest. When models with two powers of *Hb* are fitted, that with $p_1 = -2$ and $p_2 = -1$ or -0.5 lead to the smallest values of $-2 \log \hat{L}$, but neither leads to a significant improvement on the model with just one power of *Hb*. If another power of *Hb* was to be added to the model that includes *Hb* alone, we would add Hb^{-2}, but again there is no need to do this

Table 3.13 *Values of* $-2\log\hat{L}$ *on fitting fractional polynomials in* Hb *of order* $m = 1, 2$ *to the data from Example 1.3.*

$m = 1$		$m = 2$								
p_1	$-2\log\hat{L}$	p_1	p_2	$-2\log\hat{L}$	p_1	p_2	$-2\log\hat{L}$	p_1	p_2	$-2\log\hat{L}$
−2	204.42	−2	−1	202.69	−1	1	202.81	0	2	202.94
−1	203.77	−2	−0.5	202.69	−1	2	202.94	0	3	203.04
−0.5	203.48	−2	0	202.71	−1	3	203.10	0.5	1	202.86
0	203.23	−2	0.5	202.74	−0.5	0	202.75	0.5	2	202.93
0.5	203.05	−2	1	202.79	−0.5	0.5	202.78	0.5	3	202.99
1	202.94	−2	2	202.94	−0.5	1	202.83	1	2	202.92
2	202.94	−2	3	203.14	−0.5	2	202.94	1	3	202.94
3	203.20	−1	−0.5	202.71	−0.5	3	203.07	2	3	202.80
		−1	0	202.73	0	0.5	202.81			
		−1	0.5	202.76	0	1	202.84			

as no model with two powers of *Hb* is a significant improvement on the model with *Hb* alone. We conclude that a linear term in *Hb* suffices, confirming the results of the analysis in Example 3.8.

3.9 Interpretation of parameter estimates

When a Cox regression model is used in the analysis of survival data, the coefficients of the explanatory variables in the model can be interpreted as logarithms of the ratio of the hazard of death to the baseline hazard. This means that estimates of this hazard ratio, and corresponding confidence intervals, can easily be found from the fitted model. The interpretation of parameters corresponding to different types of term in the Cox regression model is described in the following sections.

3.9.1 Models with a variate

Suppose that a Cox regression model contains a single continuous variable X, so that the hazard function for the ith of n individuals, for whom X takes the value x_i, is

$$h_i(t) = e^{\beta x_i} h_0(t).$$

The coefficient of x_i in this model can then be interpreted as the logarithm of a hazard ratio. Specifically, consider the ratio of the hazard of death for an individual for whom the value $x + 1$ is recorded on X, relative to one for whom the value x is obtained. This is

$$\frac{\exp\{\beta(x+1)\}}{\exp(\beta x)} = e^{\beta},$$

and so $\hat{\beta}$ in the fitted Cox regression model is the estimated change in the logarithm of the hazard ratio when the value of X is increased by one unit.

Using a similar argument, the estimated change in the log-hazard ratio when the value of the variable X is increased by r units is $r\hat{\beta}$, and the corresponding estimate of the hazard ratio is $\exp(r\hat{\beta})$. The standard error of the estimated log-hazard ratio will be $r\,\mathrm{se}\,(\hat{\beta})$, from which confidence intervals for the true hazard ratio can be derived.

The above argument shows that when a continuous variable X is included in a Cox regression model, the hazard ratio when the value of X is changed by r units does not depend on the actual value of X. For example, if X refers to the age of an individual, the hazard ratio for an individual aged 70, relative to one aged 65, would be the same as that for an individual aged 20, relative to one aged 15. This feature is a direct result of fitting X as a linear term in the Cox regression model. If there is doubt about the assumption of linearity, this can be checked using the procedure described in Section 3.8.1. Fractional polynomials in X or a non-linear transformation of X might then be used in the modelling process.

3.9.2 Models with a factor

When individuals fall into one of m groups, $m \geqslant 2$, which correspond to categories of an explanatory variable, the groups can be indexed by the levels of a factor. Under a Cox regression model, the hazard function for an individual in the jth group, $j = 1, 2, \ldots, m$, is given by

$$h_j(t) = \exp(\gamma_j)h_0(t),$$

where γ_j is the effect due to the jth level of the factor, and $h_0(t)$ is the baseline hazard function. This model is overparameterised, and so, as in Section 3.2.2, we take $\gamma_1 = 0$. The baseline hazard function then corresponds to the hazard of death at time t for an individual in the first group. The ratio of the hazards at time t for an individual in the jth group, $j \geqslant 2$, relative to an individual in the first group, is then $\exp(\gamma_j)$. Consequently, the parameter γ_j is the logarithm of this relative hazard, that is,

$$\gamma_j = \log\{h_j(t)/h_0(t)\}.$$

A model that contains the terms γ_j, $j = 1, 2, \ldots, m$, with $\gamma_1 = 0$, can be fitted by defining $m - 1$ indicator variables, $X_2, X_3, \ldots, X_m$, as shown in Section 3.2.2. Fitting this model leads to estimates $\hat{\gamma}_2, \hat{\gamma}_3, \ldots, \hat{\gamma}_m$, and their standard errors. The estimated logarithm of the relative hazard for an individual in group j, relative to an individual in group 1, is then $\hat{\gamma}_j$.

A $100(1 - \alpha)\%$ confidence interval for the true log-hazard ratio is the interval from $\hat{\gamma}_j - z_{\alpha/2}\,\mathrm{se}\,(\hat{\gamma}_j)$ to $\hat{\gamma}_j + z_{\alpha/2}\,\mathrm{se}\,(\hat{\gamma}_j)$, where $z_{\alpha/2}$ is the upper $\alpha/2$-point of the standard normal distribution. A corresponding confidence interval for the hazard ratio itself is obtained by exponentiating these confidence limits.

Example 3.10 Treatment of hypernephroma

Data on the survival times of patients with hypernephroma were given in Table 3.6. In this example, we will only consider the data from those patients on whom a nephrectomy has been performed, given in columns 4 to 6 of Table 3.6. The survival times of this set of patients are classified according to their age group. If the effect due to the jth age group is denoted by α_j, $j = 1, 2, 3$, the Cox regression model for the hazard at time t for a patient in the jth age group is such that

$$h_j(t) = \exp(\alpha_j)h_0(t).$$

This model can be fitted by defining two indicator variables, A_2 and A_3, where A_2 is unity if the patient is aged between 60 and 70, and A_3 is unity if the patient is more than 70 years of age, as in Example 3.4. This corresponds to taking $\alpha_1 = 0$.

The value of $-2 \log \hat{L}$ for the null model is 128.901, and when the term α_j is added, the value of this statistic reduces to 122.501. This reduction of 6.400 on 2 d.f. is significant at the 5% level ($P = 0.041$), and so we conclude that the hazard function does depend on which age group the patient is in.

The coefficients of the indicator variables A_2 and A_3 are estimates of α_2 and α_3, respectively, and are given in Table 3.14. Since the constraint $\alpha_1 = 0$ has been used, $\hat{\alpha}_1 = 0$.

Table 3.14 *Parameter estimates and their standard errors on fitting a Cox regression model to the data from Example 3.4.*

Parameter	Estimate	se (Estimate)
α_2	−0.065	0.498
α_3	1.824	0.682

The hazard ratio for a patient aged 60–70, relative to one aged less than 60, is $e^{-0.065} = 0.94$, while that for a patient whose age is greater than 70, relative to one aged less than 60, is $e^{1.824} = 6.20$. These results suggest that the hazard of death at any given time is greatest for patients who are older than 70, but that there is little difference in the hazard functions for patients in the other two age groups.

The standard error of the parameter estimates in Table 3.14 can be used to obtain a confidence interval for the true hazard ratios. A 95% confidence interval for the log-hazard ratio for a patient whose age is between 60 and 70, relative to one aged less than 60, is the interval with limits $-0.065 \pm (1.96 \times 0.498)$, that is, the interval $(-1.041, 0.912)$. The corresponding 95% confidence interval for the hazard ratio itself is $(0.35, 2.49)$. This confidence interval includes unity, which suggests that the hazard function for an individual whose age is between 60 and 70 is similar to that for a patient aged less than 60. Similarly, a 95% confidence interval for the hazard for a patient aged greater than 70, relative to one aged less than 60, is found to be (1.63, 23.59). This interval does not include unity, and so an individual whose age is greater than 70 has a significantly greater hazard of death, at any given time, than patients aged less than 60.

In some applications, the hazard ratio relative to the level of a factor other than the first may be required. In these circumstances, the levels of the factor, and associated indicator variables, could be redefined so that some other level of the factor corresponds to the required baseline level, and the model refitted. The required estimates can also be found directly from the estimates obtained when the first level of the original factor is taken as the baseline, although this is more difficult.

The hazard functions for individuals at levels j and j' of the factor are $\exp(\alpha_j)h_0(t)$ and $\exp(\alpha_{j'})h_0(t)$, respectively, and so the hazard ratio for an individual at level j, relative to one at level j', is $\exp(\alpha_j - \alpha_{j'})$. The log-hazard ratio is then $\alpha_j - \alpha_{j'}$, which is estimated by $\hat{\alpha}_j - \hat{\alpha}_{j'}$. To obtain the standard error of this estimate, we use the result that the variance of the difference $\hat{\alpha}_j - \hat{\alpha}_{j'}$ is given by

$$\operatorname{var}(\hat{\alpha}_j - \hat{\alpha}_{j'}) = \operatorname{var}(\hat{\alpha}_j) + \operatorname{var}(\hat{\alpha}_{j'}) - 2\operatorname{cov}(\hat{\alpha}_j, \hat{\alpha}_{j'}).$$

In view of this, an estimate of the covariance between $\hat{\alpha}_j$ and $\hat{\alpha}_{j'}$, as well as estimates of their variance, will be needed to compute the standard error of $(\hat{\alpha}_j - \hat{\alpha}_{j'})$. The calculations are illustrated in Example 3.11.

Example 3.11 Treatment of hypernephroma

Consider again the subset of the data from Example 3.4, corresponding to those patients who have had a nephrectomy. Suppose that an estimate of the hazard ratio for an individual aged greater than 70, relative to one aged between 60 and 70, is required. Using the estimates in Table 3.14, the estimated log-hazard ratio is $\hat{\alpha}_3 - \hat{\alpha}_2 = 1.824 + 0.065 = 1.889$, and so the estimated hazard ratio is $e^{1.889} = 6.61$. This suggests that the hazard of death at any given time for someone aged greater than 70 is more than six and a half times that for someone aged between 60 and 70.

The variance of $\hat{\alpha}_3 - \hat{\alpha}_2$ is

$$\operatorname{var}(\hat{\alpha}_3) + \operatorname{var}(\hat{\alpha}_2) - 2\operatorname{cov}(\hat{\alpha}_3, \hat{\alpha}_2),$$

and the variance-covariance matrix of the parameter estimates gives the required variances and covariance. This matrix can be obtained from statistical software used to fit the Cox regression model, and is found to be

$$\begin{matrix} A_2 \\ A_3 \end{matrix} \begin{pmatrix} 0.2484 & 0.0832 \\ 0.0832 & 0.4649 \end{pmatrix}, \\ \qquad\quad A_2 \qquad\quad A_3$$

from which $\operatorname{var}(\hat{\alpha}_2) = 0.2484$, $\operatorname{var}(\hat{\alpha}_3) = 0.4649$ and $\operatorname{cov}(\hat{\alpha}_2, \hat{\alpha}_3) = 0.0832$.

Of course, the variances are simply the squares of the standard errors in Table 3.14. It then follows that

$$\text{var}\,(\hat{\alpha}_3 - \hat{\alpha}_2) = 0.4649 + 0.2484 - (2 \times 0.0832) = 0.5469,$$

and so the standard error of $\hat{\alpha}_2 - \hat{\alpha}_3$ is 0.740. Consequently a 95% confidence interval for the log-hazard ratio is $(0.440, 3.338)$ and that for the hazard ratio itself is $(1.55, 8.18)$.

An easier way of obtaining the estimated value of the hazard ratio for an individual who is aged greater than 70, relative to one aged between 60 and 70, and the standard error of the estimate, is to redefine the levels of the factor associated with age group. Suppose that the data are now arranged so that the first level of the factor corresponds to the age range 60–70, level 2 corresponds to patients aged greater than 70 and level 3 to those aged less than 60. Choosing indicator variables to be such that the effect due to the first level of the redefined factor is set equal to zero leads to the variables B_2 and B_3 defined in Table 3.15.

Table 3.15 *Indicator variables for age group.*

Age group	B_2	B_3
<60	0	1
60–70	0	0
>70	1	0

The estimated log-hazard ratio is now simply the estimated coefficient of B_2, and its standard error can be read directly from standard computer output.

The manner in which the coefficients of indicator variables are interpreted is crucially dependent upon the coding that has been used for them. This means that when a Cox regression model is fitted using a statistical package that enables factors to be fitted directly, it is essential to know how indicator variables used within the package have been defined.

As a further illustration of this point, suppose that individuals fall into one of m groups and that the coding used for the $m-1$ indicator variables, $X_2, X_3, \ldots, X_m$, is such that the sum of the main effects of A, $\sum_{j=1}^{m} \alpha_j$, is equal to zero. The values of the indicator variables corresponding to an m-level factor A, are then as shown in Table 3.16.

With this choice of indicator variables, a Cox regression model that contains this factor can be expressed in the form

$$h_j(t) = \exp(\alpha_2 x_2 + \alpha_3 x_3 + \cdots + \alpha_m x_m) h_0(t),$$

where x_j is the value of X_j for an individual for whom the factor A is at the jth level, $j = 2, 3, \ldots, m$. The hazard of death at a given time for an individual at the first level of the factor is

$$\exp\{-(\alpha_2 + \alpha_3 + \cdots + \alpha_m)\} h_0(t),$$

Table 3.16 *Indicator variables for a factor where the main effects sum to zero.*

Level of A	X_2	X_3	...	X_m
1	-1	-1	...	-1
2	1	0	...	0
3	0	1	...	0
. . .	. . .	. . .	. . .	. . .
m	0	0	...	1

while that for an individual at the jth level of the factor is $\exp(\alpha_j)h_0(t)$, for $j \geqslant 2$. The ratio of the hazards for an individual in group j, $j \geqslant 2$, relative to that of an individual in the first group, is then

$$\exp(\alpha_j + \alpha_2 + \alpha_3 + \cdots + \alpha_m).$$

For example, if $m = 4$ and $j = 3$, the hazard ratio is $\exp(\alpha_2 + 2\alpha_3 + \alpha_4)$, and the variance of the corresponding estimated log-hazard ratio is

$$\begin{aligned} &\text{var}\,(\hat{\alpha}_2) + 4\,\text{var}\,(\hat{\alpha}_3) + \text{var}\,(\hat{\alpha}_4) + 4\,\text{cov}\,(\hat{\alpha}_2, \hat{\alpha}_3) \\ &\quad + 4\,\text{cov}\,(\hat{\alpha}_3, \hat{\alpha}_4) + 2\,\text{cov}\,(\hat{\alpha}_2, \hat{\alpha}_4). \end{aligned}$$

Each of the terms in this expression can be found from the variance-covariance matrix of the parameter estimates after fitting a Cox regression model, and a confidence interval for the hazard ratio obtained. However, this particular coding of the indicator variables does make it much more complicated to interpret the individual parameter estimates in a fitted model.

3.9.3 Models with combinations of terms

In previous sections, we have only considered the interpretation of parameter estimates in Cox regression models that contain a single term. More generally, a fitted model will contain terms corresponding to a number of variates, factors or combinations of the two. With suitable coding of indicator variables corresponding to factors in the model, the parameter estimates can again be interpreted as logarithms of hazard ratios.

When a model contains more than one variable, the parameter estimate associated with a particular effect is said to be *adjusted* for the other variables in the model, and so the estimates are log-hazard ratios, adjusted for the other terms in the model. The Cox regression model can therefore be used to estimate hazard ratios, taking account of other variables included in the model.

When interactions between factors, or mixed terms involving factors and variates, are fitted, the estimated log-hazard ratios for a particular factor will differ according to the level of any factor, or the value of any variate with which it interacts. In this situation, the value of any such factor level or variate will need to be made clear when the estimated hazard ratios for the factor of primary interest are presented.

Instead of giving algebraic details on how hazard ratios can be estimated after fitting models with different combinations of terms, the general approach will be illustrated in two examples. The first of these involves both factors and variates, while the second includes an interaction between two factors.

Example 3.12 Comparison of two treatments for prostatic cancer
In Example 3.6, the most important prognostic variables in the study on the survival of prostatic cancer patients were found to be size of tumour (*Size*) and the Gleason index of tumour stage (*Index*). The indicator variable *Treat*, which represents the treatment effect, is also included in a Cox regression model, since the aim of the study is to quantify the treatment effect. The model for the ith individual can then be expressed in the form

$$h_i(t) = \exp\{\beta_1 \, Size_i + \beta_2 \, Index_i + \beta_3 \, Treat_i\} h_0(t),$$

for $i = 1, 2, \ldots, 38$. Estimates of the β-coefficients and their standard errors on fitting this model are given in Table 3.17.

Table 3.17 *Estimated coefficients of the explanatory variables on fitting a Cox regression model to the data from Example 1.4.*

Variable	$\hat{\beta}$	se $(\hat{\beta})$
Size	0.083	0.048
Index	0.710	0.338
Treat	−1.113	1.203

The estimated log-hazard ratio for an individual on the active treatment DES (*Treat* = 1), relative to an individual on the placebo (*Treat* = 0), with the same values of *Size* and *Index* as the individual on DES, is $\hat{\beta}_3 = -1.113$. Consequently the estimated hazard ratio is $e^{-1.113} = 0.329$. The value of this hazard ratio is unaffected by the actual values of *Size* and *Index*. However, since these two explanatory variables were included in the model, the estimated hazard ratio is adjusted for these variables.

For comparison, if a model that only contains *Treat* is fitted, the estimated coefficient of *Treat* is −1.978. The estimated hazard ratio for an individual on DES, relative to one on the placebo, unadjusted for *Size* and *Index*, is now $e^{-1.978} = 0.14$. This shows that unless proper account is taken of the effect of size of tumour and index of tumour grade, the extent of the treatment effect is overestimated.

Now consider the hazard ratio for an individual on a particular treatment with a given value of the variable *Index* and a tumour of a given size, relative to an individual on the same treatment with the same value of *Index*, but whose size of tumour is one unit less. This is $e^{0.083} = 1.09$. Since this is greater than unity, we conclude that, other things being equal, the greater the size of the tumour, the greater that hazard of death at any given time. Similarly, the hazard ratio for an individual on a given treatment with a given value of *Size*, relative to one on the same treatment with the same value of *Size*, whose value of *Index* is one unit less, is $e^{0.710} = 2.03$. This again means that the greater the value of the Gleason index, the greater is the hazard of death at any given time. In particular, an increase of one unit in the value of *Index* doubles the hazard of death.

Example 3.13 Treatment of hypernephroma
Consider again the full set of data on survival times following treatment for hypernephroma, given in Table 3.6. In Example 3.4, the most appropriate Cox regression model was found to contain terms α_j, $j = 1, 2, 3$, corresponding to age group, and terms ν_k, $k = 1, 2$, corresponding to whether or not a nephrectomy was performed. For illustrative purposes, in this example we will consider the model that also contains the interaction between these two factors, even though it was found not to be significant. Under this model, the hazard function for an individual in the jth age group and the kth level of nephrectomy status is

$$h(t) = \exp\{\alpha_j + \nu_k + (\alpha\nu)_{jk}\}h_0(t), \tag{3.16}$$

where $(\alpha\nu)_{jk}$ is the term corresponding to the interaction.

Consider the ratio of the hazard of death at time t for a patient in the jth age group, $j = 1, 2, 3$, and the kth level of nephrectomy status, $k = 1, 2$, relative to an individual in the first age group who has not had a nephrectomy, which is

$$\frac{\exp\{\alpha_j + \nu_k + (\alpha\nu)_{jk}\}}{\exp\{\alpha_1 + \nu_1 + (\alpha\nu)_{11}\}}.$$

As in Example 3.4, the model in Equation (3.16) is fitted by including the indicator variables A_2, A_3, and N in the model, together with the products A_2N and A_3N. The estimated coefficients of these variables are then $\hat{\alpha}_2$, $\hat{\alpha}_3$, $\hat{\nu}_2$, $\widehat{(\alpha\nu)}_{22}$, and $\widehat{(\alpha\nu)}_{32}$, respectively. From the coding of the indicator variables that has been used, the estimates $\hat{\alpha}_1$, $\hat{\nu}_1$, $\widehat{(\alpha\nu)}_{11}$ and $\widehat{(\alpha\nu)}_{12}$ are all zero. The estimated hazard ratio for an individual in the jth age group, $j = 1, 2, 3$, and the kth level of nephrectomy status, $k = 1, 2$, relative to one in the first age group who has not had a nephrectomy, is then just

$$\exp\{\hat{\alpha}_j + \hat{\nu}_k + \widehat{(\alpha\nu)}_{jk}\}.$$

The non-zero parameter estimates are $\hat{\alpha}_2 = 0.005$, $\hat{\alpha}_3 = 0.065$, $\hat{\nu}_2 = -1.943$, $\widehat{(\alpha\nu)}_{22} = -0.051$, and $\widehat{(\alpha\nu)}_{32} = 2.003$, and the estimated hazard ratios are summarised in Table 3.18.

Inclusion of the combination of factor levels for which the estimated hazard ratio is 1.000 in tables such as Table 3.18, emphasises that the hazards are relative to those for individuals in the first age group who have not had a nephrectomy. This table shows that individuals aged less than or equal to 70,

Table 3.18 *Estimated hazard ratios on fitting a model that contains an interaction to the data from Example 3.4.*

Age group	No nephrectomy	Nephrectomy
<60	1.000	0.143
60–70	1.005	0.137
>70	1.067	1.133

who have had a nephrectomy, have a much reduced hazard of death, compared to those in the other age group and those who have not had a nephrectomy.

Confidence intervals for the corresponding true hazard ratios can be found using the method described in Section 3.9.2. As a further illustration, a confidence interval will be obtained for the hazard ratio for individuals who have had a nephrectomy in the second age group relative to those in the first. The log-hazard ratio is now $\hat{\alpha}_2 + \widehat{(\alpha\nu)}_{22}$, and so the estimated hazard ratio is 0.955. The variance of this estimate is given by

$$\text{var}\,(\hat{\alpha}_2) + \text{var}\,\{\widehat{(\alpha\nu)}_{22}\} + 2\,\text{cov}\,\{\hat{\alpha}_2, \widehat{(\alpha\nu)}_{22}\}.$$

From the variance-covariance matrix of the parameter estimates after fitting the model in Equation (3.16), $\text{var}\,(\hat{\alpha}_2) = 0.697$, $\text{var}\,\{\widehat{(\alpha\nu)}_{22}\} = 0.942$, and the covariance term is $\text{cov}\,\{\hat{\alpha}_2, \widehat{(\alpha\nu)}_{22}\} = -0.695$. Consequently, the variance of the estimated log-hazard ratio is 0.248, and so a 95% confidence interval for the true log-hazard ratio ranges from -0.532 to 0.441. The corresponding confidence interval for the true hazard ratio is $(0.59, 1.55)$. This interval includes unity, and so the hazard ratio of 0.955 is not significantly different from unity at the 5% level. Confidence intervals for the hazard ratios in Table 3.18 can be found in a similar manner.

3.10* Estimating the hazard and survivor functions

So far in this chapter, we have only considered the estimation of the β-parameters in the linear component of a Cox regression model. As we have seen, this is all that is required in order to draw inferences about the effect of explanatory variables in the model on the hazard function. Once a suitable model for a set of survival data has been identified, the hazard function, and the corresponding survivor function, can be estimated. These estimates can then be used to summarise the survival experience of individuals in the study.

Suppose that the linear component of a Cox regression model contains p explanatory variables, $X_1, X_2, \ldots, X_p$, and that the estimated coefficients of these variables are $\hat{\beta}_1, \hat{\beta}_2, \ldots, \hat{\beta}_p$. The estimated hazard function for the ith of n individuals in the study is then given by

$$\hat{h}_i(t) = \exp(\hat{\boldsymbol{\beta}}'\boldsymbol{x}_i)\hat{h}_0(t), \qquad (3.17)$$

where $\boldsymbol{x}_i$ is the vector of values of the explanatory variables for the ith individual, $i = 1, 2, \ldots, n$, $\hat{\boldsymbol{\beta}}$ is the vector of estimated coefficients, and $\hat{h}_0(t)$ is the estimated baseline hazard function. Using this equation, the hazard function for an individual can be estimated once an estimate of $h_0(t)$ has been found. The relationship between the hazard, cumulative hazard and survivor functions can then be used to give estimates of the cumulative hazard function and the survivor function.

An estimate of the baseline hazard function was derived by Kalbfleisch and Prentice (1973) using an approach based on the method of maximum likelihood. Suppose that there are r distinct death times which, when arranged in increasing order, are $t_{(1)} < t_{(2)} < \cdots < t_{(r)}$, and that there are d_j deaths and n_j individuals at risk at time $t_{(j)}$. The estimated baseline hazard function at time $t_{(j)}$ is then given by

$$\hat{h}_0(t_{(j)}) = 1 - \hat{\xi}_j, \tag{3.18}$$

where $\hat{\xi}_j$ is the solution of the equation

$$\sum_{l \in D(t_{(j)})} \frac{\exp(\hat{\boldsymbol{\beta}}' \boldsymbol{x}_l)}{1 - \hat{\xi}_j^{\exp(\hat{\boldsymbol{\beta}}' \boldsymbol{x}_l)}} = \sum_{l \in R(t_{(j)})} \exp(\hat{\boldsymbol{\beta}}' \boldsymbol{x}_l), \tag{3.19}$$

for $j = 1, 2, \ldots, r$. In Equation (3.19), $D(t_{(j)})$ is the set of all d_j individuals who die at the jth ordered death time, $t_{(j)}$, and as in Section 3.3, $R(t_{(j)})$ is the set of all n_j individuals at risk at time $t_{(j)}$. The estimates of the βs, which form the vector $\hat{\boldsymbol{\beta}}$, are those which maximise the likelihood function in Equation (3.4). The derivation of this estimate of $h_0(t)$ is quite complex, and so it will not be reproduced here.

In the particular case where there are no tied death times, that is, where $d_j = 1$ for $j = 1, 2, \ldots, r$, the left-hand side of Equation (3.19) will be a single term. This equation can then be solved to give

$$\hat{\xi}_j = \left(1 - \frac{\exp(\hat{\boldsymbol{\beta}}' \boldsymbol{x}_{(j)})}{\sum_{l \in R(t_{(j)})} \exp(\hat{\boldsymbol{\beta}}' \boldsymbol{x}_l)} \right)^{\exp(-\hat{\boldsymbol{\beta}}' \boldsymbol{x}_{(j)})},$$

where $\boldsymbol{x}_{(j)}$ is the vector of explanatory variables for the individual who dies at time $t_{(j)}$.

When there are tied observations, that is, when one or more of the d_j are greater than unity, the summation on the left-hand side of Equation (3.19) is the sum of a series of fractions in which $\hat{\xi}_j$ occurs in the denominators, raised to different powers. Equation (3.19) cannot then be solved explicitly, and an iterative scheme is required.

We now make the assumption that the hazard of death is constant between adjacent death times. An appropriate estimate of the baseline hazard function in this interval is then obtained by dividing the estimated hazard in Equation (3.18) by the time interval, to give the step-function

$$\hat{h}_0(t) = \frac{1 - \hat{\xi}_j}{t_{(j+1)} - t_{(j)}}, \tag{3.20}$$

for $t_{(j)} \leqslant t < t_{(j+1)}$, $j = 1, 2, \ldots, r-1$, with $\hat{h}_0(t) = 0$ for $t < t_{(1)}$.

The quantity $\hat{\xi}_j$ can be regarded as an estimate of the probability that an individual survives through the interval from $t_{(j)}$ to $t_{(j+1)}$. The baseline survivor function can then be estimated by

$$\hat{S}_0(t) = \prod_{j=1}^{k} \hat{\xi}_j, \tag{3.21}$$

for $t_{(k)} \leqslant t < t_{(k+1)}$, $k = 1, 2, \ldots, r-1$, and so this estimate is also a step-function. The estimated value of the baseline survivor function is unity for $t < t_{(1)}$, and zero for $t \geqslant t_{(r)}$, unless there are censored survival times greater than $t_{(r)}$. If this is the case, $\hat{S}_0(t)$ can be taken to be $\hat{S}_0(t_{(r)})$ until the largest censored time, but the estimated survivor function is undefined beyond that time.

The baseline cumulative hazard function is, from Equation (1.8), given by $H_0(t) = -\log S_0(t)$, and so an estimate of this function is

$$\hat{H}_0(t) = -\log \hat{S}_0(t) = -\sum_{j=1}^{k} \log \hat{\xi}_j, \tag{3.22}$$

for $t_{(k)} \leqslant t < t_{(k+1)}$, $k = 1, 2, \ldots, r-1$, with $\hat{H}_0(t) = 0$ for $t < t_{(1)}$.

The estimates of the baseline hazard, survivor and cumulative hazard functions in Equations (3.20), (3.21) and (3.22) can be used to obtain the corresponding estimates for an individual with a vector of explanatory variables $\boldsymbol{x}_i$. In particular, from Equation (3.17), the hazard function is estimated by $\exp(\hat{\boldsymbol{\beta}}'\boldsymbol{x}_i)\hat{h}_0(t)$. Next, integrating both sides of Equation (3.17), we get

$$\int_0^t \hat{h}_i(u)\,du = \exp(\hat{\boldsymbol{\beta}}'\boldsymbol{x}_i)\int_0^t \hat{h}_0(u)\,du, \tag{3.23}$$

so that the estimated cumulative hazard function for the ith individual is given by

$$\hat{H}_i(t) = \exp(\hat{\boldsymbol{\beta}}'\boldsymbol{x}_i)\hat{H}_0(t). \tag{3.24}$$

On multiplying each side of Equation (3.23) by -1 and exponentiating, and making use of Equation (1.6), we find that the estimated survivor function for the ith individual is

$$\hat{S}_i(t) = \left\{\hat{S}_0(t)\right\}^{\exp(\hat{\boldsymbol{\beta}}'\boldsymbol{x}_i)}, \tag{3.25}$$

for $t_{(k)} \leqslant t < t_{(k+1)}$, $k = 1, 2, \ldots, r-1$. Note that once the estimated survivor function, $\hat{S}_i(t)$, has been obtained, an estimate of the cumulative hazard function is simply $-\log \hat{S}_i(t)$.

3.10.1 The special case of no covariates

When there are no covariates, so that we have just a single sample of survival times, Equation (3.19) becomes

$$\frac{d_j}{1-\hat{\xi}_j} = n_j,$$

from which

$$\hat{\xi}_j = \frac{n_j - d_j}{n_j}.$$

Then, the estimated baseline hazard function at time $t_{(j)}$ is $1 - \hat{\xi}_j$, which is d_j/n_j. The corresponding estimate of the survivor function from Equation (3.21) is $\prod_{j=1}^{k} \hat{\xi}_j$, that is,

$$\prod_{j=1}^{k} \left(\frac{n_j - d_j}{n_j} \right),$$

which is the Kaplan-Meier estimate of the survivor function given earlier in Equation (2.4). This shows that the estimate of the survivor function given in Equation (3.25) generalises the Kaplan-Meier estimate to the case where the hazard function depends on explanatory variables.

Furthermore, the estimate of the hazard function in Equation (3.20) reduces to $d_j/\{n_j(t_{(j+1)} - t_{(j)})\}$, which is the estimate of the hazard function given in Equation (2.13) of Chapter 2.

3.10.2 Some approximations to estimates of baseline functions

When there are tied survival times, the estimated baseline hazard can only be found by using an iterative method to solve Equation (3.19). This iterative process can be avoided by using an approximation to the summation on the left-hand side of Equation (3.19).

The term

$$\hat{\xi}_j^{\exp(\hat{\boldsymbol{\beta}}'\boldsymbol{x}_l)},$$

in the denominator of the left-hand side of Equation (3.19), can be written as

$$\exp\left\{ e^{\hat{\boldsymbol{\beta}}'\boldsymbol{x}_l} \log \hat{\xi}_j \right\},$$

and taking the first two terms in the expansion of the exponent gives

$$\exp\left\{ e^{\hat{\boldsymbol{\beta}}'\boldsymbol{x}_l} \log \hat{\xi}_j \right\} \approx 1 + e^{\hat{\boldsymbol{\beta}}'\boldsymbol{x}_l} \log \hat{\xi}_j.$$

Writing $1 - \tilde{\xi}_j$ for the estimated baseline hazard at time $t_{(j)}$, obtained using this approximation, and substituting $1 + e^{\hat{\boldsymbol{\beta}}'\boldsymbol{x}_l} \log \tilde{\xi}_j$ for $\hat{\xi}_j^{\exp(\hat{\boldsymbol{\beta}}'\boldsymbol{x}_l)}$ in Equation (3.19), we find that $\tilde{\xi}_j$ is such that

$$-\sum_{l \in D(t_{(j)})} \frac{1}{\log \tilde{\xi}_j} = \sum_{l \in R(t_{(j)})} \exp(\hat{\boldsymbol{\beta}}'\boldsymbol{x}_l).$$

Therefore,

$$\frac{-d_j}{\log \tilde{\xi}_j} = \sum_{l \in R(t_{(j)})} \exp(\hat{\boldsymbol{\beta}}'\boldsymbol{x}_l),$$

since d_j is the number of deaths at the jth ordered death time, $t_{(j)}$, and so

$$\tilde{\xi}_j = \exp\left(\frac{-d_j}{\sum_{l \in R(t_{(j)})} \exp(\hat{\boldsymbol{\beta}}'\boldsymbol{x}_l)}\right). \tag{3.26}$$

From Equation (3.21), an estimate of the survivor function, based on the values of $\tilde{\xi}_j$, is given by

$$\tilde{S}_0(t) = \prod_{j=1}^{k} \exp\left(\frac{-d_j}{\sum_{l \in R(t_{(j)})} \exp(\hat{\boldsymbol{\beta}}'\boldsymbol{x}_l)}\right), \tag{3.27}$$

for $t_{(k)} \leqslant t < t_{(k+1)}$, $k = 1, 2, \ldots, r-1$. From this definition, the estimated survivor function is not necessarily zero at the longest survival time, when that time is uncensored, unlike the estimate in Equation (3.21). The estimate of the baseline cumulative hazard function derived from $\tilde{S}_0(t)$ is

$$\tilde{H}_0(t) = -\log \tilde{S}_0(t) = \sum_{j=1}^{k} \frac{d_j}{\sum_{l \in R(t_{(j)})} \exp(\hat{\boldsymbol{\beta}}'\boldsymbol{x}_l)}, \tag{3.28}$$

for $t_{(k)} \leqslant t < t_{(k+1)}$, $k = 1, 2, \ldots, r-1$. This estimate is often referred to as the *Nelson-Aalen estimate* or the *Breslow estimate* of the baseline cumulative hazard function.

When there are no covariates, the estimated baseline survivor function in Equation (3.27) becomes

$$\prod_{j=1}^{k} \exp(-d_j/n_j), \tag{3.29}$$

since n_j is the number of individuals at risk at time $t_{(j)}$. This is the Nelson-Aalen estimate of the survivor function given in Equation (2.5) of Chapter 2, and the corresponding estimate of the baseline cumulative hazard function is $\sum_{j=1}^{k} d_j/n_j$, as in Section 2.3.3 of Chapter 2.

A further approximation is found from noting that the expression

$$\frac{-d_j}{\sum_{l \in R(t_{(j)})} \exp(\hat{\boldsymbol{\beta}}'\boldsymbol{x}_l)},$$

in the exponent of Equation (3.26), will tend to be small, unless there are large numbers of ties at particular death times. Taking the first two terms of the expansion of this exponent, and denoting this new approximation to ξ_j by ξ_j^* gives

$$\xi_j^* = 1 - \frac{d_j}{\sum_{l \in R(t_{(j)})} \exp(\hat{\boldsymbol{\beta}}' \boldsymbol{x}_l)}.$$

Adapting Equation (3.20), the estimated baseline hazard function in the interval from $t_{(j)}$ to $t_{(j+1)}$ is then given by

$$h_0^*(t) = \frac{d_j}{(t_{(j+1)} - t_{(j)}) \sum_{l \in R(t_{(j)})} \exp(\hat{\boldsymbol{\beta}}' \boldsymbol{x}_l)}, \tag{3.30}$$

for $t_{(j)} \leqslant t < t_{(j+1)}$, $j = 1, 2, \ldots, r-1$. Using ξ_j^* in place of $\hat{\xi}_j$ in Equation (3.21), the corresponding estimated baseline survivor function is

$$S_0^*(t) = \prod_{j=1}^{k} \left(1 - \frac{d_j}{\sum_{l \in R(t_{(j)})} \exp(\hat{\boldsymbol{\beta}}' \boldsymbol{x}_l)} \right),$$

and a further approximate estimate of the baseline cumulative hazard function is $H_0^*(t) = -\log S_0^*(t)$. Notice that the cumulative hazard function in Equation (3.28) at time t can be expressed in the form

$$\tilde{H}_0(t) = \sum_{j=1}^{k} (t_{(j+1)} - t_{(j)}) h_0^*(t),$$

where $h_0^*(t)$ is given in Equation (3.30). Consequently, differences in successive values of the estimated baseline cumulative hazard function in Equation (3.28) provide an approximation to the baseline hazard function, at times $t_{(1)}, t_{(2)}, \ldots, t_{(r)}$, that can easily be computed.

In the particular case where there are no covariates, the estimates $h_0^*(t)$, $S_0^*(t)$ and $H_0^*(t)$ are the same as those given in Section 3.10.1. Equations similar to Equations (3.24) and (3.25) can be used to estimate the cumulative hazard and survivor functions for an individual whose vector of explanatory variables is $\boldsymbol{x}_i$.

In practice, it will often be computationally advantageous to use either $\tilde{S}_0(t)$ or $S_0^*(t)$ in place of $\hat{S}_0(t)$. When the number of tied survival times is small, all three estimates will tend to be very similar. Moreover, since the estimates are generally used as descriptive summaries of the survival data, small differences between the estimates are unlikely to be of practical importance.

Once an estimate of the survivor function has been obtained, the median and other percentiles of the survival time distribution can be found from tabular or graphical displays of the function for individuals with particular values of explanatory variables. The method used is very similar to that described in Section 2.4, and is illustrated in the following example.

Example 3.14 Treatment of hypernephroma

In Example 3.4, a Cox regression model was fitted to the data on the survival times of patients with hypernephroma. The hazard function was found to depend on the age group of a patient, and whether or not a nephrectomy had been performed. The estimated hazard function for the ith patient was found to be

$$\hat{h}_i(t) = \exp\{0.013\, A_{2i} + 1.342\, A_{3i} - 1.412\, N_i\}\hat{h}_0(t),$$

where A_{2i} is unity if the patient is aged between 60 and 70 and zero otherwise, A_{3i} is unity if the patient is aged over 70 and zero otherwise, and N_i is unity if the patient has had a nephrectomy and zero otherwise. The estimated baseline hazard function is therefore the estimated hazard of death at time t, for an individual whose age is less than 60 and who has not had a nephrectomy.

In Table 3.19, the estimated baseline hazard function, $\hat{h}_0(t)$, cumulative hazard function, $\hat{H}_0(t)$, and survivor function, $\hat{S}_0(t)$, obtained using Equations (3.18), (3.22) and (3.21), respectively, are tabulated.

Table 3.19 *Estimates of the baseline hazard, survivor and cumulative hazard functions for the data from Example 3.4.*

Time	$\hat{h}_0(t)$	$\hat{S}_0(t)$	$\hat{H}_0(t)$
0	0.000	1.000	0.000
5	0.050	0.950	0.051
6	0.104	0.852	0.161
8	0.113	0.755	0.281
9	0.237	0.576	0.552
10	0.073	0.534	0.628
12	0.090	0.486	0.722
14	0.108	0.433	0.836
15	0.116	0.383	0.960
17	0.132	0.333	1.101
18	0.285	0.238	1.436
21	0.185	0.194	1.641
26	0.382	0.120	2.123
35	0.232	0.092	2.387
36	0.443	0.051	2.972
38	0.279	0.037	3.299
48	0.299	0.026	3.655
52	0.560	0.011	4.476
56	0.382	0.007	4.958
68	0.421	0.004	5.504
72	0.467	0.002	6.134
84	0.599	0.001	7.045
108	0.805	0.000	8.692
115	–	0.000	–

From this table, we see that the general trend is for the estimated baseline hazard function to increase with time. From the manner in which the estimated baseline hazard function has been computed, the estimates only apply at the death times of the patients in the study. However, if the assumption of a constant hazard in each time interval is made, by dividing the estimated hazard by the corresponding time interval, the risk of death per unit time can be found. This leads to the estimate in Equation (3.20). A graph of this hazard function is shown in Figure 3.4.

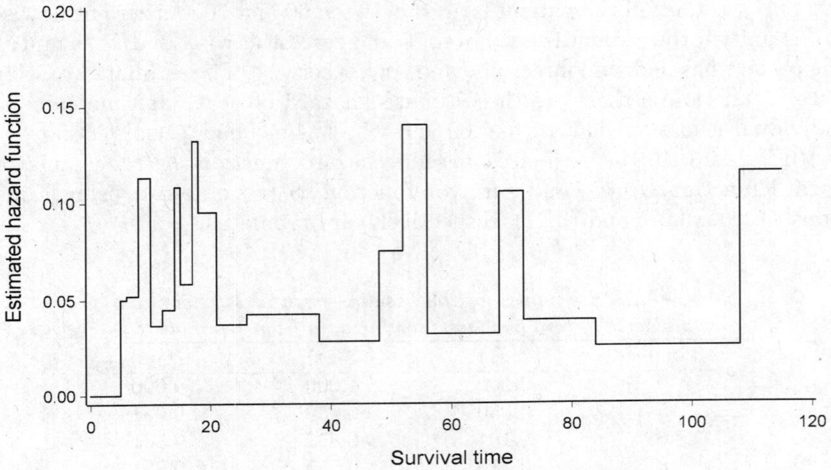

Figure 3.4 *Estimated baseline hazard function, per unit time, assuming constant hazard between adjacent death times.*

This graph shows that the risk of death per unit time is roughly constant over the duration of the study. Table 3.19 also shows that the values of $\hat{h}_0(t)$ are very similar to differences in the values of $\hat{H}_0(t)$ between successive observations, as would be expected.

We now consider the estimation of the median survival time, defined as the smallest observed survival time for which the estimated survivor function is less than 0.5. From Table 3.19, the estimated median survival time for patients aged less than 60 who have not had a nephrectomy is 12 months.

By raising the estimate of the baseline survivor function to a suitable power, the estimated survivor functions for patients in other age groups, and for patients who have had a nephrectomy, can be obtained using Equation (3.25). Thus, the estimated survivor function for the ith individual is given by

$$\hat{S}_i(t) = \left\{\hat{S}_0(t)\right\}^{\exp\{0.013A_{2i}+1.342A_{3i}-1.412N_i\}}.$$

For an individual aged less than 60 who has had a nephrectomy, $A_2 = 0$, $A_3 = 0$, and $N = 1$, so that the estimated survivor function for this individual becomes

$$\left\{\hat{S}_0(t)\right\}^{\exp\{-1.412\}}.$$

This function is plotted in Figure 3.5, together with the estimated baseline survivor function, which is for an individual in the same age group but who has not had a nephrectomy.

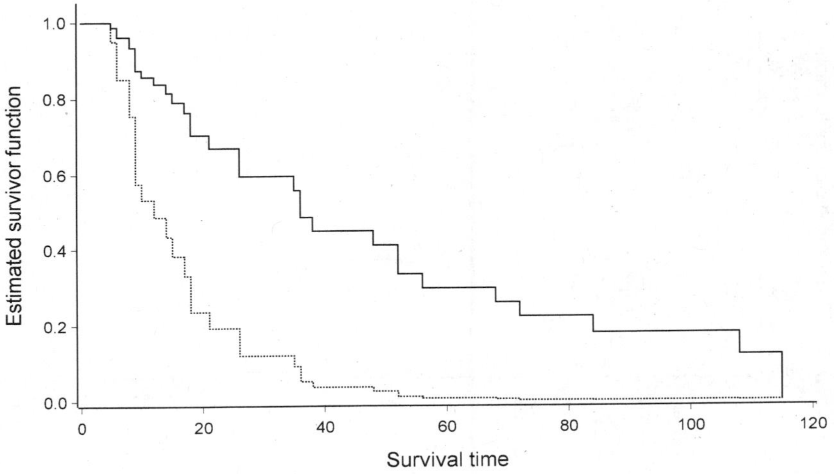

Figure 3.5 *Estimated survivor functions for patients aged less than 60, with (—) and without (⋯⋯) a nephrectomy.*

This figure shows that the probability of surviving beyond any given time is greater for those who have had a nephrectomy, confirming that a nephrectomy improves the prognosis for patients with hypernephroma.

Note that because of the assumption of proportional hazards, the two estimated survivor functions in Figure 3.5 cannot cross. Moreover, the estimated survivor function for those who have had a nephrectomy lies above that of those on whom a nephrectomy has not been performed. This is a direct consequence of the estimated hazard ratio for those who have had the operation, relative to those who have not, being less than unity.

An estimate of the median survival time for this type of patient can be obtained from the tabulated values of the estimated survivor function, or from the graph in Figure 3.5. We find that the estimated median survival time for a patient aged less than 60 who has had a nephrectomy is 36 months. Other percentiles of the distribution of survival times can be estimated using a similar approach.

In a similar manner, the survivor functions for patients in the different age groups can be compared, either for those who have had or not had a nephrectomy. For example, for patients who have had a nephrectomy, the estimated survivor functions for patients in the three age groups are respectively $\{\hat{S}_0(t)\}^{\exp\{-1.412\}}$, $\{\hat{S}_0(t)\}^{\exp\{-1.412+0.013\}}$ and $\{\hat{S}_0(t)\}^{\exp\{-1.412+1.342\}}$. These estimated survivor functions are shown in Figure 3.6, which clearly shows that patients aged over 70 have a poorer prognosis than those in the other two age groups.

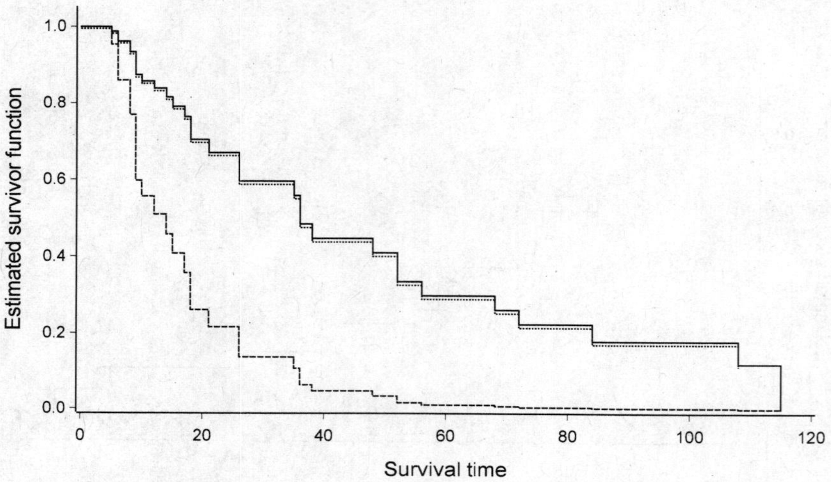

Figure 3.6 *Estimated survivor functions for patients aged less than 60 (—), between 60 and 70 (·······) and greater than 70 (- - -), who have had a nephrectomy.*

3.11 Risk adjusted survivor function

Once a Cox regression model has been fitted, the estimated survivor function can be obtained for each individual. It might then be of interest to see how the fitted survivor functions compare with the unadjusted Kaplan-Meier estimate of the survivor function. The impact of the risk adjustment can then be determined. To do this, a *risk adjusted survivor function* is obtained by averaging the individual estimated values of the survivor function at each event time in the data set.

Formally, suppose that a Cox regression model is fitted to survival data from n individuals, in which the hazard of death for the ith individual, $i = 1, 2, \ldots, n$, at time t is

$$h_i(t) = \exp(\boldsymbol{\beta}'\boldsymbol{x}_i)h_0(t),$$

where $\boldsymbol{\beta}'\boldsymbol{x}_i = \beta_1 x_{1i} + \beta_2 x_{2i} + \cdots + \beta_p x_{pi}$, $x_{1i}, x_{2i}, \ldots, x_{pi}$ are the values of p explanatory variables measured on each individual, and $h_0(t)$ is the baseline hazard function. The corresponding survivor function for the ith individual is

$$S_i(t) = \{S_0(t)\}^{\exp(\boldsymbol{\beta}'\boldsymbol{x}_i)},$$

and the model fitting process leads to estimates of the p β-parameters, $\hat{\beta}_1, \hat{\beta}_2, \ldots, \hat{\beta}_p$, and the baseline survivor function, $\hat{S}_0(t)$. The *average survivor function* at a given time t is then

$$\hat{S}(t) = \frac{1}{n}\sum_{i=1}^{n} \hat{S}_i(t), \tag{3.31}$$

where

$$\hat{S}_i(t) = \left\{\hat{S}_0(t)\right\}^{\exp(\hat{\boldsymbol{\beta}}'\boldsymbol{x}_i)}$$

is the estimated survivor function for the ith individual. Risk adjusted estimates of survival rates, the median and other percentiles of the survival time distribution can then be obtained from $\hat{S}(t)$.

Example 3.15 Survival of multiple myeloma patients
In Example 3.5, a Cox regression model that contained the explanatory variables *Hb* and *Bun* was found to be appropriate in modelling data on the survival times of patients suffering from multiple myeloma, introduced in Example 1.3. The estimated survivor function for the ith patient, $i = 1, 2, \ldots, 48$, is

$$\hat{S}_i(t) = \left\{\hat{S}_0(t)\right\}^{\exp(\hat{\eta}_i)},$$

where the risk score, $\hat{\eta}_i$, is given by $\hat{\eta}_i = -0.134 Hb_i + 0.019 Bun_i$. The estimated survivor function is then obtained at each of the event times in the data set, for each of the 48 patients. Averaging the estimates across the 48 patients, for each event time, leads to the risk adjusted survivor function. This is plotted in Figure 3.7, together with the unadjusted Kaplan-Meier estimate of the survivor function. The unadjusted and risk adjusted estimates of the survivor function are very close, so that in this example, the risk adjustment process makes very little difference to estimates of survival rates or the median survival time.

3.11.1 Risk adjusted survivor function for groups of individuals

In many circumstances, it is of interest to estimate the survivor functions for certain groups of individuals after adjustment has been made for differences between these groups in terms of the values of measured explanatory variables. For example, consider a study on disease-free survival following treatment with one or other of two treatment regimens. If such a study were carried out as a randomised controlled trial, it is likely that the values of measured explanatory variables would be balanced between the treatment groups. It may then be sufficient to summarise the data using the unadjusted Kaplan-Meier estimate of the survivor function for each group, supplemented by unadjusted and adjusted hazard ratios for the treatment effect. However, suppose that the data were obtained in an observational study, where values of the explanatory

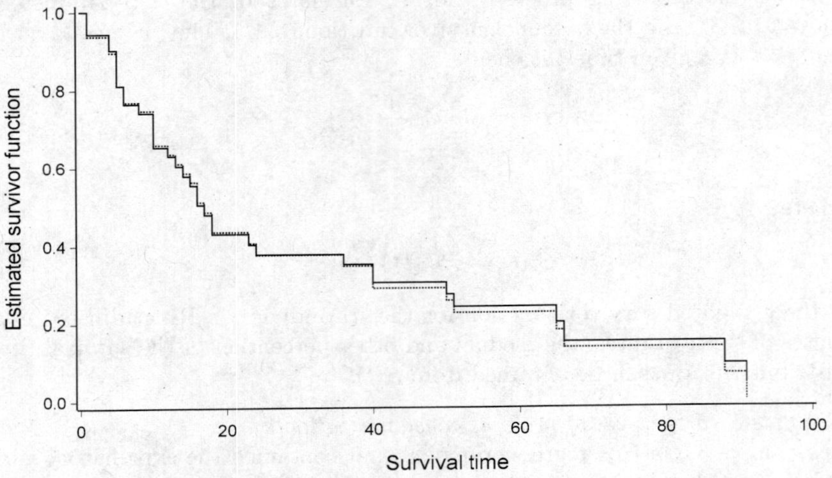

Figure 3.7 *Unadjusted (⋯⋯) and risk adjusted (—) estimated survivor functions for the data on the survival of multiple myeloma patients.*

variables were not evenly distributed across the two treatment groups. In this situation, the unadjusted estimates of the two survivor functions may be misleading. A risk adjustment process will then be needed to take account of any imbalance between the characteristics of individuals in the two groups, before conclusions can be drawn about the treatment effect.

If differences between the treatment groups can be assumed to be independent of time, the group effect can be added to the survival model, and the risk adjusted survivor function for the individuals in each treatment group can be calculated using Equation (3.31). However, in many applications, such as when comparing survival rates between institutions, to be considered in Chapter 11, this assumption cannot be made. The Cox regression model is then extended to have a different baseline hazard function for each group.

Suppose that in a study to compare the survival rates of individuals in g groups, a Cox regression model containing relevant explanatory variables has been fitted, excluding the group effect. The model for the hazard of death for the ith individual, $i = 1, 2, \ldots, n_j$, in the jth group, $j = 1, 2, \ldots, g$, at time t is then

$$h_{ij}(t) = \exp(\boldsymbol{\beta}'\boldsymbol{x}_{ij})h_{0j}(t),$$

where $\boldsymbol{\beta}'\boldsymbol{x}_{ij} = \beta_1 x_{1ij} + \beta_2 x_{2ij} + \cdots + \beta_p x_{pij}$, $x_{1ij}, x_{2ij}, \ldots, x_{pij}$ are the values of p explanatory variables measured on each individual, and $h_{0j}(t)$ is the baseline hazard function for the jth group. In this model, the coefficients of the p explanatory variables, $\beta_1, \beta_2, \ldots, \beta_p$, are constant over the g groups, but there is a different baseline hazard function for each group. This is a *stratified*

Cox regression model in which the g groups define the separate strata. These models are considered in greater detail in Chapter 11.

On fitting the stratified model, the corresponding estimated survivor function for the ith patient in the jth group is

$$\hat{S}_{ij}(t) = \left\{ \hat{S}_{0j}(t) \right\}^{\exp(\hat{\boldsymbol{\beta}}' \boldsymbol{x}_{ij})},$$

where $\hat{S}_{0j}(t)$ is the estimated baseline survivor function for individuals in the jth group. If the groups can be assumed to act proportionately on the hazard function, a common baseline hazard would be fitted and a group effect included in the model. Then, $h_{0j}(t)$ is replaced by $\exp(g_j)h_0(t)$, where g_j is the effect of the jth group. In general, it is less restrictive to allow the group effects to vary over time by using a stratified model.

The risk adjusted survivor function for each group can be found from the stratified model by averaging the values of the estimated survivor functions at each of the event times, across the individuals in each group. The average risk adjusted survivor function at time t is then

$$\hat{S}_j(t) = \frac{1}{n_j} \sum_{i=1}^{n_j} \hat{S}_{ij}(t),$$

for individuals in the jth group.

An alternative approach is to average the values of each explanatory variable for individuals in each group, and to then use these values to estimate the group-specific survivor functions. Writing $\bar{\boldsymbol{x}}_j$ for the vector of average values of the p variables across the individuals in the jth group, the corresponding estimated survivor function for an 'average individual' in group j is

$$\tilde{S}_j(t) = \left\{ \hat{S}_{0j}(t) \right\}^{\exp(\hat{\boldsymbol{\beta}}' \bar{\boldsymbol{x}}_j)}.$$

Although this approach is widely used, it can be criticised on a number of grounds. Averaging the values of explanatory variables is not appropriate for categorical variables. For example, suppose that the two levels of a variable associated with the presence or absence of diabetes are coded as 1 and 0, respectively, and that 10% of the individuals on whom data are available are diabetic. Setting the average of the indicator variable to be 0.1 does not lead to a meaningful interpretation of the survivor function at this value of diabetic status. Also, even with continuous explanatory variables, the set of average values of the explanatory variables within a group may not correspond to a realistic combination of values, and the survivor function for an average individual may be very different from the patterns of the individual survivor functions.

Example 3.16 Comparison of two treatments for prostatic cancer
Consider the data from Example 1.4 on the survival times of 38 prostatic

cancer patients in two treatment groups. In Example 3.6, the explanatory variables *Size* and *Index* were found to affect the hazard of death, and so a stratified Cox regression model that contains these two variables is fitted. The estimated survivor function for the ith patient in the jth treatment group, for $j = 1$ (placebo) and 2 (DES), is

$$\hat{S}_{ij}(t) = \left\{\hat{S}_{0j}(t)\right\}^{\exp(\hat{\eta}_{ij})},$$

where

$$\hat{\eta}_{ij} = 0.0673\, Size_{ij} + 0.6532\, Index_{ij},$$

and $\hat{S}_{0j}(t)$ is the estimated baseline survivor function for the jth treatment group. Averaging the estimated survivor functions at each event time over the patients in each group gives the risk adjusted survivor functions shown in Figure 3.8. Also shown in this figure are the unadjusted Kaplan-Meier estimates of the survivor functions for each group.

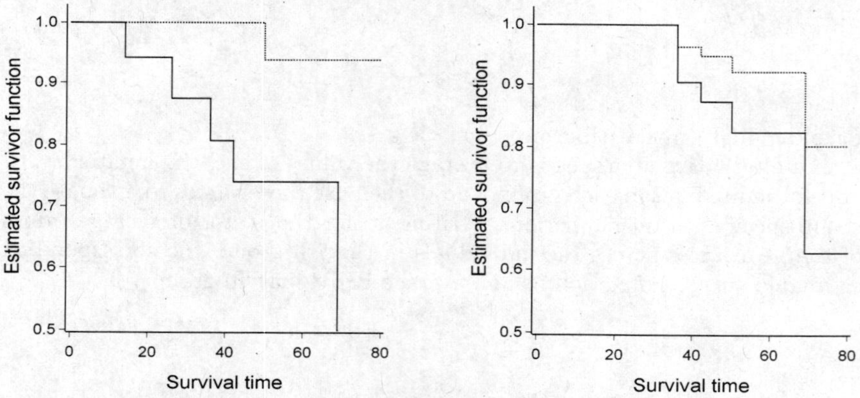

Figure 3.8 *(i) Unadjusted and (ii) risk adjusted survivor functions for prostatic cancer patients on DES (·······) and placebo (—).*

This figure shows how the risk adjustment process has diminished the treatment difference. Of course, this is also seen by comparing the unadjusted hazard ratio for a patient on DES relative to placebo (0.14) with the corresponding value adjusted for tumour size and Gleason index (0.33), although this latter analysis assumes proportional hazards for the two treatments.

3.12* Explained variation in the Cox regression model

In linear regression analysis, the proportion of variation in the response variable that is accounted for by the explanatory variables is widely used to summarise the explanatory power of a model. This statistic is usually denoted by R^2. For a general linear model with p explanatory variables, where the expectation of the ith value of a response variable Y, $i = 1, 2, \ldots, n$, is given by

$$\mathrm{E}\,(Y_i) = \beta_0 + \beta_1 x_{1i} + \cdots + \beta_p x_{pi},$$

the R^2 statistic is defined as

$$R^2 = \frac{\text{Model SS}}{\text{Total SS}} = \frac{\text{Model SS}}{\text{Model SS} + \text{Residual SS}}.$$

In this equation, the variation in the response variable that is explained by the model is summarised in the Model sum of squares (SS), $\sum_i (\hat{y}_i - \bar{y})^2$, and expressed as a proportion of the total variation in the data, represented by the Total SS, $\sum_i (y_i - \bar{y})^2$, where $\bar{y} = n^{-1} \sum_i y_i$ and $\hat{y}_i$ is the model-based estimate of $\mathrm{E}\,(Y_i)$, the ith fitted value, given by

$$\hat{y}_i = \hat{\beta}_0 + \hat{\beta}_1 x_{1i} + \cdots + \hat{\beta}_p x_{pi}.$$

The Total SS can be partitioned into the Model SS and the Residual SS, $\sum_i (y_i - \hat{y}_i)^2$, which represents the unexplained variation. The larger the value of R^2, the greater the proportion of variation in the response variable that is accounted for by the model.

The R^2 statistic for the general linear model can also be expressed in the form

$$R^2 = \frac{\hat{V}_M}{\hat{V}_M + \hat{\sigma}^2}, \tag{3.32}$$

where $\hat{V}_M$ = Model SS$/(n - 1)$ is an estimate of the variation in the data explained by the model, and $\hat{\sigma}^2$ is an estimate of the residual variation. Note that in this formulation, $\hat{\sigma}^2$ = Residual SS$/(n - 1)$, rather than the usual unbiased estimator with divisor $n - p - 1$. The quantity $\hat{V}_M$ in Equation (3.32) can be expressed in matrix form as $\hat{\boldsymbol{\beta}}' \boldsymbol{S} \hat{\boldsymbol{\beta}}$, where $\hat{\boldsymbol{\beta}}$ is the vector of estimated coefficients for the p explanatory variables in the fitted regression model, and $\boldsymbol{S}$ is the variance-covariance matrix of the explanatory variables. This matrix is formed from the sample variance of each of the p explanatory variables, $(n - 1)^{-1} \sum_i (x_{ij} - \bar{x}_j)^2$, on its diagonals, and the sample covariance terms, $(n - 1)^{-1} \sum_i (x_{ij} - \bar{x}_j)(x_{ij'} - \bar{x}_{j'})$, as the off-diagonal terms, for $i = 1, 2, \ldots, n$ and $j, j' = 1, 2, \ldots, p$ for $j \neq j'$, and where $\bar{x}_j$ is the sample mean of the jth variable.

In the analysis of survival data, a large number of different measures of the proportion of variation in the data that is explained by a fitted Cox regression model have been proposed. However, published reviews of these measures, based on extensive simulation studies, suggest that three particular statistics have desirable properties. All of them take values between 0 and 1, are largely independent of the degree of censoring, are not affected by the scale of the survival data, and increase in value as explanatory variables are added to the model. These are described in the next section.

3.12.1 Measures of explained variation

Consider a Cox regression model for the hazard of death at time t in the ith individual, $h_i(t) = \exp(\boldsymbol{\beta}'\boldsymbol{x}_i)h_0(t)$, where $\boldsymbol{x}_i$ is the vector of values of p explanatory variables, $\boldsymbol{\beta}$ is the vector of their unknown coefficients, and $h_0(t)$ is the baseline hazard function. One of the earliest suggestions for an R^2 type statistic, due to Kent and O'Quigley (1988), is similar in form to the R^2 statistic for linear regression analysis in Equation (3.32). This statistic is defined by

$$R_P^2 = \frac{\hat{V}_P}{\hat{V}_P + \pi^2/6},$$

where $\hat{V}_P = \hat{\boldsymbol{\beta}}'\boldsymbol{S}\hat{\boldsymbol{\beta}}$ is an estimate of the variation in the risk score, $\hat{\boldsymbol{\beta}}'\boldsymbol{x}_i$, between the n individuals, $\hat{\boldsymbol{\beta}}$ is the vector of parameter estimates in the fitted Cox regression model, and $\boldsymbol{S}$ is the variance-covariance matrix of the explanatory variables. The reason for including the term $\pi^2/6$ in place of $\hat{\sigma}^2$ in Equation (3.32) will be explained later in Section 5.8 of Chapter 5.

The statistic R_D^2, proposed by Royston and Sauerbrei (2004), is also based on an estimate of the variation in the risk score between individuals. To obtain this statistic, the values of the risk score for the fitted Cox regression model, $\hat{\boldsymbol{\beta}}'\boldsymbol{x}_i$, are first ordered from smallest value to largest, so that the ith of the n ordered values is $\hat{\eta}_{(i)} = \hat{\boldsymbol{\beta}}'\boldsymbol{x}_{(i)}$, where $\hat{\eta}_{(1)} < \hat{\eta}_{(2)} < \cdots < \hat{\eta}_{(n)}$. The ith of these ordered values is then associated with a quantity $z_{(i)}$ that is an approximation to the expected value of the ith order statistic of a standard normal distribution in a sample of n observations. This is usually referred to as a *normal score*, and the most widely used score is $z_{(i)} = \Phi^{-1}\{(i - 3/8)/(n + 1/4)\}$, where $\Phi^{-1}(\cdot)$ is the inverse standard normal distribution function. The values $\hat{\eta}_{(i)}$ are then regressed on the $z_{(i)}$, and the resulting estimate of the coefficient of $z_{(i)}$ in the linear regression model, labelled D_0, is then scaled to give $D = D_0\sqrt{(\pi/8)}$. The R_D^2 measure of explained variation for a Cox regression model is then

$$R_D^2 = \frac{D^2}{D^2 + \pi^2/6}.$$

This has a similar form to the R_P^2 statistic, and indeed, D^2 can also be regarded as an estimate of the variation between the values of the risk score.

Another statistic from Kent and O'Quigley (1988) is based on the 'distance' between the model of interest and the model that has no explanatory variables. This latter model is known as the null model, and is such that the hazard function for each individual is simply the baseline hazard, $h_0(t)$. This statistic is

$$R_W^2 = 1 - \exp(-\tilde{W}),$$

where $\tilde{W}$, the distance measure, is an estimate of the expected value of the likelihood ratio statistic, defined as $W = -2\,\mathrm{E}\{\log L(0) - \log L(\hat{\boldsymbol{\beta}})\}$, for comparing the maximised log-likelihood under the fitted model, $\log L(\hat{\boldsymbol{\beta}})$ with that of the null model, $\log L(0)$. This is given by

$$\tilde{W} = 2\left[(1-\tilde{\omega})\Psi(1) + \log\Gamma(\tilde{\omega}) + \log\left\{n^{-1}\sum_{i=1}^{n}\exp(-\tilde{\omega}z_i)\right\}\right],$$

where $z_i = \hat{\boldsymbol{\beta}}'(\boldsymbol{x}_i - \bar{\boldsymbol{x}})$, $\hat{\boldsymbol{\beta}}$ is the vector of parameter estimates in the fitted Cox regression model, $\bar{\boldsymbol{x}}$ is the vector of mean values of the p explanatory variables, and $\Gamma(\tilde{\omega}) = \int_0^\infty u^{\tilde{\omega}-1}e^{-u}\,du$ is a gamma function. Also, $\tilde{\omega}$ is the value of ω that satisfies the non-linear equation

$$\Psi(1) - \Psi(\omega) + \sum_{i=1}^{n}\frac{\exp(-\omega z_i)}{\sum_{l=1}^{n}\exp(-\omega z_l)}z_i = 0,$$

where $\Psi(\omega)$ is the digamma function, defined by the series expansion

$$\Psi(\omega) = -\lambda + \sum_{j=0}^{\infty}\frac{\omega-1}{(1+j)(\omega+j)},$$

so that $\Psi(1) = -\lambda$, and $\lambda = 0.577216$ is Euler's constant. This is a complicated statistic to calculate, but it has been included here as it performs well, and can now be obtained using several software packages for survival analysis.

3.12.2 Measures of predictive ability

In addition to measures of explained variation, statistics that summarise the agreement or *concordance* between the ranks of observed and predicted survival times are useful in assessing the predictive ability of a model. These statistics summarise the potential of a fitted model to discriminate between individuals, by separating those with longer survival times from those with shorter times. As for measures of explained variation, these statistics take values between 0 and 1, corresponding to perfect discordance and perfect concordance. Values around 0.5 are obtained when a model has no predictive ability, and models with a reasonable degree of predictive ability would lead to a value greater than 0.7.

A particular measure of concordance is the c-statistic described by Harrell, Lee and Mark (1996). This statistic is an estimate of the probability that, for any two individuals, the one with the shortest survival time is the one with the greatest hazard of death. To calculate this statistic, consider all possible pairs of survival times, where either both members of the pair have died, or where one member of the pair dies before the censored survival time of the other. Pairs in which both individuals have censored survival times, or where the survival time of one exceeds the censored survival time of the other, are not included. If in a pair where both individuals have died, the model-based predicted survival time is greater for the individual who lived longer, the two individuals are said to be *concordant*. In a proportional hazards model, an individual in a pair who is predicted to have the greatest survival time will be the one with the lower hazard of death at a given time, the higher estimated survivor function at a given time, or the lower value of the risk score. For pairs where just one individual dies, and one individual has a time that is censored after the survival time of the other member of the pair, the individual with the censored time has survived longer than the other, and so it can be determined whether the two members of such a pair are concordant. The c-statistic is obtained by dividing the number of concordant pairs by the number of all possible pairs being considered.

Since pairs where both individuals are censored, or where the censored survival time of one occurs before the death time of the other, the c-statistic is affected by the pattern of censoring. This considerable disadvantage is overcome in a statistic proposed by Gönen and Heller (2005). Their measure of concordance is an estimate of the probability that, for any two individuals, the survival time of one exceeds the survival time of the other, conditional on the individual with the longer survival time having the lower risk score.

To obtain this statistic, let $\hat{\eta}_i = \hat{\boldsymbol{\beta}}'\boldsymbol{x}_i$ be the risk score for the ith individual. A pair of survival times, (T_i, T_j), say, is then concordant if the individual with the lower risk score has the longer survival time. The probability of concordance is then $K = \text{P}(T_i > T_j \mid \eta_i \leqslant \eta_j)$, and an estimate of this concordance probability, $\hat{K}$, is the Gönen and Heller measure of the predictive value of a model. This estimate is given by

$$\hat{K} = \frac{2}{n(n-1)} \sum\sum_{i<j} \left\{ \frac{I\{(\hat{\eta}_j - \hat{\eta}_i) < 0\}}{1 + \exp(\hat{\eta}_j - \hat{\eta}_i)} + \frac{I\{(\hat{\eta}_i - \hat{\eta}_j) < 0\}}{1 + \exp(\hat{\eta}_i - \hat{\eta}_j)} \right\},$$

where the indicator function $I(\cdot)$ is such that $I\{X < 0\} = 1$ if $X < 0$ and zero otherwise. In addition, the standard error of $\hat{K}$ can be obtained, so that the precision of $\hat{K}$ can be assessed, although details will not be given here.

3.12.3 Model validation

The methods described in Sections 3.12.1 and 3.12.2 to determine the variation in a set of survival data that is explained by a fitted Cox regression model, and the predictive ability of the model, can lead to an over-optimistic assessment of the strength of a model if the same data has been used both to fit the model and to validate it. For this reason, measures of explained variation and predictive ability are best determined from fitting the model to data that has not been used in the modelling process. If an independent data set, such as data from another region or country is available, then these data should be used for the validation process. This is referred to as *external validation.* This is often not possible and a data-splitting procedure, based on partitioning the data at random into a modelling and a validation data set, may be used. The model is then determined from the modelling data set and validated on the remaining data, leading to an *internal validation* process. Depending on the size of the data set, up to 50% of the data may be set aside for validation purposes, although for smaller sets of data, this proportion may be somewhere between 20% and 40%. In any case, this validation data set should contain a sufficient number of events, and a general guideline is that at least 100 events are needed.

Example 3.17 Survival of multiple myeloma patients
In this example, the three different R^2 measures will be compared for the data on the survival times of multiple myeloma patients, presented in Example 1.3. In Example 3.5, the most satisfactory Cox regression model for the hazard of death contained the explanatory variables *Hb* (serum haemoglobin) and *Bun* (blood urea nitrogen). The values of the different statistics are shown in Table 3.20 for both the selected model that contains *Hb* and *Bun*, and the full model that contains *Age*, *Sex*, *Bun*, *Ca*, *Hb*, *Pcells* and *Protein*.

Table 3.20 *Measures of explained variation on fitting the selected and full models.*

Measure	R^2 (selected model)	R^2 (full model)
R_P^2	0.27	0.31
R_D^2	0.25	0.29
R_W^2	0.30	0.34

The three different measures of explained variation have broadly similar values for both models, and the difference between their values for the selected and full models is the same for each statistic. On the basis of the R_W^2 statistic, we conclude that 30% of the variation in the survival times is explained by the levels of serum haemoglobin and blood urea nitrogen.

Turning to measures of predictive ability, the value of Harrell's c-statistic is 0.66 for the selected model and 0.70 for the full model. Gönen and Heller's measure of concordance is 0.67 (se = 0.044) for the selected model and 0.68 (se = 0.044) for the full model. In this example, the two measure of the discriminatory power of either model are very similar because there is relatively little censoring, and so most of the pairs of survival times can be used in the computation of the c-statistic. There is also very little difference in the value of either statistic for the selected and full model, confirming that the predictive ability of the selected model is comparable to that of the full model. However a value of 0.67 for the Gönen and Heller statistic indicates that the model is not particularly good at discriminating between the survival times of the individuals in this study.

3.13* Proportional hazards modelling and the log-rank test

The Cox regression model can be used to test the null hypothesis that there is no difference between the hazard functions for two groups of survival times, as illustrated in Example 3.3. This modelling approach therefore provides an alternative to the log-rank test in this situation. However, there is a close connection between the two procedures, which is explored in greater detail in this section.

Following the notation used in Section 2.6.2, and summarised in Table 2.7, the two groups will be labelled Group I and Group II, respectively. The numbers of individuals in the two groups who die at the jth ordered death time, $t_{(j)}$, $j = 1, 2, \ldots, r$, will be denoted by d_{1j} and d_{2j}, respectively. Similarly, the numbers of individuals at risk in the two groups at time $t_{(j)}$, that is, the numbers who are alive and uncensored just prior to this time, will be denoted n_{1j} and n_{2j}, respectively.

Now let X be an indicator variable that is unity when an individual is in Group I and zero when an individual is in Group II. The Cox regression model for the ith individual can be written as

$$h_i(t) = e^{\beta x_i} h_0(t),$$

where x_i is the value of X for the ith individual, $i = 1, 2, \ldots, n$. When there are no tied observations, that is, when $d_j = d_{1j} + d_{2j} = 1$, this model can be fitted by finding that value $\hat{\beta}$ which maximises the likelihood function in Equation (3.4). Denoting the value of X for the individual who dies at $t_{(j)}$ by $x_{(j)}$, the likelihood function is given by

$$L(\beta) = \prod_{j=1}^{r} \frac{\exp(\beta x_{(j)})}{\sum_{l=1}^{n_j} \exp(\beta x_l)}, \tag{3.33}$$

since there are $n_j = n_{1j} + n_{2j}$ individuals in the risk set, $R(t_{(j)})$, at time $t_{(j)}$, and the corresponding log-likelihood function is

$$\log L(\beta) = \sum_{j=1}^{r} \beta x_{(j)} - \sum_{j=1}^{r} \log \left\{ \sum_{l=1}^{n_j} \exp(\beta x_l) \right\}.$$

Since $x_{(j)}$ is zero for individuals in Group II, the first summation in this expression is over the death times in Group I, and so is simply $d_1\beta$, where $d_1 = \sum_{j=1}^{r} d_{1j}$ is the total number of deaths in Group I. Also,

$$\sum_{l=1}^{n_j} \exp(\beta x_l) = n_{1j}e^{\beta} + n_{2j},$$

and so

$$\log L(\beta) = d_1\beta - \sum_{j=1}^{r} \log \left\{ n_{1j}e^{\beta} + n_{2j} \right\}. \tag{3.34}$$

The maximum likelihood estimate of β can be found by maximising this expression with respect to β, using a non-linear optimisation routine. Then, the null hypotheses that $\beta = 0$ can be tested by comparing the value of $-2 \log L(\hat{\beta})$ with $-2 \log L(0)$. This latter quantity is simply $2 \sum_{j=1}^{r} \log n_j$.

Computation of $\hat{\beta}$ can be avoided by using a *score test* of the null hypothesis that $\beta = 0$. This test procedure, which is outlined in Appendix A, is based on the test statistic

$$\frac{u^2(0)}{i(0)},$$

where

$$u(\beta) = \frac{\partial \log L(\beta)}{\partial \beta}$$

is the efficient score, and

$$i(\beta) = -\frac{\partial^2 \log L(\beta)}{\partial \beta^2}$$

is Fisher's (observed) information function. Under the null hypothesis that $\beta = 0$, $u^2(0)/i(0)$ has a chi-squared distribution on one degree of freedom.

Now, from Equation (3.34),

$$\frac{\partial \log L(\beta)}{\partial \beta} = \sum_{j=1}^{r} \left(d_{1j} - \frac{n_{1j}e^{\beta}}{n_{1j}e^{\beta} + n_{2j}} \right),$$

and

$$\begin{aligned}\frac{\partial^2 \log L(\beta)}{\partial \beta^2} &= -\sum_{j=1}^{r} \frac{(n_{1j}e^{\beta} + n_{2j})n_{1j}e^{\beta} - (n_{1j}e^{\beta})^2}{(n_{1j}e^{\beta} + n_{2j})^2} \\ &= -\sum_{j=1}^{r} \frac{n_{1j}n_{2j}e^{\beta}}{(n_{1j}e^{\beta} + n_{2j})^2}.\end{aligned}$$

The efficient score and information function, evaluated at $\beta = 0$, are therefore given by

$$u(0) = \sum_{j=1}^{r} \left(d_{1j} - \frac{n_{1j}}{n_{1j} + n_{2j}} \right),$$

and

$$i(0) = \sum_{j=1}^{r} \frac{n_{1j}n_{2j}}{(n_{1j} + n_{2j})^2}.$$

These are simply the expressions for U_L and V_L given in Equations (2.20) and (2.22) of Chapter 2, for the special case where there are no ties, that is, where $d_j = 1$ for $j = 1, 2, \ldots, r$.

When there are tied observations, the likelihood function in Equation (3.33) has to be replaced by one that allows for ties. In particular, if the likelihood function in Equation (3.12) is used, the efficient score and information function are exactly those given in Equations (2.20) and (2.22). Hence, when there are tied survival times, the log-rank test corresponds to using the score test for the discrete proportional hazards model due to Cox (1972). In practice, the P-value that results from this score test will not usually differ much from that obtained from comparing the values of the statistic $-2\log\hat{L}$ for the models with and without a term corresponding to the treatment effect. This was noted in the discussion of Example 3.3. Of course, one advantage of using the Cox regression model in the analysis of such data is that it leads directly to an estimate of the hazard ratio.

3.14 Further reading

Comprehensive introductions to statistical modelling in the context of linear regression analysis are given by Draper and Smith (1998) and Montgomery, Peck and Vining (2012). McCullagh and Nelder (1989) include a chapter on models for survival data in their encyclopaedic survey of generalised linear modelling.

The proportional hazards model for survival data, in which the baseline hazard function remains unspecified, was proposed by Cox (1972). This paper introduced the notion of partial likelihood, which was subsequently considered in greater detail by Cox (1975). See also the contributions to the discussion of Cox (1972) by Kalbfleisch and Prentice (1972) and Breslow (1972). A detailed review of the model, and extensions of it, is contained in Therneau and Grambsch (2000).

Introductions to the Cox regression model intended for medical researchers have been given by Christensen (1987), Elashoff (1983) and Tibshirani (1982). More recent accounts are given in the textbooks referenced in Section 1.5 of Chapter 1. In particular, Hosmer, Lemeshow and May (2008) include a careful discussion on model development and the interpretation of model-based parameter estimates.

A detailed treatment of ties in survival data is given in Kalbfleisch and Prentice (2002) and Lawless (2002); see also Breslow (1972) and Peto (1972). The estimate of the baseline survivor function, denoted by $\hat{S}_0(t)$ in Section 3.10, was introduced by Kalbfleisch and Prentice (1973) and is also described in Kalbfleisch and Prentice (2002). The estimate $S_0^*(t)$ was presented by Breslow (1972, 1974), although it was derived using a different argument from that used in Section 3.10.2.

Model formulation and strategies for model selection are discussed in books on linear regression analysis, and also in Chapter 5 of Chatfield (1995), Chapter 4 of Cox and Snell (1981), and Appendix 2 of Cox and Snell (1989). Miller (2002) describes a wide range of procedures for identifying suitable subsets of variables to use in linear regression modelling. What has come to be known as Akaike's information criterion was introduced by Akaike (1974). It is widely used in times series analysis and described in books on this subject, such as Chatfield (2004). The use of the *BIC* statistic in modelling survival data was described by Volinsky and Raftery (2000). The hierarchic principle is fully discussed by Nelder (1977), and in Chapter 3 of McCullagh and Nelder

(1989). Harrell (2001) addresses many practical issues in model building and illustrates the process using two extensive case studies involving survival data.

The lasso was first proposed by Tibshirani (1996), and Tibshirani (1997) showed how the method can be used for variable selection in the Cox model. An efficient algorithm for computing the lasso estimates was described by Goeman (2010). This algorithm is now implemented in the R package `penalized` for fitting penalised Cox regression models; see Goeman, Meijer and Chaturvedi (2013). The piecewise linearity property of the lasso was established by Efron et al. (2004), and Yuan and Lin (2006) introduced the group lasso to handle categorical variables.

The use of fractional polynomials in regression modelling was described by Royston and Altman (1994); see also Sauerbrei and Royston (1999). The Box-Tidwell transformation, referred to in the context of fractional polynomials, was introduced by Box and Tidwell (1962).

Methods for the calculation of the adjusted survivor function have been reviewed by Nieto and Coresh (1996) and in his comments on this paper, Zahl (1997) outlines some related approaches. The method is also described in Zhang et al. (2007), who present a SAS macro for its implementation. Neuberger et al. (1986) used the method based on averaging the values of explanatory variables to summarise observational data from a liver transplant programme, which was subsequently referred to in Thomsen et al. (1991).

A considerable number of measures of explained variation have been proposed, and there have been several reviews that compare and contrast their properties. The most extensive reviews are those of Schemper and Stare (1996), Hielscher et al. (2010) and the two consecutive papers of Choodari-Oskooei, Royston and Parmar (2012). The R^2 measures described in this chapter were introduced by Kent and O'Quigley (1988) and Royston and Sauerbrei (2004). The links between these and other measures of explained variation are also described in Royston (2006). Heinzl (2000) describes SAS macros for the calculation of Kent and O'Quigley's R_W^2 statistic. Harrell's c-statistic is described in Harrell, Lee and Mark (1996), and a preferred measure of concordance was introduced by Gönen and Heller (2005). One further measure of explained variation, due to Stare, Perme and Henderson (2011), can be used in proportional hazards modelling, and has the advantage of being applicable to some of the other models presented in later chapters. This statistic is based on explaining variability in the ranks of observations, and R software for calculating the statistic is available.

One issue that has not been discussed in this chapter is how to handle missing values of explanatory variables. A method of *multiple imputation* based on *fully conditional specification*, also known as *multiple imputation by chained equations*, is a widely used technique for dealing with this common problem. The multiple imputation process involves generating a number of sets of imputed values for each explanatory variable with missing values. The parameter estimates on fitting a given model to each imputed data set are then combined to give overall estimates, with standard errors that allow for uncertainty in the imputed values. Advances in software development mean that this technique can now be used routinely in conjunction with commonly available software packages, including SAS, Stata and R. The tutorial paper of White, Royston and Wood (2011) describes the method, its limitations and possible dangers, and also includes a comprehensive reference list.

Chapter 4

Model checking in the Cox regression model

After a model has been fitted to an observed set of survival data, the adequacy of the model needs to be assessed. Indeed, the use of diagnostic procedures for model checking is an essential part of the modelling process.

In some situations, careful inspection of an observed set of data may lead to the identification of certain features, such as individuals with unusually large or small survival times. However, unless there are only one or two explanatory variables, a visual examination of the data may not be very revealing. The situation is further complicated by censoring, in that the occurrence of censored survival times make it difficult to judge aspects of model adequacy, even in the simplest of situations. Visual inspection of the data should therefore be supplemented by diagnostic procedures for detecting inadequacies in a fitted model.

Once a model has been fitted, there are a number of aspects of the fit of a model that need to be studied. For example, the model must include an appropriate set of explanatory variables from those measured in the study, and we will need to check that the correct functional form of these variables has been used. It might be important to identify observed survival times that are greater than would have been anticipated, or individuals whose explanatory variables have an undue impact on particular hazard ratios. Also, some means of checking the assumption of proportional hazards might be required.

Many model-checking procedures are based on quantities known as *residuals*. These are values that can be calculated for each individual in the study, and have the feature that their behaviour is known, at least approximately, when the fitted model is satisfactory. A number of residuals have been proposed for use in connection with the Cox regression model, and this chapter begins with a review of some of these. The use of residuals in assessing specific aspects of model adequacy is then discussed in subsequent sections.

4.1 Residuals for the Cox regression model

Throughout this section, we will suppose that the survival times of n individuals are available, where r of these are death times and the remaining $n - r$

are right-censored. We further suppose that a Cox regression model has been fitted to the survival times, and that the linear component of the model contains p explanatory variables, $X_1, X_2, \ldots, X_p$. The fitted hazard function for the ith individual, $i = 1, 2, \ldots, n$, is therefore

$$\hat{h}_i(t) = \exp(\hat{\boldsymbol{\beta}}'\boldsymbol{x}_i)\hat{h}_0(t),$$

where $\hat{\boldsymbol{\beta}}'\boldsymbol{x}_i = \hat{\beta}_1 x_{1i} + \hat{\beta}_2 x_{2i} + \cdots + \hat{\beta}_p x_{pi}$ is the value of the risk score for that individual and $\hat{h}_0(t)$ is the estimated baseline hazard function.

4.1.1 Cox-Snell residuals

The residual that is most widely used in the analysis of survival data is the *Cox-Snell residual*, so called because it is a particular example of the general definition of residuals given by Cox and Snell (1968).

The Cox-Snell residual for the ith individual, $i = 1, 2, \ldots, n$, is given by

$$r_{Ci} = \exp(\hat{\boldsymbol{\beta}}'\boldsymbol{x}_i)\hat{H}_0(t_i), \tag{4.1}$$

where $\hat{H}_0(t_i)$ is an estimate of the baseline cumulative hazard function at time t_i, the observed survival time of that individual. In practice, the Nelson-Aalen estimate given in Equation (3.28) is generally used. Note that from Equation (3.24), the Cox-Snell residual, r_{Ci}, is the value of $\hat{H}_i(t_i) = -\log \hat{S}_i(t_i)$, where $\hat{H}_i(t_i)$ and $\hat{S}_i(t_i)$ are the estimated values of the cumulative hazard and survivor functions of the ith individual at t_i.

This residual can be derived from a general result in mathematical statistics on the distribution of a function of a random variable. According to this result, if T is the random variable associated with the survival time of an individual, and $S(t)$ is the corresponding survivor function, then the random variable $Y = -\log S(T)$ has an exponential distribution with unit mean, irrespective of the form of $S(t)$. The proof of this result is outlined in the following paragraph, which can be omitted without loss of continuity.

From a general result, if $f_X(x)$ is the probability density function of the random variable X, the density of the random variable $Y = g(X)$ is given by

$$f_Y(y) = f_X\{g^{-1}(y)\} / \left|\frac{\mathrm{d}y}{\mathrm{d}x}\right|,$$

where $f_X\{g^{-1}(y)\}$ is the density of X expressed in terms of y. Using this result, the probability density function of the random variable $Y = -\log S(T)$ is given by

$$f_Y(y) = f_T\left\{S^{-1}(e^{-y})\right\} / \left|\frac{\mathrm{d}y}{\mathrm{d}t}\right|, \tag{4.2}$$

where $f_T(t)$ is the probability density function of T. Now,

$$\frac{\mathrm{d}y}{\mathrm{d}t} = \frac{\mathrm{d}\{-\log S(t)\}}{\mathrm{d}t} = \frac{f_T(t)}{S(t)},$$

and when the absolute value of this function is expressed in terms of y, the derivative becomes

$$\frac{f_T\{S^{-1}(e^{-y})\}}{S\{S^{-1}(e^{-y})\}} = \frac{f_T\{S^{-1}(e^{-y})\}}{e^{-y}}.$$

Finally, on substituting for the derivative in Equation (4.2), we find that

$$f_Y(y) = e^{-y},$$

which, from Equation (5.3), is the probability density function of an exponential random variable, Y, with unit mean.

The next and crucial step in the argument is as follows. If the model fitted to the observed data is satisfactory, a model-based estimate of the survivor function for the ith individual at t_i, the survival time of that individual, will be close to the corresponding true value $S_i(t_i)$. This suggests that if the correct model has been fitted, the values $\hat{S}_i(t_i)$ will have properties similar to those of $S_i(t_i)$. Then, the negative logarithms of the estimated survivor functions, $-\log \hat{S}_i(t_i)$, $i = 1, 2, \ldots, n$, will behave as n observations from a unit exponential distribution. These estimates are the Cox-Snell residuals.

If the observed survival time for an individual is right-censored, then the corresponding value of the residual is also right-censored. The residuals will therefore be a censored sample from the unit exponential distribution, and a test of this assumption provides a test of model adequacy, to which we return in Section 4.2.1.

The Cox-Snell residuals, r_{Ci}, have properties that are quite dissimilar to those of residuals used in linear regression analysis. In particular, they will not be symmetrically distributed about zero and they cannot be negative. Furthermore, since the Cox-Snell residuals are assumed to have an exponential distribution when an appropriate model has been fitted, they have a highly skew distribution and the mean and variance of the ith residual will both be unity.

4.1.2 Modified Cox-Snell residuals

Censored observations lead to residuals that cannot be regarded on the same footing as residuals derived from uncensored observations. We might therefore seek to modify the Cox-Snell residuals so that explicit account can be taken of censoring.

Suppose that the ith survival time is a censored observation, t_i^*, and let t_i be the actual, but unknown, survival time, so that $t_i > t_i^*$. The Cox-Snell residual for this individual, evaluated at the censored survival time, is then given by

$$r_{Ci} = \hat{H}_i(t_i^*) = -\log \hat{S}_i(t_i^*),$$

where $\hat{H}_i(t_i^*)$ and $\hat{S}_i(t_i^*)$ are the estimated cumulative hazard and survivor functions, respectively, for the ith individual at the censored survival time.

If the fitted model is correct, then the values r_{Ci} can be taken to have a unit exponential distribution. The cumulative hazard function of this distribution increases linearly with time, and so the greater the value of the survival time t_i for the ith individual, the greater the value of the Cox-Snell residual for that individual. It then follows that the residual for the ith individual at the actual (unknown) failure time, $\hat{H}_i(t_i)$, will be greater than the residual evaluated at the observed censored survival time.

To take account of this, Cox-Snell residuals can be modified by the addition of a positive constant Δ, which can be called the *excess residual.* Modified Cox-Snell residuals are therefore of the form

$$r'_{Ci} = \begin{cases} r_{Ci} & \text{for uncensored observations,} \\ r_{Ci} + \Delta & \text{for censored observations,} \end{cases}$$

where r_{Ci} is the Cox-Snell residual for the ith observation, defined in Equation (4.1). It now remains to identify a suitable value for Δ. For this, we use the *lack of memory property* of the exponential distribution.

To demonstrate this property, suppose that the random variable T has an exponential distribution with mean λ^{-1}, and consider the probability that T exceeds $t_0 + t_1$, $t_1 \geqslant 0$, conditional on T being at least equal to t_0. From the standard result for conditional probability given in Section 3.3.1, this probability is

$$\text{P}(T \geqslant t_0 + t_1 \mid T \geqslant t_0) = \frac{\text{P}(T \geqslant t_0 + t_1 \text{ and } T \geqslant t_0)}{\text{P}(T \geqslant t_0)}.$$

The numerator of this expression is simply $\text{P}(T \geqslant t_0 + t_1)$, and so the required probability is the ratio of the probability of survival beyond $t_0 + t_1$ to the probability of survival beyond t_0, that is $S(t_0 + t_1)/S(t_0)$. The survivor function for the exponential distribution is given by $S(t) = e^{-\lambda t}$, as in Equation (5.2) of Chapter 5, and so

$$\text{P}(T \geqslant t_0 + t_1 \mid T \geqslant t_0) = \frac{\exp\{-\lambda(t_0 + t_1)\}}{\exp(-\lambda t_0)} = e^{-\lambda t_1},$$

which is the survivor function of an exponential random variable at time t_1, that is $\text{P}(T \geqslant t_1)$. This result means that, conditional on survival to time t_0, the excess survival time beyond t_0 also has an exponential distribution with mean λ^{-1}. In other words, the probability of survival beyond time t_0 is not affected by the knowledge that the individual has already survived to time t_0.

From this result, since r_{Ci} has a unit exponential distribution, the excess residual, Δ, will also have a unit exponential distribution. The expected value of Δ is therefore unity, suggesting that Δ may be taken to be unity, and this leads to modified Cox-Snell residuals, given by

$$r'_{Ci} = \begin{cases} r_{Ci} & \text{for uncensored observations,} \\ r_{Ci} + 1 & \text{for censored observations.} \end{cases} \tag{4.3}$$

The ith modified Cox-Snell residual can be expressed in an alternative form by introducing an event indicator, δ_i, which takes the value zero if the observed survival time of the ith individual is censored and unity if it is uncensored. Then, Equation (4.3), the modified Cox-Snell residual is given by

$$r'_{Ci} = 1 - \delta_i + r_{Ci}. \tag{4.4}$$

Note that from the definition of this type of residual, r'_{Ci} must be greater than unity for a censored observation. Also, as for the unmodified residuals, the r'_{Ci} can take any value between zero and infinity, and they will have a skew distribution.

On the basis of empirical evidence, Crowley and Hu (1977) found that the addition of unity to a Cox-Snell residual for a censored observation inflated the residual to too great an extent. They therefore suggested that the median value of the excess residual be used rather than the mean. For the unit exponential distribution, the survivor function is $S(t) = e^{-t}$, and so the median, $t(50)$, is such that $e^{-t(50)} = 0.5$, whence $t(50) = \log 2 = 0.693$. Thus, a second version of the modified Cox-Snell residual has

$$r''_{Ci} = \begin{cases} r_{Ci} & \text{for uncensored observations,} \\ r_{Ci} + 0.693 & \text{for censored observations.} \end{cases} \tag{4.5}$$

However, if the proportion of censored observations is not too great, the sets of modified residuals from Equations (4.3) and (4.5) will not appear too different.

4.1.3 Martingale residuals

The modified residuals r'_{Ci} defined in Equation (4.4) have a mean of unity for uncensored observations. Accordingly, these residuals might be further refined by relocating the r'_{Ci} so that they have a mean of zero when an observation is uncensored. If in addition the resulting values are multiplied by -1, we obtain the residuals

$$r_{Mi} = \delta_i - r_{Ci}. \tag{4.6}$$

These residuals are known as *martingale residuals*, since they can also be derived using what are known as *martingale methods*, referred to later in Section 13.1 of Chapter 13. In this derivation, the r_{Ci} are based on the Nelson-Aalen estimate of the cumulative hazard function.

Martingale residuals take values between $-\infty$ and unity, with the residuals for censored observations, where $\delta_i = 0$, being negative. It can also be shown that these residuals sum to zero and, in large samples, the martingale residuals are uncorrelated with one another and have an expected value of zero. In this respect, they have properties similar to those possessed by residuals encountered in linear regression analysis.

Another way of looking at the martingale residuals is to note that the quantity r_{Mi} in Equation (4.6) is the difference between the observed number of deaths for the ith individual in the interval $(0, t_i)$ and the corresponding estimated expected number on the basis of the fitted model. To see this, note that the observed number of deaths is unity if the survival time t_i is uncensored, and zero if censored, that is δ_i. The second term in Equation (4.6) is an estimate of $H_i(t_i)$, the cumulative hazard of death for the ith individual over the interval $(0, t_i)$. From Section 1.3.3 of Chapter 1, this can be interpreted as the expected number of deaths in that interval. This shows another similarity between the martingale residuals and residuals from other areas of data analysis.

4.1.4 Deviance residuals

Although martingale residuals share many of the properties possessed by residuals encountered in other situations, such as in linear regression analysis, they are not symmetrically distributed about zero, even when the fitted model is correct. This skewness makes plots based on the residuals difficult to interpret. The deviance residuals, which were introduced by Therneau et al. (1990), are much more symmetrically distributed about zero. They are defined by

$$r_{Di} = \text{sgn}(r_{Mi}) \left[-2 \left\{r_{Mi} + \delta_i \log(\delta_i - r_{Mi})\right\}\right]^{\frac{1}{2}}, \tag{4.7}$$

where r_{Mi} is the martingale residual for the ith individual, and the function $\text{sgn}(\cdot)$ is the sign function. This is the function that takes the value $+1$ if its argument is positive and -1 if negative. Thus, $\text{sgn}(r_{Mi})$ ensures that the deviance residuals have the same sign as the martingale residuals.

The original motivation for these residuals is that they are components of the *deviance*. The deviance is a statistic that is used to summarise the extent to which the fit of a model of current interest deviates from that of a model which is a perfect fit to the data. This latter model is called the *saturated* or *full* model, and is a model in which the β-coefficients are allowed to be different for each individual. The statistic is given by

$$D = -2\left\{\log \hat{L}_c - \log \hat{L}_f\right\},$$

where $\hat{L}_c$ is the maximised partial likelihood under the current model and $\hat{L}_f$ is the maximised partial likelihood under the full model. The smaller the value of the deviance, the better the model. The deviance can be regarded as a generalisation of the residual sum of squares used in modelling normal data to the analysis of non-normal data, and features prominently in generalised linear modelling. Note that differences in deviance between two alternative models are the same as differences in the values of the statistic $-2 \log \hat{L}$ introduced in Chapter 3. The deviance residuals are then such that $D = \sum r_{Di}^2$, so that observations that correspond to relatively large deviance residuals are those that are not well fitted by the model.

Another way of viewing the deviance residuals is that they are martingale residuals that have been transformed to produce values that are symmetric about zero when the fitted model is appropriate. To see this, first recall that the martingale residuals r_{Mi} can take any value in the interval $(-\infty, 1)$. For large negative values of r_{Mi}, the term in square brackets in Equation (4.7) is dominated by r_{Mi}. Taking the square root of this quantity has the effect of bringing the residual closer to zero. Thus, martingale residuals in the range $(-\infty, 0)$ are shrunk toward zero. Now consider martingale residuals in the interval $(0, 1)$. The term $\delta_i \log(\delta_i - r_{Mi})$ in Equation (4.7) will only be non-zero for uncensored observations, and will then have the value $\log(1 - r_{Mi})$. As r_{Mi} gets closer to unity, $1 - r_{Mi}$ gets closer to zero and $\log(1 - r_{Mi})$ takes large negative values. The quantity in square brackets in Equation (4.7) is then dominated by this logarithmic term, and so the deviance residuals are expanded toward $+\infty$ as the martingale residual reaches its upper limit of unity.

One final point to note is that although these residuals can be expected to be symmetrically distributed about zero when an appropriate model has been fitted, they do not necessarily sum to zero.

4.1.5 Schoenfeld residuals*

Two disadvantages of the residuals described in Sections 4.1.1 to 4.1.4 are that they depend heavily on the observed survival time and require an estimate of the cumulative hazard function. Both of these disadvantages are overcome in a residual proposed by Schoenfeld (1982). These residuals were originally termed *partial residuals*, for reasons given in the sequel, but are now commonly known as *Schoenfeld residuals*. This residual differs from those considered previously in one important respect. This is that there is not a single value of the residual for each individual, but a set of values, one for each explanatory variable included in the fitted Cox regression model.

The ith Schoenfeld residual for X_j, the jth explanatory variable in the model, is given by

$$r_{Sji} = \delta_i \{x_{ji} - \hat{a}_{ji}\}, \tag{4.8}$$

where x_{ji} is the value of the jth explanatory variable, $j = 1, 2, \ldots, p$, for the ith individual in the study,

$$\hat{a}_{ji} = \frac{\sum_{l \in R(t_i)} x_{jl} \exp(\hat{\boldsymbol{\beta}}' \boldsymbol{x}_l)}{\sum_{l \in R(t_i)} \exp(\hat{\boldsymbol{\beta}}' \boldsymbol{x}_l)}, \tag{4.9}$$

and $R(t_i)$ is the set of all individuals at risk at time t_i.

Note that non-zero values of these residuals only arise for uncensored observations. Moreover, if the largest observation in a sample of survival times is uncensored, the value of $\hat{a}_{ji}$ for that observation, from Equation (4.9), will be equal to x_{ji} and so $r_{Sji} = 0$. To distinguish residuals that are genuinely zero from those obtained from censored observations, the latter are usually expressed as missing values.

The ith Schoenfeld residual, for the explanatory variable X_j, is an estimate of the ith component of the first derivative of the logarithm of the partial likelihood function with respect to β_j, which, from Equation (3.6), is given by

$$\frac{\partial \log L(\boldsymbol{\beta})}{\partial \beta_j} = \sum_{i=1}^{n} \delta_i \left\{ x_{ji} - a_{ji} \right\}, \tag{4.10}$$

where

$$a_{ji} = \frac{\sum_l x_{jl} \exp(\boldsymbol{\beta}'\boldsymbol{x}_l)}{\sum_l \exp(\boldsymbol{\beta}'\boldsymbol{x}_l)}. \tag{4.11}$$

The ith term in this summation, evaluated at $\hat{\boldsymbol{\beta}}$, is then the Schoenfeld residual for X_j, given in Equation (4.8). Since the estimates of the β's are such that

$$\frac{\partial \log L(\boldsymbol{\beta})}{\partial \beta_j}\bigg|_{\hat{\boldsymbol{\beta}}} = 0,$$

the Schoenfeld residuals must sum to zero. These residuals also have the property that, in large samples, the expected value of r_{Sji} is zero, and they are uncorrelated with one another.

It turns out that a scaled version of the Schoenfeld residuals, proposed by Grambsch and Therneau (1994), is more effective in detecting departures from the assumed model. Let the vector of Schoenfeld residuals for the ith individual be denoted $\boldsymbol{r}_{Si} = (r_{S1i}, r_{S2i}, \ldots, r_{Spi})'$. The scaled, or weighted, Schoenfeld residuals, r^*_{Sji}, are then the components of the vector

$$\boldsymbol{r}^*_{Si} = d \operatorname{var}(\hat{\boldsymbol{\beta}}) \boldsymbol{r}_{Si},$$

where d is the number of deaths among the n individuals, and $\operatorname{var}(\hat{\boldsymbol{\beta}})$ is the variance-covariance matrix of the parameter estimates in the fitted Cox regression model. These scaled Schoenfeld residuals are therefore quite straightforward to compute.

4.1.6 Score residuals*

There is one other type of residual that is useful in some aspects of model checking, and which, like the Schoenfeld residual, is obtained from the first derivative of the logarithm of the partial likelihood function with respect to the parameter β_j, $j = 1, 2, \ldots, p$. However, the derivative in Equation (4.10) is now expressed in a quite different form, namely

$$\frac{\partial \log L(\boldsymbol{\beta})}{\partial \beta_j} = \sum_{i=1}^{n} \left\{ \delta_i (x_{ji} - a_{ji}) + \exp(\boldsymbol{\beta}'\boldsymbol{x}_i) \sum_{t_r \leqslant t_i} \frac{(a_{jr} - x_{ji})\delta_r}{\sum_{l \in R(t_r)} \exp(\boldsymbol{\beta}'\boldsymbol{x}_l)} \right\}, \tag{4.12}$$

where x_{ji} is the ith value of the jth explanatory variable, δ_i is the event indicator which is zero for censored observations and unity otherwise, a_{ji} is given in Equation (4.11), and $R(t_r)$ is the risk set at time t_r. In this formulation, the contribution of the ith observation to the derivative only depends on information up to time t_i. In other words, if the study was actually concluded at time t_i, the ith component of the derivative would be unaffected. Residuals are then obtained as the estimated value of the n components of the derivative. From Appendix A, the first derivative of the logarithm of the partial likelihood function, with respect to β_j, is the efficient score for β_j, written $u(\beta_j)$. These residuals are therefore known as *score residuals*, and are denoted by r_{Uji}.

From Equation (4.12), the ith score residual, $i = 1, 2, \ldots, n$, for the jth explanatory variable in the model, X_j, is given by

$$r_{Uji} = \delta_i(x_{ji} - \hat{a}_{ji}) + \exp(\hat{\boldsymbol{\beta}}'\boldsymbol{x}_i) \sum_{t_r \leqslant t_i} \frac{(\hat{a}_{jr} - x_{ji})\delta_r}{\sum_{l \in R(t_r)} \exp(\hat{\boldsymbol{\beta}}'\boldsymbol{x}_l)}.$$

Using Equation (4.8), this may be written in the form

$$r_{Uji} = r_{Sji} + \exp(\hat{\boldsymbol{\beta}}'\boldsymbol{x}_i) \sum_{t_r \leqslant t_i} \frac{(\hat{a}_{jr} - x_{ji})\delta_r}{\sum_{l \in R(t_r)} \exp(\hat{\boldsymbol{\beta}}'\boldsymbol{x}_l)}, \qquad (4.13)$$

which shows that the score residuals are modifications of the Schoenfeld residuals. As for the Schoenfeld residuals, the score residuals sum to zero, but will not necessarily be zero when an observation is censored.

In this section, a number of residuals have been defined. We conclude with an example that illustrates the calculation of these different types of residual and that shows similarities and differences between them. This example will be used in many illustrations in this chapter, mainly because the relatively small number of observations allows the values of the residuals and other diagnostics to be readily tabulated. However, the methods of this chapter are generally more informative in larger data sets.

Example 4.1 Infection in patients on dialysis
In the treatment of certain disorders of the kidney, dialysis may be used to remove waste materials from the blood. One problem that can occur in patients on dialysis is the occurrence of an infection at the site at which the catheter is inserted. If any such infection occurs, the catheter must be removed, and the infection cleared up. In a study to investigate the incidence of infection, described by McGilchrist and Aisbett (1991), the time from insertion of the catheter until infection was recorded for a group of kidney patients. Sometimes, the catheter has to be removed for reasons other than infection, giving rise to right-censored observations. The data in this example relate to the 13 patients suffering from diseases of the kidney coded as type 3 in their paper.

Table 4.1 gives the number of days from insertion of the catheter until its removal following the first occurrence of an infection, together with the value of a variable that indicates the infection status of an individual. This variable takes the value zero if the catheter was removed for a reason other than the occurrence of an infection, and unity otherwise. The data set also includes the age of each patient in years and a variable that denotes their sex (1 = male, 2 = female).

Table 4.1 *Times to removal of a catheter following a kidney infection.*

Patient	Time	Status	Age	Sex
1	8	1	28	1
2	15	1	44	2
3	22	1	32	1
4	24	1	16	2
5	30	1	10	1
6	54	0	42	2
7	119	1	22	2
8	141	1	34	2
9	185	1	60	2
10	292	1	43	2
11	402	1	30	2
12	447	1	31	2
13	536	1	17	2

When a Cox regression model is fitted to these data, the estimated hazard function for the ith patient, $i = 1, 2, \ldots, 13$, is found to be

$$\hat{h}_i(t) = \exp\{0.030\, Age_i - 2.711\, Sex_i\}\, \hat{h}_0(t), \tag{4.14}$$

where Age_i and Sex_i refer to the age and sex of the ith patient.

The variable *Sex* is certainly important, since when *Sex* is added to the model that contains *Age* alone, the decrease in the value of the $-2\log\hat{L}$ statistic is 6.445 on 1 d.f. This change is highly significant ($P = 0.011$). On the other hand, there is no statistical evidence for including the variable *Age* in the model, since the change in the value of the $-2\log\hat{L}$ statistic on adding *Age* to the model that contains *Sex* is 1.320 on 1 d.f. ($P = 0.251$). However, it can be argued that from a clinical viewpoint, the hazard of infection may well depend on age. Consequently, both variables will be retained in the model.

The values of different types of residual for the model in Equation (4.14) are displayed in Table 4.2. In this table, r_{Ci}, r_{Mi} and r_{Di} are the Cox-Snell residuals, martingale residuals and deviance residuals, respectively. Also r_{S1i} and r_{S2i} are the values of Schoenfeld residuals for the variables *Age* and *Sex*, respectively, r^*_{S1i} and r^*_{S2i} are the corresponding scaled Schoenfeld residuals, and r_{U1i}, r_{U2i} are the score residuals.

The values in this table were computed using the Nelson-Aalen estimate of the baseline cumulative hazard function given in Equation (3.28). Had the estimate $\hat{H}_0(t)$, in Equation (3.22), been used, different values for all but the

Table 4.2 *Different types of residual after fitting a Cox regression model.*

Patient	r_{Ci}	r_{Mi}	r_{Di}	r_{S1i}	r_{S2i}	r^*_{S1i}	r^*_{S2i}	r_{U1i}	r_{U2i}
1	0.280	0.720	1.052	−1.085	−0.242	0.033	−3.295	−0.781	−0.174
2	0.072	0.928	1.843	14.493	0.664	0.005	7.069	13.432	0.614
3	1.214	−0.214	−0.200	3.129	−0.306	0.079	−4.958	−0.322	0.058
4	0.084	0.916	1.765	−10.222	0.434	−0.159	8.023	−9.214	0.384
5	1.506	−0.506	−0.439	−16.588	−0.550	−0.042	−5.064	9.833	0.130
6	0.265	−0.265	−0.728	–	–	–	–	−3.826	−0.145
7	0.235	0.765	1.168	−17.829	0.000	−0.147	3.083	−15.401	−0.079
8	0.484	0.516	0.648	−7.620	0.000	−0.063	1.318	−7.091	−0.114
9	1.438	−0.438	−0.387	17.091	0.000	0.141	−2.955	−15.811	−0.251
10	1.212	−0.212	−0.199	10.239	0.000	0.085	−1.770	1.564	−0.150
11	1.187	−0.187	−0.176	2.857	0.000	0.024	−0.494	6.575	−0.101
12	1.828	−0.828	−0.670	5.534	0.000	0.046	−0.957	4.797	−0.104
13	2.195	−1.195	−0.904	0.000	0.000	0.000	0.000	16.246	−0.068

Schoenfeld residuals would be obtained. In addition, because the corresponding estimate of the survivor function is zero at the longest removal time, which is that for patient number 13, values of the Cox-Snell, martingale and deviance residuals would not then be defined for this patient, and the martingale residuals would no longer sum to zero.

In this data set, there is just one censored observation, which is for patient number 6. The modified Cox-Snell residuals will then be the same as the Cox-Snell residuals for all patients except number 6. For this patient, the values of the two forms of modified residuals are $r'_{C6} = 1.265$ and $r''_{C6} = 0.958$. Also, the Schoenfeld residuals are not defined for the patient with a censored removal time, and are zero for the patient that has the longest period of time before removal of the catheter.

The skewness of the Cox-Snell and martingale residuals is clearly shown in Table 4.2, as is the fact that the Cox-Snell residuals are centred on unity while the martingale and deviance residuals are centred on zero. Note also that the martingale, Schoenfeld and score residuals sum to zero, as they should do.

One unusual feature about the residuals in Table 4.2 is the large number of zeros for the values of the Schoenfeld residual corresponding to *Sex*. The reason for this is that for infection times greater than 30 days, the value of the variable *Sex* is always equal to 2. This means that the value of the term $\hat{a}_{ji}$ for this variable, given in Equation (4.9), is equal to 2 for a survival time greater than 30 days, and so the corresponding Schoenfeld residual defined in Equation (4.8) is zero.

We now consider how residuals obtained after fitting a Cox regression model can be used to throw light on the extent to which the fitted model provides an appropriate description of the observed data. We will then be in a position to study the residuals obtained in Example 4.1 in greater detail.

4.2 Assessment of model fit

A number of plots based on residuals can be used in the graphical assessment of the adequacy of a fitted model. Unfortunately, many graphical procedures that are analogues of residual plots used in linear regression analysis have not proved to be very helpful. This is because plots of residuals against quantities such as the observed survival times, or the rank order of these times, often exhibit a definite pattern, even when the correct model has been fitted. Traditionally, plots of residuals have been based on the Cox-Snell residuals, or adjusted versions of them described in Section 4.1.2. The use of these residuals is therefore reviewed in the next section, and this is followed by a description of how some other types of residuals may be used in the graphical assessment of the fit of a model.

4.2.1 Plots based on the Cox-Snell residuals

In Section 4.1.1, the Cox-Snell residuals were shown to have an exponential distribution with unit mean, if the fitted model is correct. They therefore have a mean and variance of unity, and are asymmetrically distributed about the mean. This means that simple plots of the residuals, such as plots of the residuals against the observation number, known as *index plots*, will not lead to a symmetric display. The residuals are also correlated with the survival times, and so plots of these residuals against quantities such as the observed survival times, or the rank order of these times, are also unhelpful.

One particular plot of these residuals, which can be used to assess the overall fit of the model, leads to an assessment of whether the residuals are a plausible sample from a unit exponential distribution. This plot is based on the fact that if a random variable T has an exponential distribution with unit mean, then the survivor function of T is e^{-t}; see Section 5.1.1 of Chapter 5. Accordingly, a plot of the cumulative hazard function $H(t) = -\log S(t)$ against t, known as a *cumulative hazard plot*, will give a straight line through the origin with unit slope.

This result can be used to examine whether the residuals have a unit exponential distribution. After computing the Cox-Snell residuals, r_{Ci}, the Kaplan-Meier estimate of the survivor function of these values is found. This estimate is computed in a similar manner to the Kaplan-Meier estimate of the survivor function for survival times, except that the data on which the estimate is based are now the residuals r_{Ci}. Residuals obtained from censored survival times are themselves taken to be censored. Denoting the estimate by $\hat{S}(r_{Ci})$, the values of $\hat{H}(r_{Ci}) = -\log \hat{S}(r_{Ci})$ are plotted against r_{Ci}. This gives a cumulative hazard plot of the residuals. A straight line with unit slope and zero intercept will then indicate that the fitted survival model is satisfactory. On the other hand, a plot that displays a systematic departure from a straight line, or yields a line that does not have approximately unit slope or zero intercept, might suggest that the model needs to be modified in some way. Equivalently, a *log-cumulative hazard plot* of the residuals, that is a plot of $\log \hat{H}(r_{Ci})$ against $\log r_{Ci}$ may be used. This plot is discussed in more detail in Section 4.4.1.

Example 4.2 Infection in patients on dialysis
Consider again the data on the time to the occurrence of an infection in kidney patients, described in Example 4.1. In this example, we first examine whether the Cox-Snell residuals are a plausible sample of observations from a unit exponential distribution. For this, the Kaplan-Meier estimate of the survivor function of the Cox-Snell residuals, $\hat{S}(r_{Ci})$, is obtained. The cumulative hazard function of the residuals, $\hat{H}(r_{Ci})$, derived from $-\log \hat{S}(r_{Ci})$, is then plotted against the corresponding residual to give a cumulative hazard plot of the residuals. The details of this calculation are summarised in Table 4.3, and the cumulative hazard plot is shown in Figure 4.1. The residual for patient number 6 does not lead to values of $\hat{S}(r_{C6})$ and $\hat{H}(r_{C6})$ because this observation is censored.

Table 4.3 *Calculation of the cumulative hazard function of the Cox-Snell residuals.*

r_{Ci}	$\hat{S}(r_{Ci})$	$\hat{H}(r_{Ci})$
0.072	0.9231	0.080
0.084	0.8462	0.167
0.235	0.7692	0.262
0.265	–	–
0.280	0.6838	0.380
0.484	0.5983	0.514
1.187	0.5128	0.668
1.212	0.4274	0.850
1.214	0.3419	1.073
1.438	0.2564	1.361
1.506	0.1709	1.767
1.828	0.0855	2.459
2.195	0.0000	–

The relatively small number of observations in this data set makes it difficult to interpret plots of residuals. However, the plotted points in Figure 4.1 are fairly close to a straight line through the origin, which has approximately unit slope. This could suggest that the model fitted to the data given in Table 4.1 is satisfactory.

On the face of it, this procedure would appear to have some merit, but cumulative hazard plots of the Cox-Snell residuals have not proved to be very useful in practice. In an earlier section it was argued that since the values $-\log S(t_i)$ have a unit exponential distribution, the Cox-Snell residuals, which are estimates of these quantities, should have an approximate unit exponential distribution when the fitted model is correct. This result is then used when interpreting a cumulative hazard plot of the residuals. Unfortu-

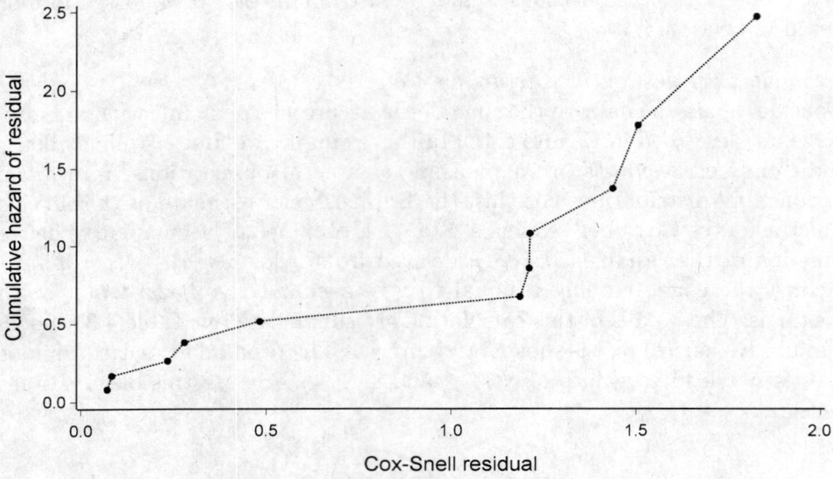

Figure 4.1 *Cumulative hazard plot of the Cox-Snell residuals.*

nately this approximation is not very reliable, particularly in small samples. This is because estimates of the βs, and also of the baseline cumulative hazard function, $H_0(t)$, are needed in the computation of the r_{Ci}. The substitution of estimates means that the actual distribution of the residuals is not necessarily unit exponential, but their exact distribution is not known. In fact, the distribution of Cox-Snell residuals for $n = 3$ was shown by Lagakos (1981) to be quite dissimilar to a unit exponential sample.

On other occasions, a straight line plot may be obtained when the model fitted is known to be incorrect. Indeed, practical experience suggests that a fitted model has to be seriously wrong before anything other than a straight line of unit slope is seen in the cumulative hazard plot of the Cox-Snell residuals.

In the particular case of the null model, that is, the model that contains no explanatory variates, the cumulative hazard plot will be a straight line with unit slope and zero intercept, even if some explanatory variables should actually be included in the model. The reason for this is that when no covariates are included, the Cox-Snell residual for the ith individual reduces to $-\log \hat{S}_0(t_i)$. From Equation (3.29) in Chapter 3, in the absence of ties this is approximately $\sum_{j=1}^{k} 1/n_j$ at the kth uncensored survival time, $k = 1, 2, \ldots, r-1$, where n_j is the number at risk at time t_j. This summation is simply $\sum_{j=1}^{k} 1/(n-j+1)$, which is the expected value of the kth order statistic in a sample of size n from a unit exponential distribution.

In view of the limitations of the Cox-Snell residuals in assessing model adequacy, diagnostic procedures based on other types of residuals that are of practical use, are described in the following section.

4.2.2 Plots based on the martingale and deviance residuals

The martingale residuals, introduced in Section 4.1.3, can be interpreted as the difference between the observed and expected number of deaths in the time interval $(0, t_i)$, for the ith individual. Accordingly, these residuals highlight individuals who, on the basis of the assumed model, have died too soon or lived too long. Large negative residuals will correspond to individuals who have a long survival time, but covariate values that suggest they should have died earlier. On the other hand, a residual close to unity, the upper limit of a martingale residual, will be obtained when an individual has an unexpectedly short survival time. An index plot of the martingale residuals will highlight individuals whose survival time is not well fitted by the model. Such observations may be termed *outliers*. The data from individuals for whom the residual is unusually large in absolute value, will need to be the subject of further scrutiny. Plots of these residuals against the survival time, the rank order of the survival times, or explanatory variables, may indicate whether there are particular times, or values of the explanatory variables, where the model does not fit well.

Since the deviance residuals are more symmetrically distributed than the martingale residuals, plots based on these residuals tend to be easier to interpret. Consequently, an index plot of the deviance residuals may also be used to identify individuals whose survival times are out of line.

In a fitted Cox regression model, the hazard of death for the ith individual at any time depends on the values of explanatory variables for that individual, $\boldsymbol{x}_i$, through the function $\exp(\hat{\boldsymbol{\beta}}'\boldsymbol{x}_i)$. This means that individuals for whom $\hat{\boldsymbol{\beta}}'\boldsymbol{x}_i$ has a large negative value have a lower than average risk of death, and individuals for whom $\hat{\boldsymbol{\beta}}'\boldsymbol{x}_i$ has a large positive value have a higher than average risk. The quantity $\hat{\boldsymbol{\beta}}'\boldsymbol{x}_i$ is the risk score, introduced in Section 3.1 of Chapter 3, and provides information about whether an individual might be expected to survive for a short or long time. By reconciling information about individuals whose survival times are out of line, with the values of their risk score, useful information can be obtained about the characteristics of observations that are not well fitted by the model. In this context, a plot of the deviance residuals against the risk score is a particularly helpful diagnostic.

Example 4.3 Infection in patients on dialysis
Consider again the data on times to infection in kidney patients. From the values of the martingale and deviance residuals given in Table 4.2, we see that patient 2 has the largest positive residual, suggesting that the time to removal of the catheter is shorter for this patient than might have been expected on the basis of the fitted model. The table also shows that the two types of residual do not rank the observations in the same order. For example, the second largest negative martingale residual is found for patient 12, whereas patient 6 has the second largest negative deviance residual. However, the observations that have the most extreme values of the martingale and deviance residuals will

tend to be the same, as in this example. Index plots of the martingale and deviance residuals are shown in Figure 4.2.

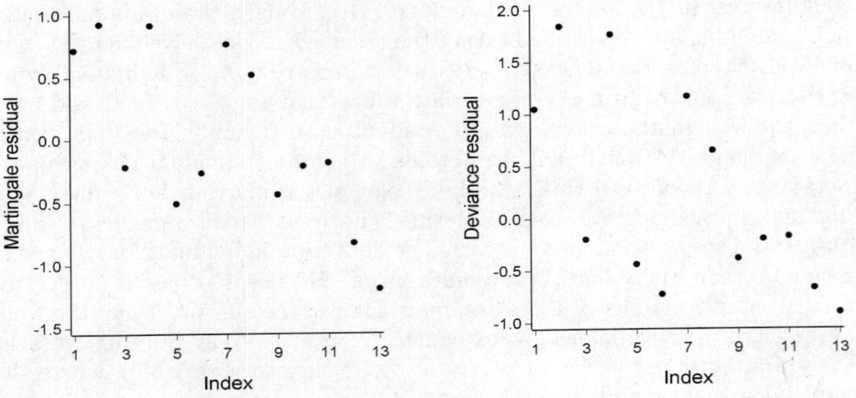

Figure 4.2 *Index plots of the martingale and deviance residuals.*

The plots are quite similar, but the distribution of the deviance residuals is seen to be more symmetric. The plots also show that there are no patients who have residuals that are unusually large in absolute value. Figure 4.3 gives a plot of the deviance residuals against the risk scores, that are found from the values of $0.030\, Age_i - 2.711\, Sex_i$, for $i = 1, 2, \ldots, 13$.

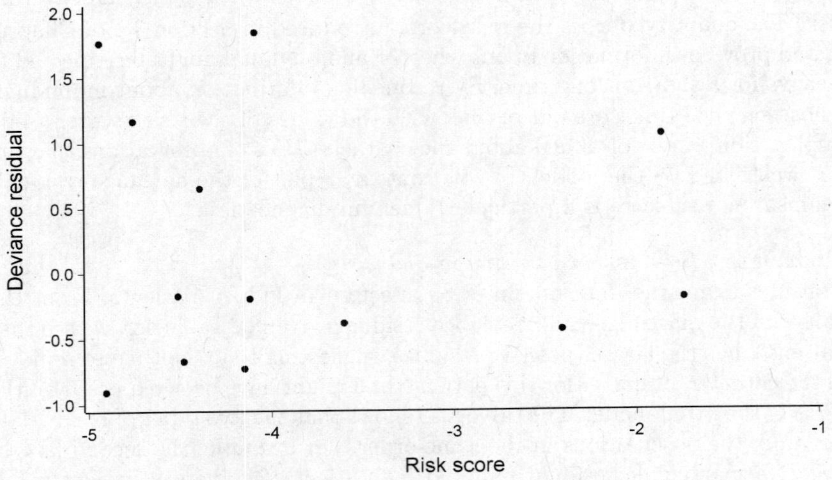

Figure 4.3 *Plot of the deviance residuals against the values of the risk score.*

This figure shows that patients with the largest deviance residuals have low risk scores. This indicates that these patients are at relatively low risk of an early catheter removal, and yet their removal time is sooner than expected.

4.2.3 Checking the functional form of covariates

Although the model-based approach to the analysis of survival data, described in Chapter 3, identifies a particular set of covariates on which the hazard function depends, it will be important to check that the correct functional form has been adopted for these variables. An improvement in the fit of a model may well be obtained by using some transformation of the values of a variable instead of the original values. For example, it might be that a better fitting model is obtained by using a non-linear function of the age of an individual at baseline, or the logarithm of a biochemical variable such as serum bilirubin level. Similarly, an explanatory variable such as serum cholesterol level may only begin to exert an effect on survival when it exceeds some threshold value, after which time the hazard of death might increase with increasing values of that variable.

A straightforward means of assessing this aspect of model adequacy is based on the martingale residuals obtained from fitting the null model, that is, the model that contains no covariates. These residuals are then plotted against the values of each covariate in the model. It has been shown by Therneau et al. (1990) that this plot should display the functional form required for the covariate. In particular, a straight line plot indicates that a linear term is needed.

As an extension to this approach, if the functional form of certain covariates can be assumed to be known, martingale residuals may be calculated from the fitted Cox regression model that contains these covariates alone. The resulting martingale residuals are then plotted against the covariates whose functional form needs to be determined.

The graphs obtained in this way are usually quite 'noisy' and their interpretation is much helped by superimposing a smoothed curve that is fitted to the scatterplot. There are a number of such *smoothers* in common use, including *smoothing splines*. However, the most widely used smoothers are the *LOWESS* (locally weighted scatterplot smoothing) and *LOESS* (locally estimated scatterplot smoothing) methods, introduced by Cleveland (1979) and implemented in many software packages.

Even with a smoother, it can be difficult to discern a specific functional form when a non-linear pattern is seen in the plot. If a specific transformation is suggested, such as the logarithmic transformation, the covariate can be so transformed, and the martingale residuals for the null model plotted against the transformed variate. A straight line would then confirm that an appropriate transformation has been applied.

Example 4.4 Infection in patients on dialysis
In this example, we illustrate the use of martingale residuals in assessing whether the age effect is linear in the Cox regression model fitted to the data of Example 4.1. First, the martingale residuals for the null model are obtained and these are plotted against the corresponding values of the age of a patient in Figure 4.4.

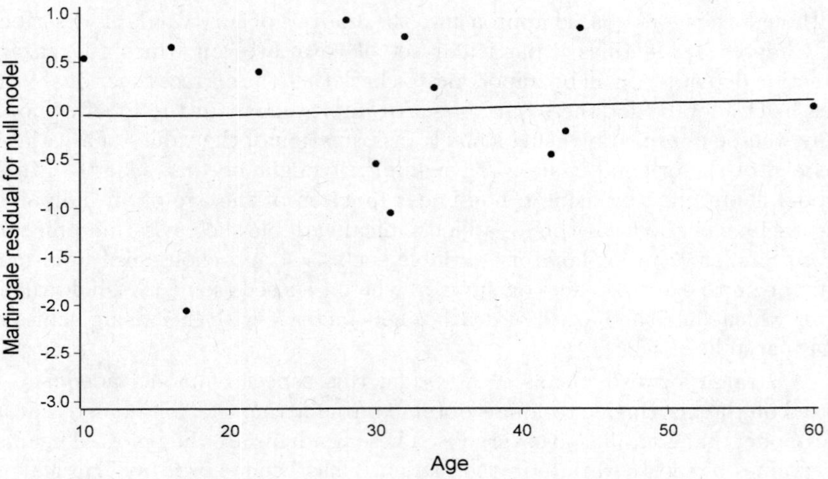

Figure 4.4 *Plot of the martingale residuals for the null model against Age, with a smoothed curve superimposed.*

There is too little data to say much about this graph, but the smoothed curve indicates that there is no need for anything other than a linear term in *Age*. In fact, the age effect is not actually significant, and so it is not surprising that the smoothed curve is roughly horizontal.

We end this section with a further illustrative example.

Example 4.5 Survival of multiple myeloma patients
In this example we return to the data on the survival times of 48 patients with multiple myeloma, described in Example 1.3. In Example 3.5, a Cox regression model that contained the explanatory variables *Hb* (serum haemoglobin) and *Bun* (blood urea nitrogen) was found to be a suitable model for the hazard function. We now perform an analysis of the residuals in order to study the adequacy of this fitted model.

First, a cumulative hazard plot of the Cox-Snell residuals is shown in Figure 4.5. The line made by the plotted points in Figure 4.5 is reasonably straight, and has a unit slope and zero intercept. On the basis of this plot, there is no reason to doubt the adequacy of the fitted model. However, as

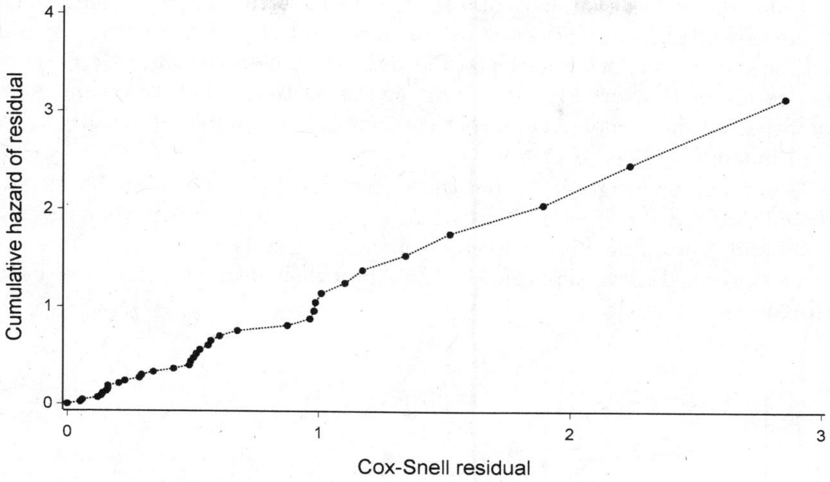

Figure 4.5 *Cumulative hazard plot of the Cox-Snell residuals.*

pointed out in Section 4.2.1, this plot is not very sensitive to departures from the fitted model.

To further assess the fit of the model, the deviance residuals are plotted against the corresponding risk scores in Figure 4.6.

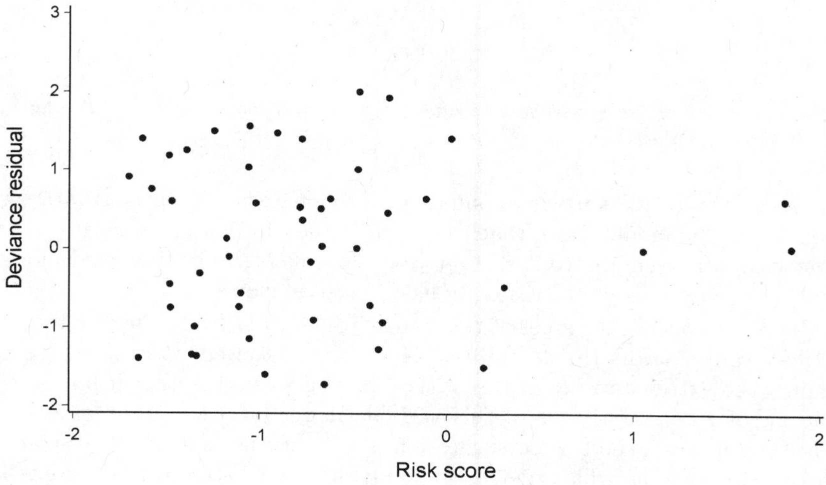

Figure 4.6 *Deviance residuals plotted against the risk score.*

This plot shows that patients 41 and 38 have the largest values of the deviance residuals, but these are not much separated from values of the residuals for some of the other patients. Patients with the three largest risk scores have residuals that are close to zero, suggesting that these observations are well fitted by the model. Again, there is no reason to doubt the validity of the fitted model.

In order to investigate whether the correct functional form for the variates *Hb* and *Bun* has been used, martingale residuals are calculated for the null model and plotted against the values of these variables. The resulting plots, with a smoothed curve superimposed to aid in their interpretation, are shown in Figures 4.7 and 4.8.

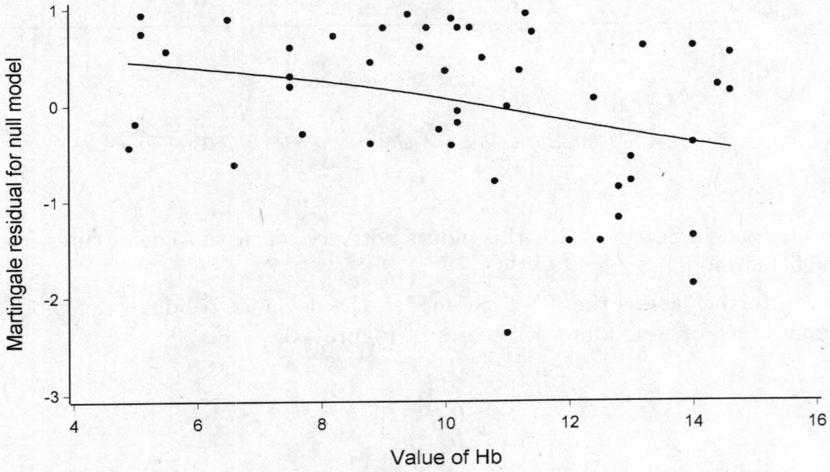

Figure 4.7 *Plot of the martingale residuals for the null model against the values of Hb, with a smoothed curve superimposed.*

The plots for *Hb* and *Bun* confirm that linear terms in each variable are required in the model. Note that the slope of the plot for *Hb* in Figure 4.7 is negative, corresponding to the negative coefficient of *Hb* in the fitted model, while the plot for *Bun* in Figure 4.8 has a positive slope.

In this data set, the values of *Bun* range from 6 to 172, and the distribution of their values across the 48 subjects is positively skewed. In order to guard against the extreme values of this variate having an undue impact on the coefficient of *Bun*, logarithms of this variable might be used in the modelling process. Although there is no suggestion of this in Figure 4.8, for illustrative purposes, we will use this type of plot to investigate whether a model containing log *Bun* rather than *Bun* is acceptable. Figure 4.9 shows the martingale residuals for the null model plotted against the values of log *Bun*.

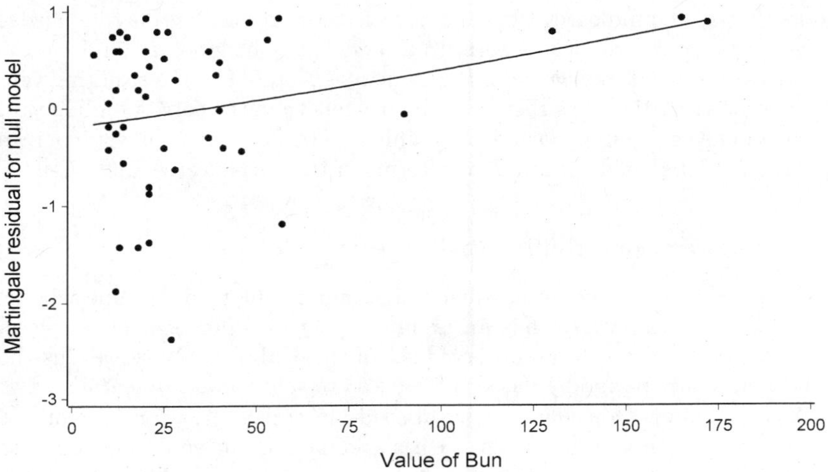

Figure 4.8 *Plot of the martingale residuals for the null model against the values of Bun, with a smoothed curve superimposed.*

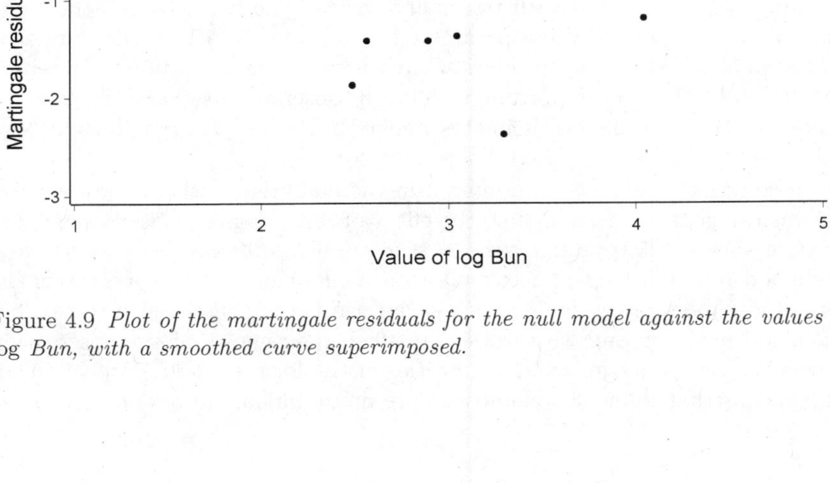

Figure 4.9 *Plot of the martingale residuals for the null model against the values of* log *Bun, with a smoothed curve superimposed.*

The smoothed curve in this figure does suggest that it is not appropriate to use a linear term in log *Bun*. Indeed, if it were decided to use log *Bun* in the model, Figure 4.9 indicates that a quadratic term in log *Bun* may be needed. In fact, adding this quadratic term to a model that includes *Hb* and log *Bun* leads to a significant reduction in the value of $-2\log\hat{L}$, but the resulting value of this statistic, 201.458, is then only slightly less than the corresponding value for the model containing *Hb* and *Bun*, which is 202.938. This analysis confirms that the model should contain linear terms in the variables *Hb* and *Bun*.

4.3 Identification of influential observations

In the assessment of model adequacy, it is important to determine whether any particular observation has an undue impact on inferences made on the basis of a model fitted to an observed set of survival data. Observations that do have an effect on model-based inferences are said to be *influential*.

As an example, consider a survival study in which a new treatment is to be compared with a standard. In such a comparison, it would be important to determine if the hazard of death on the new treatment, relative to that on the standard, was substantially affected by any one individual. In particular, it might be that when the data record for one individual is removed from the database, the relative hazard is increased or reduced by a substantial amount. If this happens, the data from such an individual would need to be subject to particular scrutiny.

Conclusions from a survival analysis are often framed in terms of estimates of quantities such as the relative hazard and median survival time, which depend on the estimated values of the β-parameters in the fitted Cox regression model. It is therefore of particular interest to examine the influence of each observation on these estimates. We can do this by examining the extent to which the estimated parameters in the fitted model are affected by omitting in turn the data record for each individual in the study. In some circumstances, estimates of a subset of the parameters may be of special importance, such as parameters associated with treatment effects. The study of influence may then be limited to just these parameters. On many occasions, the influence that each observation has on the estimated hazard function will be of interest, and it would then be important to identify observations that influence the complete set of parameter estimates under the model. These two aspects of influence are discussed in the following sections.

In contrast to models encountered in the analysis of other types of data, such as the general linear model, the effect of removing one observation from a set of survival data is not easy to study. This is mainly because the log-likelihood function for the Cox regression model cannot be expressed as the sum of a number of terms, in which each term is the contribution to the log-likelihood made by each observation. Instead, the removal of one observation affects the risk sets over which quantities of the form $\exp(\boldsymbol{\beta}'\boldsymbol{x})$ are summed. This means that influence diagnostics are quite difficult to derive and so the following sections of this chapter simply give the relevant results. References to the articles that contain derivations of the quoted formulae are included in the final section of this chapter.

4.3.1 Influence of observations on a parameter estimate*

Suppose that we wish to determine whether any particular observation has an untoward effect on $\hat{\beta}_j$, the jth parameter estimate, $j = 1, 2, \ldots, p$, in a fitted Cox regression model. One way of doing this would be to fit the model to all n observations in the data set, and to then fit the same model to the sets of $n - 1$ observations obtained by omitting each of the n observations in turn. The actual effect that omitting each observation has on the parameter estimate could then be determined. This procedure is computationally expensive, unless the number of observations is not too large, and so we use instead an approximation to the amount by which $\hat{\beta}_j$ changes when the ith observation is omitted, for $i = 1, 2, \ldots, n$. Suppose that the value of the jth parameter estimate on omitting the ith observation is denoted by $\hat{\beta}_{j(i)}$. Cain and Lange (1984) showed that an approximation to $\hat{\beta}_j - \hat{\beta}_{j(i)}$ is based on the score residuals, described in Section 4.1.6.

Let $\boldsymbol{r}_{Ui}$ denote the vector of values of the score residuals for the ith observation, so that $\boldsymbol{r}'_{Ui} = (r_{U1i}, r_{U2i}, \ldots, r_{Upi})$, where r_{Uji}, $j = 1, 2, \ldots, p$, is the ith score residual for the jth explanatory variable, given in Equation (4.13). An approximation to $\hat{\beta}_j - \hat{\beta}_{j(i)}$, the change in $\hat{\beta}_j$ on omitting the ith observation, is then the jth component of the vector

$$\boldsymbol{r}'_{Ui} \operatorname{var}(\hat{\boldsymbol{\beta}}),$$

$\operatorname{var}(\hat{\boldsymbol{\beta}})$ being the variance-covariance matrix of the vector of parameter estimates in the fitted Cox regression model. The jth element of this vector, which is called a *delta-beta*, will be denoted by $\Delta_i\hat{\beta}_j$, so that $\Delta_i\hat{\beta}_j \approx \hat{\beta}_j - \hat{\beta}_{j(i)}$. Use of this approximation means that the values of $\Delta_i\hat{\beta}_j$ can be computed from quantities available after fitting the model to the full data set.

Observations that influence a particular parameter estimate, the jth say, will be such that the values of $\Delta_i\hat{\beta}_j$, the delta-betas for these observations, are larger in absolute value than for other observations in the data set. Index plots of the delta-betas for each explanatory variable in the model will then reveal whether there are observations that have an undue impact on the parameter estimate for any particular explanatory variable. In addition, a plot of the values of $\Delta_i\hat{\beta}_j$ against the rank order of the survival times yields information about the relation between survival time and influence.

The delta-betas may be standardised by dividing $\Delta_i\hat{\beta}_j$ by the standard error of $\hat{\beta}_j$ to give a *standardised delta-beta*. The standardised delta-beta can be interpreted as the change in the value of the statistic $\hat{\beta}/\operatorname{se}(\hat{\beta})$, on omitting the ith observation. Since this statistic can be used in assessing whether a particular parameter has a value significantly different from zero (see Section 3.4

of Chapter 3), the standardised delta-beta can be used to provide information on how the significance of the parameter estimate is affected by the removal of the ith observation from the database. Again, an index plot is the most useful way of displaying the standardised delta-betas.

The statistic $\Delta_i \hat{\beta}_j$ is an approximation to the actual change in the parameter estimate when the ith observation is omitted from the fit. The approximation is generally adequate in the sense that observations that have an influence on a parameter estimate will be highlighted. However, the actual effect of omitting any particular observation on model-based inferences will need to be studied. The agreement between the actual and approximate delta-betas in a particular situation is illustrated in Example 4.6.

Example 4.6 Infection in patients on dialysis
In this example, we return to the data on the times to infection following commencement of dialysis. To investigate the influence that the data from each of the 13 patients in the study has on the estimated value of the coefficients of the variables *Age* and *Sex* in the linear component of the fitted Cox regression model, the approximate unstandardised delta-betas, $\Delta_i \hat{\beta}_1$ and $\Delta_i \hat{\beta}_2$, are obtained. These are given in Table 4.4.

Table 4.4 *Approximate delta-betas for Age ($\hat{\beta}_1$), and Sex ($\hat{\beta}_2$).*

Observation	$\Delta_i \hat{\beta}_1$	$\Delta_i \hat{\beta}_2$
1	0.0020	−0.1977
2	0.0004	0.5433
3	−0.0011	0.0741
4	−0.0119	0.5943
5	0.0049	0.0139
6	−0.0005	−0.1192
7	−0.0095	0.1270
8	−0.0032	−0.0346
9	−0.0073	−0.0734
10	0.0032	−0.2023
11	0.0060	−0.2158
12	0.0048	−0.1939
13	0.0122	−0.3157

The largest delta-beta for *Age* occurs for patient number 13, but there are other delta-betas with similar values. The actual change in the parameter estimate on omitting the data for this patient is 0.0195, and so omission of this observation reduces the hazard of infection relative to the baseline hazard. The standard error of the parameter estimate for *Age* in the full data set is 0.026, and so the maximum amount by which this estimate is changed when one observation is deleted is about three-quarters of a standard error. When the data from patient 13 is omitted, the age effect becomes less significant, but the difference is unlikely to be of practical importance.

There are two large delta-betas for *Sex* that are quite close to one another. These correspond to the observations from patients 2 and 4. The actual change in the parameter estimate when each observation is omitted in turn is 0.820 and 0.818, and so the approximate delta-betas underestimate the actual change. The standard error of the estimated coefficient of *Sex* in the full data set is 1.096, and so again the change in the estimate on deleting an observation is less than one standard error. The effect of deleting either of these two observations is to increase the hazard for males relative to females, so that the sex effect is slightly more significant.

The approximate delta-betas can be compared with the actual values. In this example, the agreement is generally quite good, although there is a tendency for the actual changes in the parameter estimates to be underestimated by the approximation. The largest difference between the actual and approximate value of the delta-beta for *Age* is 0.010, which occurs for patient number 8. That for *Sex* is 0.276, which occurs for patient number 2. These differences are about a quarter of the value of the standard error of each parameter estimate.

4.3.2 Influence of observations on the set of parameter estimates*

It may happen that the structure of the fitted model is particularly sensitive to one or more observations in the data set. Such observations can be detected using diagnostics that are designed to highlight observations that influence the complete set of parameter estimates in the risk score. These diagnostics therefore reflect the influence that individual observations have on the risk score, and give information that is additional to that provided by the delta-betas. In particular, excluding a given observation from the data set may not have a great influence on any particular parameter estimate, and so will not be revealed from a study of the delta-beta statistics. However, the change in the set of parameter estimates might be such that the form of the estimated hazard function, or values of summary statistics based on the fitted model, change markedly when that observation is removed. Statistics for assessing the influence of observations on the set of parameter estimates also have the advantage that there is a single value of the diagnostic for each observation. This makes them easier to use than diagnostics such as the delta-betas.

A number of diagnostics for assessing the influence of each observation on the set of parameter estimates have been proposed. In this section, two will be described, but references to others will be given in the concluding section of this chapter.

One way of assessing the influence of each observation on the overall fit of the model is to examine the amount by which the value of minus twice the logarithm of the maximised partial likelihood, $-2\log\hat{L}$, under a fitted model, changes when each observation in turn is left out. Write $\log L(\hat{\boldsymbol{\beta}})$ for the value of the maximised log-likelihood when the model is fitted to all n observations, and $\log L(\hat{\boldsymbol{\beta}}_{(i)})$ for the value of the maximised log-likelihood of the n observations when the parameter estimates are computed after omitting the ith observation from the fit. The diagnostic

$$2\left\{\log L(\hat{\boldsymbol{\beta}}) - \log L(\hat{\boldsymbol{\beta}}_{(i)})\right\}$$

can then be useful in the study of influence.

Pettitt and Bin Daud (1989) show that an approximation to this *likelihood displacement* is

$$LD_i = \boldsymbol{r}'_{Ui} \operatorname{var}(\hat{\boldsymbol{\beta}})\, \boldsymbol{r}_{Ui}, \tag{4.15}$$

where $\boldsymbol{r}_{Ui}$ is the $p \times 1$ vector of score residuals, whose jth component is given in Equation (4.13), and $\operatorname{var}(\hat{\boldsymbol{\beta}})$ is the variance-covariance matrix of $\hat{\boldsymbol{\beta}}$, the vector of parameter estimates. The values of this statistic may therefore be straightforwardly obtained from terms used in computing the delta-betas for each explanatory variable in the model. An index plot, or a plot of the likelihood displacements against the rank order of the survival times, provides an informative visual summary of the values of the diagnostic. Observations that have relatively large values of the diagnostic are influential. Plots against explanatory variables are not recommended, since, as demonstrated by Pettitt and Bin Daud (1989), these plots can have a deterministic pattern, even when the fitted model is correct.

Another diagnostic that can be used to assess the impact of each observation on the set of parameter estimates is based on the $n \times n$ symmetric matrix

$$\boldsymbol{B} = \boldsymbol{\Theta}' \operatorname{var}(\hat{\boldsymbol{\beta}})\, \boldsymbol{\Theta},$$

where $\boldsymbol{\Theta}'$ is the $n \times p$ matrix formed from the vectors $\boldsymbol{r}_{Ui}$, for $i = 1, 2, \ldots, p$. An argument from linear algebra shows that the absolute values of the elements of the $n \times 1$ eigenvector associated with the largest eigenvalue of the matrix $\boldsymbol{B}$, standardised to have unit length by dividing each component by the square root of the sum of squares of all the components of the eigenvector, is a measure of the sensitivity of the fit of the model to each of the n observations in the data set. Denoting this eigenvector by $\boldsymbol{l}_{\max}$, the ith element of $\boldsymbol{l}_{\max}$ is a measure of the influence of the ith observation on the set of parameter estimates. The sign of this diagnostic is immaterial, and so plots based on the absolute values, $|\boldsymbol{l}_{\max}|$ are commended for general use. Denoting the ith element of $|\boldsymbol{l}_{\max}|$ by $|\boldsymbol{l}_{\max}|_i$, $i = 1, 2, \ldots, n$, index plots of these values, plots against the rank order of the survival times, and against explanatory variables in the model, can all be useful in the assessment of influence.

The standardisation to unit length means that the squares of the values $|\boldsymbol{l}_{\max}|_i$ must sum to 1.0. Observations for which the squares of the elements of the eigenvector account for a substantial proportion of the total sum of squares of unity will then be those that are most influential. Large elements of this eigenvector will therefore correspond to observations that have most effect on the value of the likelihood function. A final point to note is that unlike other diagnostics, a plot of the values of $|\boldsymbol{l}_{\max}|_i$ against explanatory variables will not have a deterministic pattern if the fitted model is correct. This means that plots of $|\boldsymbol{l}_{\max}|_i$ against explanatory variables can be useful in assessing whether there are particular ranges of values of the variates over which the model does not fit well.

Example 4.7 Infection in patients on dialysis
The data first given in Example 4.1 will again be used to illustrate the use of diagnostics designed to reveal observations that influence the complete set of parameter estimates. In Table 4.5, the approximate likelihood displacements from Equation (4.15), and the values of $|\boldsymbol{l}_{\max}|_i$ are given.

Table 4.5 *Values of the approximate likelihood displacement, LD_i, and the elements of $|\boldsymbol{l}_{\max}|$.*

Observation	LD_i	$\lvert\boldsymbol{l}_{\max}\rvert_i$
1	0.033	0.161
2	0.339	0.309
3	0.005	0.068
4	0.338	0.621
5	0.050	0.104
6	0.019	0.058
7	0.136	0.291
8	0.027	0.054
9	0.133	0.124
10	0.035	0.193
11	0.061	0.264
12	0.043	0.224
13	0.219	0.464

The observations that most affect the value of the maximised log-likelihood when they are omitted are those corresponding to patients 2 and 4. The value of the likelihood displacement diagnostic is also quite large for patient number 13. This means that the set of parameter estimates are most affected by the removal of either of these three patients from the database.

The fourth element of $|\boldsymbol{l}_{\max}|$, $|\boldsymbol{l}_{\max}|_4$, is the largest in absolute value, and indicates that omitting the data from patient number 4 has the greatest effect on the pair of parameter estimates. The elements corresponding to patients 2 and 13 are also large relative to the other values, suggesting that the data for these patients are also influential. The sum of the squares of elements 2, 4 and 13 of $|\boldsymbol{l}_{\max}|$ is 0.70. The total of the sums of squares of the elements is 1.00, and so cases 2, 4 and 13 account for nearly three-quarters of the variability in the vales $|\boldsymbol{l}_{\max}|_i$. Note that the analysis of the delta-betas in Example 4.6 showed that the observations from patients 2 and 4 most influence the parameter estimate for *Sex*, while the observation for patient 13 has a greater effect on the estimate for *Age*.

In summary, the observations from patients 2, 4 and 13 affect the form of the hazard function to the greatest extent. Omitting each of these in turn gives the following estimates of the linear component in the hazard functions for the ith individual.

Omitting patient number 2: $0.031\, Age_i - 3.530\, Sex_i$

Omitting patient number 4: $0.045\, Age_i - 3.529\, Sex_i$

Omitting patient number 13: $0.011\, Age_i - 2.234\, Sex_i$

For comparison, the linear component for the full data set is

$$0.030\, Age_i - 2.711\, Sex_i.$$

To illustrate the magnitude of the change in estimated hazard ratios, consider the relative hazard of infection at time t for a patient aged 50 years relative to one aged 40 years. For the full data set, this is $e^{0.304} = 1.355$. This value increases to 1.365 and 1.564 when patients 2 and 4, respectively, are omitted, and decreases to 1.114 when patient 13 is omitted. The effect on the hazard function of removing these patients from the database is therefore not particularly marked.

In the same way, the hazard of infection at time t for a male patient ($Sex = 1$) relative to a female ($Sex = 2$) is $e^{2.711}$, that is, 5.041 for the full data set. When observations 2, 4, and 13 are omitted in turn, the hazard ratio for males relative to females is 4.138, 4.097 and 9.334, respectively. Omission of the data from patient number 13 appears to have a great effect on the estimated hazard ratio. However, some caution is needed in interpreting this result. Since there are very few males in the data set, the estimated hazard ratio is imprecisely estimated. In fact, a 95% confidence interval for the hazard ratio, when the data from patient 13 are omitted, ranges from 0.012 to 82.96!

4.3.3 Treatment of influential observations

Once observations have been found to be unduly influential, it is difficult to offer any firm advice on what should be done about them. So much depends on the scientific background to the study.

When possible, the origin of influential observations should be checked. Errors in transcribing and recording categorical and numerical data frequently occur. If any mistakes are found, the data need to be corrected and the analysis repeated. If the observed value of a survival time, or other explanatory variables, is unrealistic, and correction is not possible, the corresponding observation should be omitted from the database before repeating the analysis.

In many situations it will not be possible to confirm that the data corresponding to an influential observation are valid. Certainly, influential observations should not then be rejected outright. In these circumstances, the most appropriate course of action will be to establish the actual effect on the inferences to be drawn from the analysis. For example, if a median survival time is being used to summarise survival data, or a relative hazard is being used to summarise a treatment effect, the values of these statistics with and without the influential values can be contrasted. If the difference between the results is so small as to not be of practical importance, the queried observations can be retained. On the other hand, if the effect of removing the influential observations is large enough to be of practical importance, analyses based on both the full and reduced data sets will need to be reported. The outcome of consultations with the scientists involved in the study will then be a vital ingredient in the process of deciding on the course of future action.

Example 4.8 Survival of multiple myeloma patients

The effect of individual observations on the estimated values of the parameters of a Cox regression model fitted to the data from Example 1.3 will now be investigated. Plots of the approximate unstandardised delta-betas for *Hb* and *Bun* against the rank order of the survival times are shown in Figures 4.10 and 4.11.

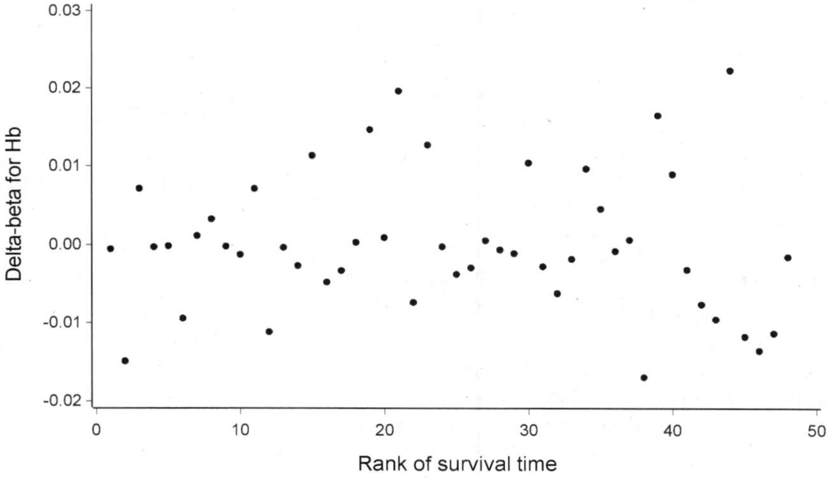

Figure 4.10 *Plot of the delta-betas for Hb against rank order of survival time.*

From Figure 4.10, no one observation stands out as having a delta-beta for *Hb* that is different from the rest. However, Figure 4.11 shows that the two observations with the shortest survival times have relatively large positive or large negative delta-betas for *Bun*. These correspond to patients 32 and 38 in the data given in Table 1.3. Patient 32 has a survival time of just one month, and the second largest value of *Bun*. Deletion of this observation from the database decreases the parameter estimate for *Bun*. Patient number 38 also survived for just one month after trial entry, but has a value of *Bun* that is

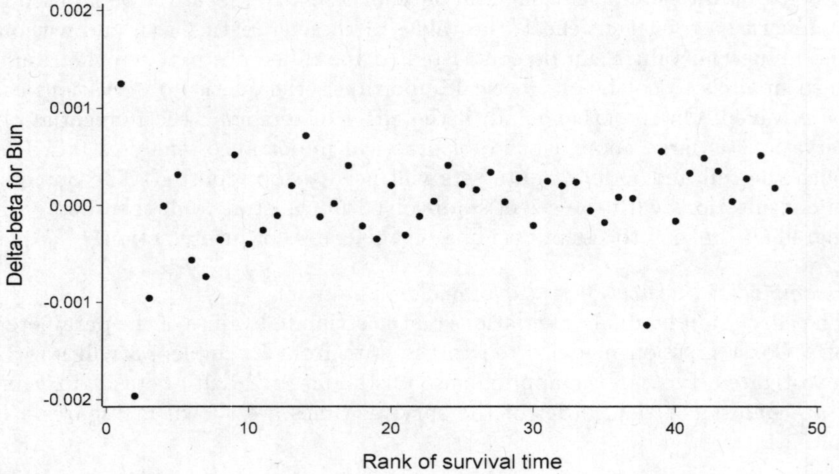

Figure 4.11 *Plot of the delta-betas for Bun against rank order of survival time.*

rather low for someone surviving for such a short time. If the data from this patient are omitted, the coefficient of *Bun* in the model is increased.

To identify observations that influence the set of parameter estimates, a plot of the absolute values of the elements of the diagnostic $\boldsymbol{l}_{\max}$ against the rank order of the survival times is shown in Figure 4.12.

The observation with the largest value of $|\boldsymbol{l}_{\max}|$ corresponds to patient 13. This patient has an unusually small value of *Hb*, and a value of *Bun* that is a little high, for someone who has survived as long as 65 months. If this observation is omitted from the data set, the coefficient of *Bun* remains the same, but that of *Hb* is reduced from -0.134 to -0.157. The effect of *Hb* on the hazard of death is then a little more significant. In summary, the record for patient 13 has little effect on the form of the estimated hazard function.

4.4 Testing the assumption of proportional hazards

So far in this chapter we have concentrated on how the adequacy of the linear component of a survival model can be examined. A crucial assumption made when using the Cox regression model is that of proportional hazards. Hazards are said to be proportional if ratios of hazards are independent of time. If there are one or more explanatory variables in the model whose coefficients vary with time, or if there are explanatory variables that are time-dependent, the proportional hazards assumption will be violated. We therefore require techniques that can be used to detect whether there is some form of time dependency in particular covariates, after allowing for the effects of explanatory variables that are known, or expected to be, independent of time.

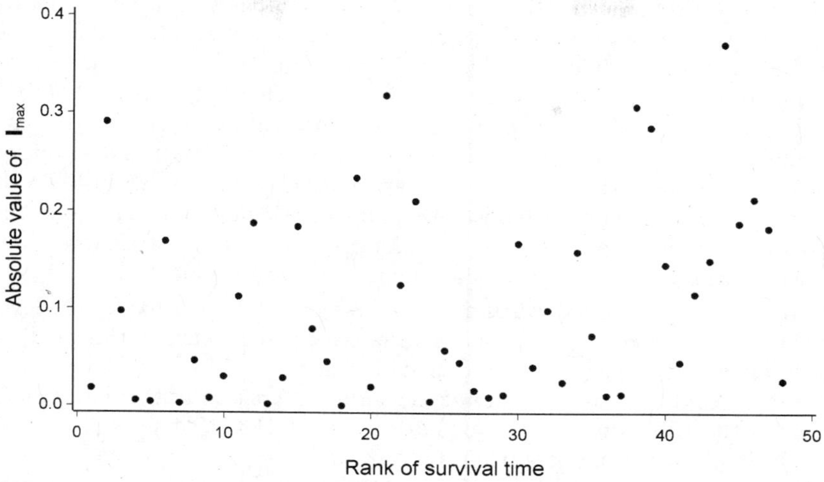

Figure 4.12 *Plot of the absolute values of the elements of* $\boldsymbol{l}_{\max}$ *against rank order of survival time.*

In this section, a straightforward plot that can be used in advance of model fitting is first described, and this is followed by a description of how diagnostics and test statistics derived from a fitted model can be used in examining the proportional hazards assumption.

4.4.1 The log-cumulative hazard plot

In the Cox regression model, the hazard of death at any time t for the ith of n individuals is given by

$$h_i(t) = \exp(\boldsymbol{\beta}'\boldsymbol{x}_i)h_0(t), \tag{4.16}$$

where $\boldsymbol{x}_i$ is the vector of values of explanatory variables for that individual, $\boldsymbol{\beta}$ is the corresponding vector of coefficients, and $h_0(t)$ is the baseline hazard function. Integrating both sides of this equation over t gives

$$\int_0^t h_i(u)\,\mathrm{d}u = \exp(\boldsymbol{\beta}'\boldsymbol{x}_i)\int_0^t h_0(u)\,\mathrm{d}u,$$

and so, using Equation (1.7),

$$H_i(t) = \exp(\boldsymbol{\beta}'\boldsymbol{x}_i)H_0(t),$$

where $H_i(t)$ and $H_0(t)$ are the cumulative hazard functions. Taking logarithms of each side of this equation, we get

$$\log H_i(t) = \boldsymbol{\beta}'\boldsymbol{x}_i + \log H_0(t),$$

from which it follows that differences in the log-cumulative hazard functions do not depend on time. This means that if the log-cumulative hazard functions for individuals with different values of their explanatory variables are plotted against time, the curves so formed will be parallel if the proportional hazards model in Equation (4.16) is valid. This provides the basis of a widely used diagnostic for assessing the validity of the proportional hazards assumption. It turns out that plotting the log-cumulative hazard functions against the logarithm of t, rather than t itself, is a useful diagnostic in parametric modelling, and so this form of plot is generally used; see Section 5.2 of Chapter 5 for further details on the use of this log-cumulative hazard plot.

To use this plot, the survival data are first grouped according to the levels of one or more factors. If continuous variables are to feature in this analysis, their values will first need to be grouped in some way to give a categorical variable. The Kaplan-Meier estimate of the survivor function of the data in each group is then obtained. A log-cumulative hazard plot, that is, a plot of the logarithm of the estimated cumulative hazard function against the logarithm of the survival time, will yield parallel curves if the hazards are proportional across the different groups. This method is informative, and simple to operate when there is a small number of factors, and a reasonable number of observations at each level. On the other hand, the plot will be based on very few observations at the later survival times, and in more highly structured data sets, a different approach needs to be taken.

Example 4.9 Survival of multiple myeloma patients
We again use the data on the survival times of 48 patients with multiple myeloma to illustrate the log-cumulative hazard plot. In particular we will investigate whether the assumption of proportional hazards is valid for the variable *Hb*, which is associated with the serum haemoglobin level. Because this is a continuous variable, we first need to categorise the values of *Hb*. This will be done in the same manner as in Example 3.8 of Chapter 3, where four groups were defined with values of *Hb* which are such that $Hb \leqslant 7$, $7 < Hb \leqslant 10$, $10 < Hb \leqslant 13$ and $Hb > 13$. The patients are then grouped according to their haemoglobin level, and the Kaplan-Meier estimate of the survivor function is obtained for each of the four groups. From this estimate, the estimated log-cumulative hazard is formed using the relation $\hat{H}(t) = -\log \hat{S}(t)$, from Equation (1.8) of Chapter 1, and plotted against the values of $\log t$. The resulting log-cumulative hazard plot is shown in Figure 4.13.

This figure indicates that the plots for $Hb \leqslant 7$, $7 < Hb \leqslant 10$ and $Hb > 13$ are roughly parallel. The plot for $10 < Hb \leqslant 13$ is not in line with the others, although this impression results from relatively large cumulative hazard estimates at the longest survival times experienced by patients in this group. This plot takes no account of the values of the other variable, *Bun*, and it could be that the survival times of the individuals in the third *Hb* group have been affected by their *Bun* values. Overall, there is little reason to doubt the proportional hazards assumption.

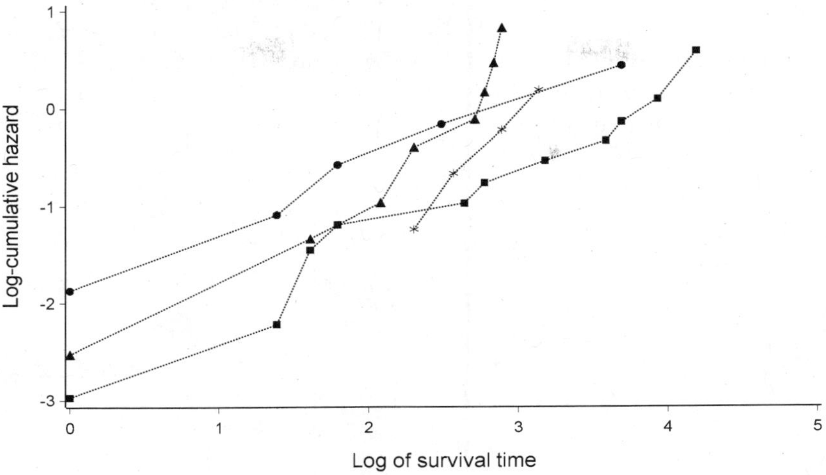

Figure 4.13 *Log-cumulative hazard plot for multiple myeloma patients in four groups defined by Hb* $\leqslant 7$ *(●),* $7 <$ *Hb* $\leqslant 10$ *(■),* $10 <$ *Hb* $\leqslant 13$ *(▲) and Hb* > 13 *(∗).*

4.4.2 Use of Schoenfeld residuals*

The Schoenfeld residuals, defined in Section 4.1.5, are particularly useful in evaluating the assumption of proportional hazards after fitting a Cox regression model. Grambsch and Therneau (1994) have shown that the expected value of the ith scaled Schoenfeld residual, $i = 1, 2, \ldots, n$, for the jth explanatory variable in the model, X_j, $j = 1, 2, \ldots, p$, denoted r^*_{Sji}, is given by

$$\mathrm{E}\,(r^*_{Sji}) \approx \beta_j(t_i) - \hat{\beta}_j, \tag{4.17}$$

where $\beta_j(t)$ is taken to be a time-varying coefficient of X_j, $\beta_j(t_i)$ is the value of this coefficient at the survival time of the ith individual, t_i, and $\hat{\beta}_j$ is the estimated value of β_j in the fitted Cox regression model. Note that these residuals are only defined at death times.

Equation (4.17) suggests that a plot of the values of $r^*_{Sji} + \hat{\beta}_j$, or equivalently just the scaled Schoenfeld residuals, r^*_{Sji}, against the observed survival times should give information about the form of the time-dependent coefficient of X_j, $\beta_j(t)$. In particular, a horizontal line will suggest that the coefficient of X_j is constant, and the proportional hazards assumption is satisfied. A smoothed curve can be superimposed on this plot to aid interpretation, as in the plots of martingale residuals against the values of explanatory variables in Section 4.2.3.

Example 4.10 Infection in patients on dialysis

The data on catheter removal times for patients on dialysis, first given in Example 4.1, are now used to illustrate the use of the scaled Schoenfeld residuals in assessing non-proportional hazards. The scaled Schoenfeld residuals for the variables *Age* and *Sex* were given in Table 4.2, and plotting these values against the removal times gives the graphs shown in Figure 4.14. The smoothed curves deviate little from horizontal lines, and in neither plot is there any suggestion of non-proportional hazards.

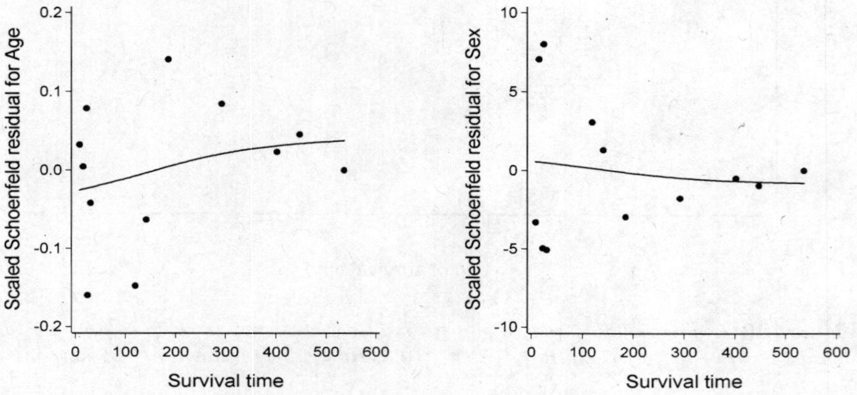

Figure 4.14 *Plot of scaled Schoenfeld residuals for Age and Sex.*

4.4.3 Tests for non-proportional hazards*

The graphical method for assessing the assumption of proportional hazards, described in Section 4.4.2, leads to a formal test procedure. From the result given in Equation (4.17), the expected value of the ith scaled Schoenfeld residual, $i = 1, 2, \ldots, n$, for the jth explanatory variable, X_j, $j = 1, 2, \ldots, p$, depends on $\beta_j(t_i)$, the value of a time-varying coefficient of X_j at time t_i. A test of the proportional hazards assumption can then be based on testing whether there is a linear relationship between $\mathrm{E}\,(r^*_{Sji})$ and some function of time. If there is evidence that $\mathrm{E}\,(r^*_{Sji})$ is time-dependent, the hypothesis of proportional hazards would be rejected.

For a particular explanatory variable X_j, linear dependence of the coefficient of X_j on time can be expressed by taking $\beta_j(t_i) = \beta_j + \nu_j(t_i - \bar{t})$, where ν_j is an unknown regression coefficient. This leads to a linear regression model with $\mathrm{E}\,(r^*_{Sji}) = \nu_j(t_i - \bar{t})$, and a test of whether the slope ν_j is zero leads to a test of whether the coefficient of X_j is time-dependent and hence of proportional hazards with respect to X_j. Letting $\tau_i, \tau_2, \ldots, \tau_d$ be the d observed death times across all n individuals in the data set, Grambsch and Therneau (1994) show that an appropriate test statistic is

$$\frac{\{\sum_{i=1}^{d}(\tau_i - \bar{\tau})r^*_{Sji}\}^2}{d\,\mathrm{var}\,(\hat{\beta}_j)\sum_{i=1}^{d}(\tau_i - \bar{\tau})^2}, \tag{4.18}$$

where $\bar{\tau} = d^{-1} \sum_{i=1}^{d} \tau_i$ is the sample mean of the observed death times. Under the null hypothesis that the slope is zero, this statistic has a χ^2 distribution on 1 d.f., and significantly large values of Expression (4.18) lead to rejection of the proportional hazards assumption for the jth explanatory variable.

An overall or global test of the proportional hazards assumption across all the p explanatory variables included in a Cox regression model is obtained by aggregating the individual test statistics in Expression (4.18). This leads to the statistic

$$\frac{(\boldsymbol{\tau} - \bar{\tau})' \boldsymbol{S} \operatorname{var}(\hat{\boldsymbol{\beta}}) \boldsymbol{S}' (\boldsymbol{\tau} - \bar{\tau})}{\sum_{i=1}^{d} (\tau_i - \bar{\tau})^2 / d}, \tag{4.19}$$

where $\boldsymbol{\tau} = (\tau_1, \tau_2, \ldots, \tau_d)'$ is the vector formed from the d event times and $\boldsymbol{S}$ is the $d \times p$ matrix whose columns are the (unscaled) Schoenfeld residuals for the j explanatory variable, so that $\boldsymbol{S} = (r_{Sj1}, r_{Sj2}, \ldots, r_{Sjd})'$, and $\operatorname{var}(\hat{\boldsymbol{\beta}})$ is the variance-covariance matrix of the estimated coefficients of the explanatory variables in the fitted Cox regression model. The test statistic in Expression (4.19) has a χ^2 distribution on p d.f. when the assumption of proportional hazards across all p explanatory variables is true. This test is known as the *Grambsch and Therneau test of proportional hazards*, and is sometimes more enigmatically referred to as the *zph* test.

The test statistics in Expressions (4.18) and (4.19) can be adapted to other time-scales by replacing the τ_i, $i = 1, 2, \ldots, d$, by transformed values of the death times. For example, using logarithms of the death times, rather than the times themselves, would allow linearity in the coefficient of X_j to be assessed on a logarithmic scale. The τ_i can also be replaced by the rank order of the death times, or by the Kaplan-Meier estimate of the survivor function at each event time. Plots of scaled Schoenfeld residuals against time, discussed in Section 4.4.2, may indicate which of these possible options is the most appropriate.

Example 4.11 Infection in patients on dialysis

We now illustrate tests of proportional hazards using the data on catheter removal times for patients on dialysis. The variances of the estimated coefficients of the variables *Age* and *Sex* in the fitted Cox regression model are 0.000688 and 1.20099, respectively, the sum of squares of the 12 event times is 393418.92, and the numerator of Expression (4.18) is calculated from the scaled Schoenfeld residuals in Table 4.2. The values of the test statistic are 0.811 ($P = 0.368$) and 0.224 ($P = 0.636$) for *Age* and *Sex*, respectively. In neither case is there evidence against the proportional hazards assumption, as might have been expected from the graphical analysis in Example 4.10.

Matrix multiplication is required to obtain the numerator of the global test for proportional hazards in Expression (4.19), and leads to 26578.805, from which the Grambsch and Therneau test statistic is 0.811. This has a χ^2 distribution on 2 d.f. leading to a P-value of 0.667. Again there is no reason to doubt the validity of the proportional hazards assumption.

4.4.4* *Adding a time-dependent variable*

Specific forms of departure from proportional hazards can be investigated by adding a *time-dependent variable* to the Cox regression model. Full details on the use of time-dependent variables in modelling survival data are given in Chapter 8, but in this section, the procedure is described in a particular context.

Consider a survival study in which each patient has been allocated to one of two groups, corresponding to a standard treatment and a new treatment. Interest may then centre on whether the ratio of the hazard of death at time t in one treatment group relative to the other, is independent of survival time. A proportional hazards model for the hazard function of the ith individual in the study is then

$$h_i(t) = \exp(\beta_1 x_{1i}) h_0(t), \tag{4.20}$$

where x_{1i} is the value of an indicator variable X_1 that is zero for the standard treatment and unity for the new treatment. The relative hazard of death at any time for a patient on the new treatment, relative to one on the standard, is then e^{β_1}, which is independent of the survival time.

Now define a time-dependent explanatory variable X_2, where $X_2 = X_1 t$. If this variable is added to the model in Equation (4.20), the hazard of death at time t for the ith individual becomes

$$h_i(t) = \exp(\beta_1 x_{1i} + \beta_2 x_{2i}) h_0(t), \tag{4.21}$$

where $x_{2i} = x_{1i} t$ is the value of $X_1 t$ for the ith individual. The relative hazard at time t is now

$$\exp(\beta_1 + \beta_2 t), \tag{4.22}$$

since $X_2 = t$ under the new treatment, and zero otherwise. This hazard ratio depends on t, and the model in Equation (4.21) is no longer a proportional hazards model. In particular, if $\beta_2 < 0$, the relative hazard decreases with time. This means that the hazard of death on the new treatment, relative to that on the standard, decreases with time. If $\beta_1 < 0$, the superiority of the new treatment becomes more apparent as time goes on. On the other hand, if $\beta_2 > 0$, the relative hazard of death on the new treatment increases with time, reflecting an increasing risk of death on the new treatment relative to the standard. In the particular case where $\beta_2 = 0$, the relative hazard is constant at e^{β_1}. This means that a test of the hypothesis that $\beta_2 = 0$ is a test of the assumption of proportional hazards. The situation is illustrated in Figure 4.15.

In order to aid both the computation and interpretation of the parameters in the model of Equation (4.21), the variable X_2 can be defined in terms of the deviation from some time, t_0. The estimated values of β_1 and β_2 will then tend to be less highly correlated, and the numerical algorithm for maximising the appropriate likelihood function will be more stable. If X_2 is taken to be

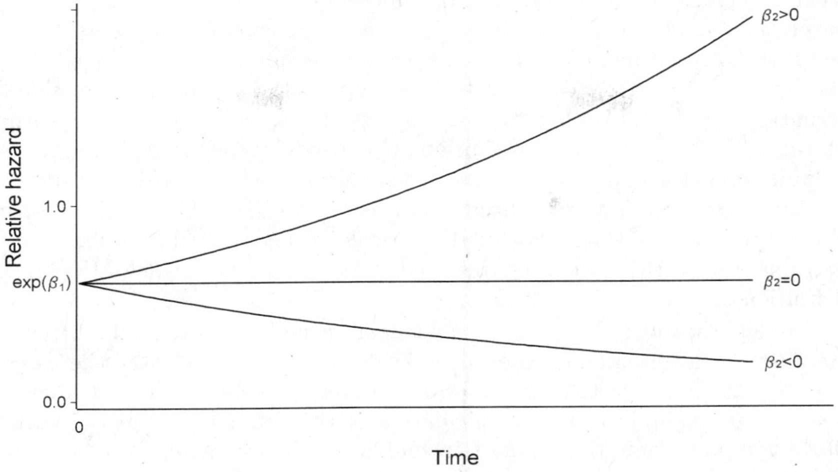

Figure 4.15 *Plot of the relative hazard,* $\exp(\beta_1 + \beta_2 t)$, *against t, for different values of* β_2.

such that $X_2 = X_1(t - t_0)$, the value of X_2 is $t - t_0$ for the new treatment and zero for the standard. The relative hazard now becomes

$$\exp\{\beta_1 + \beta_2(t - t_0)\}.$$

In the model of Equation (4.21), with $x_{2i} = x_{1i}(t - t_0)$, the quantity e^{β_1} is the hazard of death at time t_0 for an individual on the new treatment relative to one on the standard. In practical applications, t_0 will generally be chosen to provide a convenient interpretation for the time at which this relative hazard is applicable. For example, taking t_0 to be the mean or median survival time means that $\exp(\hat{\beta}_1)$ is the estimated relative hazard of death at this time.

A similar model can be used to detect whether the coefficient of a continuous variate has a coefficient that depends on time. Suppose that X is such a variate, and we wish to examine whether there is any evidence that the coefficient of X is linearly dependent on time. To do this, the term Xt is added to the model that includes X. The hazard of death at time t for the ith individual is then

$$h_i(t) = \exp(\beta_1 x_i + \beta_2 x_i t) h_0(t),$$

where x_i is the value of X for that individual. The hazard of death at time t for an individual for whom $X = x_i + 1$, relative to an individual for whom $X = x_i$, is then $\exp(\beta_1 + \beta_2 t)$, as in Equation (4.22).

The time-dependent variables considered in this section are such that their coefficients are linearly dependent on time. A similar approach can be used when a coefficient that is a non-linear function of time is anticipated. For example, $\log t$ might be used in place of t in the definition of the time-dependent variable X_2, used in Equation (4.21). In this version of the model, a test of the hypothesis that $\beta_2 = 0$ is a test of proportional hazards, where the alternative hypothesis is that the hazard ratio is dependent on the logarithm of time. Using $\log t$ in the definition of a time-dependent variable is also helpful when the numerical values of the survival times are large, such as when survival in a long-term study is measured in days. There may then be computational problems associated with calculating the value of $\exp(\beta_2 x_{2i})$ in Equation (4.21), which are resolved by using $\log t$ in place of t in the definition of X_2.

Models that include the time-dependent variable X_2 cannot be fitted by treating X_2 in the same manner as other explanatory variables in the model. The reason for this is that this variable will have different values at different death times, complicating the calculation of the denominator of the partial likelihood function in Equation (3.4). Full details on the fitting process will be deferred to Chapter 8. However, inferences about the effect of time-dependent variables on the hazard function can be evaluated as for other variables. In particular, the change in the value of the $-2 \log \hat{L}$ statistic can be compared to percentage points of the chi-squared distribution to test the significance of the variable. This is therefore a formal test of proportional hazards.

Example 4.12 Infection in patients on dialysis
The data on catheter removal times, used in Examples 4.10 and 4.11, will now be used to illustrate how the proportional hazards assumption can be tested using time-dependent variates.

We begin by fitting the Cox regression model containing just *Age* and *Sex*, which leads to a value of $-2 \log \hat{L}$ of 34.468. We now define terms that are the products of these variables with time, namely $Tage = Age \times t$ and $Tsex = Sex \times t$. These variables are then added to the model. Note that we cannot simply form these products from the observed survival times of the patients, since the model-fitting process requires that these values be computed for different values of t; see Chapter 8 for details on this.

When the variable *Tage* is added to the model that contains *Age* and *Sex*, the value of $-2 \log \hat{L}$ reduces to 32.006, but this reduction is not significant at the 5% level ($P = 0.117$). The reduction in $-2 \log \hat{L}$ when *Tsex* is added to the model that has *Age* and *Sex* is only 0.364 ($P = 0.546$). This analysis confirms that there is no reason to doubt the assumption of proportional hazards in respect of the variables *Age* and *Sex*.

4.5 Recommendations

In this chapter, a variety of diagnostics have been presented. Which should be used on a routine basis and which are needed when a more thorough assessment of model adequacy is required?

In terms of assessing the overall fit of a model, a plot of the deviance residuals against the risk score gives information on observations that are not well fitted by the model, and their relation to the set of values of the explanatory variables. This diagnostic is generally more informative than the cumulative, or log-cumulative, hazard plot of the Cox-Snell residuals. Plots of residuals against the survival times, the rank order of the survival times, or explanatory variables may also be useful.

Plots of residuals might be supplemented by influence diagnostics. When the inference to be drawn from a model centres on one or two particular parameters, the delta-beta statistic for those parameters, will be the most relevant. Plots of these values against the rank order of survival times will then be useful. To investigate whether there are observations that have an influence on the set of parameter estimates, or risk score, the diagnostic based on the absolute values of the elements of $\boldsymbol{l}_{\max}$ is probably the most suitable. Plots of these values against the rank order of survival times will be informative, but plots against particular explanatory variables might also be revealing. An initial assessment of the validity of the proportional hazards assumption can be made from log-cumulative hazard plots. However, plots based on the scaled Schoenfeld residuals, and associated tests of non-proportionality are more helpful. The Grambsch and Therneau test can be used for an overall test of the proportional hazards assumption.

Once a suitable model has been determined, and satisfactory results have been obtained from the model checking process, the final stage in the model building process is to review the model critically, in conjunction with subject matter experts. This may lead to further revisions to the model to ensure that it will be accepted as an appropriate summary of the underlying survival data.

4.6 Further reading

General introductions to model checking in linear models are included in Draper and Smith (1998) and Montgomery, Peck and Vining (2012). Cook and Weisberg (1982) give a more detailed account of the theory underlying residuals and influence diagnostics in a number of situations. Atkinson (1985) describes model checking in linear models from a practical viewpoint, and McCullagh and Nelder (1989) and Aitkin et al. (1989) discuss this topic in the context of generalised linear models.

Many textbooks devoted to the analysis of survival data, and particularly those of Cox and Oakes (1984), Hosmer, Lemeshow and May (2008), Lawless (2002), and Kalbfleisch and Prentice (2002), include sections on the use of residuals. Hinkley, Reid and Snell (1991) and Hastie and Tibshirani (1990) also include brief discussions on methods for assessing the adequacy of models fitted to survival data.

Early articles on the use of residuals in checking the adequacy of survival models include Kay (1977) and Crowley and Hu (1977). These papers include a discussion on the Cox-Snell residuals, which are based on the general definition of residuals given by Cox and Snell (1968). Crowley and Storer (1983) showed empirically that the cumulative hazard plot of the residuals is not particularly good at identifying inadequacies in the fitted model. See also Crowley and Storer (1983) for a practical application of the methods. Reviews of diagnostic procedures in survival analysis were given in the mid-1980s by Kay (1984) and Day (1985).

Martingale residuals were proposed by Barlow and Prentice (1988). Essentially the same residuals were proposed by Lagakos (1981) and their use is discussed by Therneau, Grambsch and Fleming (1990) and Henderson and Milner (1991). Deviance residuals were also introduced in Therneau, Grambsch and Fleming (1990). The Schoenfeld residuals for the Cox model were proposed by Schoenfeld (1982). In accounts of survival analysis based on the theory of counting processes, Fleming and Harrington (2005) and Therneau and Grambsch (2000) show how different types of residual can be used, and give detailed practical examples. Two other types of residual, introduced by Nardi and Schemper (1999), are particularly suitable for the detection of outlying survival times.

Influence diagnostics for the Cox regression model have been considered by many authors, but the major papers are those of Cain and Lange (1984), Reid and Crépeau (1985), Storer and Crowley (1985), Pettitt and Bin Daud (1989) and Weissfeld (1990). Pettitt and Bin Daud (1990) show how time-dependence in the Cox proportional hazards model can be detected by smoothing the Schoenfeld residuals. The LOWESS smoother was introduced by Cleveland (1979), and the algorithm is also presented in Collett (2003).

Some other graphical methods for evaluating survival models, not mentioned in this chapter, have been proposed by Cox (1979) and Arjas (1988). Gray (1990) describes the use of smoothed estimates of cumulative hazard functions in evaluating the fit of a Cox model.

Most of the diagnostic procedures presented in this chapter rely on an informal evaluation of tabular or graphical presentations of particular statistics. In addition to these procedures, a variety of significance tests have been proposed that can be used to assess the goodness of fit of the model. Examples include the methods of Schoenfeld (1980), Andersen (1982), Nagelkerke, Oosting and Hart (1984), Ciampi and Etezadi-Amoli (1985), Moreau, O'Quigley and Mesbah (1985), Gill and Schumacher (1987), O'Quigley and Pessione (1989), Quantin et al. (1996), Grønnesby and Borgan (1996), and Verweij, van Houwelingen and Stijnen (1998). Reviews of some of these goodness of fit tests for the Cox regression model are included in Lin and Wei (1991) and Quantin et al. (1996). Many of these tests involve statistics that are quite complicated, and the procedures are not widely available in computer software for survival analysis. A more simple procedure for evaluating the overall fit of a model has been proposed by May and Hosmer (1998).

Chapter 5

Parametric proportional hazards models

When the Cox regression model is used in the analysis of survival data, there is no need to assume a particular form of probability distribution for the survival times. As a result, the hazard function is not restricted to a specific functional form, and the model has flexibility and widespread applicability. On the other hand, if the assumption of a particular probability distribution for the data is valid, inferences based on such an assumption will be more precise. In particular, estimates of quantities such as relative hazards and median survival times will tend to have smaller standard errors than they would in the absence of a distributional assumption. Models in which a specific probability distribution is assumed for the survival times are known as *parametric models*, and parametric versions of the proportional hazards model, described in Chapter 3, are the subject of this chapter.

A probability distribution that plays a central role in the analysis of survival data is the Weibull distribution, introduced by W. Weibull in 1951 in the context of industrial reliability testing. Indeed, this distribution is as central to the parametric analysis of survival data as the normal distribution is in linear modelling. Proportional hazards models based on the Weibull distribution are therefore considered in some detail.

5.1 Models for the hazard function

Once a distributional model for survival times has been specified in terms of a probability density function, the corresponding survivor and hazard functions can be obtained from the relations

$$S(t) = 1 - \int_0^t f(u)\,\mathrm{d}u,$$

and

$$h(t) = \frac{f(t)}{S(t)} = -\frac{\mathrm{d}}{\mathrm{d}t}\{\log S(t)\},$$

where $f(t)$ is the probability density function of the survival times. These relationships were derived in Section 1.3. An alternative approach is to specify a functional form for the hazard function, from which the survivor function and probability density functions can be determined from the equations

$$S(t) = \exp\{-H(t)\}, \tag{5.1}$$

and

$$f(t) = h(t)S(t) = -\frac{\mathrm{d}S(t)}{\mathrm{d}t},$$

where

$$H(t) = \int_0^t h(u)\,\mathrm{d}u$$

is the integrated hazard function.

5.1.1 *The exponential distribution*

The simplest model for the hazard function is to assume that it is constant over time. The hazard of death at any time after the time origin of the study is then the same, irrespective of the time that has elapsed. Under this model, the hazard function may be written as

$$h(t) = \lambda,$$

for $0 \leqslant t < \infty$. The parameter λ is a positive constant that can be estimated by fitting the model to observed survival data. From Equation (5.1), the corresponding survivor function is

$$\begin{aligned} S(t) &= \exp\left\{-\int_0^t \lambda\,\mathrm{d}u\right\}, \\ &= e^{-\lambda t}, \end{aligned} \tag{5.2}$$

and so the implied probability density function of the survival times is

$$f(t) = \lambda e^{-\lambda t}, \tag{5.3}$$

for $0 \leqslant t < \infty$. This is the probability density function of a random variable T that has an *exponential distribution* with a mean of λ^{-1}. It is sometimes convenient to write $\mu = \lambda^{-1}$, so that the hazard function is μ^{-1}, and the survival time distribution has a mean of μ. However, the former specification of the hazard function will generally be used in this book.

The median of the exponential distribution, $t(50)$, is such that $S\{t(50)\} = 0.5$, that is,

$$\exp\{-\lambda t(50)\} = 0.5,$$

so that

$$t(50) = \frac{1}{\lambda}\log 2.$$

More generally, the pth percentile of the survival time distribution is the value $t(p)$ such that $S\{t(p)\} = 1 - (p/100)$, and using Equation (5.2), this is

$$t(p) = \frac{1}{\lambda} \log \left(\frac{100}{100 - p} \right).$$

A plot of the hazard function for three values of λ, namely 1.0, 0.1 and 0.01, is given in Figure 5.1, and the corresponding probability density functions are shown in Figure 5.2. For these values of λ, the means of the corresponding exponential distributions are 1, 10 and 100, and the median survival times are 0.69, 6.93 and 69.31, respectively.

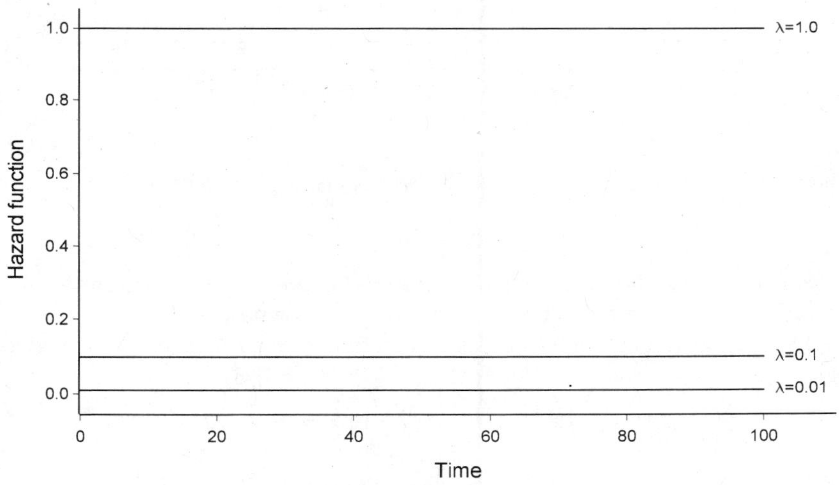

Figure 5.1 *Hazard functions for exponential distributions with* $\lambda =$ *1.0, 0.1 and 0.01.*

5.1.2 *The Weibull distribution*

In practice, the assumption of a constant hazard function, or equivalently of exponentially distributed survival times, is rarely tenable. A more general form of hazard function is such that

$$h(t) = \lambda\gamma t^{\gamma-1}, \tag{5.4}$$

for $0 \leqslant t < \infty$, a function that depends on two parameters λ and γ, which are both greater than zero. In the particular case where $\gamma = 1$, the hazard function takes a constant value λ, and the survival times have an exponential distribution. For other values of γ, the hazard function increases or decreases monotonically, that is, it does not change direction. The shape of the hazard function depends critically on the value of γ, and so γ is known as the *shape*

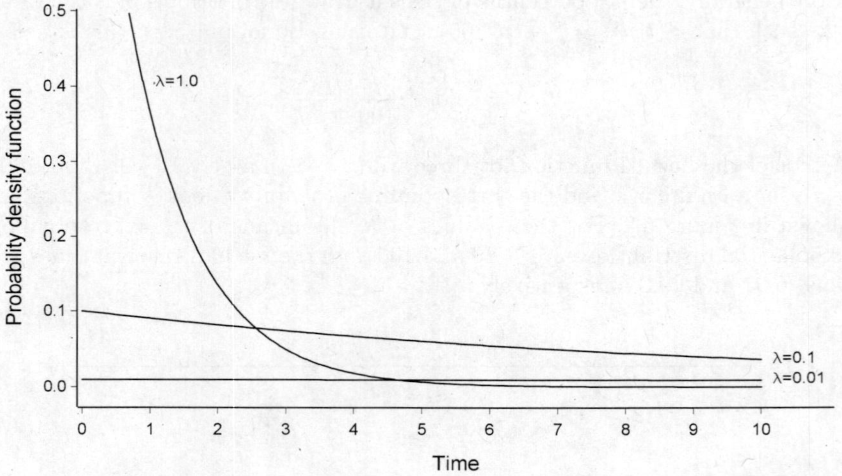

Figure 5.2 *Probability density functions for exponential distributions with* $\lambda =$ *1.0, 0.1 and 0.01.*

parameter, while the parameter λ is a *scale parameter*. The general form of this hazard function for different values of γ is shown in Figure 5.3.

For this particular choice of hazard function, the survivor function is given by

$$S(t) = \exp\left\{-\int_0^t \lambda\gamma u^{\gamma-1}\,\mathrm{d}u\right\} = \exp(-\lambda t^{\gamma}). \tag{5.5}$$

The corresponding probability density function is then

$$f(t) = \lambda\gamma t^{\gamma-1}\exp(-\lambda t^{\gamma}),$$

for $0 \leqslant t < \infty$, which is the density of a random variable that has a *Weibull distribution* with scale parameter λ and shape parameter γ. This distribution will be denoted $W(\lambda, \gamma)$. The right-hand tail of this distribution is longer than the left-hand one, and so the distribution is positively skewed.

The mean, or expected value, of a random variable T that has a $W(\lambda, \gamma)$ distribution can be shown to be given by

$$\mathrm{E}\,(T) = \lambda^{-1/\gamma}\Gamma(\gamma^{-1} + 1),$$

where $\Gamma(x)$ is the gamma function defined by the integral

$$\Gamma(x) = \int_0^\infty u^{x-1}e^{-u}\,\mathrm{d}u.$$

The value of this integral is $(x-1)!$, and so for integer values of x it can easily

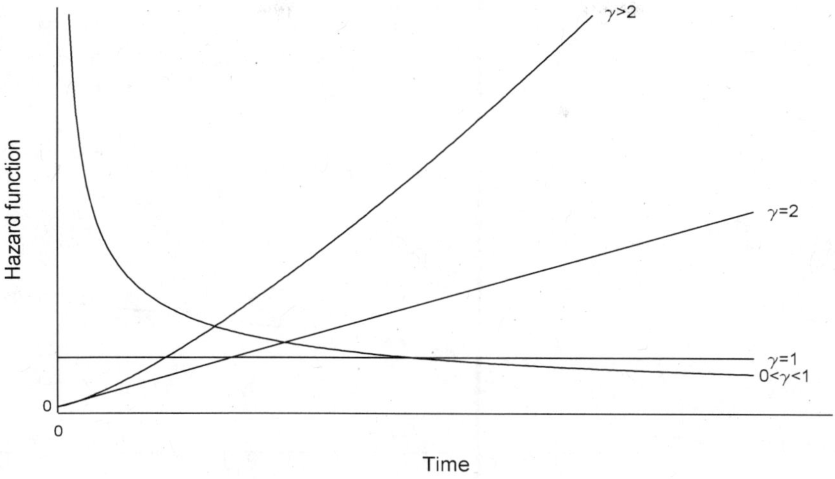

Figure 5.3 *The form of the Weibull hazard function,* $h(t) = \lambda\gamma t^{\gamma-1}$*, for different values of* γ*.*

be calculated. The function is also defined for non-integer values of x, and can then be evaluated as a standard function in many software packages.

Since the Weibull distribution is skewed, a more appropriate, and more tractable, summary of the location of the distribution is the median survival time. This is the value $t(50)$ such that $S\{t(50)\} = 0.5$, so that

$$\exp\{-\lambda[t(50)]^{\gamma}\} = 0.5,$$

and

$$t(50) = \left\{\frac{1}{\lambda}\log 2\right\}^{1/\gamma}.$$

More generally, the pth percentile of the Weibull distribution, $t(p)$, is such that

$$t(p) = \left\{\frac{1}{\lambda}\log\left(\frac{100}{100-p}\right)\right\}^{1/\gamma}. \tag{5.6}$$

The median and other percentiles of the Weibull distribution are therefore much simpler to compute than the mean of the distribution.

The hazard function and corresponding probability density function for Weibull distributions with a median of 20, and shape parameters $\gamma = 0.5$, 1.5 and 3.0, are shown in Figures 5.4 and 5.5, respectively. The corresponding value of the scale parameter, λ, for these three Weibull distributions is 0.15, 0.0078 and 0.000087, respectively.

Since the Weibull hazard function can take a variety of forms, depending on the value of the shape parameter, γ, and appropriate summary statistics can

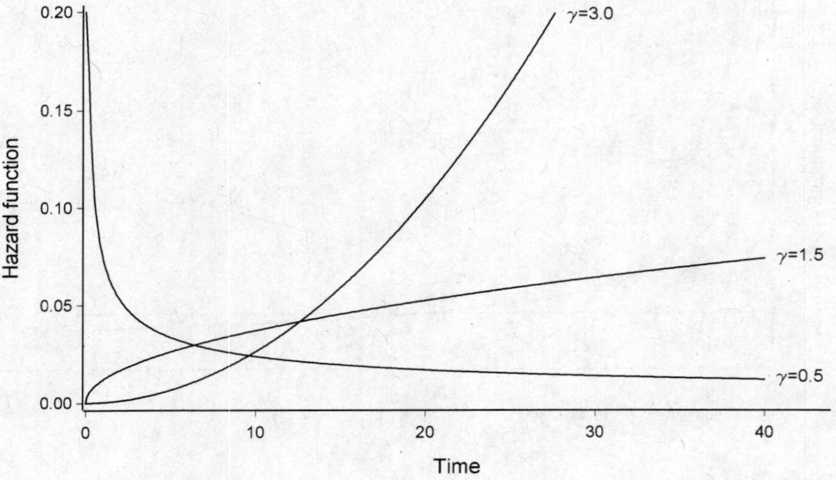

Figure 5.4 *Hazard functions for a Weibull distribution with a median of 20 and* $\gamma =$ *0.5, 1.5 and 3.0.*

Figure 5.5 *Probability density functions for a Weibull distribution with a median of 20 and* $\gamma =$ *0.5, 1.5 and 3.0.*

be easily obtained, this distribution is widely used in the parametric analysis of survival data.

5.2 Assessing the suitability of a parametric model

Prior to fitting a model based on an assumed parametric form for the hazard function, a preliminary study of the validity of this assumption should be carried out. One approach would be to estimate the hazard function using the methods outlined in Section 2.3. If the hazard function was reasonably constant over time, this would indicate that the exponential distribution might be a suitable model for the data. On the other hand, if the hazard function increased or decreased monotonically with increasing survival time, a model based on the Weibull distribution would be indicated.

A more informative way of assessing whether a particular distribution for the survival times is plausible is to compare the survivor function for the data with that of a chosen model. This is greatly helped by transforming the survivor function to produce a plot that should give a straight line if the assumed model is appropriate.

Suppose that a single sample of survival data is available, and that a Weibull distribution for the survival times is contemplated. Since the survivor function for a Weibull distribution, with scale parameter λ and shape parameter γ, is given by

$$S(t) = \exp\{-\lambda t^{\gamma}\},$$

taking the logarithm of $S(t)$, multiplying by -1, and taking logarithms a second time, gives

$$\log\{-\log S(t)\} = \log \lambda + \gamma \log t. \tag{5.7}$$

We now substitute the Kaplan-Meier estimate of the survivor function, $\hat{S}(t)$, for $S(t)$ in Equation (5.7). If the Weibull assumption is tenable, $\hat{S}(t)$ will be 'close' to $S(t)$, and a plot of $\log\{-\log \hat{S}(t)\}$ against $\log t$ would then give an approximately straight line. From Equation (1.8), the cumulative hazard function, $H(t)$, is $-\log S(t)$ and so $\log\{-\log S(t)\}$ is the log-cumulative hazard. A plot of the values of $\log\{-\log \hat{S}(t)\}$ against $\log t$ is a log-cumulative hazard plot, introduced in Section 4.4.1 of Chapter 4.

If the log-cumulative hazard plot gives a straight line, the plot can be used to provide a rough estimate of the two parameters of the Weibull distribution. Specifically, from Equation (5.7), the intercept and slope of the straight line will be $\log \lambda$ and γ, respectively. Thus, the slope of the line in a log-cumulative hazard plot gives an estimate of the shape parameter, and the exponent of the intercept provides an estimate of the scale parameter. Note that if the slope of the log-cumulative hazard plot is close to unity, the survival times could be modelled using an exponential distribution.

Example 5.1 Time to discontinuation of the use of an IUD
In Example 2.3, the Kaplan-Meier estimate of the survivor function, $\hat{S}(t)$, for

the data on the time to discontinuation of an intrauterine device was obtained. A log-cumulative hazard plot for these data, that is, a plot of $\log\{-\log \hat{S}(t)\}$ against $\log t$, is shown in Figure 5.6.

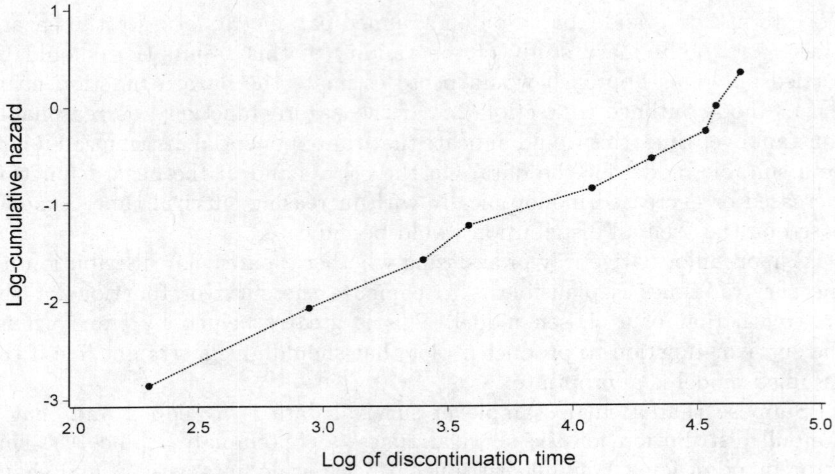

Figure 5.6 *Log-cumulative hazard plot for the data from Example 1.1.*

The plot indicates that there is a straight line relationship between the log-cumulative hazard and $\log t$, confirming that the Weibull distribution is an appropriate model for the discontinuation times. From the graph, the intercept of the line is approximately -6.0 and the slope is approximately 1.25. Approximate estimates of the parameters of the Weibull distribution are therefore $\lambda^* = \exp(-6.0) = 0.002$ and $\gamma^* = 1.25$. The estimated value of γ, the shape parameter of the Weibull distribution, is quite close to unity, suggesting that the discontinuation times might be adequately modelled by an exponential distribution.

These informal estimates of λ and γ can be used to estimate the parameters of the distribution, and hence functions of these estimates, such as the median of the survival time distribution. However, this graphical approach does not lead to a measure of the precision with which the quantities have been estimated. In view of this limitation, a more formal way of fitting parametric models to survival data is developed in the next section.

5.3 Fitting a parametric model to a single sample

Parametric models can be fitted to an observed set of survival data using the method of maximum likelihood, outlined in Section 3.3. Consider first the situation where actual survival times have been observed for n individuals, so that there are no censored observations. If the probability density function of the random variable associated with survival time is $f(t)$, the likelihood of the n observations $t_1, t_2, \ldots, t_n$ is simply the product

$$\prod_{i=1}^{n} f(t_i).$$

This likelihood will be a function of the unknown parameters in the probability density function, and the maximum likelihood estimates of these parameters are those values for which the likelihood function is a maximum. In practice, it is generally more convenient to work with the logarithm of the likelihood function. Those values of the unknown parameters in the density function that maximise the log-likelihood are of course the same values that maximise the likelihood function itself.

We now consider the more usual situation where the survival data includes one or more censored survival times. Specifically, suppose that r of the n individuals die at times $t_1, t_2, \ldots, t_r$, and that the survival times of the remaining $n - r$ individuals, $t_1^*, t_2^*, \ldots, t_{n-r}^*$, are right-censored. The r death times contribute a term of the form

$$\prod_{j=1}^{r} f(t_j)$$

to the overall likelihood function. Naturally, we cannot ignore information about the survival experience of the $n - r$ individuals for whom a censored survival time has been recorded. If a survival time is censored at time t^*, say, we know that the lifetime of the individual is at least t^*, and the probability of this event is $\mathrm{P}(T \geqslant t^*)$, which is $S(t^*)$. Thus, each censored observation contributes a term of this form to the likelihood of the n observations. The total likelihood function is therefore

$$\prod_{j=1}^{r} f(t_j) \prod_{l=1}^{n-r} S(t_l^*), \tag{5.8}$$

in which the first product is taken over the r death times and the second over the $n - r$ censored survival times.

More compactly, suppose that the data are regarded as n pairs of observations, where the pair for the ith individual is (t_i, δ_i), $i = 1, 2, \ldots, n$. In this notation, δ_i is an indicator variable that takes the value zero when the survival time t_i is censored, and unity when t_i is an uncensored survival time. The likelihood function can then be written as

$$\prod_{i=1}^{n} \{f(t_i)\}^{\delta_i} \{S(t_i)\}^{1-\delta_i}. \tag{5.9}$$

This function, which is equivalent to that in Expression (5.8), can then be maximised with respect to the unknown parameters in the density and survivor functions.

An alternative expression for this likelihood function can be obtained by writing Expression (5.9) in the form

$$\prod_{i=1}^{n} \left\{ \frac{f(t_i)}{S(t_i)} \right\}^{\delta_i} S(t_i),$$

so that, from Equation (1.4) of Chapter 1, this becomes

$$\prod_{i=1}^{n} \{h(t_i)\}^{\delta_i} S(t_i). \tag{5.10}$$

This version of the likelihood function is particularly useful when the probability density function has a complicated form, as it often does. Estimates of the unknown parameters in this likelihood function are then found by maximising the logarithm of the likelihood function.

5.3.1 Likelihood function for randomly censored data*

A more careful derivation of the likelihood function in Equation (5.9) is given in this section, which shows the relevance of the assumption of independent censoring, referred to in Section 1.1.2 of Chapter 1.

Suppose that survival data for a sample of n individuals is a mixture of event times and right-censored observations. Denote the observed time for the ith individual by t_i, and let δ_i be the corresponding event indicator, $i = 1, 2, \ldots, n$, so that $\delta_i = 1$ if t_i is an event time, and $\delta_i = 0$ if the time is censored.

The random variable associated with the event time of the ith individual will be denoted by T_i. The censoring times will be assumed to be random, and C_i will denote the random variable associated with the time to censoring. The value t_i is then an observation on the random variable $\tau_i = \min(T_i, C_i)$. The density and survivor functions of T_i will be denoted by $f_{T_i}(t)$ and $S_{T_i}(t)$, respectively. Also, $f_{C_i}(t)$ and $S_{C_i}(t)$ will be used to denote the density and survivor functions of the random variable associated with the censoring time, C_i.

We now consider the probability distribution of the pair (τ_i, δ_i) for censored and uncensored observations, respectively. Consider first the case of a censored observation, so that $\delta_i = 0$. The joint distribution of τ_i and δ_i is described by

$$\mathrm{P}(\tau_i = t, \delta_i = 0) = \mathrm{P}(C_i = t, T_i > t).$$

This joint probability is a mixture of continuous and discrete components, but to simplify the presentation, $\mathrm{P}(T_i = t)$, for example, will be understood to be the probability density function of T_i. The distribution of the event time, T_i, is now assumed to be independent of that of the censoring time, C_i. Then,

$$\begin{aligned}
\mathrm{P}(C_i = t, T_i > t) &= \mathrm{P}(C_i = t)\,\mathrm{P}(T_i > t), \\
&= f_{C_i}(t) S_{T_i}(t),
\end{aligned}$$

so that

$$\mathrm{P}(\tau_i = t, \delta_i = 0) = f_{C_i}(t) S_{T_i}(t).$$

Similarly, for an uncensored observation,

$$\begin{aligned}
\mathrm{P}(\tau_i = t, \delta_i = 1) &= \mathrm{P}(T_i = t, C_i > t), \\
&= \mathrm{P}(T_i = t)\,\mathrm{P}(C_i > t), \\
&= f_{T_i}(t) S_{C_i}(t),
\end{aligned}$$

again assuming that the distributions of C_i and T_i are independent. Putting these two results together, the joint probability, or likelihood, of the n observations, $t_1, t_2, \ldots, t_n$, is therefore

$$\prod_{i=1}^{n} \{f_{T_i}(t_i) S_{C_i}(t_i)\}^{\delta_i} \{f_{C_i}(t_i) S_{T_i}(t_i)\}^{1-\delta_i},$$

which can be written as

$$\prod_{i=1}^{n} f_{C_i}(t_i)^{1-\delta_i} S_{C_i}(t_i)^{\delta_i} \times \prod_{i=1}^{n} f_{T_i}(t_i)^{\delta_i} S_{T_i}(t_i)^{1-\delta_i}.$$

On the assumption of independent censoring, the first product in this expression will not involve any parameters that are relevant to the distribution of the survival times, and so can be regarded as a constant. The likelihood of the observed data is then proportional to

$$\prod_{i=1}^{n} f_{T_i}(t_i)^{\delta_i} S_{T_i}(t_i)^{1-\delta_i},$$

which was given in Expression (5.9) of this chapter.

It can also be shown that when the study has a fixed duration, so that individuals who have not experienced an event by the end of the study are censored, the same likelihood function is obtained. Details are not given here, but see Klein and Moeschberger (2005) or Lawless (2002), for example.

5.4* Fitting exponential and Weibull models

We now consider fitting exponential and Weibull distributions to a single sample of survival data.

5.4.1 *Fitting the exponential distribution*

Suppose that the survival times of n individuals, $t_1, t_2, \ldots, t_n$, are assumed to have an exponential distribution with mean λ^{-1}. Further suppose that the data give the actual death times of r individuals, and that the remaining $n-r$ survival times are right-censored.

For the exponential distribution,

$$f(t) = \lambda e^{-\lambda t}, \qquad S(t) = e^{-\lambda t},$$

and on substituting into Expression (5.9), the likelihood function for the n observations is given by

$$L(\lambda) = \prod_{i=1}^{n} \left(\lambda e^{-\lambda t_i}\right)^{\delta_i} \left(e^{-\lambda t_i}\right)^{1-\delta_i},$$

where δ_i is zero if the survival time of the ith individual is censored and unity otherwise. After some simplification,

$$L(\lambda) = \prod_{i=1}^{n} \lambda^{\delta_i} e^{-\lambda t_i},$$

and the corresponding log-likelihood function is

$$\log L(\lambda) = \sum_{i=1}^{n} \delta_i \log \lambda - \lambda \sum_{i=1}^{n} t_i.$$

Since the data contain r deaths, $\sum_{i=1}^{n} \delta_i = r$ and the log-likelihood function becomes

$$\log L(\lambda) = r \log \lambda - \lambda \sum_{i=1}^{n} t_i.$$

We now need to identify the value $\hat{\lambda}$, for which the log-likelihood function is a maximum. Differentiation with respect to λ gives

$$\frac{\mathrm{d} \log L(\lambda)}{\mathrm{d}\lambda} = \frac{r}{\lambda} - \sum_{i=1}^{n} t_i,$$

and equating the derivative to zero and evaluating it at $\hat{\lambda}$ gives

$$\hat{\lambda} = r \Big/ \sum_{i=1}^{n} t_i \qquad (5.11)$$

for the maximum likelihood estimator of λ.

The mean of an exponential distribution is $\mu = \lambda^{-1}$, and so the maximum likelihood estimator of μ is

$$\hat{\mu} = \hat{\lambda}^{-1} = \frac{1}{r} \sum_{i=1}^{n} t_i.$$

This estimator of μ is the total time survived by the n individuals in the data set divided by the number of deaths observed. The estimator therefore has intuitive appeal as an estimate of the mean lifetime from censored survival data.

The standard error of either $\hat{\lambda}$ or $\hat{\mu}$ can be obtained from the second derivative of the log-likelihood function, using a result from the theory of maximum likelihood estimation given in Appendix A. Differentiating $\log L(\lambda)$ a second time gives

$$\frac{\mathrm{d}^2 \log L(\lambda)}{\mathrm{d}\lambda^2} = -\frac{r}{\lambda^2},$$

and so the asymptotic variance of $\hat{\lambda}$ is

$$\operatorname{var}(\hat{\lambda}) = \left\{ -\operatorname{E}\left(\frac{\mathrm{d}^2 \log L(\lambda)}{\mathrm{d}\lambda^2} \right) \right\}^{-1} = \frac{\lambda^2}{r}.$$

Consequently, the standard error of $\hat{\lambda}$ is given by

$$\operatorname{se}(\hat{\lambda}) = \hat{\lambda}/\sqrt{r}. \tag{5.12}$$

This result could be used to obtain a confidence interval for the mean survival time. In particular, the limits of a $100(1-\alpha)\%$ confidence interval for λ are $\hat{\lambda} \pm z_{\alpha/2} \operatorname{se}(\hat{\lambda})$, where $z_{\alpha/2}$ is the upper $\alpha/2$-point of the standard normal distribution.

In presenting the results of a survival analysis, the estimated survivor and hazard functions, and the median and other percentiles of the distribution of survival times, are useful. Once an estimate of λ has been found, all these functions can be estimated using the results given in Section 5.1.1. In particular, under the assumed exponential distribution, the estimated hazard function is $\hat{h}(t) = \hat{\lambda}$ and the estimated survivor function is $\hat{S}(t) = \exp(-\hat{\lambda}t)$. In addition, the estimated pth percentile is given by

$$\hat{t}(p) = \frac{1}{\hat{\lambda}} \log\left(\frac{100}{100-p} \right), \tag{5.13}$$

and the estimated median survival time is

$$\hat{t}(50) = \hat{\lambda}^{-1} \log 2. \tag{5.14}$$

The standard error of an estimate of the pth percentile of the distribution of survival times can be found using the result for the approximate variance of a function of a random variable given in Equation (2.8) of Chapter 2. According to this result, an approximation to the variance of a function $g(\hat{\lambda})$ of $\hat{\lambda}$ is such that

$$\operatorname{var}\{g(\hat{\lambda})\} \approx \left\{ \frac{\mathrm{d}g(\hat{\lambda})}{\mathrm{d}\hat{\lambda}} \right\}^2 \operatorname{var}(\hat{\lambda}). \tag{5.15}$$

Using this result, the approximate variance of the estimated pth percentile is given by

$$\text{var}\,\{\hat{t}(p)\} \approx \left\{-\frac{1}{\hat{\lambda}^2}\log\left(\frac{100}{100-p}\right)\right\}^2 \text{var}\,(\hat{\lambda}).$$

Taking the square root, we get

$$\text{se}\,\{\hat{t}(p)\} = \frac{1}{\hat{\lambda}^2}\log\left(\frac{100}{100-p}\right)\text{se}\,(\hat{\lambda}),$$

and on substituting for $\text{se}\,(\hat{\lambda})$ from Equation (5.12) and $\hat{t}(p)$ from Equation (5.13), we find

$$\text{se}\,\{\hat{t}(p)\} = \hat{t}(p)/\sqrt{r}. \tag{5.16}$$

In particular, the standard error of the estimated median survival time is

$$\text{se}\,\{\hat{t}(50)\} = \hat{t}(50)/\sqrt{r}. \tag{5.17}$$

Confidence intervals for a true percentile are best obtained from exponentiating the confidence limits for the logarithm of the percentile. This procedure ensures that confidence limits for the percentile will be non-negative. Again making use of the result in Equation (5.15), the standard error of $\log\hat{t}(p)$ is given by

$$\text{se}\,\{\log\hat{t}(p)\} = \hat{t}(p)^{-1}\,\text{se}\,\{\hat{t}(p)\},$$

and after substituting for $\text{se}\,\{\hat{t}(p)\}$ from Equation (5.16), this standard error becomes

$$\text{se}\,\{\log\hat{t}(p)\} = 1/\sqrt{r}.$$

Using this result, $100(1-\alpha)\%$ confidence limits for the 100pth percentile are $\exp\{\log\hat{t}(p) \pm z_{\alpha/2}/\sqrt{r}\}$, that is, $\hat{t}(p)\exp\{\pm z_{\alpha/2}/\sqrt{r}\}$, where $z_{\alpha/2}$ is the upper $\alpha/2$-point of the standard normal distribution.

Example 5.2 Time to discontinuation of the use of an IUD

In this example, the data of Example 1.1 on the times to discontinuation of an IUD for 18 women are analysed under the assumption of a constant hazard of discontinuation. An exponential distribution is therefore fitted to the discontinuation times. For these data, the total of the observed and right-censored discontinuation times is 1046 days, and the number of uncensored times is 9. Therefore, using Equation (5.11), $\hat{\lambda} = 9/1046 = 0.0086$, and the standard error of $\hat{\lambda}$ from Equation (5.12) is $\text{se}\,(\hat{\lambda}) = 0.0086/\sqrt{9} = 0.0029$. The estimated hazard function is therefore $\hat{h}(t) = 0.0086$, $t > 0$, and the estimated survivor function is $\hat{S}(t) = \exp(-0.0086\,t)$. The estimated hazard and survivor functions are shown in Figures 5.7 and 5.8, respectively.

Estimates of the median and other percentiles of the distribution of discontinuation times can be found from Figure 5.8, but more accurate estimates are obtained from Equation (5.13). In particular, using Equation (5.14), the

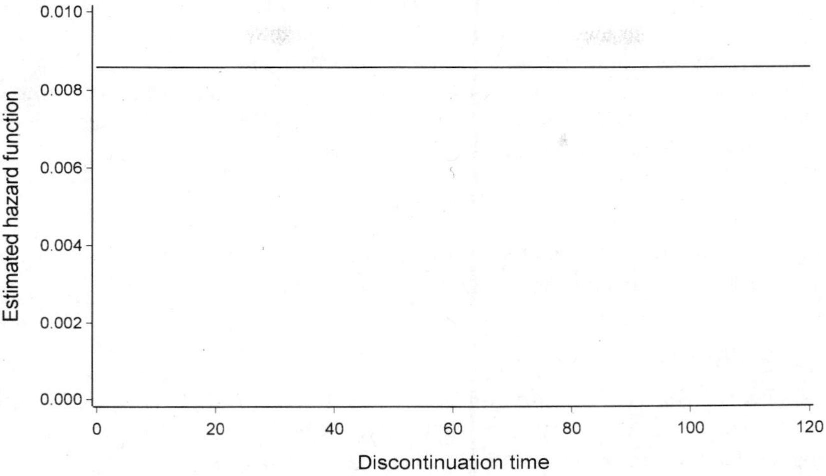

Figure 5.7 *Estimated hazard function on fitting the exponential distribution.*

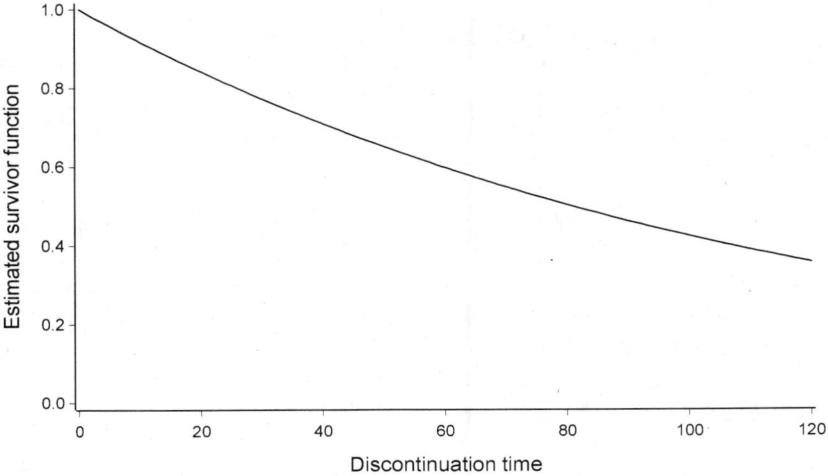

Figure 5.8 *Estimated survivor function on fitting the exponential distribution.*

median discontinuation time is 81 days, and an estimate of the 90th percentile of the distribution of discontinuation times is, from Equation (5.13), $\hat{t}(90) = \log 10/0.0086 = 267.61$. This means that on the assumption that the risk of discontinuing the use of an IUD is independent of time, 90% of women will have a discontinuation time of less than 268 days.

From Equation (5.17), the standard error of the estimated median time to discontinuation is $80.56/\sqrt{9}$, that is, 26.85 days. The limits of a 95% confidence interval for the true median discontinuation time are

$$80.56 \exp\{\pm 1.96/\sqrt{9}\},$$

and so the interval is from 42 days to 155 days. Confidence intervals for other percentiles can be calculated in a similar manner.

5.4.2 Fitting the Weibull distribution

The survival times of n individuals are now taken to be a censored sample from a Weibull distribution with scale parameter λ and shape parameter γ. Suppose that there are r deaths among the n individuals and $n - r$ right-censored survival times. We can again use Expression (5.9) to obtain the likelihood of the sample data. The probability density, survivor and hazard function of a $W(\lambda, \gamma)$ distribution are given by

$$f(t) = \lambda\gamma t^{\gamma-1}\exp(-\lambda t^{\gamma}), \quad S(t) = \exp(-\lambda t^{\gamma}), \quad h(t) = \lambda\gamma t^{\gamma-1},$$

and so, from Expression (5.9), the likelihood of the n survival times is

$$\prod_{i=1}^{n}\left\{\lambda\gamma t_i^{\gamma-1}\exp(-\lambda t_i^{\gamma})\right\}^{\delta_i}\left\{\exp(-\lambda t_i^{\gamma})\right\}^{1-\delta_i},$$

where δ_i is zero if the ith survival time is censored and unity otherwise. Equivalently, from Expression (5.10), the likelihood function is

$$\prod_{i=1}^{n}\left\{\lambda\gamma t_i^{\gamma-1}\right\}^{\delta_i}\exp(-\lambda t_i^{\gamma}).$$

This is regarded as a function of λ and γ, the unknown parameters in the Weibull distribution, and so can be written $L(\lambda, \gamma)$. The corresponding log-likelihood function is given by

$$\log L(\lambda, \gamma) = \sum_{i=1}^{n}\delta_i \log(\lambda\gamma) + (\gamma - 1)\sum_{i=1}^{n}\delta_i \log t_i - \lambda\sum_{i=1}^{n} t_i^{\gamma},$$

and noting that $\sum_{i=1}^{n}\delta_i = r$, the log-likelihood becomes

$$\log L(\lambda, \gamma) = r\log(\lambda\gamma) + (\gamma - 1)\sum_{i=1}^{n}\delta_i \log t_i - \lambda\sum_{i=1}^{n} t_i^{\gamma}.$$

The maximum likelihood estimates of λ and γ are found by differentiating this function with respect to λ and γ, equating the derivatives to zero, and evaluating them at $\hat{\lambda}$ and $\hat{\gamma}$. The resulting equations are

$$\frac{r}{\hat{\lambda}} - \sum_{i=1}^{n} t_i^{\hat{\gamma}} = 0, \tag{5.18}$$

and

$$\frac{r}{\hat{\gamma}} + \sum_{i=1}^{n} \delta_i \log t_i - \hat{\lambda} \sum_{i=1}^{n} t_i^{\hat{\gamma}} \log t_i = 0. \tag{5.19}$$

From Equation (5.18),

$$\hat{\lambda} = r \Big/ \sum_{i=1}^{n} t_i^{\hat{\gamma}}, \tag{5.20}$$

and on substituting for $\hat{\lambda}$ in Equation (5.19), we get the equation

$$\frac{r}{\hat{\gamma}} + \sum_{i=1}^{n} \delta_i \log t_i - \frac{r}{\sum_i t_i^{\hat{\gamma}}} \sum_{i=1}^{n} t_i^{\hat{\gamma}} \log t_i = 0. \tag{5.21}$$

This is a non-linear equation in $\hat{\gamma}$, which can only be solved numerically using an iterative procedure. Once the estimate, $\hat{\gamma}$, which satisfies Equation (5.21), has been found, Equation (5.20) can be used to obtain $\hat{\lambda}$.

In practice, a numerical method, such as the Newton-Raphson procedure, is used to find the values $\hat{\lambda}$ and $\hat{\gamma}$ which maximise the likelihood function simultaneously. This procedure was described in Section 3.3.3 of Chapter 3, in connection with fitting the Cox regression model. In that section it was noted that an important by-product of the Newton-Raphson procedure is an approximation to the variance-covariance matrix of the parameter estimates, from which their standard errors can be obtained.

Once estimates of the parameters λ and γ have been found from fitting the Weibull distribution to the observed data, percentiles of the survival time distribution can be estimated using Equation (5.6). The estimated pth percentile of the distribution is

$$\hat{t}(p) = \left\{ \frac{1}{\hat{\lambda}} \log\left(\frac{100}{100-p} \right) \right\}^{1/\hat{\gamma}}, \tag{5.22}$$

and so the estimated median survival time is given by

$$\hat{t}(50) = \left\{ \frac{1}{\hat{\lambda}} \log 2 \right\}^{1/\hat{\gamma}}. \tag{5.23}$$

An expression for the standard error of a percentile of the Weibull distribution, and a corresponding confidence interval, is derived in Section 5.4.3.

5.4.3 Standard error of a percentile of the Weibull distribution

The standard error of the estimated pth percentile of the Weibull distribution with scale parameter λ and shape parameter γ, $\hat{t}(p)$, is most easily found from the variance of $\log \hat{t}(p)$. Now, from Equation (5.22),

$$\log \hat{t}(p) = \frac{1}{\hat{\gamma}} \log \left\{ \hat{\lambda}^{-1} \log \left(\frac{100}{100 - p} \right) \right\},$$

and so

$$\log \hat{t}(p) = \frac{1}{\hat{\gamma}} \left\{ c_p - \log \hat{\lambda} \right\},$$

where

$$c_p = \log \log \left(\frac{100}{100 - p} \right).$$

This is a function of two parameter estimates, $\hat{\lambda}$ and $\hat{\gamma}$.

To obtain the variance of $\log \hat{t}(p)$, we use the general result that the approximate variance of a function $g(\hat{\theta}_1, \hat{\theta}_2)$ of two parameter estimates, $\hat{\theta}_1$, $\hat{\theta}_2$, is

$$\left(\frac{\partial g}{\partial \hat{\theta}_1} \right)^2 \operatorname{var}(\hat{\theta}_1) + \left(\frac{\partial g}{\partial \hat{\theta}_2} \right)^2 \operatorname{var}(\hat{\theta}_2) + 2 \left(\frac{\partial g}{\partial \hat{\theta}_1} \frac{\partial g}{\partial \hat{\theta}_2} \right) \operatorname{cov}(\hat{\theta}_1, \hat{\theta}_2). \qquad (5.24)$$

This is an extension of the result given in Equation (2.8) of Chapter 2 for the approximate variance of a function of a single random variable. Using Equation (5.24),

$$\operatorname{var}\left\{ \log \hat{t}(p) \right\} \approx \left(\frac{\partial \log \hat{t}(p)}{\partial \hat{\lambda}} \right)^2 \operatorname{var}(\hat{\lambda}) + \left(\frac{\partial \log \hat{t}(p)}{\partial \hat{\gamma}} \right)^2 \operatorname{var}(\hat{\gamma})$$
$$+ 2 \frac{\partial \log \hat{t}(p)}{\partial \hat{\lambda}} \frac{\partial \log \hat{t}(p)}{\partial \hat{\gamma}} \operatorname{cov}(\hat{\lambda}, \hat{\gamma}).$$

Now, the derivatives of $\log \hat{t}(p)$ with respect to $\hat{\lambda}$ and $\hat{\gamma}$ are given by

$$\frac{\partial \log \hat{t}(p)}{\partial \hat{\lambda}} = -\frac{1}{\hat{\lambda}\hat{\gamma}},$$
$$\frac{\partial \log \hat{t}(p)}{\partial \hat{\gamma}} = -\frac{c_p - \log \hat{\lambda}}{\hat{\gamma}^2},$$

and so the approximate variance of $\log \hat{t}(p)$ is

$$\frac{1}{\hat{\lambda}^2 \hat{\gamma}^2} \operatorname{var}(\hat{\lambda}) + \frac{\left(c_p - \log \hat{\lambda} \right)^2}{\hat{\gamma}^4} \operatorname{var}(\hat{\gamma}) + \frac{2 \left(c_p - \log \hat{\lambda} \right)}{\hat{\lambda} \hat{\gamma}^3} \operatorname{cov}(\hat{\lambda}, \hat{\gamma}). \qquad (5.25)$$

The variance of $\hat{t}(p)$ itself is found from the result in Equation (2.8) of Chapter 2, from which

$$\operatorname{var}\{\hat{t}(p)\} \approx \hat{t}(p)^2 \operatorname{var}\{\log \hat{t}(p)\}, \qquad (5.26)$$

and using Expression (5.25),

$$\text{var}\,\{\hat{t}(p)\} \approx \frac{\hat{t}(p)^2}{\hat{\lambda}^2\hat{\gamma}^4}\left\{\hat{\gamma}^2\,\text{var}\,(\hat{\lambda}) + \hat{\lambda}^2\left(c_p - \log\hat{\lambda}\right)^2\,\text{var}\,(\hat{\gamma}) + 2\hat{\lambda}\hat{\gamma}\left(c_p - \log\hat{\lambda}\right)\,\text{cov}\,(\hat{\lambda},\hat{\gamma})\right\}.$$

The standard error of $\hat{t}(p)$ is the square root of this expression, given by

$$\text{se}\,\{\hat{t}(p)\} = \frac{\hat{t}(p)}{\hat{\lambda}\hat{\gamma}^2}\left\{\hat{\gamma}^2\,\text{var}\,(\hat{\lambda}) + \hat{\lambda}^2\left(c_p - \log\hat{\lambda}\right)^2\,\text{var}\,(\hat{\gamma}) + 2\hat{\lambda}\hat{\gamma}\left(c_p - \log\hat{\lambda}\right)\,\text{cov}\,(\hat{\lambda},\hat{\gamma})\right\}^{\frac{1}{2}}. \qquad (5.27)$$

Note that for the special case of the exponential distribution, where the shape parameter, γ, is equal to unity, the standard error of the estimated pth percentile from Equation (5.27) is

$$\frac{\hat{t}(p)}{\hat{\lambda}}\,\text{se}\,(\hat{\lambda}).$$

Now, using Equation (5.12) of Chapter 5,

$$\text{se}\,(\hat{\lambda}) = \hat{\lambda}/\sqrt{r},$$

where r is the number of death times in the data set, and so

$$\text{se}\,\{\hat{t}(p)\} = \hat{t}(p)/\sqrt{r},$$

as in Equation (5.16).

A $100(1-\alpha)\%$ confidence interval for the pth percentile of a Weibull distribution is found from the corresponding confidence limits for $\log t(p)$. These limits are

$$\log\hat{t}(p) \pm z_{\alpha/2}\,\text{se}\,\{\log\hat{t}(p)\},$$

where $\text{se}\,\{\log\hat{t}(p)\}$ is, from Equation (5.26), given by

$$\text{se}\,\{\log\hat{t}(p)\} = \frac{1}{\hat{t}(p)}\,\text{se}\,\{\hat{t}(p)\}, \qquad (5.28)$$

and $z_{\alpha/2}$ is the upper $\alpha/2$-point of the standard normal distribution. The corresponding $100(1-\alpha)\%$ confidence interval for the pth percentile, $t(p)$, is then $\hat{t}(p)\exp\left[\pm z_{\alpha/2}\,\text{se}\,\{\log\hat{t}(p)\}\right]$.

Example 5.3 Time to discontinuation of the use of an IUD
In Example 5.1, it was found that an exponential distribution provides a satisfactory model for the data on the discontinuation times of 18 IUD users. For comparison, a Weibull distribution will be fitted to the same data set. This

distribution is fitted using computer software, and from the resulting output, the estimated scale parameter of the distribution is found to be $\hat{\lambda} = 0.000454$, while the estimated shape parameter is $\hat{\gamma} = 1.676$. The standard errors of these estimates are given by $\text{se}(\hat{\lambda}) = 0.000965$ and $\text{se}(\hat{\gamma}) = 0.460$, respectively. Note that approximate confidence limits for the shape parameter, γ, found using $\hat{\gamma} \pm 1.96\,\text{se}(\hat{\gamma})$, include unity, suggesting that the exponential distribution would provide a satisfactory model for the discontinuation times.

The estimated hazard and survivor functions are obtained by substituting these estimates into Equations (5.4) and (5.5), whence

$$\hat{h}(t) = \hat{\lambda}\hat{\gamma}t^{\hat{\gamma}-1},$$

and

$$\hat{S}(t) = \exp\left(-\hat{\lambda}t^{\hat{\gamma}}\right).$$

These two functions are shown in Figures 5.9 and 5.10.

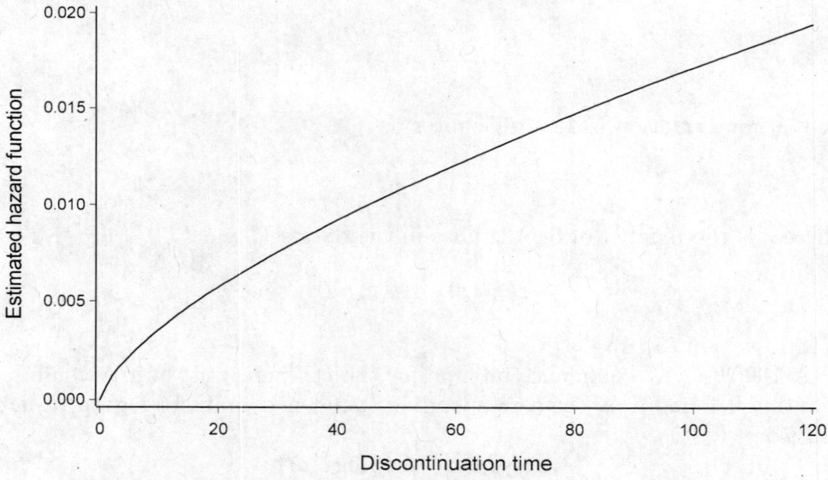

Figure 5.9 *Estimated hazard function on fitting the Weibull distribution.*

Although percentiles of the discontinuation time can be read from the estimated survivor function in Figure 5.10, they are better estimated using Equation (5.22). Hence, under the Weibull distribution, the median discontinuation time can be estimated using Equation (5.23), and is given by

$$\hat{t}(50) = \left\{\frac{1}{0.000454}\log 2\right\}^{1/1.676} = 79.27.$$

As a check, notice that this is perfectly consistent with the value of the discontinuation time corresponding to $\hat{S}(t) = 0.5$ in Figure 5.10. The standard

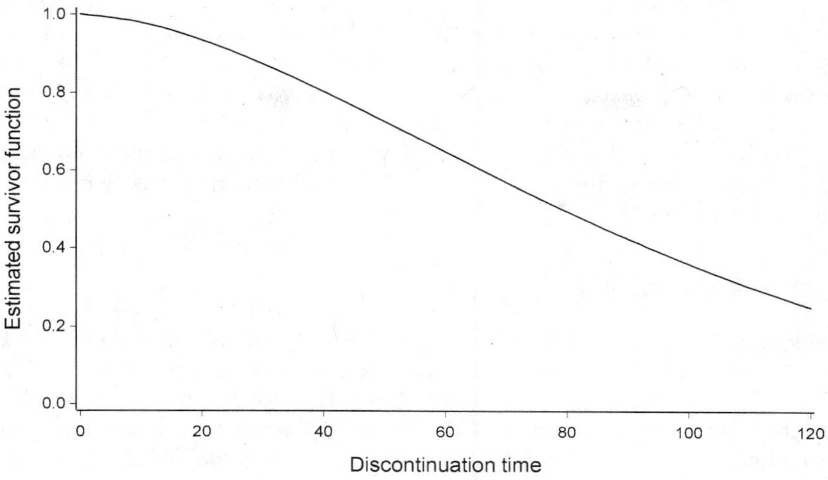

Figure 5.10 *Estimated survivor function on fitting the Weibull distribution.*

error of this estimate, from Equation (5.27) is, after much arithmetic, found to be

$$\text{se}\,\{\hat{t}(50)\} = 15.795.$$

In order to obtain a 95% confidence interval for the median discontinuation time, the standard error of $\log \hat{t}(50)$ is required. From Equation (5.28),

$$\text{se}\,\{\log \hat{t}(50)\} = \frac{15.795}{79.272} = 0.199,$$

and so the required confidence limits for the log median discontinuation time are $\log 79.272 \pm 1.96 \times 0.199$, that is, $(3.982, 4.763)$. The corresponding interval estimate for the true median discontinuation time, found from exponentiating these limits, is $(53.64, 117.15)$. This means that there is a 95% chance that the interval from 54 days to 117 days includes the true value of the median discontinuation time. This interval is rather wide because of the small number of actual discontinuation times in the data set.

It is interesting to compare these results with those found in Example 5.2, where the discontinuation times were modelled using an exponential distribution. The estimated median survival times are very similar, at 80.6 days for the exponential and 79.3 days for the Weibull model. However, the standard error of the estimated median survival time is 26.8 days when the times are assumed to have an exponential distribution, and only 15.8 days under the Weibull model. The median is therefore estimated more precisely when the discontinuation times are assumed to have a Weibull distribution.

Other percentiles of the discontinuation time distribution, and accompanying standard errors and confidence intervals, can be found in a similar fashion. For example, the 90th percentile, that is, the time beyond which 10% of those in the study continue with the use of the IUD, is 162.23 days, and 95% confidence limits for the true percentile are from 95.41 to 275.84 days. Notice that the width of this confidence interval is larger than that for the median discontinuation time, reflecting the fact that the median is more precisely estimated than other percentiles.

5.5 A model for the comparison of two groups

We saw in Section 3.1 that a convenient general model for comparing two groups of survival times is the proportional hazards model. Here, the two groups will be labelled Group I and Group II, and X will be an indicator variable that takes the value zero if an individual is in Group I and unity if an individual is in Group II. Under the proportional hazards model, the hazard of death at time t for the ith individual is given by

$$h_i(t) = e^{\beta x_i} h_0(t), \tag{5.29}$$

where x_i is the value of X for the ith individual. Consequently, the hazard at time t for an individual in Group I is $h_0(t)$, and that for an individual in Group II is $\psi h_0(t)$, where $\psi = \exp(\beta)$. The quantity β is then the logarithm of the ratio of the hazard for an individual in Group II, to that of an individual in Group I.

We will now make the additional assumption that the survival times for the individuals in Group I have a Weibull distribution with scale parameter λ and shape parameter γ. Using Equation (5.29), the hazard function for the individuals in this group is $h_0(t)$, where $h_0(t) = \lambda\gamma t^{\gamma-1}$. Now, also from Equation (5.29), the hazard function for those in Group II is $\psi h_0(t)$, that is, $\psi\lambda\gamma t^{\gamma-1}$. This is the hazard function for a Weibull distribution with scale parameter $\psi\lambda$ and shape parameter γ. We therefore have the result that if the survival times of individuals in one group have a Weibull distribution with shape parameter γ, and the hazard of death at time t for an individual in the second group is proportional to that of an individual in the first, the survival times of those in the second group will also have a Weibull distribution with shape parameter γ. The Weibull distribution is then said to have the *proportional hazards property*. This property is another reason for the importance of the Weibull distribution in the analysis of survival data.

5.5.1 *The log-cumulative hazard plot*

When a single sample of survival times has a Weibull distribution $W(\lambda, \gamma)$, the log-cumulative hazard plot, described in Section 5.2, will give a straight line with intercept $\log \lambda$ and slope γ. It then follows that if the survival times in a second group have a $W(\psi\lambda, \gamma)$ distribution, as they would under the proportional hazards model in Equation (5.29), the log-cumulative hazard plot will give a straight line, also of slope γ, but with intercept $\log \psi + \log \lambda$. If the estimated log-cumulative hazard function is plotted against the logarithm of the survival time for individuals in two groups, parallel straight lines would mean that the assumptions of a proportional hazards model and Weibull survival times were tenable. The vertical separation of the two lines provides an estimate of $\beta = \log \psi$, the logarithm of the relative hazard.

If the two lines in a log-cumulative hazard plot are essentially straight, but not parallel, this means that the shape parameter, γ, is different in the two groups, and the hazards are no longer proportional. If the lines are not particularly straight, the Weibull model may not be appropriate. However, if the curves can be taken to be parallel, this would mean that the proportional hazards model is valid, and the Cox regression model discussed in Chapter 3 might be more satisfactory.

Example 5.4 Prognosis for women with breast cancer
In this example, we investigate whether the Weibull proportional hazards model is likely to be appropriate for the data of Example 1.2 on the survival times of breast cancer patients. These data relate to women classified according to whether their tumours were positively or negatively stained. The Kaplan-Meier estimate of the survivor functions for the women in each group were shown in Figure 2.9. From these estimates, the log-cumulative hazards can be estimated and plotted against $\log t$. The resulting log-cumulative hazard plot is shown in Figure 5.11.

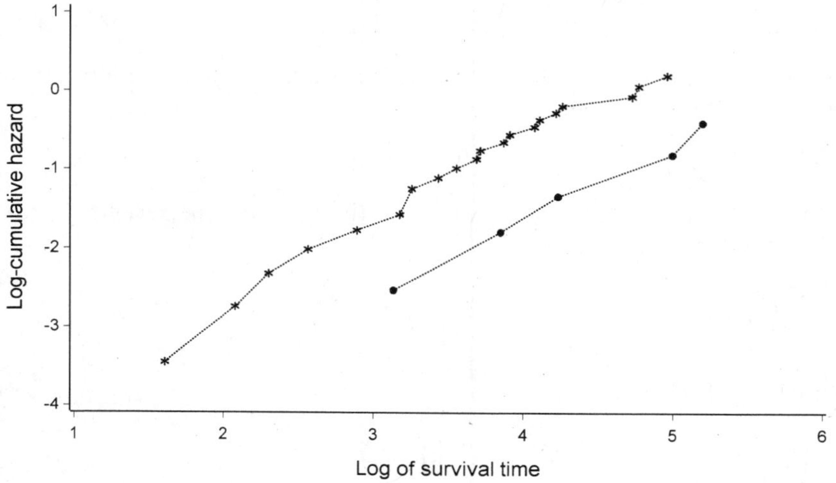

Figure 5.11 *Log-cumulative hazard plot for women with tumours that were positively stained (∗) and negatively stained (•).*

In this figure, the lines corresponding to the two staining groups are reasonably straight. This means that the assumption of Weibull distributions for the survival times of the women in each group is quite plausible. Moreover, the gradients of the two lines are very similar, which means that the proportional hazards model is valid. The vertical separation of the two lines provides an estimate of the log relative hazard. From Figure 5.11, the vertical distance between the two straight lines is approximately 1.0, and so a rough estimate of the hazard ratio is $e^{1.0} = 2.72$. Women in the positively stained group would appear to have nearly three times the risk of death at any time compared to those in the negatively stained group. More accurate estimates of the relative hazard will be obtained from fitting exponential and Weibull models to the data of this example, in Examples 5.5 and 5.6.

5.5.2 Fitting the model*

The proportional hazards model in Equation (5.29) can be fitted using the method of maximum likelihood. To illustrate the process, we consider the situation where the survival times in each group have an exponential distribution.

Suppose that the observations from n_1 individuals in Group I can be expressed as (t_{i1}, δ_{i1}), $i = 1, 2, \ldots, n_1$, where δ_{i1} takes the value zero if the survival time of the ith individual in that group is censored, and unity if that time is a death time. Similarly, let $(t_{i'2}, \delta_{i'2})$, $i' = 1, 2, \ldots, n_2$, be the observations from the n_2 individuals in Group II. For individuals in Group I, the hazard function will be taken to be λ, and the probability density function and survivor function are given by

$$f(t_{i1}) = \lambda e^{-\lambda t_{i1}}, \qquad S(t_{i1}) = e^{-\lambda t_{i1}}.$$

For those in Group II, the hazard function is $\psi\lambda$, and the probability density function and survivor function are

$$f(t_{i'2}) = \psi\lambda e^{-\psi\lambda t_{i'2}}, \qquad S(t_{i'2}) = e^{-\psi\lambda t_{i'2}}.$$

Using Equation (5.9), the likelihood of the $n_1 + n_2$ observations, $L(\psi, \lambda)$, is

$$\prod_{i=1}^{n_1} \left\{\lambda e^{-\lambda t_{i1}}\right\}^{\delta_{i1}} \left\{e^{-\lambda t_{i1}}\right\}^{1-\delta_{i1}} \prod_{i'=1}^{n_2} \left\{\psi\lambda e^{-\psi\lambda t_{i'2}}\right\}^{\delta_{i'2}} \left\{e^{-\psi\lambda t_{i'2}}\right\}^{1-\delta_{i'2}},$$

which simplifies to

$$\prod_{i=1}^{n_1} \lambda^{\delta_{i1}} e^{-\lambda t_{i1}} \prod_{i'=1}^{n_2} (\psi\lambda)^{\delta_{i'2}} e^{-\psi\lambda t_{i'2}}.$$

If the numbers of actual death times in the two groups are r_1 and r_2, respectively, then $r_1 = \sum_i \delta_{i1}$ and $r_2 = \sum_{i'} \delta_{i'2}$, and the log-likelihood function is given by

$$\log L(\psi, \lambda) = r_1 \log \lambda - \lambda \sum_{i=1}^{n_1} t_{i1} + r_2 \log(\psi\lambda) - \psi\lambda \sum_{i'=1}^{n_2} t_{i'2}.$$

Now write T_1 and T_2 for the total known time survived by the individuals in Groups I and II, respectively. Then, T_1 and T_2 are the totals of uncensored and censored survival times in each group, so that the log-likelihood function becomes

$$\log L(\psi, \lambda) = (r_1 + r_2) \log \lambda + r_2 \log \psi - \lambda(T_1 + \psi T_2).$$

In order to obtain the values $\hat{\psi}, \hat{\lambda}$ for which this function is a maximum, we differentiate with respect to ψ and λ, and set the derivatives equal to zero. The resulting equations that are satisfied by $\hat{\psi}, \hat{\lambda}$ are

$$\frac{r_2}{\hat{\psi}} - \hat{\lambda} T_2 = 0, \tag{5.30}$$

$$\frac{r_1 + r_2}{\hat{\lambda}} - (T_1 + \hat{\psi} T_2) = 0. \tag{5.31}$$

From Equation (5.30),

$$\hat{\lambda} = \frac{r_2}{\hat{\psi} T_2},$$

and on substituting for $\hat{\lambda}$ in Equation (5.31) we get

$$\hat{\psi} = \frac{r_2 T_1}{r_1 T_2}. \tag{5.32}$$

Then, from Equation (5.30),

$$\hat{\lambda} = r_1 / T_1.$$

Both of these estimates have an intuitive justification. The estimated value of λ is the reciprocal of the average time survived by individuals in Group I, while the estimated relative hazard, $\hat{\psi}$, is the ratio of the average times survived by the individuals in the two groups.

The asymptotic variance-covariance matrix of the parameter estimates is the inverse of the information matrix, whose elements are found from the second derivatives of the log-likelihood function; see Appendix A. We have that

$$\frac{\mathrm{d}^2 \log L(\psi, \lambda)}{\mathrm{d}\psi^2} = -\frac{r_2}{\psi^2}, \quad \frac{\mathrm{d}^2 \log L(\psi, \lambda)}{\mathrm{d}\lambda^2} = -\frac{r_1 + r_2}{\lambda^2}, \quad \frac{\mathrm{d}^2 \log L(\psi, \lambda)}{\mathrm{d}\lambda \mathrm{d}\psi} = -T_2,$$

and the information matrix is the matrix of negative expected values of these partial derivatives. The only second derivative for which expectations need to be obtained is the derivative with respect to λ and ψ, for which $\mathrm{E}(T_2)$

is required. This is straightforward when the survival times have an exponential distribution, but as shown in Section 5.1.2, the expected value of a survival time that has a Weibull distribution is much more difficult to calculate. For this reason, the information matrix is usually approximated by using the observed values of the negative second partial derivatives. The observed information matrix is thus

$$\boldsymbol{I}(\psi, \lambda) = \begin{pmatrix} r_2/\psi^2 & T_2 \\ T_2 & (r_1 + r_2)/\lambda^2 \end{pmatrix},$$

and the inverse of this matrix is

$$\frac{1}{(r_1 + r_2)r_2 - T_2^2\psi^2\lambda^2} \begin{pmatrix} (r_1 + r_2)\psi^2 & -T_2\psi^2\lambda^2 \\ -T_2\psi^2\lambda^2 & r_2\lambda^2 \end{pmatrix}.$$

The standard errors of $\hat{\psi}$ and $\hat{\lambda}$ are found by substituting $\hat{\psi}$ and $\hat{\lambda}$ for ψ and λ in this matrix, and taking square roots. Thus, the standard error of $\hat{\psi}$ is given by

$$\text{se}\,(\hat{\psi}) = \sqrt{\frac{(r_1 + r_2)\hat{\psi}^2}{(r_1 + r_2)r_2 - T_2^2\hat{\psi}^2\hat{\lambda}^2}}.$$

On substituting for $\hat{\psi}$ and $\hat{\lambda}$ in the denominator of this expression, this standard error simplifies to

$$\hat{\psi}\sqrt{\frac{r_1 + r_2}{r_1 r_2}}. \tag{5.33}$$

Similarly, the standard error of $\hat{\lambda}$ turns out to be given by

$$\text{se}\,(\hat{\lambda}) = \hat{\lambda}/\sqrt{r_1}.$$

The standard error of these estimates cannot be used directly in the construction of confidence intervals for ψ and λ. The reason for this is that the values of both parameters must be positive and their estimated values will tend to have skewed distributions. This means that the assumption of normality, used in constructing a confidence interval, would not be justified. The distribution of the logarithm of an estimate of either ψ or λ is much more likely to be symmetric, and so confidence limits for the logarithm of the parameter are found using the standard error of the logarithm of the parameter estimate. The resulting confidence limits are then exponentiated to give an interval estimate for the parameter itself.

The standard error of the logarithm of a parameter estimate can be found using the general result given in Equation (5.15). Thus, the approximate variance of $\log\hat{\psi}$ is

$$\text{var}\,(\log\hat{\psi}) \approx \hat{\psi}^{-2}\,\text{var}\,(\hat{\psi}),$$

and so the standard error of $\log\hat{\psi}$ is given by

$$\text{se}\,(\log\hat{\psi}) \approx \hat{\psi}^{-1}\,\text{se}\,(\hat{\psi}) = \sqrt{\frac{r_1 + r_2}{r_1 r_2}}. \tag{5.34}$$

A $100(1-\alpha)\%$ confidence interval for the logarithm of the relative hazard has limits $\log\hat{\psi} \pm z_{\alpha/2}\,\text{se}\,(\log\hat{\psi})$, and confidence limits for the hazard ratio ψ are found by exponentiating these limits for $\log\psi$. If required, a confidence interval for λ can be found in a similar manner.

Example 5.5 Prognosis for women with breast cancer

The theoretical results developed in this section will now be illustrated using the data on the survival times of breast cancer patients. The survival times for the women in each group are assumed to have exponential distributions, so that the hazard of death, at any time, for a woman in the negatively stained group is a constant value, λ, while that for a woman in the positively stained group is $\psi\lambda$, where ψ is the hazard ratio.

From the data given in Table 1.2 of Chapter 1, the numbers of death times in the negatively and positively stained groups are, respectively, $r_1 = 5$ and $r_2 = 21$. Also, the total time survived in each group is $T_1 = 1652$ and $T_2 = 2679$ months. Using Equation (5.32), the estimated hazard of death for a woman in the positively stained group, relative to one in the negatively stained group, is

$$\hat{\psi} = \frac{21 \times 1652}{5 \times 2679} = 2.59,$$

so that a woman in the positively stained group has about two and a half times the risk of death at any given time, compared to a woman whose tumour was negatively stained. This is consistent with the estimated value of ψ of 2.72 from the graphical procedure used in Example 5.4.

Next, using Equation (5.33), the standard error of the estimated hazard ratio is given by

$$\text{se}\,(\hat{\psi}) = 2.59\sqrt{\frac{5+21}{5 \times 21}} = 1.289.$$

In order to obtain a 95% confidence interval for the true relative hazard, the standard error of $\log\hat{\psi}$ is required. Using Equation (5.34), this is found to be given by $\text{se}\,(\log\hat{\psi}) = 0.498$, and so 95% confidence limits for $\log\psi$ are $\log(2.59) \pm 1.96\,\text{se}\,(\log\hat{\psi})$, that is, $0.952 \pm (1.96 \times 0.498)$. The confidence interval for the log relative hazard is $(-0.024, 1.927)$, and the corresponding interval estimate for the relative hazard itself is $(e^{-0.024}, e^{1.927})$, that is, $(0.98, 6.87)$. This interval only just includes unity, and suggests that women with positively stained tumours have a poorer prognosis than those whose tumours were negatively stained. This result is consistent with the result of the log-rank test in Example 2.12, where a P-value of 0.061 was obtained on testing the hypothesis of no group difference.

In practice, computer software is used to fit a parametric models to two groups of survival data, assuming proportional hazards. When the model in Equation (5.29) is fitted, estimates of β, λ and γ, and their standard errors, can be obtained from the resulting output. Further calculation may then be needed to obtain an estimate of the relative hazard, and the standard error of this estimate. In particular, the estimated hazard ratio would be obtained as $\hat{\psi} = \exp(\hat{\beta})$ and se$(\hat{\psi})$ found from the equation

$$\text{se}\,(\hat{\psi}) = \exp(\hat{\beta})\,\text{se}\,(\hat{\beta}),$$

a result that follows from Equation (5.15).

The median and other percentiles of the survival time distributions in the two groups can be estimated from the values of $\hat{\lambda}$ and $\hat{\psi}$. For example, from Equation (5.22), the estimated pth percentile for those in Group I is found from

$$\hat{t}(p) = \left\{ \frac{1}{\hat{\lambda}} \log \left(\frac{100}{100 - p} \right) \right\}^{1/\hat{\gamma}},$$

and that for individuals in Group II is

$$\hat{t}(p) = \left\{ \frac{1}{\hat{\psi}\hat{\lambda}} \log \left(\frac{100}{100 - p} \right) \right\}^{1/\hat{\gamma}}.$$

An expression similar to that in (5.27) can be used to obtain the standard error of an estimated percentile for individuals in each group, once the variances and covariances of the parameter estimates in the model have been found. Specific results for the standard error of percentiles of the survival time distributions in each of the two groups will not be given. Instead, the general expression for the standard error of the pth percentile after fitting a Weibull model, given in Equation (5.27), may be used.

Example 5.6 Prognosis for women with breast cancer

In Example 5.4, a Weibull proportional hazards model was found to be appropriate for the data on the survival times of two groups of breast cancer patients. Under this model, the hazard of death at time t is $\lambda\gamma t^{\gamma-1}$ for a negatively stained patient and $\psi\lambda\gamma t^{\gamma-1}$ for a patient who is positively stained.

The estimated value of the shape parameter of the fitted Weibull distribution is $\hat{\gamma} = 0.937$. The estimated scale parameter for women in Group I is $\hat{\lambda} = 0.00414$ and that for women in Group II is $\hat{\lambda}\hat{\psi} = 0.0105$. The estimated hazard ratio under this Weibull model is $\hat{\psi} = 2.55$, which is not very different from the value obtained in Example 5.5, on the assumption of exponentially distributed survival times.

Putting $\hat{\gamma} = 0.937$ and $\hat{\lambda} = 0.00414$ in Equation (5.23) gives 235.89 for the median survival time of those in Group I. The estimated median survival time for women in Group II is found by putting $\hat{\gamma} = 0.937$ and $\hat{\lambda} = 0.0105$ in that equation, and gives 87.07 for the estimated median survival time. The median survival time of women whose tumour was positively stained is about one-third that of those whose tumour was negatively stained.

Using the general result for the standard error of the median survival time, given in Equation (5.27), the standard error of the two medians is found by taking $p = 50$, $\hat{\gamma} = 0.937$ and $\hat{\lambda} = 0.00414$ and 0.0105 in turn. They turn out to be 114.126 and 20.550, respectively.

As in Section 5.4.3, 95% confidence limits for the true median survival times for each group of women are best obtained by working with the logarithm of the median. The standard error of $\log \hat{t}(50)$ is found using Equation (5.28), from which

$$\text{se}\,\{\hat{t}(50)\} = \frac{1}{\hat{t}(50)}\,\text{se}\,\{\hat{t}(50)\}.$$

Confidence limits for $\log t(50)$ are then exponentiated to give the corresponding confidence limits for $t(50)$ itself.

In this example, 95% confidence intervals for the true median survival times of the two groups of women are $(91.4, 608.9)$ and $(54.8, 138.3)$, respectively. Notice that the confidence interval for the median survival time of patients with positive staining is much narrower than that for women with negative staining. This is due to there being a relatively small number of uncensored survival times in the women whose tumours were negatively stained.

5.6 The Weibull proportional hazards model

The model in Equation (5.29) for the comparison of two groups of survival data can easily be generalised to give a model that is similar in form to the Cox regression model described in Section 3.1.2. Suppose that the values $x_1, x_2, \ldots, x_p$ of p explanatory variables, $X_1, X_2, \ldots, X_p$, are recorded for each of n individuals. Under the proportional hazards model, the hazard of death at time t for the ith individual is

$$h_i(t) = \exp(\beta_1 x_{1i} + \beta_2 x_{2i} + \cdots + \beta_p x_{pi}) h_0(t), \tag{5.35}$$

for $i = 1, 2, \ldots, n$. Although this model has a similar appearance to that given in Equation (3.3), there is one fundamental difference, which concerns the specification of the baseline hazard function $h_0(t)$. In the Cox regression model, the form of $h_0(t)$ is unspecified, and the shape of the function is essentially determined by the actual data. In the model being considered in this section, the survival times are assumed to have a Weibull distribution, and this imposes a particular parametric form on $h_0(t)$.

Consider an individual for whom the values of the p explanatory variables in the model of Equation (5.35) are all equal to zero. The hazard function for such an individual is $h_0(t)$. If the survival time of this individual has a Weibull distribution with scale parameter λ and shape parameter γ, then their hazard function is such that

$$h_0(t) = \lambda\gamma t^{\gamma-1}.$$

Using Equation (5.35), the hazard function for the ith individual in the study is then given by

$$h_i(t) = \exp(\boldsymbol{\beta}'\boldsymbol{x}_i)\lambda\gamma t^{\gamma-1}, \tag{5.36}$$

where $\boldsymbol{\beta}'\boldsymbol{x}_i$ stands for $\beta_1 x_{1i} + \beta_2 x_{2i} + \cdots + \beta_p x_{pi}$. From the form of this hazard function, we can see that the survival time of the ith individual in the study has a Weibull distribution with scale parameter $\lambda \exp(\boldsymbol{\beta}'\boldsymbol{x}_i)$ and shape parameter γ. This again is a manifestation of the proportional hazards property of the Weibull distribution. This result shows that the effect of the explanatory variates in the model is to alter the scale parameter of the distribution, while the shape parameter remains constant.

The survivor function corresponding to the hazard function given in Equation (5.36) is found using Equation (1.6), and turns out to be

$$S_i(t) = \exp\left\{-\exp(\boldsymbol{\beta}'\boldsymbol{x}_i)\lambda t^{\gamma}\right\}. \tag{5.37}$$

5.6.1* *Fitting the model*

The Weibull proportional hazards model is fitted by constructing the likelihood function of the n observations, and maximising this function with respect to the unknown parameters, $\beta_1, \beta_2, \ldots, \beta_p$, λ and γ. Since the hazard function and survivor function differ for each individual, the likelihood function in Expression (5.10) is now written as

$$\prod_{i=1}^{n} \{h_i(t_i)\}^{\delta_i} S_i(t_i). \tag{5.38}$$

The logarithm of the likelihood function, rather than the likelihood itself, is maximised with respect to the unknown parameters, and from Expression (5.38), this is

$$\sum_{i=1}^{n} [\delta_i \log h_i(t_i) + \log S_i(t_i)].$$

On substituting for $h_i(t_i)$ and $S_i(t_i)$ from Equations (5.36) and (5.37), the log-likelihood becomes

$$\sum_{i=1}^{n} \left[\delta_i\{\boldsymbol{\beta}'\boldsymbol{x}_i + \log(\lambda\gamma) + (\gamma - 1)\log t_i\} - \lambda \exp(\boldsymbol{\beta}'\boldsymbol{x}_i) t^{\gamma}\right],$$

which can be written as

$$\sum_{i=1}^{n} \left[\delta_i\{\boldsymbol{\beta}'\boldsymbol{x}_i + \log(\lambda\gamma) + \gamma \log t_i\} - \lambda \exp(\boldsymbol{\beta}'\boldsymbol{x}_i) t^{\gamma}\right] - \sum_{i=1}^{n} \delta_i \log t_i. \tag{5.39}$$

The final term in this expression, $-\sum_{i=1}^{n} \delta_i \log t_i$, does not involve any of the unknown parameters, and can be omitted from the likelihood. The resulting log-likelihood function is then

$$\sum_{i=1}^{n} \left[\delta_i\{\boldsymbol{\beta}'\boldsymbol{x}_i + \log(\lambda\gamma) + \gamma \log t_i\} - \lambda \exp(\boldsymbol{\beta}'\boldsymbol{x}_i) t^{\gamma}\right], \tag{5.40}$$

which differs from that obtained from the full log-likelihood, given in Expression (5.39), by the value of $\sum_{i=1}^{n} \delta_i \log t_i$. When computer software is used to fit the Weibull proportional hazards model, the log-likelihood is generally computed from Expression (5.40). This expression will also be used in the examples given in this book.

Computer software for fitting parametric proportional hazards models generally includes the standard errors of the parameter estimates, from which confidence intervals for relative hazards and the median and other percentiles of the survival time distribution can be found. Specifically, suppose that the estimates of the parameters in the model of Equation (5.36) are $\hat{\beta}_1, \hat{\beta}_2, \ldots, \hat{\beta}_p, \hat{\lambda}$ and $\hat{\gamma}$. The estimated survivor function for the ith individual in the study, for whom the values of the explanatory variables in the model are $x_{1i}, x_{2i}, \ldots, x_{pi}$, is then

$$\hat{S}_i(t) = \exp\left\{-\exp(\hat{\beta}_1 x_{1i} + \hat{\beta}_2 x_{2i} + \cdots + \hat{\beta}_p x_{pi})\hat{\lambda} t^{\hat{\gamma}}\right\},$$

and the corresponding estimated hazard function is

$$\hat{h}_i(t) = \exp(\hat{\beta}_1 x_{1i} + \hat{\beta}_2 x_{2i} + \cdots + \hat{\beta}_p x_{pi})\hat{\lambda}\hat{\gamma} t^{\hat{\gamma}-1}.$$

Both of these functions can be estimated and plotted against t, for individuals with particular values of the explanatory variables in the model.

Generalising the result in Equation (5.22) to the situation where the Weibull scale parameter is $\lambda \exp(\boldsymbol{\beta}'\boldsymbol{x}_i)$, the estimated pth percentile of the survival time distribution for an individual, whose vector of explanatory variables is $\boldsymbol{x}_i$, is

$$\hat{t}(p) = \left\{\frac{1}{\hat{\lambda}\exp(\hat{\boldsymbol{\beta}}'\boldsymbol{x}_i)} \log\left(\frac{100}{100-p}\right)\right\}^{1/\hat{\gamma}}. \tag{5.41}$$

The estimated median survival time for such an individual is therefore

$$\hat{t}(50) = \left\{\frac{\log 2}{\hat{\lambda}\exp(\hat{\boldsymbol{\beta}}'\boldsymbol{x}_i)}\right\}^{1/\hat{\gamma}}. \tag{5.42}$$

The standard error of $\hat{t}(p)$ and corresponding interval estimates for $t(p)$, are derived in Section 5.6.2.

5.6.2 Standard error of a percentile in the Weibull model*

As in Section 5.4.3, the standard error of the estimated pth percentile of the survival time distribution for the Weibull proportional hazards model, $\hat{t}(p)$, given in Equation (5.41), is found from the variance of $\log \hat{t}(p)$. Writing

$$c_p = \log\log\left(\frac{100}{100-p}\right),$$

we have from Equation (5.41),

$$\log \hat{t}(p) = \frac{1}{\hat{\gamma}}\left(c_p - \log\hat{\lambda} - \hat{\boldsymbol{\beta}}'\boldsymbol{x}_i\right). \tag{5.43}$$

This is a function of the $p+2$ parameter estimates $\hat{\lambda}$, $\hat{\gamma}$ and $\hat{\beta}_1, \hat{\beta}_2, \ldots, \hat{\beta}_p$, and the approximate variance of this function can be found using a further generalisation of the result in Equation (5.24). This generalisation is best expressed in matrix form.

Suppose that $\hat{\boldsymbol{\theta}}$ is a vector formed from k parameter estimates, $\hat{\theta}_1$, $\hat{\theta}_2, \ldots, \hat{\theta}_k$, and that $g(\hat{\boldsymbol{\theta}})$ is a function of these k estimates. The approximate variance of $g(\hat{\boldsymbol{\theta}})$ is then given by

$$\text{var}\,\{g(\hat{\boldsymbol{\theta}})\} \approx \boldsymbol{d}(\hat{\boldsymbol{\theta}})'\,\text{var}\,(\hat{\boldsymbol{\theta}})\,\boldsymbol{d}(\hat{\boldsymbol{\theta}}), \tag{5.44}$$

where $\text{var}\,(\hat{\boldsymbol{\theta}})$ is the $k \times k$ variance-covariance matrix of the estimates in $\hat{\boldsymbol{\theta}}$, and $\boldsymbol{d}(\hat{\boldsymbol{\theta}})$ is the k-component vector whose ith element is

$$\left.\frac{\partial g(\hat{\boldsymbol{\theta}})}{\partial \hat{\theta}_i}\right|_{\hat{\boldsymbol{\theta}}},$$

for $i = 1, 2, \ldots, k$.

We now write $\boldsymbol{V}$ for the $(p+2) \times (p+2)$ variance-covariance matrix of $\hat{\lambda}$, $\hat{\gamma}$ and $\hat{\beta}_1, \hat{\beta}_2, \ldots, \hat{\beta}_p$. Next, from Equation (5.43), the derivatives of $\log \hat{t}(p)$ with respect to these parameter estimates are

$$\begin{aligned}
\frac{\partial \log \hat{t}(p)}{\partial \hat{\lambda}} &= -\frac{1}{\hat{\lambda}\hat{\gamma}}, \\
\frac{\partial \log \hat{t}(p)}{\partial \hat{\gamma}} &= -\frac{c_p - \log\hat{\lambda} - \hat{\boldsymbol{\beta}}'\boldsymbol{x}_i}{\hat{\gamma}^2}, \\
\frac{\partial \log \hat{t}(p)}{\partial \hat{\beta}_j} &= -\frac{x_{ji}}{\hat{\gamma}},
\end{aligned}$$

for $j = 1, 2, \ldots, p$, where x_{ji} is the jth component of $\boldsymbol{x}_i$. The vector $\boldsymbol{d}(\hat{\boldsymbol{\theta}})$ in Equation (5.44) can be expressed as $-\hat{\gamma}^{-1}\boldsymbol{d}_0$, where $\boldsymbol{d}_0$ is a vector with components $\hat{\lambda}^{-1}$, $\hat{\gamma}^{-1}\{c_p - \log\hat{\lambda} - \hat{\boldsymbol{\beta}}'\boldsymbol{x}_i\}$, and $x_{1i}, x_{2i}, \ldots, x_{pi}$. Then, the standard error of $\log \hat{t}(p)$ is given by

$$\text{se}\,\left\{\log \hat{t}(p)\right\} = \hat{\gamma}^{-1}\sqrt{\left(\boldsymbol{d}_0'\boldsymbol{V}\boldsymbol{d}_0\right)}, \tag{5.45}$$

from which the standard error of $\hat{t}(p)$ itself is obtained using

$$\text{se}\,\{\hat{t}(p)\} = \hat{t}(p)\,\text{se}\,\left\{\log \hat{t}(p)\right\}. \tag{5.46}$$

Notice that for the null model that contains no explanatory variables, the standard error of $\hat{t}(p)$ in Equation (5.46) reduces to the result in Equation (5.27).

Confidence limits for $\log t(p)$, can be found from the standard error of $\log \hat{t}(p)$, shown in Equation (5.45), and a confidence interval for $t(p)$ is obtained by exponentiating these limits.

5.6.3* Log-linear form of the model

Most computer software for fitting the Weibull proportional hazards model uses a different form of the model from that adopted in this chapter. The reason for this will be given in the next chapter, but for the moment we note that the model can be formulated as a log-linear model for T_i, the random variable associated with the survival time of the ith individual. In this version of the model,

$$\log T_i = \mu + \alpha_1 x_{1i} + \alpha_2 x_{2i} + \cdots + \alpha_p x_{pi} + \sigma\epsilon_i, \tag{5.47}$$

where $\alpha_1, \alpha_2, \ldots, \alpha_p$ are the coefficients of the p explanatory variables in the model, whose values are $x_{1i}, x_{2i}, \ldots, x_{pi}$ for the ith of n individuals, μ and σ are unknown parameters, and ϵ_i is a random variable that has a probability distribution that leads to T_i having a Weibull distribution. In this form of the model, the survivor function of T_i, given in Equation (5.37), is expressed as

$$S_i(t) = \exp\left\{-\exp\left(\frac{\log t - \mu - \alpha_1 x_{1i} - \alpha_2 x_{2i} - \cdots - \alpha_p x_{pi}}{\sigma}\right)\right\}.$$

The correspondence between these two representations of the model is such that

$$\lambda = \exp(-\mu/\sigma), \quad \gamma = \sigma^{-1}, \quad \beta_j = -\alpha_j/\sigma,$$

for $j = 1, 2, \ldots, p$, and μ, σ are often termed the *intercept* and *scale parameter*, respectively; see Sections 6.4 and 6.5 of Chapter 6 for full details.

Generally speaking, it will be more straightforward to use the log-linear form of the model to estimate the hazard and survivor functions, percentiles of the survival time distribution, and their standard errors. The relevant expressions are given as Equations (6.16), (6.17) and (6.19) in Section 6.5 of Chapter 6.

However, the log-linear representation of the model makes it difficult to obtain confidence intervals for a log-hazard ratio, β, in a proportional hazards model, since only the standard error of the estimate of α is given in the output. In particular, on fitting the Weibull proportional hazards model, the output provides the estimated value of $\alpha = -\sigma\beta$, $\hat{\alpha}$, and the standard error of $\hat{\alpha}$. The corresponding estimate of β is easily found from $\hat{\beta} = -\hat{\alpha}/\hat{\sigma}$, but the standard error of $\hat{\beta}$ is more complicated to calculate.

To obtain the standard error of $\hat{\beta}$, we can use the result given in Equation (5.24) of Section 5.4.3. Using this result, the approximate variance of the function

$$g(\hat{\alpha}, \hat{\sigma}) = -\frac{\hat{\alpha}}{\hat{\sigma}}$$

is

$$\left(\frac{\partial g}{\partial \hat{\alpha}}\right)^2 \text{var}\,(\hat{\alpha}) + \left(\frac{\partial g}{\partial \hat{\sigma}}\right)^2 \text{var}\,(\hat{\sigma}) + 2\left(\frac{\partial g}{\partial \hat{\alpha}}\frac{\partial g}{\partial \hat{\sigma}}\right) \text{cov}\,(\hat{\alpha}, \hat{\sigma}). \tag{5.48}$$

The derivatives of $g(\hat{\alpha}, \hat{\sigma})$, with respect to $\hat{\alpha}$ and $\hat{\sigma}$, are given by

$$\frac{\partial g}{\partial \hat{\alpha}} = -\frac{1}{\hat{\sigma}}, \qquad \frac{\partial g}{\partial \hat{\sigma}} = \frac{\hat{\alpha}}{\hat{\sigma}^2},$$

and so using Expression (5.48),

$$\text{var}\left(-\frac{\hat{\alpha}}{\hat{\sigma}}\right) \approx \left(-\frac{1}{\hat{\sigma}}\right)^2 \text{var}\,(\hat{\alpha}) + \left(\frac{\hat{\alpha}}{\hat{\sigma}^2}\right)^2 \text{var}\,(\hat{\sigma}) + 2\left(-\frac{1}{\hat{\sigma}}\right)\left(\frac{\hat{\alpha}}{\hat{\sigma}^2}\right) \text{cov}\,(\hat{\alpha}, \hat{\sigma}).$$

After some algebra, the approximate variance becomes

$$\frac{1}{\hat{\sigma}^4}\left\{\hat{\sigma}^2 \,\text{var}\,(\hat{\alpha}) + \hat{\alpha}^2 \,\text{var}\,(\hat{\sigma}) - 2\hat{\alpha}\hat{\sigma}\,\text{cov}\,(\hat{\alpha}, \hat{\sigma})\right\}, \tag{5.49}$$

and the square root of this is the standard error of $\hat{\beta}$.

Example 5.7 Prognosis for women with breast cancer
The computation of a standard error of a log-hazard ratio is now illustrated using the data on the survival times of two groups breast cancer patients. In this example, computer output from fitting the log-linear form of the Weibull proportional hazards model is used to illustrate the estimation of the hazard ratio, and calculation of the standard error of the estimate.

On fitting the model that contains the treatment effect, represented by a variable X, where $X = 0$ for a woman with negative staining and $X = 1$ for positive staining, we find that the estimated coefficient of X is $\hat{\alpha} = -0.9967$. Also, the estimates of μ and σ are given by $\hat{\mu} = 5.8544$ and $\hat{\sigma} = 1.0668$, respectively. The estimated log-hazard ratio for a woman with positive staining, ($X = 1$) relative to a woman with negative staining ($X = 0$) is

$$\hat{\beta} = -\frac{-0.9967}{1.0668} = 0.9343.$$

The corresponding hazard ratio is 2.55, as in Example 5.6.

The standard errors of $\hat{\alpha}$ and $\hat{\sigma}$ are generally included in standard computer output, and are 0.5441 and 0.1786, respectively. The estimated variances of $\hat{\alpha}$ and $\hat{\sigma}$ are therefore 0.2960 and 0.0319, respectively. The covariance between $\hat{\alpha}$ and $\hat{\sigma}$ can be found from computer software, although it is not usually part of the default output. It is found to be -0.0213.

Substituting for $\hat{\alpha}$, $\hat{\sigma}$ and their variances and covariance in Expression (5.49), we get

$$\text{var}\,(\hat{\beta}) \approx 0.2498,$$

and so the standard error of $\hat{\beta}$ is given by $\text{se}\,(\hat{\beta}) = 0.4998$. This can be used in the construction of confidence intervals for the corresponding true hazard ratio.

5.6.4 Exploratory analyses

In Sections 5.2 and 5.5.1, we saw how a log-cumulative hazard plot could be used to assess whether survival data can be modelled by a Weibull distribution, and whether the proportional hazards assumption is valid. These procedures work perfectly well when we are faced with a single sample of survival data, or data where the number of groups is small and there is a reasonably large number of individuals in each group. But in situations where there are a small number of death times distributed over a relatively large number of groups, it may not be possible to estimate the survivor function, and hence the log-cumulative hazard function, for each group.

As an example, consider the data on the survival times of patients with hypernephroma, given in Table 3.6. Here, individuals are classified according to age group and whether or not a nephrectomy has been performed, giving six combinations of age group and nephrectomy status. To examine the assumption of a Weibull distribution for the survival times in each group, and the assumption of proportional hazards across the groups, a log-cumulative hazard plot would be required for each group. The number of patients in each age group who have not had a nephrectomy is so small that the survivor function cannot be properly estimated in these groups. If there were more individuals in the study who had died and not had a nephrectomy, it would be possible to construct a log-cumulative hazard plot. If this plot featured six parallel straight lines, the Weibull proportional hazards model is likely to be satisfactory.

When a model contains continuous variables, their values will first need to be grouped before a log-cumulative hazard plot can be obtained. This may also result in there being insufficient numbers of individuals in some groups to enable the log-cumulative hazard function to be estimated.

The only alternative to using each combination of factor levels in constructing a log-cumulative hazard plot is to ignore some of the factors. However, the resulting plot can be very misleading. For example, suppose that patients are classified according to the levels of two factors, A and B. The log-cumulative hazard plot obtained by grouping the individuals according to the levels of A ignoring B, or according to the levels of B ignoring A, may not give cause to doubt the Weibull or proportional hazards assumptions. However, if the log-cumulative hazard plot is obtained for individuals at each combination of levels of A and B, the plot may not feature a series of four parallel lines. By the same token, the log-cumulative hazard plot obtained when either A or B is ignored may not show sets of parallel straight lines, but when a plot is obtained for all combinations of A and B, parallel lines may result. This feature is illustrated in the following example.

Example 5.8 A numerical illustration

Suppose that a number of individuals are classified according to the levels of two factors, A and B, each with two levels, and that their survival times are as shown in Table 5.1.

Table 5.1 *Artificial data on the survival times of 37 patients classified according to the levels of two factors, A and B.*

$A = 1$		$A = 2$	
$B = 1$	$B = 2$	$B = 1$	$B = 2$
59	10	88	25*
20	4	70*	111
71	16	54	152
33	18	139	86
25	19	31	212
25	35	59	187*
15	11	111	54
53		149	357
47		30	301
		44	195
		25	

* Censored survival times.

The log-cumulative hazard plot shown in Figure 5.12 is derived from the individuals classified according to the two levels of A, ignoring the level of factor B. The plot in Figure 5.13 is from individuals classified according to the two levels of B, ignoring the level of factor A.

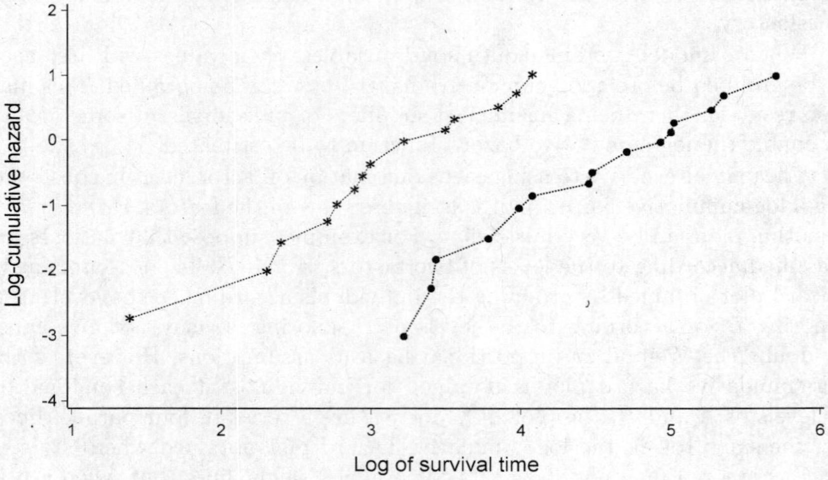

Figure 5.12 *Log-cumulative hazard plot for individuals for whom $A = 1$ (∗) and $A = 2$ (•).*

From Figure 5.12 there is no reason to doubt the assumption of a Weibull distribution for the survival times at the two levels of A, and the assumption of proportional hazards is clearly tenable. However, the crossed lines on the plot

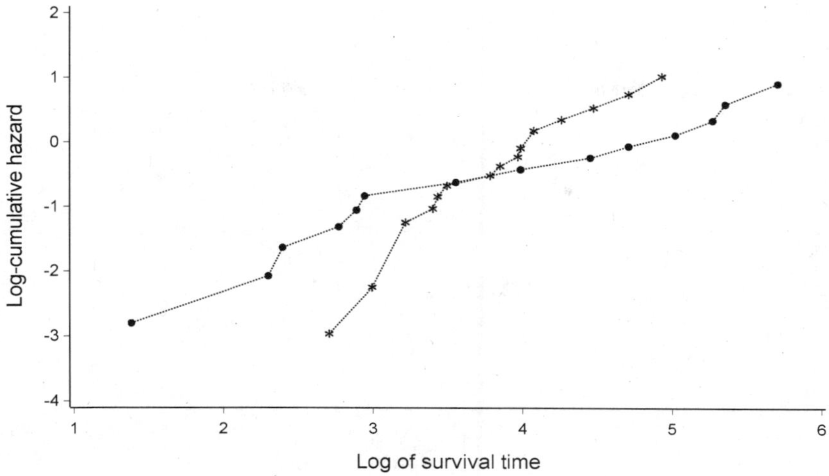

Figure 5.13 *Log-cumulative hazard plot for individuals for whom* $B = 1$ *(∗) and* $B = 2$ *(•).*

shown as Figure 5.13 strongly suggest that the hazards are not proportional when individuals are classified according to the levels of B. A different picture emerges when the 37 survival times are classified according to the levels of both A and B. The log-cumulative hazard plot based on the four groups is shown in Figure 5.14. The four parallel lines show that there is no doubt about the validity of the proportional hazards assumption across the groups.

In this example, the reason why the log-cumulative hazard plot for B ignoring A is misleading is that there is an interaction between A and B. An examination of the data reveals that, on average, the difference in the survival times of patients for whom $B = 1$ and $B = 2$ is greater when $A = 2$ than when $A = 1$.

Even when a log-cumulative hazard plot gives no reason to doubt the assumption of a Weibull proportional hazards model, the validity of the fitted model will need to be examined using the methods to be described in Chapter 7. When it is not possible to use a log-cumulative hazard plot to explore whether a Weibull distribution provides a reasonable model for the survival times, a procedure based on the Cox regression model, described in Chapter 3, might be helpful. Essentially, a Cox regression model that includes all the relevant explanatory variables is fitted, and the baseline hazard function is estimated, using the procedure described in Section 3.10. A plot of this function may suggest whether or not the assumption of a Weibull distribution is tenable. In particular, if the estimated baseline hazard function in the Cox model is increasing or decreasing, the Weibull model may provide a more con-

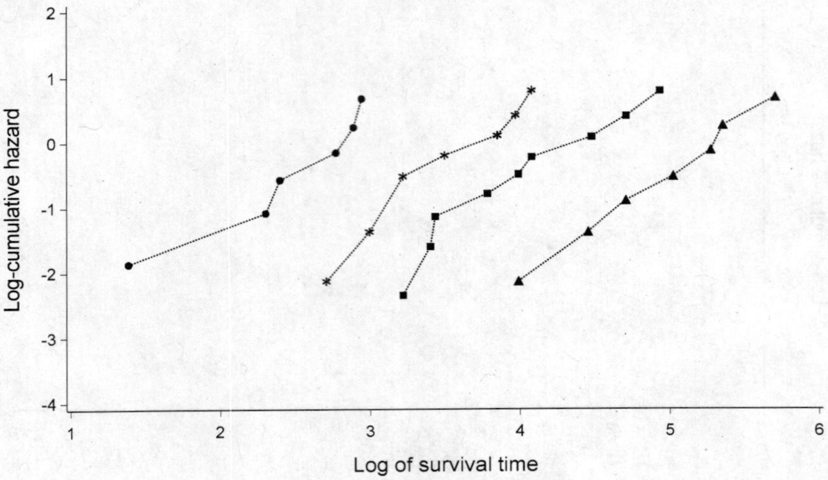

Figure 5.14 *Log-cumulative hazard plot for individuals in the groups defined by the four combinations of levels of A and B.*

cise summary of the baseline hazard function than the Cox regression model. Because the estimated baseline hazard function for a fitted Cox model can be somewhat irregular, comparing the estimated baseline cumulative hazard or the baseline survivor function, under the fitted Cox regression model, with that of the Weibull model may be more fruitful.

5.7 Comparing alternative Weibull models

In order to ascertain which explanatory variables should be included in a Weibull proportional hazards model, alternative models need to be compared. Comparisons between different Weibull models can be made using methods analogous to those for the Cox regression model described in Section 3.5.

Suppose that one model contains a subset of the explanatory variables in another, so that the two models are nested. The two models can then be compared on the basis of the statistic $-2\log\hat{L}$, where $\hat{L}$ is the maximised value of the likelihood function under the fitted model. For a model that contains p explanatory variables, the sample likelihood is a function of $p+2$ unknown parameters, $\beta_1, \beta_2, \ldots, \beta_p, \lambda$ and γ. The maximised likelihood is then the value of this function when these parameters take their estimates, $\hat{\beta}_1, \hat{\beta}_2, \ldots, \hat{\beta}_p, \hat{\lambda}$ and $\hat{\gamma}$.

More specifically, suppose that one model, Model (1), say, contains p explanatory variables, $X_1, X_2, \ldots, X_p$, and another model, Model (2), contains an additional q explanatory variables, $X_{p+1}, X_{p+2}, \ldots, X_{p+q}$. The estimated hazard functions for the ith of n individuals under these two models are as shown below:

$$\text{Model (1):} \quad h_i(t) = \exp\{\hat{\beta}_1 x_{1i} + \hat{\beta}_2 x_{2i} + \cdots + \hat{\beta}_p x_{pi}\}\hat{\lambda}\hat{\gamma}t^{\hat{\gamma}-1}$$

$$\text{Model (2):} \quad h_i(t) = \exp\{\hat{\beta}_1 x_{1i} + \hat{\beta}_2 x_{2i} + \cdots + \hat{\beta}_{p+q} x_{p+q,i}\}\hat{\lambda}\hat{\gamma}t^{\hat{\gamma}-1}$$

where $x_{1i}, x_{2i}, \ldots, x_{p+q,i}$ are the values of the $p+q$ explanatory variables for the ith individual. The maximised likelihoods under Model (1) and Model (2) will be denoted by $\hat{L}_1$ and $\hat{L}_2$, respectively. The difference between the values of $-2\log\hat{L}_1$ and $-2\log\hat{L}_2$, that is, $-2\{\log\hat{L}_1 - \log\hat{L}_2\}$, then has an approximate chi-squared distribution with q degrees of freedom, under the null hypothesis that the coefficients of the additional q variates in Model (2) are all equal to zero. If the difference between the values of $-2\log\hat{L}$ for these two models is significantly large when compared with percentage points of the chi-squared distribution, we would deduce that the extra q terms are needed in the model, in addition to the p that are already included. Since differences between values of $-2\log\hat{L}$ are used in comparing models, it does not matter whether the maximised log-likelihood, used in computing the value of $-2\log\hat{L}$, is based on Expression (5.39) or (5.40).

The description of the modelling process in Sections 3.5–3.8 applies equally well to models based on the Weibull proportional hazards model, and so will not be repeated here. However, the variable selection strategy will be illustrated using two examples.

Example 5.9 Treatment of hypernephroma

Data on the survival times of 36 patients, classified according to their age group and whether or not they have had a nephrectomy, were introduced in Example 3.4 of Chapter 3. In that example, the data were analysed using the Cox proportional hazards model. Here, the analysis is repeated using the Weibull proportional hazards model. As in Example 3.4, the effect of the jth age group will be denoted by α_j, and that associated with whether or not a nephrectomy was performed by ν_k. There are then five possible models for the hazard function of the ith individual, $h_i(t)$, which are as follows:

$$\text{Model (1):} \quad h_i(t) = h_0(t)$$

$$\text{Model (2):} \quad h_i(t) = \exp\{\alpha_j\}h_0(t)$$

$$\text{Model (3):} \quad h_i(t) = \exp\{\nu_k\}h_0(t)$$

$$\text{Model (4):} \quad h_i(t) = \exp\{\alpha_j + \nu_k\}h_0(t)$$

$$\text{Model (5):} \quad h_i(t) = \exp\{\alpha_j + \nu_k + (\alpha\nu)_{jk}\}h_0(t)$$

In these models, $h_0(t) = \lambda\gamma t^{\gamma-1}$ is the baseline hazard function, and the parameters λ and γ have to be estimated along with those in the linear component of the model. These five models have the interpretations given in Example 3.4. They can be fitted by constructing indicator variables corresponding to the factors age group and nephrectomy status, as shown in Example 3.4, or by using software that allows factors to be fitted directly.

Once a Weibull proportional hazards model has been fitted to the data, values of $-2\log\hat{L}$ can be found. These are given in Table 5.2 for the five models of interest.

Table 5.2 *Values of* $-2\log\hat{L}$ *on fitting five Weibull models to the data on hypernephroma.*

Model	Terms in model	$-2\log\hat{L}$
(1)	null model	104.886
(2)	α_j	96.400
(3)	ν_k	94.384
(4)	$\alpha_j + \nu_k$	87.758
(5)	$\alpha_j + \nu_k + (\alpha\nu)_{jk}$	83.064

The values of the $-2\log\hat{L}$ statistic in Table 5.2, and other examples in this book, have been computed using the log-likelihood in Expression (5.40). Accordingly these values may differ from the values given by some computer software packages by an amount equal to $2\sum_{i=1}^{n}\delta_i \log t_i$, which in this case has the value 136.3733.

The reduction in the value of $-2\log\hat{L}$ on adding the interaction term to Model (4) is 4.69 on two degrees of freedom. This reduction is just about significant at the 10% level ($P = 0.096$) and so there is some suggestion of an interaction between age group and nephrectomy status. For comparison, note that when the Cox regression model was fitted in Example 3.4, the interaction was not significant ($P = 0.220$).

The interaction can be investigated in greater detail by examining the hazard ratios under the model. Under Model (5), the estimated hazard function for the ith individual is

$$\hat{h}_i(t) = \exp\{\hat{\alpha}_j + \hat{\nu}_k + \widehat{(\alpha\nu)}_{jk}\}\hat{h}_0(t),$$

where

$$\hat{h}_0(t) = \hat{\lambda}\hat{\gamma}t^{\hat{\gamma}-1}$$

is the estimated baseline hazard function. The logarithm of the hazard ratio for an individual in the jth age group, $j = 1, 2, 3$, and kth level of nephrectomy status, $k = 1, 2$, relative to an individual in the youngest age group who has not had a nephrectomy, is therefore

$$\hat{\alpha}_j + \hat{\nu}_k + \widehat{(\alpha\nu)}_{jk} - \hat{\alpha}_1 - \hat{\nu}_1 - \widehat{(\alpha\nu)}_{11}, \tag{5.50}$$

since the baseline hazard functions cancel out.

As in Example 3.4, models can be fitted to the data by defining indicator variables A_2 and A_3 for age group and N for nephrectomy status. As in that example, A_2 is unity for an individual in the second age group and zero otherwise, A_3 is unity for an individual in the third age group and zero otherwise, and N is unity if a nephrectomy has been performed and zero otherwise. Thus, fitting the term α_j corresponds to fitting the variables A_2 and A_3, fitting ν_k corresponds to fitting N, and fitting the interaction term $(\alpha\nu)_{jk}$ corresponds to fitting the products $A_2N = A_2 \times N$ and $A_3N = A_3 \times N$. In particular, to fit Model (5), the five variables A_2, A_3, N, A_2N, A_3N are included in the model. With this choice of indicator variables, $\hat{\alpha}_1 = 0$, $\hat{\nu}_1 = 0$ and $\widehat{(\alpha\nu)}_{jk} = 0$ when either i or j is unity. The remaining values of $\hat{\alpha}_j, \hat{\nu}_k$ and $\widehat{(\alpha\nu)}_{jk}$ are the coefficients of A_2, A_3, N, A_2N, A_3N and are given in Table 5.3.

Table 5.3 *Parameter estimates on fitting a Weibull model to the data on hypernephroma.*

Parameter	Estimate
α_2	−0.085
α_3	0.115
ν_2	−2.436
$(\alpha\nu)_{22}$	0.121
$(\alpha\nu)_{32}$	2.538

Many computer packages set up indicator variables internally, and so estimates such as those in the above table can be obtained directly from the output. However, to repeat an earlier warning, when packages are used to fit factors, the coding used to define the indicator variables must be known if the output is to be properly interpreted.

When the indicator variables specified above are used, the logarithm of the hazard ratio given in Equation (5.50) reduces to

$$\hat{\alpha}_j + \hat{\nu}_k + \widehat{(\alpha\nu)}_{jk},$$

for $j = 1, 2, 3$, $k = 1, 2$. Table 5.4 gives the hazards for the individuals, relative to the baseline hazard. The baseline hazard corresponds to an individual in the youngest age group who has not had a nephrectomy, and so a hazard ratio of unity for these individuals is recorded in Table 5.4.

Table 5.4 *Hazard ratios for individuals classified by age group and nephrectomy status.*

Age group	No nephrectomy	Nephrectomy
<60	1.00	0.09
60–70	0.92	0.09
>70	1.12	1.24

This table helps to explain the interaction between age group and nephrectomy status, in that the effect of a nephrectomy is not the same for individuals in each of the three age groups. For patients in the two youngest age groups, a nephrectomy substantially reduces the hazard of death at any given time. Performing a nephrectomy on patients aged over 70 does not have much effect on the risk of death. We also see that for those patients who have not had a nephrectomy, age does not much affect the hazard of death.

Estimated median survival times can be found in a similar way. Using Equation (5.42), the median survival time for a patient in the jth age group, $j = 1, 2, 3$, and the kth level of nephrectomy status, $k = 1, 2$, becomes

$$\hat{t}(50) = \left\{ \frac{\log 2}{\hat{\lambda} \exp\{\hat{\alpha}_j + \hat{\nu}_k + \widehat{(\alpha\nu)}_{jk}\}} \right\}^{1/\hat{\gamma}}.$$

When the model containing the interaction term is fitted to the data, the estimated values of the parameters in the baseline hazard function are $\hat{\lambda} = 0.0188$ and $\hat{\gamma} = 1.5538$. Table 5.5 gives the estimated median survival times, in months, for individuals with each combination of age group and nephrectomy status.

Table 5.5 *Median survival times for individuals classified by age group and nephrectomy status.*

Age group	No nephrectomy	Nephrectomy
<60	10.21	48.94
60–70	10.78	47.81
>70	9.48	8.87

This table shows that a nephrectomy leads to more than a fourfold increase in the median survival time in patients aged up to 70 years. The median survival time of patients aged over 70 is not much affected by the performance of a nephrectomy.

We end this example with a note of caution. For some combinations of age group and nephrectomy status, particularly the groups of individuals who have not had a nephrectomy, the estimated hazard ratios and median survival times are based on small numbers of survival times. As a result, the standard errors of estimates of such quantities, which have not been given here, will be large.

Example 5.10 Chemotherapy in ovarian cancer patients

Following surgical treatment of ovarian cancer, patients may undergo a course of chemotherapy. In a study of two different forms of chemotherapy treatment, Edmunson et al. (1979) compared the anti-tumour effects of cyclophosphamide alone and cyclophosphamide combined with adriamycin. The trial involved 26 women with minimal residual disease and who had experienced surgical excision of all tumour masses greater than 2 cm in diameter. Following surgery, the patients were further classified according to whether the residual disease was completely or partially excised. The age of the patient and their performance status were also recorded at the start of the trial. The response variable was the survival time in days following randomisation to one or other of the two chemotherapy treatments. The variables in the data set are therefore as follows:

Time:	Survival time in days
Status:	Event indicator (0 = censored, 1 = uncensored)
Treat:	Treatment (1 = single, 2 = combined)
Age:	Age of patient in years
Rdisease:	Extent of residual disease (1 = incomplete, 2 = complete)
Perf:	Performance status (1 = good, 2 = poor)

The data, which were obtained from Therneau (1986), are given in Table 5.6.

Table 5.6 *Survival times of ovarian cancer patients.*

Patient	*Time*	*Status*	*Treat*	*Age*	*Rdisease*	*Perf*
1	156	1	1	66	2	2
2	1040	0	1	38	2	2
3	59	1	1	72	2	1
4	421	0	2	53	2	1
5	329	1	1	43	2	1
6	769	0	2	59	2	2
7	365	1	2	64	2	1
8	770	0	2	57	2	1
9	1227	0	2	59	1	2
10	268	1	1	74	2	2
11	475	1	2	59	2	2
12	1129	0	2	53	1	1
13	464	1	2	56	2	2
14	1206	0	2	44	2	1
15	638	1	1	56	1	2
16	563	1	2	55	1	2
17	1106	0	1	44	1	1
18	431	1	1	50	2	1
19	855	0	1	43	1	2
20	803	0	1	39	1	1
21	115	1	1	74	2	1
22	744	0	2	50	1	1
23	477	0	1	64	2	1
24	448	0	1	56	1	2
25	353	1	2	63	1	2
26	377	0	2	58	1	1

In modelling these data, the factors *Treat*, *Rdisease* and *Perf* each have two levels, and will be fitted as variates that take the values given in Table 5.6. This does of course mean that the baseline hazard function is not directly interpretable, since there can be no individual for whom the values of all these variates are zero. From both a computational and interpretive viewpoint, it is more convenient to relocate the values of the variables *Age*, *Rdisease*, *Perf* and *Treat*. If the variable *Age* − 50 is used in place of *Age*, and unity is subtracted from *Rdisease*, *Perf* and *Treat*, the baseline hazard then corresponds to the hazard for an individual of age 50 with incomplete residual disease, good performance status, and who has been allocated to the cyclophosphamide group. However, the original variables will be used in this example.

We begin by identifying which prognostic factors are associated with the survival times of the patients. The values of the statistic $-2\log\hat{L}$ on fitting a range of models to these data are given in Table 5.7.

Table 5.7 *Values of* $-2\log\hat{L}$ *on fitting models to the data in Table 5.6.*

Variables in model	$-2\log\hat{L}$
none	59.534
Age	43.566
Rdisease	55.382
Perf	58.849
Age, Rdisease	41.663
Age, Perf	43.518
Age, Treat	41.126
Age, Treat, Treat × *Age*	39.708

When Weibull models that contain just one of *Age*, *Rdisease* and *Perf* are fitted, we find that both *Age* and *Rdisease* lead to reductions in the value of $-2\log\hat{L}$ that are significant at the 5% level. After fitting *Age*, the variables *Rdisease* and *Perf* further reduce $-2\log\hat{L}$ by 1.903 and 0.048, respectively, neither of which is significant at the 10% level. Also, when *Age* is added to the model that already includes *Rdisease*, the reduction in $-2\log\hat{L}$ is 13.719 on 1 d.f., which is highly significant ($P < 0.001$). This leads us to the conclusion that *Age* is the only prognostic variable that needs to be incorporated in the model.

The term associated with the treatment effect is now added to the model. The value of $-2\log\hat{L}$ is then reduced by 2.440 on 1 d.f. This reduction of 2.440 is not quite large enough for it to be significant at the 10% level ($P = 0.118$). There is therefore only very slight evidence of a difference in the effect of the two chemotherapy treatments on the hazard of death.

For comparison, when *Treat* alone is added to the null model, the value of $-2\log\hat{L}$ is reduced from 59.534 to 58.355. This reduction of 1.179 is certainly not significant when compared to percentage points of the chi-squared distribution on 1 d.f. Ignoring *Age* therefore leads to an underestimate of the magnitude of the treatment effect.

To explore whether the treatment difference is consistent over age, the interaction term formed as the product of *Age* and *Treat* is added to the model.

On doing so, $-2\log\hat{L}$ is only reduced by 1.419. This reduction is nowhere near being significant and so there is no need to include an interaction term in the model.

The variable *Treat* will be retained in the model, since interest centres on the magnitude of the treatment effect. The fitted model for the hazard of death at time t for the ith individual is then found to be

$$\hat{h}_i(t) = \exp\{0.144\, Age_i - 1.023\, Treat_i\}\hat{\lambda}\hat{\gamma}t^{\hat{\gamma}-1},$$

where $\hat{\lambda} = 5.645 \times 10^{-9}$ and $\hat{\gamma} = 1.822$. In this model, *Treat* $= 1$ for cyclophosphamide alone and *Treat* $= 2$ for the combination of cyclophosphamide with adriamycin. The hazard for a patient on the single treatment, relative to one on the combined treatment, is therefore estimated by

$$\hat{\psi} = \exp\{(-1.023 \times 1) - (-1.023 \times 2)\} = 2.78.$$

This means that a patient receiving the single chemotherapy treatment is nearly three times more likely to die at any given time than a patient on the combined treatment. Expressed in this way, the benefits of the combined chemotherapy treatment appear substantial. However, when account is taken of the inherent variability of the data on which these results are based, this relative hazard is only significantly greater than unity at the 12% level ($P = 0.118$).

The median survival time can be estimated for patients of a given age on a given treatment from the equation

$$\hat{t}(50) = \left\{\frac{\log 2}{\hat{\lambda}\exp(0.144\, Age - 1.023\, Treat)}\right\}^{1/\hat{\gamma}}.$$

For example, a woman aged 60 (*Age* $= 60$) who is given cyclophosphamide alone (*Treat* $= 1$) has an estimated median survival time of 423 days, whereas someone of the same age on the combination of the two chemotherapy treatments has an estimated median survival time of 741 days. Confidence intervals for these estimates can be found using the method illustrated in Example 5.6.

5.8* Measures of explained variation in the Weibull model

Measures of explained variation in the Cox regression model were described in Section 3.12 of Chapter 3. In Equation (3.32) of that section, the R^2 measure of explained variation for the general linear model was expressed as

$$R^2 = \frac{\hat{V}_M}{\hat{V}_M + \hat{\sigma}^2},$$

where $\hat{V}_M$ is an estimate of variation in the data due to the fitted model and $\hat{\sigma}^2$ is the residual variation. Now, V_M can be expressed as $\hat{\boldsymbol{\beta}}'\boldsymbol{S}\hat{\boldsymbol{\beta}}$, where $\boldsymbol{S}$ is the variance-covariance matrix of the explanatory variables; see Section 3.12 of Chapter 3. It then follows that R^2 is a sample estimate of the quantity

$$\rho^2 = \frac{\boldsymbol{\beta}'\boldsymbol{S}\boldsymbol{\beta}}{\boldsymbol{\beta}'\boldsymbol{S}\boldsymbol{\beta} + \sigma^2}$$

in which σ^2 is the variance of the response variable, Y.

We now adapt this measure for use in the analysis of survival data, which requires the replacement of σ^2 by a suitable quantity. To do this, we take σ^2 to be the variance of the error term, ϵ_i, in the log-linear form of the Weibull model given in Equation (5.47) of Section 5.6.3. In the particular case of Weibull survival times, ϵ_i has a distribution which is such that the variance of ϵ_i is $\pi^2/6$; further details are given in Section 6.5.1 of Chapter 6. This leads to the statistic

$$R_P^2 = \frac{\hat{\boldsymbol{\beta}}'\boldsymbol{S}\hat{\boldsymbol{\beta}}}{\hat{\boldsymbol{\beta}}'\boldsymbol{S}\hat{\boldsymbol{\beta}} + \pi^2/6},$$

that was introduced in Section 3.12.1 of Chapter 3. This measure of explained variation can be generally recommended for use with both the Cox and Weibull proportional hazards models.

The R_D^2 statistic, also described in Section 3.12.1 of Chapter 3, can be adapted for use with parametric survival models in a similar manner. This leads to

$$R_D^2 = \frac{D^2}{D^2 + \pi^2/6}.$$

where D is the scaled coefficient for the regression of the ordered values of the risk score on normal scores as before.

Example 5.11 Survival of multiple myeloma patients

To illustrate the use of measures of explained variation in a Weibull model for survival data, consider the data on the survival times of patients with multiple myeloma, for which the values of three R^2 statistics on fitting Cox regression models were given in Example 3.17. For a Weibull model containing the variables *Hb* and *Bun*, $R_P^2 = 0.25$ and $R_D^2 = 0.23$. For the model that contains all 7 variables, $R_P^2 = 0.30$ and $R_D^2 = 0.28$. These values are quite similar to those obtained on fitting corresponding Cox regression models, so that the Cox and Weibull models have similar explanatory power.

5.9 The Gompertz proportional hazards model

Although the Weibull model is the most widely used parametric proportional hazards model, the Gompertz model has found application in demography and the biological sciences. Indeed the distribution was introduced by Gompertz in 1825, as a model for human mortality.

The hazard function of the Gompertz distribution is given by

$$h(t) = \lambda e^{\theta t},$$

for $0 \leqslant t < \infty$, and $\lambda > 0$. In the particular case where $\theta = 0$, the hazard function has a constant value, λ, and the survival times then have an exponential distribution. The parameter θ determines the shape of the hazard function, positive values leading to a hazard function that increases with time. The hazard function can also be expressed as $h(t) = \exp(\alpha + \theta t)$, which shows that the log-hazard function is linear in t. On the other hand, from Equation (5.4), the Weibull log-hazard function is linear in $\log t$. Like the Weibull hazard function, the Gompertz hazard increases or decreases monotonically.

The survivor function of the Gompertz distribution is given by

$$S(t) = \exp\left\{\frac{\lambda}{\theta}(1 - e^{\theta t})\right\},$$

and the corresponding density function is

$$f(t) = \lambda e^{\theta t} \exp\left\{\frac{\lambda}{\theta}(1 - e^{\theta t})\right\}.$$

The pth percentile is such that

$$t(p) = \frac{1}{\theta} \log\left\{1 - \frac{\theta}{\lambda} \log\left(\frac{100 - p}{100}\right)\right\},$$

from which the median survival time is

$$t(50) = \frac{1}{\theta} \log\left\{1 + \frac{\theta}{\lambda} \log 2\right\}.$$

A plot of the Gompertz hazard function for distributions with a median of 20 and $\theta = -0.2, 0.02$ and 0.05 is shown in Figure 5.15. The corresponding values of λ are 0.141, 0.028 and 0.020.

It is straightforward to see that the Gompertz distribution has the proportional hazards property, described in Section 5.5.1, since if we take $h_0(t) = \lambda e^{\theta t}$, then $\psi h_0(t)$ is also a Gompertz hazard function with parameters $\psi\lambda$ and θ.

The general Gompertz proportional hazards model for the hazard of death at time t for the ith of n individuals is expressed as

$$h_i(t) = \exp(\beta_1 x_{1i} + \beta_2 x_{2i} + \cdots + \beta_p x_{pi})\lambda e^{\theta t},$$

where $x_{1i}, x_{2i}, \ldots, x_{pi}$ are the values of p explanatory variables $X_1, X_2, \ldots, X_p$ for the ith individual, $i = 1, 2, \ldots, n$, and the β's, λ and θ are unknown parameters. The model can be fitted by maximising the likelihood function given in Expression (5.9) or (5.10). The β-coefficients are interpreted as log-hazard ratios, and alternative models are compared using the approach described in Section 5.7. No new principles are involved.

Example 5.12 Chemotherapy in ovarian cancer patients

In Example 5.10 on the survival times of ovarian cancer patients, a Weibull

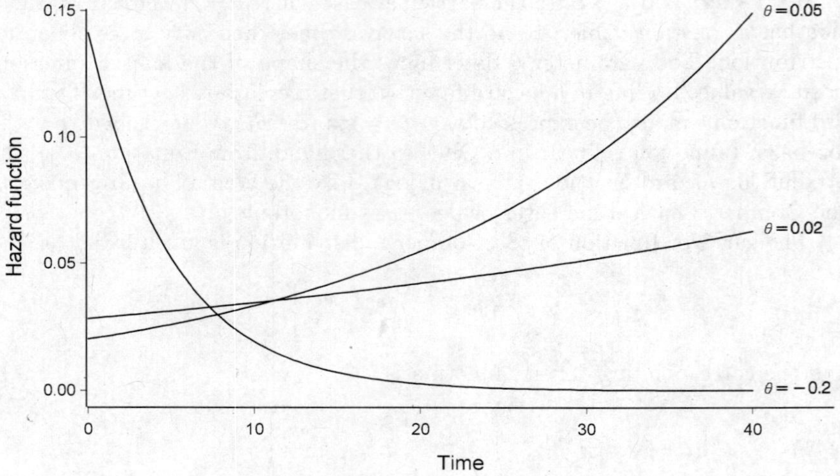

Figure 5.15 *Hazard functions for a Gompertz distribution with a median of 20 and* $\theta = -0.2$*, 0.02 and 0.05.*

proportional hazards model that contained the variables *Age* and *Treat* was fitted. For comparison, a Gompertz proportional hazards model that contains these two variables is now fitted. Under this model, the fitted hazard function for the ith patient is

$$\hat{h}_i(t) = \exp\{0.122\, Age_i - 0.848\, Treat_i\}\hat{\lambda}\exp(\hat{\theta}t),$$

where $\hat{\lambda} = 1.706 \times 10^{-6}$ and $\hat{\theta} = 0.00138$. The change in the value of $-2\log\hat{L}$ on adding *Treat* to the Gompertz proportional hazards model that contains *Age* alone is now 1.686 ($P = 0.184$). The hazard ratio for the treatment effect, which is now $\exp(0.848) = 2.34$, is therefore smaller and less significant under this model than it was for the Weibull model.

5.10 Model choice

One attraction of the proportional hazards model for survival data is that it is not necessary to adopt a specific probability distribution for the survival times. However, when a Weibull distribution is appropriate for the observed survival data, the parametric version of the proportional hazards model provides a more suitable basis for modelling the data.

Diagnostic plots based on the log-cumulative hazard function, described in Section 5.5.1, may throw light on whether the assumption of Weibull survival times is plausible, but as has already been pointed out, this technique is often not informative in the presence of explanatory variables that affect survival times. In such circumstances, to help choose between the Cox and Weibull proportional hazards models, it can be useful to fit the Cox regression model and examine the shape of the baseline hazard function. The fitted Weibull baseline cumulative hazard function, or the fitted baseline survivor function, can also be compared with the corresponding estimates for the Cox regression model, as described in Section 5.6.4.

A suitable analysis of residuals, to be discussed in Chapter 7, can be used to investigate whether one model fits better than the other. However, it will only be in exceptional circumstances that model-checking diagnostics provide convincing evidence that one or other of the two models is more acceptable.

In general, discrimination between a Cox and a Weibull proportional hazards model will be difficult unless the sample data contain a large number of death times. In cases where there is little to choose between the two models in terms of goodness of fit, the standard errors of the estimated β-parameters in the linear component of the two models can be compared. If those for the Weibull model are substantially smaller than those for the Cox model, the Weibull model would be preferred on grounds of efficiency. On the other hand, if these standard errors are similar, the Cox model is likely to be the model of choice in view of its less restrictive assumptions.

5.11 Further reading

The properties of the exponential, Weibull and Gompertz distributions are presented in Johnson and Kotz (1994). A thorough discussion of the theory of maximum likelihood estimation is included in Barnett (1999) and Cox and Hinkley (1974), and a useful summary of the main results is contained in Hinkley, Reid and Snell (1991). Numerical methods for obtaining maximum likelihood estimates, and the Newton-Raphson procedure in particular, are described by Everitt (1987) and Thisted (1988), for example; see also the description in Section 3.3.3 of Chapter 3. Byar (1982) presents a comparison of the Cox and Weibull proportional hazards models.

Papers that define and compare measures of explained variation for the Weibull model include those of Kent and O'Quigley (1988) and Royston and Sauerbrei (2004), cited in Chapter 3.

One other distribution with the proportional hazards property is the *Pareto distribution*. This model is rarely used in practice, but see Davis and Feldstein (1979) for further details.

Chapter 6

Accelerated failure time and other parametric models

Although the proportional hazards model finds widespread applicability in the analysis of survival data, there are relatively few probability distributions for the survival times that can be used with this model. Moreover, the distributions that are available, principally the Weibull and Gompertz distributions, lead to hazard functions that increase or decrease monotonically. A model that encompasses a wider range of survival time distributions is the *accelerated failure time model*. In circumstances where the proportional hazards assumption is not tenable, models based on this general family may prove to be fruitful. Again, the Weibull distribution may be adopted for the distribution of survival times in the accelerated failure time model, but some other probability distributions are also available. This chapter therefore begins with a brief survey of alternative distributions for survival data, that may be used in conjunction with an accelerated failure time model. The model itself is then considered in detail in Sections 6.3 to 6.6. One other general family of survival models, known as the *proportional odds model*, may be useful in some circumstances. This model is described in Section 6.7.

Parametric models based on standard probability distributions for survival data may not adequately summarise the pattern of an underlying baseline survivor or hazard function. An important extension to the basic proportional hazards and proportional odds models that leads to more flexible models is described and illustrated in Section 6.9.

6.1 Probability distributions for survival data

The Weibull distribution, described in Section 5.1.2, will not necessarily provide a satisfactory model for survival times in all circumstances, and so alternatives to this distribution need to be considered. Although any continuous distribution for non-negative random variables might be used, the properties of the log-logistic distribution make it a particularly attractive alternative to the Weibull distribution. The lognormal, gamma and inverse Gaussian distributions are also used in accelerated failure time modelling, and so these distributions are introduced in this section.

6.1.1 The log-logistic distribution

One limitation of the Weibull hazard function is that it is a monotonic function of time. However, situations in which the hazard function changes direction can arise. For example, following a heart transplant, a patient faces an increasing hazard of death over the first ten days or so after the transplant, while the body adapts to the new organ. The hazard then decreases with time as the patient recovers. In situations such as this, a unimodal hazard function may be appropriate.

A particular form of unimodal hazard is the function

$$h(t) = \frac{e^{\theta}\kappa t^{\kappa-1}}{1+e^{\theta}t^{\kappa}}, \tag{6.1}$$

for $0 \leqslant t < \infty$, $\kappa > 0$. This hazard function decreases monotonically if $\kappa \leqslant 1$, but if $\kappa > 1$, the hazard has a single mode. The survivor function corresponding to the hazard function in Equation (6.1) is given by

$$S(t) = \left\{1 + e^{\theta}t^{\kappa}\right\}^{-1}, \tag{6.2}$$

and the probability density function is

$$f(t) = \frac{e^{\theta}\kappa t^{\kappa-1}}{(1+e^{\theta}t^{\kappa})^2}.$$

This is the density of a random variable T that has a *log-logistic distribution*, with parameters θ, κ. The distribution is so called because the variable $\log T$ has a *logistic distribution*, a symmetric distribution whose probability density function is very similar to that of the normal distribution.

The pth percentile of the log-logistic distribution is

$$t(p) = \left(\frac{p\,e^{-\theta}}{100-p}\right)^{1/\kappa},$$

and so the median of the distribution is

$$t(50) = e^{-\theta/\kappa}.$$

The hazard functions for log-logistic distributions with a median of 20 and $\kappa = 0.5$, 2.0 and 5.0 are shown in Figure 6.1. The corresponding values of θ for these distributions are -1.5, -6.0 and -15.0, respectively.

6.1.2 The lognormal distribution

The *lognormal distribution* is also defined for random variables that take positive values, and so may be used as a model for survival data. A random variable, T, is said to have a lognormal distribution, with parameters μ and

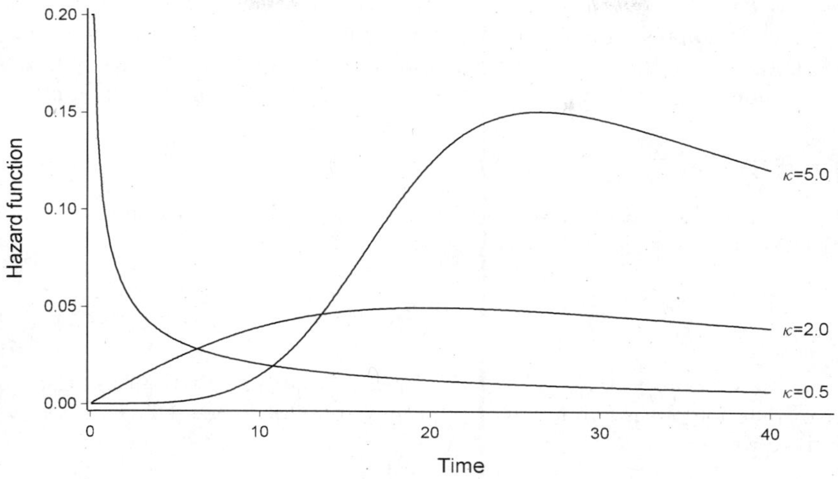

Figure 6.1 *Hazard functions for a log-logistic distribution with a median of 20 and* $\kappa =$ *0.5, 2.0 and 5.0.*

σ, if $\log T$ has a normal distribution with mean μ and variance σ^2. The probability density function of T is given by

$$f(t) = \frac{1}{\sigma\sqrt{(2\pi)}} t^{-1} \exp\left\{-(\log t - \mu)^2/2\sigma^2\right\},$$

for $0 \leqslant t < \infty$, $\sigma > 0$, from which the survivor and hazard functions can be derived. The survivor function of the lognormal distribution is

$$S(t) = 1 - \Phi\left(\frac{\log t - \mu}{\sigma}\right), \qquad (6.3)$$

where $\Phi(\cdot)$ is the standard normal distribution function, given by

$$\Phi(z) = \frac{1}{\sqrt{(2\pi)}} \int_{-\infty}^{z} \exp\left(-u^2/2\right) du.$$

The pth percentile of the distribution is then

$$t(p) = \exp\left\{\sigma\Phi^{-1}(p/100) + \mu\right\},$$

where $\Phi^{-1}(p/100)$, the pth percentile of the standard normal distribution, is sometimes called the *probit* of $p/100$. In particular, the median survival time under this distribution is simply $t(50) = e^{\mu}$.

The hazard function can be found from the relation $h(t) = f(t)/S(t)$. This function is zero when $t = 0$, increases to a maximum and then decreases to zero as t tends to infinity. The fact that the survivor and hazard functions can only be expressed in terms of integrals limits the usefulness of this model. Moreover, in view of the similarity of the normal and logistic distributions, the lognormal model will tend to be very similar to the log-logistic model.

6.1.3 The gamma distribution*

The probability density function of a *gamma distribution* with mean ρ/λ and variance ρ/λ^2 is such that

$$f(t) = \frac{\lambda^\rho t^{\rho-1} e^{-\lambda t}}{\Gamma(\rho)}, \tag{6.4}$$

for $0 \leqslant t < \infty$, $\lambda > 0$, and $\rho > 0$. As for the lognormal distribution, the survivor function of the gamma distribution can only be expressed as an integral, and we write

$$S(t) = 1 - \Gamma_{\lambda t}(\rho),$$

where $\Gamma_{\lambda t}(\rho)$ is known as the *incomplete gamma function*, given by

$$\Gamma_{\lambda t}(\rho) = \frac{1}{\Gamma(\rho)} \int_0^{\lambda t} u^{\rho-1} e^{-u} \, du.$$

The hazard function for the gamma distribution is then $h(t) = f(t)/S(t)$. This hazard function increases monotonically if $\rho > 1$ and decreases if $\rho < 1$, and tends to λ as t tends to ∞.

When $\rho = 1$, the gamma distribution reduces to the exponential distribution described in Section 5.1.1, and so this distribution, like the Weibull distribution, includes the exponential distribution as a special case. Indeed, the gamma distribution is quite similar to the Weibull, and inferences based on either model will often be very similar.

A generalisation of the gamma distribution is actually more useful than the gamma distribution itself, since it includes the Weibull and lognormal distributions as special cases. This model, known as the *generalised gamma distribution*, may therefore be used to discriminate between alternative parametric models for survival data.

The probability density function of the generalised gamma distribution is an extension of the gamma density in Equation (6.4), that includes an additional parameter, θ, where $\theta > 0$, and is defined by

$$f(t) = \frac{\theta \lambda^{\rho\theta} t^{\rho\theta-1} \exp\{-(\lambda t)^\theta\}}{\Gamma(\rho)},$$

for $0 \leqslant t < \infty$. The survivor function for this distribution is again defined in terms of the incomplete gamma function and is given by

$$S(t) = 1 - \Gamma_{(\lambda t)^\theta}(\rho),$$

and the hazard function is again found from $h(t) = f(t)/S(t)$. This distribution leads to a wide range of shapes for the hazard function, governed by the parameter θ. This parameter is therefore termed the *shape parameter* of the distribution. When $\rho = 1$, the distribution becomes the Weibull, when $\theta = 1$, the gamma, and as $\rho \to \infty$, the lognormal.

6.1.4 The inverse Gaussian distribution*

The *inverse Gaussian distribution* is a flexible model that has some important theoretical properties. The probability density function of the distribution which has mean μ and scale parameter λ is given by

$$f(t) = \left(\frac{\lambda}{2\pi t^3}\right)^{\frac{1}{2}} \exp\left\{\frac{\lambda(t-\mu^2)}{2\mu^2 t}\right\},$$

for $0 \leqslant t < \infty$, and $\lambda > 0$. The corresponding survivor function is

$$S(t) = \Phi\left\{\left(1 - t\mu^{-1}\right)\surd\left(\lambda t^{-1}\right)\right\} - \exp(2\lambda/\mu)\,\Phi\left\{-\left(1 + t\mu^{-1}\right)\surd\left(\lambda t^{-1}\right)\right\},$$

and the hazard function is found from the ratio of the density and survivor functions. However, the complicated form of the survivor function makes this distribution difficult to work with.

6.2 Exploratory analyses

When the number of observations in a single sample is reasonably large, an empirical estimate of the hazard function could be obtained using the method described in Section 2.3.1. A plot of the estimated hazard function may then suggest a suitable parametric form for the hazard function. For example, if the hazard plot is found to be unimodal, a log-logistic distribution could be used for the survival times. When the database includes a number of explanatory variables, the form of the estimated baseline hazard, cumulative hazard, or survivor functions, for a fitted Cox regression model, may also indicate whether a particular parametric model is suitable, in the manner described in Section 5.6.4 of Chapter 5.

A method for exploring the adequacy of the Weibull model in describing a single sample of survival times was described in Section 5.2. A similar procedure can be used to assess the suitability of the log-logistic distribution. The basic idea is that a transformation of the survivor function is sought, which leads to a straight line plot. From Equation (6.2), the odds of surviving beyond time t are

$$\frac{S(t)}{1 - S(t)} = e^{-\theta} t^{-\kappa},$$

and so the log-odds of survival beyond t can be expressed as

$$\log\left\{\frac{S(t)}{1 - S(t)}\right\} = -\theta - \kappa \log t.$$

If the survivor function for the data is estimated using the Kaplan-Meier estimate, and the estimated log-odds of survival beyond t are plotted against $\log t$, a straight line plot will be obtained if a log-logistic model for the survival times is suitable. Estimates of the parameters of the log-logistic distribution, θ and κ, can be obtained from the intercept and slope of the straight line plot.

The suitability of other parametric models can be investigated along similar lines. For example, from the survivor function of the lognormal distribution, given in Equation (6.3),

$$\Phi^{-1}\{1 - S(t)\} = \frac{\log t - \mu}{\sigma},$$

and so a plot of $\Phi^{-1}\{1 - \hat{S}(t)\}$ against $\log t$ should give a straight line, if the lognormal model is appropriate. The slope and intercept of this line provide estimates of σ^{-1} and $-\mu/\sigma$, respectively.

Example 6.1 Time to discontinuation of the use of an IUD
In Example 5.1, a log-cumulative hazard plot was used to evaluate the fit of the Weibull distribution to the data on times to discontinuation of an intrauterine device (IUD), given in Example 1.1. We now consider whether the log-logistic distribution is appropriate. A plot of $\log\{\hat{S}(t)/[1 - \hat{S}(t)]\}$ against $\log t$ for the data on the times to discontinuation of an IUD is shown in Figure 6.2.

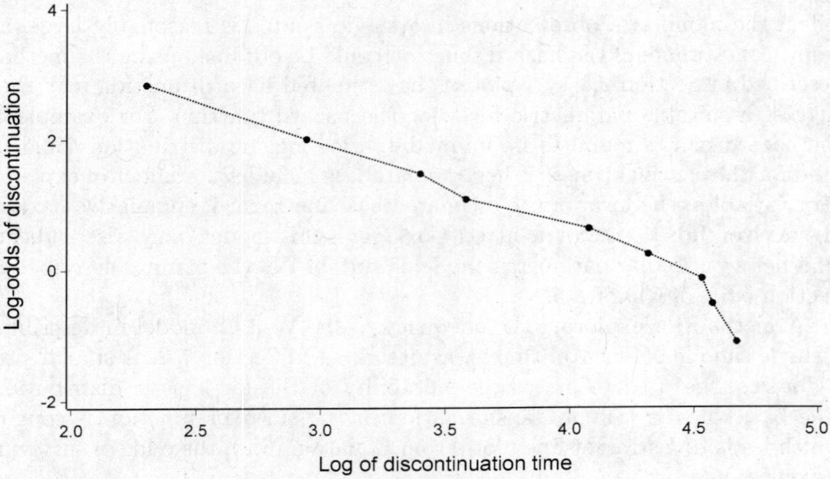

Figure 6.2 *A plot of the estimated log-odds of discontinuation after* t *against* $\log t$ *for the data from Example 1.1.*

From this plot, it appears that the relationship between the estimated log-odds of discontinuing use of the contraceptive after time t, and $\log t$, is reasonably straight. This suggests that a log-logistic model could be used to model the observed data.

Notice that there is very little difference in the extent of departures from linearity in the plots of Figures 5.6 and 6.2. This means that either the Weibull distribution or the log-logistic distribution is likely to be satisfactory, even though the estimated hazard function under these two distributions may be quite different. Indeed, when survival data are obtained for a relatively small number of individuals, as in this example, there will often be little to choose between alternative distributional models for the data. The model that is the most convenient for the purpose in hand will then be adopted.

6.3 The accelerated failure time model for comparing two groups

The accelerated failure time model is a general model for survival data, in which explanatory variables measured on an individual are assumed to act multiplicatively on the time-scale, and so affect the rate at which an individual proceeds along the time axis. This means that the models can be interpreted in terms of the speed of progression of a disease, an interpretation that has immediate intuitive appeal. Before the general form of the model is presented in Section 6.4, the model for comparing the survival times of two groups of patients is described in detail.

Suppose that patients are randomised to receive one of two treatments, a standard treatment, S, or a new treatment, N. Under an accelerated failure time model, the survival time of an individual on the new treatment is taken to be a multiple of the survival time for an individual on the standard treatment. Thus, the effect of the new treatment is to 'speed up' or 'slow down' the passage of time. Under this assumption, the probability that an individual on the new treatment survives beyond time t is the probability that an individual on the standard treatment survives beyond time t/ϕ, where ϕ is an unknown positive constant.

Now let $S_S(t)$ and $S_N(t)$ be the survivor functions for individuals in the two treatment groups. Then, the accelerated failure time model specifies that

$$S_N(t) = S_S(t/\phi),$$

for any value of the survival time t. One interpretation of this model is that the lifetime of an individual on the new treatment is ϕ times the lifetime that the individual would have experienced under the standard treatment. The parameter ϕ therefore reflects the impact of the new treatment on the baseline time-scale. When the end-point of concern is the death of a patient, values of ϕ less than unity correspond to an acceleration in the time to death of an individual assigned to the new treatment, relative to an individual on the standard treatment. The standard treatment would then be the more suitable in terms of promoting longevity. On the other hand, when the end-point is the recovery from some disease state, values of ϕ less than unity would be found when the effect of the new treatment is to speed up the recovery time.

In these circumstances, the new treatment would be superior to the standard. The quantity ϕ^{-1} is therefore termed the *acceleration factor.*

The acceleration factor can also be interpreted in terms of the median survival times of patients on the new and standard treatments, $t_N(50)$ and $t_S(50)$, say. These values are such that $S_N\{t_N(50)\} = S_S\{t_S(50)\} = 0.5$. Now, under the accelerated failure time model, $S_N\{t_N(50)\} = S_S\{t_N(50)/\phi\}$, and so it follows that $t_N(50) = \phi t_S(50)$. In other words, under the accelerated failure time model, the median survival time of a patient on the new treatment is ϕ times that of a patient on the standard treatment. In fact, the same argument can be used for any percentile of the survival time distribution. This means that the pth percentile of the survival time distribution for a patient on the new treatment, $t_N(p)$, is such that $t_N(p) = \phi t_S(p)$, where $t_S(p)$ is the pth percentile for the standard treatment. This interpretation of the acceleration factor is particularly appealing to clinicians.

From the relationship between the survivor function, probability density function and hazard function given in Equation (1.4), the relationship between the density and hazard functions for individuals in the two treatment groups is

$$f_N(t) = \phi^{-1} f_S(t/\phi),$$

and

$$h_N(t) = \phi^{-1} h_S(t/\phi).$$

Now let X be an indicator variable that takes the value zero for an individual in the group receiving the standard treatment, and unity for one who receives the new treatment. The hazard function for the ith individual can then be expressed as

$$h_i(t) = \phi^{-x_i} h_0(t/\phi^{x_i}), \tag{6.5}$$

where x_i is the value of X for the ith individual in the study. Putting $x_i = 0$ in this expression shows that the function $h_0(t)$ is the hazard function for an individual on the standard treatment. This is again referred to as the baseline hazard function. The hazard function for an individual on the new treatment is then $\phi^{-1} h_0(t/\phi)$.

The parameter ϕ must be non-negative, and so it is convenient to set $\phi = e^{\alpha}$. The accelerated failure time model in Equation (6.5) then becomes

$$h_i(t) = e^{-\alpha x_i} h_0(t/e^{\alpha x_i}), \tag{6.6}$$

so that the hazard function for an individual on the new treatment is now $e^{-\alpha} h_0(t/e^{\alpha})$.

6.3.1 Comparison with the proportional hazards model*

To illustrate the difference between a proportional hazards model and the accelerated failure time model, again suppose that the survival times of individuals in two groups, Group I and Group II, say, are to be modelled. Further suppose that for the individuals in Group I, the hazard function is given by

$$h_0(t) = \begin{cases} 0.5 \text{ if } t \leqslant 1, \\ 1.0 \text{ if } t > 1, \end{cases}$$

where the time-scale is measured in months. This type of hazard function arises from a *piecewise exponential model*, since a constant hazard in each time interval implies exponentially distributed survival times, with different means, in each interval. This model provides a simple way of representing a variable hazard function, and may be appropriate in situations where there is a constant short-term risk that increases abruptly after a threshold time.

Now let $h_P(t)$ and $h_A(t)$ denote the hazard functions for individuals in Group II under a proportional hazards model and an accelerated failure time model, respectively. Consequently, we may write

$$h_P(t) = \psi h_0(t),$$

and

$$h_A(t) = \phi^{-1} h_0(t/\phi),$$

for the two hazard functions. Using the result $S(t) = \exp\{-\int_0^t h(u)\,du\}$, the baseline survivor function is

$$S_0(t) = \begin{cases} e^{-0.5t} & \text{if } t \leqslant 1, \\ e^{-0.5-(t-1)} & \text{if } t > 1. \end{cases}$$

Since $S_0(t) > 0.61$ if $t < 1$, the median occurs in the second part of the survivor function and is when $\exp\{-0.5 - (t-1)\} = 0.5$. The median survival time for those in Group I is therefore 1.19 months.

The survivor functions for the individuals in Group II under the two models are

$$S_P(t) = [S_0(t)]^{\psi},$$

and

$$S_A(t) = S_0(t/\phi),$$

respectively.

To illustrate the difference between the hazard functions under proportional hazards and accelerated failure time models, consider the particular case where $\psi = \phi^{-1} = 2.0$. The median survival time for individuals in Group II is 0.69 months under the proportional hazards model, and 0.60 months under the accelerated failure time model. The hazard functions for the two groups under both models are shown in Figure 6.3 and the corresponding survivor functions are shown in Figure 6.4.

Under the accelerated failure time model, the increase in the hazard for Group II from 1.0 to 2.0 occurs sooner than under the proportional hazards model. The 'kink' in the survivor function also occurs earlier under the accelerated failure time model.

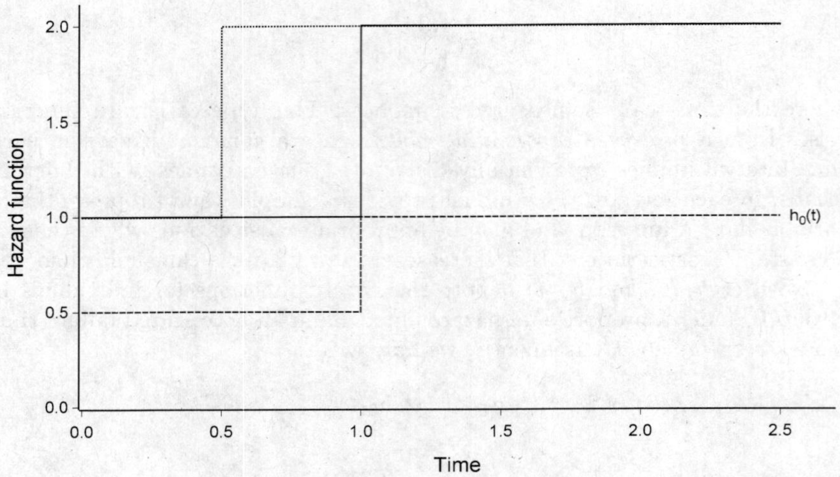

Figure 6.3 *The hazard functions for individuals in Group I, $h_0(t)$, and in Group II under (i) a proportional hazards model (—) and (ii) an accelerated failure time model ($\cdots$).*

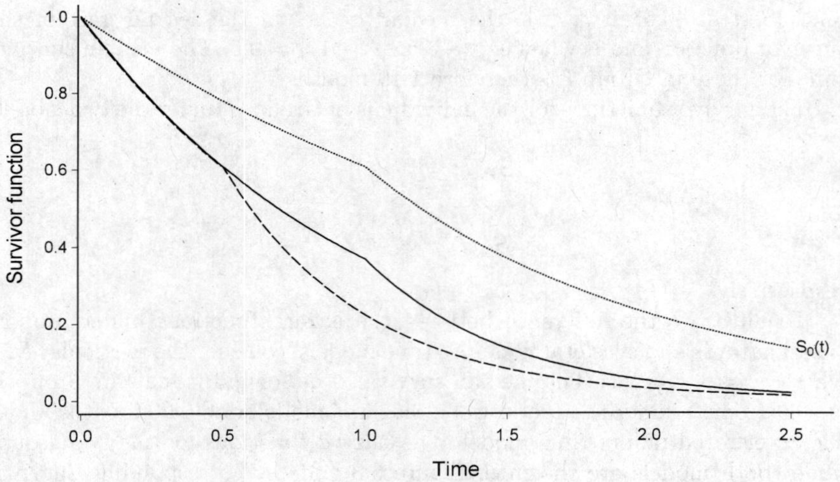

Figure 6.4 *The survivor functions for individuals in Group I, $S_0(t)$, and in Group II, under (i) a proportional hazards model (—) and (ii) an accelerated failure time model ($\cdots$).*

6.3.2 The percentile-percentile plot

The *percentile-percentile plot*, also known as the *quantile-quantile plot* or the *Q-Q plot*, provides an exploratory method for assessing the validity of an accelerated failure time model for two groups of survival data. Recall that the pth percentile of a distribution is the value $t(p)$, which is such that the estimated survivor function at time $t(p)$ is $1 - (p/100)$, for any value of p in the interval $(0, 100)$. The pth percentile is therefore such that

$$t(p) = S^{-1}\left(\frac{100 - p}{100}\right).$$

Now let $t_0(p)$ and $t_1(p)$ be the pth percentiles estimated from the survivor functions of the two groups of survival data. The values of p might be taken to be $10, 20, \ldots, 90$, so long as the number of observations in each of the two groups is not too small. The percentiles of the two groups may therefore be expressed as

$$t_0(p) = S_0^{-1}\left(\frac{100 - p}{100}\right), \quad t_1(p) = S_1^{-1}\left(\frac{100 - p}{100}\right),$$

where $S_0(t)$ and $S_1(t)$ are the survivor functions for the two groups. It then follows that

$$S_1\{t_1(p)\} = S_0\{t_0(p)\}, \tag{6.7}$$

for any given value of p.

Under the accelerated failure time model, $S_1(t) = S_0(t/\phi)$, and so the pth percentile for the second group, $t_1(p)$, is such that

$$S_1\{t_1(p)\} = S_0\{t_1(p)/\phi\}.$$

Using Equation (6.7),

$$S_0\{t_0(p)\} = S_0\{t_1(p)/\phi\},$$

and hence

$$t_0(p) = \phi^{-1}t_1(p).$$

Now let $\hat{t}_0(p)$, $\hat{t}_1(p)$ be the estimated percentiles in the two groups, so that

$$\hat{t}_0(p) = \hat{S}_0^{-1}\left(\frac{100 - p}{100}\right), \quad \hat{t}_1(p) = \hat{S}_1^{-1}\left(\frac{100 - p}{100}\right).$$

A plot of the quantity $\hat{t}_0(p)$ against $\hat{t}_1(p)$, for suitably chosen values of p, should give a straight line through the origin if the accelerated failure time model is appropriate. The slope of this line will be an estimate of the acceleration factor, ϕ^{-1}. This plot may therefore be used in an exploratory assessment of the adequacy of the accelerated failure time model. In this sense, it is an analogue of the log-cumulative hazard plot, used in Section 4.4.1 to examine the validity of the proportional hazards model.

Example 6.2 Prognosis for women with breast cancer
In this example, the data on the survival times of women with breast tumours that were negatively or positively stained, originally given as Example 1.2 in Chapter 1, is used to illustrate the percentile-percentile plot. The percentiles of the distribution of the survival times in each of the two groups can be estimated from the Kaplan-Meier estimate of the respective survivor functions. These are given in Table 6.1.

Table 6.1 *Estimated percentiles of the distributions of survival times for women with tumours that were positively or negatively stained.*

Percentile	Negative staining	Positive staining
10	47	13
20	69	26
30	148	35
40	181	48
50	–	61
60	–	113
70	–	143
80	–	–
90	–	–

The relatively small numbers of death times, and the censoring pattern in the data from the two groups of women, mean that not all of the percentiles can be estimated. The percentile-percentile plot will therefore have just four pairs of points. For illustration, this is shown in Figure 6.5. The points fall on a line that is reasonably straight, suggesting that the accelerated failure time model would not be inappropriate. However, this conclusion must be regarded with some caution in view of the limited number of points in the graph.

The slope of a straight line drawn through the points in Figure 6.5 is approximately equal to 3, which is a rough estimate of the acceleration factor. The interpretation of this is that for women whose tumours were positively stained, the disease process is speeded up by a factor of three, relative to those whose tumours were negatively stained. We can also say that the median survival time for women with negatively stained tumours is estimated to be three times that of women with positively stained tumours.

6.4 The general accelerated failure time model

The accelerated failure time model in Equation (6.6) can be generalised to the situation where the values of p explanatory variables have been recorded for each individual in a study. According to the general accelerated failure time model, the hazard function of the ith individual at time t, $h_i(t)$, is then such

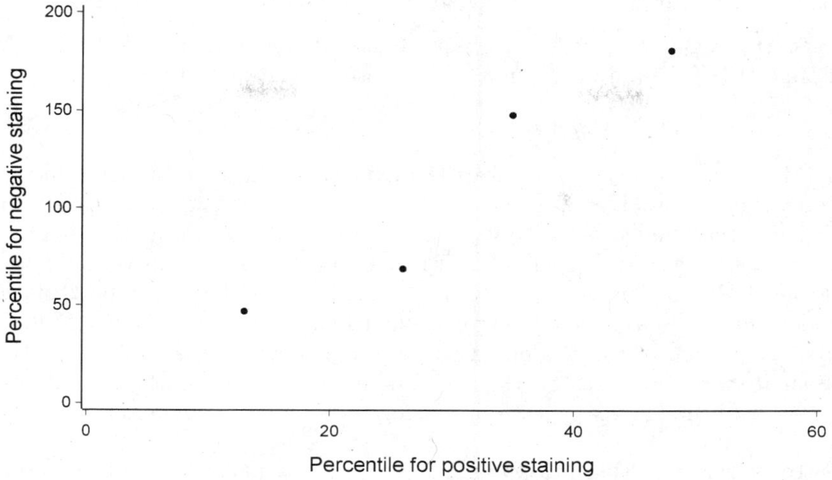

Figure 6.5 *Percentile-percentile plot for the data on the survival times of breast cancer patients.*

that

$$h_i(t) = e^{-\eta_i} h_0(t/e^{\eta_i}), \tag{6.8}$$

where

$$\eta_i = \alpha_1 x_{1i} + \alpha_2 x_{2i} + \cdots + \alpha_p x_{pi}$$

is the linear component of the model, in which x_{ji} is the value of the jth explanatory variable, X_j, $j = 1, 2, \ldots, p$, for the ith individual, $i = 1, 2, \ldots, n$. As in the proportional hazards model, the baseline hazard function, $h_0(t)$, is the hazard of death at time t for an individual for whom the values of the p explanatory variables are all equal to zero. The corresponding survivor function for the ith individual is

$$S_i(t) = S_0\{t/\exp(\eta_i)\},$$

where $S_0(t)$ is the baseline survivor function.

Parametric accelerated failure time models are unified by the adoption of a log-linear representation of the model, described in the sequel. This representation shows that the accelerated failure time model for survival data is closely related to the general linear model used in regression analysis. Moreover, this form of the model is adopted by most computer software packages for accelerated failure time modelling.

6.4.1 Log-linear form of the accelerated failure time model*

Consider a *log-linear model* for the random variable T_i, associated with the lifetime of the ith individual in a survival study, according to which

$$\log T_i = \mu + \alpha_1 x_{1i} + \alpha_2 x_{2i} + \cdots + \alpha_p x_{pi} + \sigma\epsilon_i. \tag{6.9}$$

In this model, $\alpha_1, \alpha_2, \ldots, \alpha_p$ are the unknown coefficients of the values of p explanatory variables, $X_1, X_2, \ldots, X_p$, with values $x_{1i}, x_{2i}, \ldots, x_{pi}$ for the ith individual, and μ, σ are two further parameters, known as the *intercept* and *scale parameter*, respectively. The quantity ϵ_i is a random variable used to model the deviation of the values of $\log T_i$ from the linear part of the model, and ϵ_i is assumed to have a particular probability distribution. In this formulation of the model, the α-parameters reflect the effect that each explanatory variable has on the survival times; positive values suggest that the survival time increases with increasing values of the explanatory variable, and vice versa.

To show the relationship between this representation of the model and that in Equation (6.8), consider the survivor function of T_i, the random variable associated with the survival time of the ith individual. Using Equation (6.9), this is given by

$$S_i(t) = \mathrm{P}(T_i \geqslant t) = \mathrm{P}\left\{\exp(\mu + \boldsymbol{\alpha}'\boldsymbol{x}_i + \sigma\epsilon_i) \geqslant t\right\},$$

where $\boldsymbol{\alpha}'\boldsymbol{x}_i = \alpha_1 x_{1i} + \alpha_2 x_{2i} + \cdots + \alpha_p x_{pi}$.

Now, $S_i(t)$ can be written in the form

$$S_i(t) = \mathrm{P}\left\{\exp(\mu + \sigma\epsilon_i) \geqslant t/\exp(\boldsymbol{\alpha}'\boldsymbol{x}_i)\right\},$$

and the baseline survivor function, $S_0(t)$, the survivor function of an individual for whom $\boldsymbol{x} = \mathbf{0}$, is

$$S_0(t) = \mathrm{P}\left\{\exp(\mu + \sigma\epsilon_i) \geqslant t\right\}.$$

It then follows that

$$S_i(t) = S_0\{t/\exp(\boldsymbol{\alpha}'\boldsymbol{x}_i)\}, \tag{6.10}$$

which is the general form of the survivor function for the ith individual in an accelerated failure time model. In this version of the model, the acceleration factor is $\exp(-\boldsymbol{\alpha}'\boldsymbol{x}_i)$ for the ith individual. The corresponding relationship between the hazard functions is obtained using Equation (1.5) of Chapter 1. Specifically, taking logarithms of both sides of Equation (6.10), multiplying by -1, and differentiating with respect to t, leads to

$$h_i(t) = \exp(-\boldsymbol{\alpha}'\boldsymbol{x}_i) h_0\{t/\exp(\boldsymbol{\alpha}'\boldsymbol{x}_i)\},$$

which is the model in Equation (6.8) with $\eta_i = \boldsymbol{\alpha}'\boldsymbol{x}_i$.

The log-linear formulation of the model can also be used to give a general form of the survivor function for the ith individual, which is

$$S_i(t) = \mathrm{P}(T_i \geqslant t) = \mathrm{P}(\log T_i \geqslant \log t).$$

From Equation (6.9),

$$\begin{aligned} S_i(t) &= \mathrm{P}(\mu + \alpha_1 x_{1i} + \alpha_2 x_{2i} + \cdots + \alpha_p x_{pi} + \sigma\epsilon_i \geqslant \log t), \\ &= \mathrm{P}\left(\epsilon_i \geqslant \frac{\log t - \mu - \alpha_1 x_{1i} - \alpha_2 x_{2i} - \cdots - \alpha_p x_{pi}}{\sigma}\right). \end{aligned} \tag{6.11}$$

If we now write $S_{\epsilon_i}(\epsilon)$ for the survivor function of the random variable ϵ_i in the log-linear model of Equation (6.9), the survivor function of the ith individual can, from Equation (6.11), be expressed as

$$S_i(t) = S_{\epsilon_i}\left(\frac{\log t - \mu - \alpha_1 x_{1i} - \alpha_2 x_{2i} - \cdots - \alpha_p x_{pi}}{\sigma}\right). \tag{6.12}$$

This result shows how the survivor function for T_i can be found from the survivor function of the distribution of ϵ_i. The result also demonstrates that an accelerated failure time model can be derived from many probability distributions for ϵ_i, although some are more tractable than others.

A general expression for the pth percentile of the distribution of survival times also follows from the results in this section. The pth percentile for the ith individual, $t_i(p)$, is given by

$$S_i\{t_i(p)\} = \frac{100 - p}{100},$$

and using Equation (6.11),

$$\mathrm{P}\left(\epsilon_i \geqslant \frac{\log t_i(p) - \mu - \alpha_1 x_{1i} - \alpha_2 x_{2i} - \cdots - \alpha_p x_{pi}}{\sigma}\right) = \frac{100 - p}{100}.$$

If $\epsilon_i(p)$ is used to denote the pth percentile of the distribution of ϵ_i, then

$$S_{\epsilon_i}\{\epsilon_i(p)\} = \mathrm{P}\left\{\epsilon_i \geqslant \epsilon_i(p)\right\} = \frac{100 - p}{100}.$$

Consequently,

$$\epsilon_i(p) = \frac{\log t_i(p) - \mu - \alpha_1 x_{1i} - \alpha_2 x_{2i} - \cdots - \alpha_p x_{pi}}{\sigma},$$

and so

$$t_i(p) = \exp\left\{\sigma\epsilon_i(p) + \mu + \alpha_1 x_{1i} + \alpha_2 x_{2i} + \cdots + \alpha_p x_{pi}\right\} \tag{6.13}$$

is the pth percentile of the distribution of survival times for the ith individual. Note that the percentile in Equation (6.13) can be written in the form

$$t_i(p) = \exp(\alpha_1 x_{1i} + \alpha_2 x_{2i} + \cdots + \alpha_p x_{pi}) t_0(p),$$

where $t_0(p)$ is the pth percentile for a baseline individual for whom all explanatory variables take the value zero. This confirms that the α-coefficients can be interpreted in terms of the effect of the explanatory variables on the percentiles of the distribution of survival times.

The cumulative hazard function of the distribution of T_i is given by $H_i(t) = -\log S_i(t)$, and from Equation (6.12),

$$\begin{aligned} H_i(t) &= -\log S_{\epsilon_i}\left(\frac{\log t - \mu - \alpha_1 x_{1i} - \alpha_2 x_{2i} - \cdots - \alpha_p x_{pi}}{\sigma}\right), \\ &= H_{\epsilon_i}\left(\frac{\log t - \mu - \alpha_1 x_{1i} - \alpha_2 x_{2i} - \cdots - \alpha_p x_{pi}}{\sigma}\right), \end{aligned} \tag{6.14}$$

where $H_{\epsilon_i}(\epsilon) = -\log S_{\epsilon_i}(\epsilon)$ is the cumulative hazard function of ϵ_i. The corresponding hazard function, found by differentiating $H_i(t)$ in Equation (6.14) with respect to t, is

$$h_i(t) = \frac{1}{\sigma t}\, h_{\epsilon_i}\left(\frac{\log t - \mu - \alpha_1 x_{1i} - \alpha_2 x_{2i} - \cdots - \alpha_p x_{pi}}{\sigma}\right), \tag{6.15}$$

where $h_{\epsilon_i}(\epsilon)$ is the hazard function of the distribution of ϵ_i.

The distributions of ϵ_i that are most often used in accelerated failure time modelling are such that their percentiles, $\epsilon_i(p)$, have a simple form. Models based on such distributions are described in the following section.

6.5 Parametric accelerated failure time models

Particular choices for the distribution of ϵ_i in the log-linear formulation of the accelerated failure time model, described in Section 6.4.1, lead to distributions for the random variable associated with the survival time of the ith individual. But the representation of the model in Equation (6.9) invariably leads to different parameterisations of the models from those given in Sections 5.1 and 6.1. Parametric accelerated failure time models based on the Weibull, log-logistic and lognormal distributions for the survival times are most commonly used in practice, and so these models are described in detail, and summarised in Section 6.5.4.

6.5.1 The Weibull accelerated failure time model

Suppose that survival times are assumed to have a Weibull distribution with scale parameter λ and shape parameter γ, written $W(\lambda, \gamma)$, so that the baseline hazard function is

$$h_0(t) = \lambda\gamma t^{\gamma-1}.$$

The hazard function for the ith individual is then, from Equation (6.8), given by

$$h_i(t) = e^{-\eta_i}\lambda\gamma(e^{-\eta_i}t)^{\gamma-1} = (e^{-\eta_i})^{\gamma}\lambda\gamma t^{\gamma-1},$$

so that the survival time of this individual has a $W(\lambda e^{-\gamma\eta_i}, \gamma)$ distribution. The Weibull distribution is therefore said to possess the *accelerated failure time property.* Indeed, this is the only probability distribution that has both the proportional hazards and accelerated failure time properties.

Because the Weibull distribution has both the proportional hazards property and the accelerated failure time property, there is a direct correspondence between the parameters under the two models. If the baseline hazard function is the hazard function of a $W(\lambda, \gamma)$ distribution, the survival times under the general proportional hazards model in Equation (5.35) of Chapter 5 have a $W(\lambda \exp(\boldsymbol{\beta}'\boldsymbol{x}_i), \gamma)$ distribution, while those under the accelerated failure time model have a $W(\lambda \exp(-\gamma\boldsymbol{\alpha}'\boldsymbol{x}_i), \gamma)$ distribution. It then follows that when the coefficients of the explanatory variables in the linear component of the accelerated failure time model are multiplied by $-\gamma$, we get the corresponding β-coefficients in the proportional hazards model. In the particular case of comparing two groups, an acceleration factor of $\phi^{-1} = e^{-\alpha}$ under the accelerated failure time model corresponds to a hazard ratio of $\phi^{-\gamma} = e^{-\gamma\alpha}$ in a proportional hazards model.

In terms of the log-linear representation of the model in Equation (6.9), if T_i has a Weibull distribution, then ϵ_i does in fact have a type of extreme value distribution known as the *Gumbel distribution.* This is an asymmetric distribution with mean 0.5772, which is *Euler's constant*, and variance $\pi^2/6$. The survivor function of the Gumbel distribution is given by

$$S_{\epsilon_i}(\epsilon) = \exp(-e^{\epsilon}),$$

for $-\infty < \epsilon < \infty$, and the cumulative hazard and hazard functions of this distribution are given by $H_{\epsilon_i}(\epsilon) = e^{\epsilon}$, and $h_{\epsilon_i}(\epsilon) = e^{\epsilon}$, respectively.

To show that the random variable $T_i = \exp(\mu + \boldsymbol{\alpha}'\boldsymbol{x}_i + \sigma\epsilon_i)$ has a Weibull distribution, from Equation (6.12), the survivor function of T_i is given by

$$S_i(t) = \exp\left\{-\exp\left(\frac{\log t - \mu - \alpha_1 x_{1i} - \alpha_2 x_{2i} - \cdots - \alpha_p x_{pi}}{\sigma}\right)\right\}. \tag{6.16}$$

This can be expressed in the form

$$S_i(t) = \exp\left(-\lambda_i t^{1/\sigma}\right),$$

where

$$\lambda_i = \exp\left\{-(\mu + \alpha_1 x_{1i} + \alpha_2 x_{2i} + \cdots + \alpha_p x_{pi})/\sigma\right\},$$

which, from Equation (5.5) of Chapter 5, is the survivor function of a Weibull distribution with scale parameter λ_i, and shape parameter σ^{-1}. Consequently, Equation (6.16) is the accelerated failure time representation of the survivor function of the Weibull model described in Section 5.6 of Chapter 5.

The cumulative hazard and hazard functions for the Weibull accelerated failure time model can be found directly from the survivor function in Equation (6.16), or from $H_{\epsilon_i}(\epsilon)$ and $h_{\epsilon_i}(\epsilon)$, using the general results in Equations (6.14) and (6.15). We find that the cumulative hazard function is

$$H_i(t) = -\log S_i(t) = \exp\left(\frac{\log t - \mu - \alpha_1 x_{1i} - \alpha_2 x_{2i} - \cdots - \alpha_p x_{pi}}{\sigma}\right),$$

which can also be expressed as $\lambda_i t^{1/\sigma}$, and the hazard function is given by

$$h_i(t) = \frac{1}{\sigma t} \exp\left(\frac{\log t - \mu - \alpha_1 x_{1i} - \alpha_2 x_{2i} - \cdots - \alpha_p x_{pi}}{\sigma}\right), \qquad (6.17)$$

or $h_i(t) = \lambda_i \sigma^{-1} t^{\sigma^{-1}-1}$.

We now reconcile this form of the model with that for the Weibull proportional hazards model. From Equation (5.37) of Chapter 5, the survivor function for the ith individual is

$$S_i(t) = \exp\left\{-\exp(\beta_1 x_{1i} + \beta_2 x_{2i} + \cdots + \beta_p x_{pi})\lambda t^{\gamma}\right\}, \qquad (6.18)$$

in which λ and γ are the parameters of the Weibull baseline hazard function. There is a direct correspondence between Equation (6.16) and Equation (6.18), in the sense that

$$\lambda = \exp(-\mu/\sigma), \quad \gamma = \sigma^{-1}, \quad \beta_j = -\alpha_j/\sigma,$$

for $j = 1, 2, \ldots, p$. We therefore deduce that the log-linear model where

$$\log T_i = \frac{1}{\gamma}\left\{-\log\lambda - \beta_1 x_{1i} - \beta_2 x_{2i} - \cdots - \beta_p x_{pi} + \epsilon_i\right\},$$

and in which ϵ_i has a Gumbel distribution, provides an alternative representation of the Weibull proportional hazards model.

In this form of the model, the pth percentile of the survival time distribution for the ith individual is the value $t_i(p)$, which is such that $S_i\{t_i(p)\} = 1-(p/100)$, where $S_i(t)$ is as given in Equation (6.16). Straightforward algebra leads to the result that

$$t_i(p) = \exp\left[\sigma \log\left\{-\log\left(\frac{100-p}{100}\right)\right\} + \mu + \boldsymbol{\alpha}'\boldsymbol{x}_i\right] \qquad (6.19)$$

for that individual. Equivalently, the pth percentile of the distribution of ϵ_i, $\epsilon_i(p)$, is such that

$$\exp\left\{-e^{\epsilon_i(p)}\right\} = \frac{100-p}{100},$$

so that

$$\epsilon_i(p) = \log\left\{-\log\left(\frac{100-p}{100}\right)\right\},$$

and the general result in Equation (6.13) leads directly to Equation (6.19).

The survivor function and hazard function of the Weibull model follow from Equations (6.16) and (6.17), and Equation (6.19) enables percentiles to be estimated directly.

6.5.2 *The log-logistic accelerated failure time model*

Now suppose that the survival times have a log-logistic distribution. If the baseline hazard function in the general accelerated failure time model in Equation (6.8) is derived from a log-logistic distribution with parameters θ, κ, this function is given by

$$h_0(t) = \frac{e^{\theta}\kappa t^{\kappa-1}}{1 + e^{\theta}t^{\kappa}}.$$

Under the accelerated failure time model, the hazard of death at time t for the ith individual is

$$h_i(t) = e^{-\eta_i} h_0(e^{-\eta_i}t),$$

where $\eta_i = \alpha_1 x_{1i} + \alpha_2 x_{2i} + \cdots + \alpha_p x_{pi}$ is a linear combination of the values of p explanatory variables for the ith individual. Consequently,

$$h_i(t) = \frac{e^{-\eta_i} e^{\theta}\kappa(e^{-\eta_i}t)^{\kappa-1}}{1 + e^{\theta}(e^{-\eta_i}t)^{\kappa}},$$

that is,

$$h_i(t) = \frac{e^{\theta-\kappa\eta_i}\kappa t^{\kappa-1}}{1 + e^{\theta-\kappa\eta_i}t^{\kappa}}.$$

It then follows that the survival time for the ith individual also has a log-logistic distribution with parameters $\theta - \kappa\eta_i$ and κ. The log-logistic distribution therefore has the accelerated failure time property. However, this distribution does not have the proportional hazards property.

The log-linear form of the accelerated failure time model in Equation (6.9) also provides a representation of the log-logistic distribution. Suppose that in this formulation, ϵ_i now has a logistic distribution with zero mean and variance $\pi^2/3$, so that the survivor function of ϵ_i is

$$S_{\epsilon_i}(\epsilon) = \frac{1}{1 + e^{\epsilon}}.$$

Using Equation (6.12), the survivor function of T_i is then

$$S_i(t) = \left\{1 + \exp\left(\frac{\log t - \mu - \alpha_1 x_{1i} - \alpha_2 x_{2i} - \cdots - \alpha_p x_{pi}}{\sigma}\right)\right\}^{-1}. \tag{6.20}$$

From Equation (6.2), the survivor function of T_i, when T_i has a log-logistic distribution with parameters $\theta - \kappa\eta_i$, κ, where $\eta_i = \alpha_1 x_{1i} + \alpha_2 x_{2i} + \cdots + \alpha_p x_{pi}$, is

$$S_i(t) = \frac{1}{1 + e^{\theta-\kappa\eta_i}t^{\kappa}}.$$

On comparing this expression with that for the survivor function in Equation (6.20), we see that the parameters θ and κ can be expressed in terms of μ and σ. Specifically,

$$\theta = -\mu/\sigma, \quad \kappa = \sigma^{-1},$$

and this shows that the accelerated failure time model with log-logistic survival times can also be formulated in terms of a log-linear model. This is the form of the model that is usually adopted by computer software, and so computer-based parameter estimates are usually estimates of μ and σ, rather than θ and κ.

The cumulative hazard and hazard functions of the distribution of ϵ_i are such that

$$H_{\epsilon_i}(\epsilon) = \log\left(1 + e^{\epsilon}\right),$$

and

$$h_{\epsilon_i}(\epsilon) = \left(1 + e^{-\epsilon}\right)^{-1},$$

respectively. Equations (6.14) and (6.15) may then be used to obtain the cumulative hazard, and hazard function, of T_i. In particular, the hazard function for the ith individual is

$$h_i(t) = \frac{1}{\sigma t}\left\{1 + \exp\left[-\left(\frac{\log t - \mu - \alpha_1 x_{1i} - \alpha_2 x_{2i} - \cdots - \alpha_p x_{pi}}{\sigma}\right)\right]\right\}^{-1}. \tag{6.21}$$

Estimates of quantities such as the acceleration factor, or the median survival time, can be obtained directly from the estimates of μ, σ and the α_j's. For example, the acceleration factor for the ith individual is $\exp\{-(\alpha_1 x_{1i} + \alpha_2 x_{2i} + \cdots + \alpha_p x_{pi})\}$ and the pth percentile of the survival time distribution, from Equation (6.20), or the general result in Equation (6.13), is

$$t_i(p) = \exp\left\{\sigma \log\left(\frac{p}{100 - p}\right) + \mu + \alpha_1 x_{1i} + \alpha_2 x_{2i} + \cdots + \alpha_p x_{pi}\right\}.$$

The median survival time is simply

$$t_i(50) = \exp\left\{\mu + \alpha_1 x_{1i} + \alpha_2 x_{2i} + \cdots + \alpha_p x_{pi}\right\}, \tag{6.22}$$

and so an estimate of the median can be straightforwardly obtained from the estimated values of the parameters in the model.

6.5.3 *The lognormal accelerated failure time model*

If the survival times are assumed to have a lognormal distribution, the baseline survivor function is given by

$$S_0(t) = 1 - \Phi\left(\frac{\log t - \mu}{\sigma}\right),$$

where μ and σ are two unknown parameters. Under the accelerated failure time model, the survivor function for the ith individual, is then

$$S_i(t) = S_0(e^{-\eta_i} t),$$

where $\eta_i = \alpha_1 x_{1i} + \alpha_2 x_{2i} + \cdots + \alpha_p x_{pi}$ is a linear combination of the values of p explanatory variables for the ith individual. Therefore,

$$S_i(t) = 1 - \Phi\left(\frac{\log t - \eta_i - \mu}{\sigma}\right), \tag{6.23}$$

which is the survivor function for an individual whose survival times have a lognormal distribution with parameters $\mu + \eta_i$ and σ. The lognormal distribution therefore has the accelerated failure time property.

In the log-linear formulation of the model, the random variable associated with the survival time of the ith individual has a lognormal distribution if $\log T_i$ is normally distributed. We therefore take ϵ_i in Equation (6.9) to have a standard normal distribution, so that the survivor function of ϵ_i is

$$S_{\epsilon_i}(\epsilon) = 1 - \Phi(\epsilon).$$

The cumulative hazard, and hazard function, of ϵ_i are

$$H_{\epsilon_i}(\epsilon) = -\log\{1 - \Phi(\epsilon)\},$$

and

$$h_{\epsilon_i}(\epsilon) = \frac{f_{\epsilon_i}(\epsilon)}{S_{\epsilon_i}(\epsilon)},$$

respectively, where $f_{\epsilon_i}(\epsilon)$ is the density function of a standard normal random variable, given by

$$f_{\epsilon_i}(\epsilon) = \frac{1}{\sqrt{(2\pi)}}\exp\left(-\epsilon^2/2\right).$$

The random variable T_i, in the general accelerated failure time model, then has a lognormal distribution with parameters $\mu + \boldsymbol{\alpha}'\boldsymbol{x}_i$ and σ. The survivor function of T_i is as given in Equation (6.23), and the hazard function is found from Equation (6.15).

The pth percentile of the distribution of T_i, from Equation (6.13), is

$$t_i(p) = \exp\left\{\sigma\Phi^{-1}(p/100) + \mu + \alpha_1 x_{1i} + \alpha_2 x_{2i} + \cdots + \alpha_p x_{pi}\right\},$$

and, in particular, $t(50) = \exp(\mu + \boldsymbol{\alpha}'\boldsymbol{x}_i)$ is the median survival time for the ith individual.

6.5.4 Summary

It is convenient to summarise the models and results that have been described in this section, so that the different parameterisations of the distributions used in accelerated failure time models can clearly be seen.

The general accelerated failure time model for the survival time of the ith of n individuals, for whom $x_{1i}, x_{2i}, \ldots, x_{pi}$ are the values of p explanatory variables, $X_1, X_2, \ldots, X_p$, is such that the random variable associated with the survival time, T_i, can be expressed in the form

$$\log T_i = \mu + \alpha_1 x_{1i} + \alpha_2 x_{2i} + \cdots + \alpha_p x_{pi} + \sigma \epsilon_i.$$

Particular distributions for T_i are derived from assumptions about the distribution of ϵ_i in this model. The survivor function and hazard function of the distributions of ϵ_i, that lead to commonly used accelerated failure time models for the survival times, are summarised in Table 6.2.

Table 6.2 *Summary of parametric accelerated failure time models.*

Distribution of T_i	$S_{\epsilon_i}(\epsilon)$	$h_{\epsilon_i}(\epsilon)$	Percentile, $\epsilon_i(p)$
Exponential	$\exp(-e^{\epsilon})$	e^{ϵ}	$\log\left\{-\log\left(\frac{100-p}{100}\right)\right\}$
Weibull	$\exp(-e^{\epsilon})$	e^{ϵ}	$\log\left\{-\log\left(\frac{100-p}{100}\right)\right\}$
Log-logistic	$(1+e^{\epsilon})^{-1}$	$(1+e^{-\epsilon})^{-1}$	$\log\left(\frac{p}{100-p}\right)$
Lognormal	$1-\Phi(\epsilon)$	$\frac{\exp(-\epsilon^2/2)}{\{1-\Phi(\epsilon)\}\sqrt{(2\pi)}}$	$\Phi^{-1}(p/100)$

The cumulative hazard function of ϵ_i is found from $H_{\epsilon_i}(\epsilon) = -\log S_{\epsilon_i}(\epsilon)$, and, if desired, the density function of ϵ_i is $f_{\epsilon_i}(\epsilon) = h_{\epsilon_i}(\epsilon)\, S_{\epsilon_i}(\epsilon)$. From the survivor and hazard function of ϵ_i, the survivor and hazard function of T_i can be found from

$$S_i(t) = S_{\epsilon_i}\left(\frac{\log t - \mu - \alpha_1 x_{1i} - \alpha_2 x_{2i} - \cdots - \alpha_p x_{pi}}{\sigma}\right),$$

and

$$h_i(t) = \frac{1}{\sigma t}\, h_{\epsilon_i}\left(\frac{\log t - \mu - \alpha_1 x_{1i} - \alpha_2 x_{2i} - \cdots - \alpha_p x_{pi}}{\sigma}\right),$$

results that were first given in Equations (6.12) and (6.15), respectively.

The pth percentile of the distribution of ϵ_i is also given in Table 6.2, from which $t_i(p)$, the pth percentile of the survival times for the ith individual, can be found from

$$t_i(p) = \exp\left\{\sigma \epsilon_i(p) + \mu + \alpha_1 x_{1i} + \alpha_2 x_{2i} + \cdots + \alpha_p x_{pi}\right\},$$

given as Equation (6.13).

The log-linear representation of the Weibull and log-logistic models leads to parameterisations of the survival time distributions that differ from those used in Sections 5.1 and 6.1, when the distributions were first presented. The link between the two sets of parameters is summarised in Table 6.3, which includes the number of the equation that gives the survivor function of each distribution in terms of the original parameters.

For the proportional hazards representation of the Weibull model, where

$$h_i(t) = \exp(\boldsymbol{\beta}'\boldsymbol{x}_i) h_0(t),$$

Table 6.3 *Summary of the parameterisation of accelerated failure time models.*

Distribution of T_i	Equation number	Parameterisation of survivor function	
Exponential	(5.2)	$\lambda = e^{-\mu}$,	$\gamma = 1$ $(\sigma = 1)$
Weibull	(5.5)	$\lambda = e^{-\mu/\sigma}$,	$\gamma = 1/\sigma$,
Log-logistic	(6.2)	$\theta = -\mu/\sigma$,	$\kappa = 1/\sigma$

the correspondence between β_j, and α_j in the accelerated time model, is such that $\beta_j = -\alpha_j/\sigma$, $j = 1, 2, \ldots, p$. This shows how the β-parameters in a Weibull proportional hazards model, which represent log-hazard ratios, can be obtained from the fitted α-parameters in an accelerated failure time model.

6.6* Fitting and comparing accelerated failure time models

Accelerated failure time models are fitted using the method of maximum likelihood. The likelihood function is best derived from the log-linear representation of the model, after which iterative methods are used to obtain the estimates. The likelihood of the n observed survival times, $t_1, t_2, \ldots, t_n$, is, from Expression (5.9) in Chapter 5, given by

$$L(\boldsymbol{\alpha}, \mu, \sigma) = \prod_{i=1}^{n} \{f_i(t_i)\}^{\delta_i} \{S_i(t_i)\}^{1-\delta_i},$$

where $f_i(t_i)$ and $S_i(t_i)$ are the density and survivor functions for the ith individual at t_i, and δ_i is the event indicator for the ith observation, so that δ_i is unity if the ith observation is an event and zero if it is censored. Now, from Equation (6.12),

$$S_i(t_i) = S_{\epsilon_i}(z_i),$$

where $z_i = (\log t_i - \mu - \alpha_1 x_{1i} - \alpha_2 x_{2i} - \cdots - \alpha_p x_{pi})/\sigma$, and differentiation with respect to t gives

$$f_i(t_i) = \frac{1}{\sigma t_i} f_{\epsilon_i}(z_i).$$

The likelihood function can then be expressed in terms of the survivor and density functions of ϵ_i, giving

$$L(\boldsymbol{\alpha}, \mu, \sigma) = \prod_{i=1}^{n} (\sigma t_i)^{-\delta_i} \{f_{\epsilon_i}(z_i)\}^{\delta_i} \{S_{\epsilon_i}(z_i)\}^{1-\delta_i}.$$

The log-likelihood function is then

$$\log L(\boldsymbol{\alpha}, \mu, \sigma) = \sum_{i=1}^{n} \{-\delta_i \log(\sigma t_i) + \delta_i \log f_{\epsilon_i}(z_i) + (1 - \delta_i) \log S_{\epsilon_i}(z_i)\}, \tag{6.24}$$

and the maximum likelihood estimates of the $p+2$ unknown parameters, μ, σ and $\alpha_1, \alpha_2, \ldots, \alpha_p$, are found by maximising this function using the Newton-Raphson procedure, described in Section 3.3.3.

Note that the expression for the log-likelihood function in Equation (6.24) includes the term $-\sum_{i=1}^{n} \delta_i \log t_i$, which does not involve any unknown parameters. This term may therefore be omitted from the log-likelihood function, as noted in Section 5.6.1 of Chapter 5, in the context of the Weibull proportional hazards model. Indeed, log-likelihood values given by most computer software for accelerated failure time modelling do not include the value of $-\sum_{i=1}^{n} \delta_i \log t_i$.

After fitting a model, the value of the statistic $-2\log \hat{L}$ can be computed, and used in making comparisons between nested models, just as for the proportional hazards model. Specifically, to compare two nested models, the difference in the values of the statistic $-2\log \hat{L}$ for the two models is calculated, and compared with percentage points of the chi-squared distribution, with degrees of freedom equal to the difference in the number of α-parameters included in the linear component of the model.

Once a suitable model has been identified, estimates of the survivor and hazard functions may be obtained and plotted. The fitted model can be interpreted in terms of the estimated value of the acceleration factor for particular individuals, or in terms of the median and other percentiles of the distribution of survival times. In particular, the estimated pth percentile of the distribution of survival times, for an individual whose vector of values of the explanatory variables is $\boldsymbol{x}_i$, is, from Equation (6.13), given by

$$\hat{t}_i(p) = \exp\{\hat{\sigma}\epsilon_i(p) + \hat{\mu} + \hat{\alpha}_1 x_{1i} + \hat{\alpha}_2 x_{2i} + \cdots + \hat{\alpha}_p x_{pi}\}.$$

The estimated percentiles of the assumed distribution of survival times are functions of the parameter estimates in the log-linear accelerated failure time model, and so the standard error of these estimates can be found using the general result in Equation (5.44) of Chapter 5. Specifically, the vector $\hat{\boldsymbol{\theta}}$ now has $p+2$ components, namely $\hat{\mu}, \hat{\alpha}_1, \hat{\alpha}_2, \ldots, \hat{\alpha}_p, \hat{\sigma}$, and $\text{var}\,(\hat{\boldsymbol{\theta}})$ is the variance-covariance matrix of these parameter estimates. Equation (5.44) shows how the variance of a function of the parameter estimates can be obtained from the vector of derivatives, $\boldsymbol{d}(\hat{\boldsymbol{\theta}})$, of the estimated percentiles. However, it is much more straightforward to first obtain the variance of $\log \hat{t}_i(p)$, since the derivatives of $\log \hat{t}_i(p)$, with respect to $\hat{\mu}, \hat{\alpha}_1, \hat{\alpha}_2, \ldots, \hat{\alpha}_p, \hat{\sigma}$, are then $1, x_{1i}, x_{2i}, \ldots, x_{pi}, \epsilon_i(p)$, respectively. Equation (5.46) is then used to obtain the standard error of the estimated percentile. Confidence intervals for a percentile will usually be formed from an interval estimate for $\log t_i(p)$. Most computer software for survival analysis provides the standard error of specified percentiles.

Example 6.3 Prognosis for women with breast cancer

In this example, accelerated failure time models are fitted to the data on the survival times of women with breast cancer. The Weibull accelerated failure time model is first considered. A log-linear model for the random variable associated with the survival time of the ith woman, T_i, is such that

$$\log T_i = \mu + \alpha x_i + \sigma \epsilon_i,$$

where ϵ_i has a Gumbel distribution, μ, σ and α are unknown parameters, and x_i is the value of an explanatory variable, X, associated with staining, such that $x_i = 0$ if the ith woman is negatively stained and $x_i = 1$ if positively stained. When this model is fitted, we find that $\hat{\mu} = 5.854$, $\hat{\sigma} = 1.067$, and $\hat{\alpha} = -0.997$.

The acceleration factor, $e^{-\alpha x_i}$, is estimated by $e^{0.997} = 2.71$ for a woman with positive staining. The time to death of a woman with a positively stained tumour is therefore accelerated by a factor of about 2.7 under this model. This is in broad agreement with the estimated slope of the percentile-percentile plot for this data set, found in Example 6.2.

The estimated survivor function for the ith woman is given by

$$\hat{S}_i(t) = \exp\left\{-\exp\left(\frac{\log t - \hat{\mu} - \hat{\alpha} x_i}{\hat{\sigma}}\right)\right\},$$

from Equation (6.16), and may be plotted against t for the two possible values of x_i. The median survival time of the ith woman under the Weibull accelerated failure time model, using Equation (6.19), is

$$t_i(50) = \exp\left\{\sigma \log(\log 2) + \mu + \alpha x_i\right\}.$$

The estimated median survival time for a woman with negative staining ($x_i = 0$) is 236 days, while that for women with positive staining ($x_i = 1$) is 87 days, as in Example 5.6. Note that the ratio of the two medians is 2.71, which is the acceleration factor. The median survival time for women with positively stained tumours is therefore about one-third that of women whose tumours were negatively stained.

The estimated hazard function for the ith woman is, from Equation (6.17), given by

$$\hat{h}_i(t) = \hat{\sigma}^{-1} t^{\hat{\sigma}^{-1}-1} \exp\left(\frac{-\hat{\mu} - \hat{\alpha} x_i}{\hat{\sigma}}\right),$$

that is,

$$\hat{h}_i(t) = 0.937\, t^{-0.063} \exp(-5.486 + 0.934\, x_i).$$

A plot of this function for the two groups of women is shown in Figure 6.6.

In the proportional hazards representation of the Weibull model, given in Section 5.6 of Chapter 5, the hazard of death at time t for the ith woman is

$$h_i(t) = e^{\beta x_i} h_0(t),$$

where x_i takes the value zero if the ith woman had a negatively stained tumour, and unity if the tumour was positively stained. For the Weibull distribution, the baseline hazard function is

$$h_0(t) = \lambda \gamma t^{\gamma - 1},$$

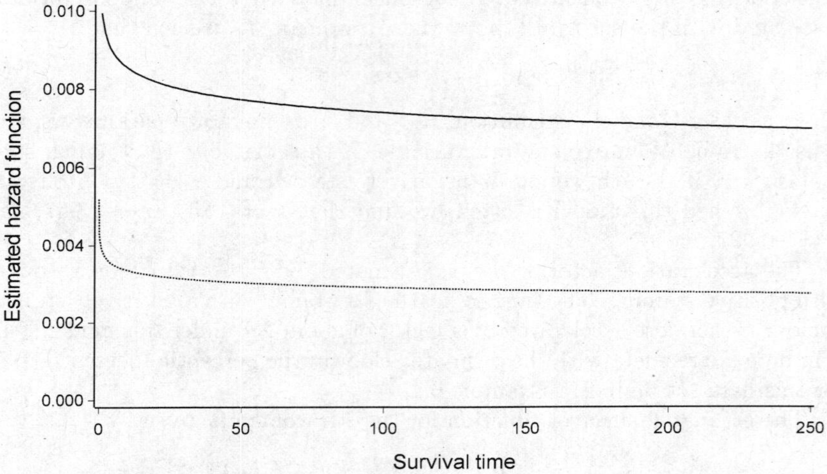

Figure 6.6 *Estimated hazard functions under the Weibull accelerated failure time model for women with positively stained (—) and negatively stained (···) tumours.*

which is the hazard function for women with negatively stained tumours, and hence

$$h_i(t) = e^{\beta x_i} \lambda \gamma t^{\gamma - 1}.$$

The corresponding estimated values of the parameters λ, γ and β are given by $\hat{\lambda} = \exp(-\hat{\mu}/\hat{\lambda}) = 0.00414$, $\hat{\gamma} = 1/\hat{\sigma} = 0.937$ and $\hat{\beta} = -\hat{\alpha}/\hat{\sigma} = 0.997$. The correspondence between the Weibull accelerated failure time model and the Weibull proportional hazards model means that the hazard ratio under the latter model is $e^{-\alpha/\sigma} = e^{\beta}$, which is estimated to be 2.55. This is in agreement with the value found in Example 5.6.

We now fit the log-logistic accelerated failure time model to the same data set. The log-linear form of the model now leads to $\hat{\mu} = 5.461$, $\hat{\sigma} = 0.805$ and $\hat{\alpha} = -1.149$. The acceleration factor is $e^{-\alpha}$, which is estimated by 3.16. This is slightly greater than that found under the Weibull accelerated failure time model.

The median survival time for the ith woman under this model is, from Equation (6.22), given by

$$\exp(\mu + \alpha x_i),$$

from which the estimated median survival time for a women with negative staining is 235 days, while that for women with positive staining is 75 days. These values are very close to those obtained under the Weibull accelerated failure time model.

The estimated hazard function for the ith woman is now

$$\hat{h}_i(t) = \frac{1}{\hat{\sigma}t}\left\{1 + \exp\left[-\left(\frac{\log t - \hat{\mu} - \hat{\alpha}x_i}{\hat{\sigma}}\right)\right]\right\}^{-1},$$

from Equation (6.21), which is

$$\hat{h}_i(t) = 1.243\, t^{-1}\left\{1 + t^{-1.243}\exp\left(6.787 - 1.428\, x_i\right)\right\}^{-1}.$$

A graph of this function for the two groups of women is shown in Figure 6.7. This can be compared with the graph in Figure 6.6.

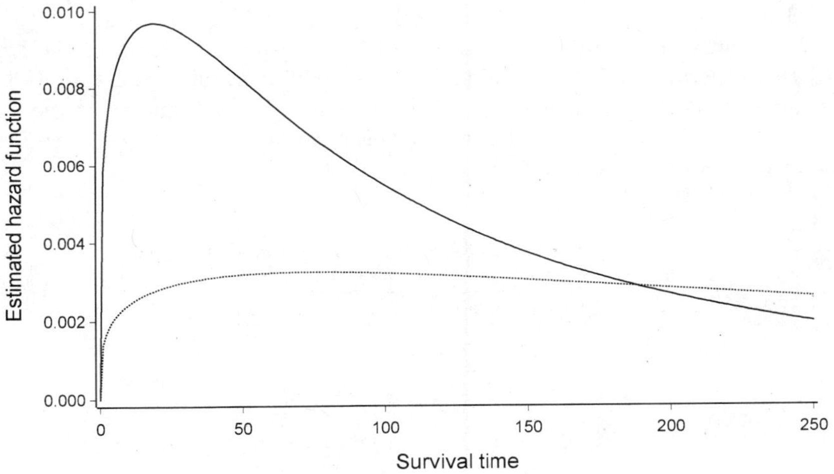

Figure 6.7 *Estimated hazard functions under the log-logistic accelerated failure time model for women with positively stained (—) and negatively stained (···) tumours.*

The hazard functions for those with negative staining are quite similar under the two models. However, the hazard function for those with positive staining under the log-logistic model is different from that under the Weibull model. The values of the statistic $-2\log\hat{L}$ for the fitted Weibull and log-logistic models are 121.77 and 118.495. On this basis, the log-logistic model is a slightly better fit. An analysis of residuals, to be discussed in Chapter 7, may help in choosing between these two models, although with this small data set, such an analysis is unlikely to be very informative.

Finally, in terms of the parameterisation of the model given in Section 6.1.1, the baseline hazard function is

$$h_0(t) = \frac{e^{\theta}\kappa t^{\kappa-1}}{1 + e^{\theta}t^{\kappa}},$$

and so the hazard function for the ith woman in the study is

$$h_i(t) = \frac{e^{\theta - \kappa \alpha x_i} \kappa t^{\kappa - 1}}{1 + e^{\theta - \kappa \alpha x_i} t^{\kappa}}.$$

The corresponding estimated values of θ and κ are given by $\hat{\theta} = -\hat{\mu}/\hat{\sigma} = -6.787$, and $\hat{\kappa} = 1/\hat{\sigma} = 1.243$.

Example 6.4 Comparison of two treatments for prostatic cancer
In a further illustration of modelling survival data using the log-logistic accelerated failure time model, the data from a clinical trial to compare two treatments for prostatic cancer are considered. These data were first given in Example 1.4, and analysed using a Cox regression model in Examples 3.6 and 3.12.

To identify the terms that should be in the linear component of the log-logistic accelerated failure time model, the procedure described in Example 3.6 can again be followed. The values of the statistic $-2 \log \hat{L}$ on fitting models with all combinations of the four prognostic variables, *Age*, *Shb*, *Size* and *Index*, are shown in Table 6.4.

Table 6.4 *Values of $-2 \log \hat{L}$ for models fitted to the data from Example 1.4.*

Variables in model	$-2 \log \hat{L}$
none	35.806
Age	35.752
Shb	35.700
Size	27.754
Index	27.965
Age + *Shb*	35.657
Age + *Size*	27.652
Age + *Index*	27.859
Shb + *Size*	27.722
Shb + *Index*	26.873
Size + *Index*	23.112
Age + *Shb* + *Size*	27.631
Age + *Shb* + *Index*	26.870
Age + *Size* + *Index*	23.002
Shb + *Size* + *Index*	22.895
Age + *Shb* + *Size* + *Index*	22.727

As in Example 3.6, the variables *Size* and *Index* are the ones that are needed in the model. When either of these variables is omitted, the corresponding increase in the value of $-2 \log \hat{L}$ is significant, and neither *Age* nor *Shb* reduce $-2 \log \hat{L}$ by a significant amount when they are added to the model.

When the term corresponding to the treatment effect, *Treat*, is added to the model that contains *Size* and *Index*, $-2 \log \hat{L}$ decreases to 21.245. When this reduction of 1.867 is compared with percentage points of a chi-squared distribution on 1 d.f., the reduction is not significant at the 10% level ($P = 0.172$). There is no evidence of any interaction between *Treat* and the prognostic variables *Size* and *Index*, and so the conclusion is that there is no statistically significant treatment effect.

The magnitude of the treatment effect can be assessed by calculating the acceleration factor. According to the log-linear form of the model, the random variable associated with the survival time of the ith patient, T_i, is such that

$$\log T_i = \mu + \alpha_1 \mathit{Size}_i + \alpha_2 \mathit{Index}_i + \alpha_3 \mathit{Treat}_i + \sigma\epsilon_i,$$

in which ϵ_i has a logistic distribution, Size_i and Index_i are the values of the tumour size and Gleason index for the ith individual, and Treat_i is zero if the ith individual is in the placebo group and unity if in the treated group. The maximum likelihood estimates of the unknown parameters in this model are given by $\hat{\mu} = 7.661$, $\hat{\sigma} = 0.338$, $\hat{\alpha}_1 = -0.029$, $\hat{\alpha}_2 = -0.293$ and $\hat{\alpha}_3 = 0.573$. The values of the α's suggests that the survival time tends to be shorter for larger values of the tumour size and tumour index, and longer for individuals assigned to the active treatment.

Using Equation (6.20), the fitted survivor function for the ith patient is

$$\hat{S}_i(t) = \left[1 + \exp\left\{\frac{\log t - \hat{\mu} - \hat{\alpha}_1 \mathit{Size}_i - \hat{\alpha}_2 \mathit{Index}_i - \hat{\alpha}_3 \mathit{Treat}_i}{\hat{\sigma}}\right\}\right]^{-1},$$

which can be written in the form

$$\hat{S}_i(t) = \left\{1 + t^{1/\hat{\sigma}} \exp\left(\hat{\zeta}_i\right)\right\}^{-1},$$

where

$$\hat{\zeta}_i = \frac{1}{\hat{\sigma}}\left\{-\hat{\mu} - \hat{\alpha}_1 \mathit{Size}_i - \hat{\alpha}_2 \mathit{Index}_i - \hat{\alpha}_3 \mathit{Treat}_i\right\},$$

that is,

$$\hat{\zeta}_i = -22.645 + 0.085\, \mathit{Size}_i + 0.865\, \mathit{Index}_i - 1.693\, \mathit{Treat}_i.$$

The corresponding estimated hazard function can be found by differentiating the estimated cumulative hazard function, $\hat{H}_i(t) = -\log \hat{S}_i(t)$, with respect to t. This gives

$$\hat{h}_i(t) = \frac{1}{\hat{\sigma} t}\left\{1 + t^{-1/\hat{\sigma}} \exp\left(-\hat{\zeta}_i\right)\right\}^{-1},$$

a result that can also be obtained directly from the hazard function given in Equation (6.21).

The estimated acceleration factor for an individual in the treated group, relative to an individual in the control group, is $e^{-0.573} = 0.56$. The interpretation of this result is that after allowing for the size and index of the tumour, the effect of the treatment with diethylstilbestrol is to slow down the progression of the cancer by a factor of about 2. This effect might be of clinical importance, even though it is not statistically significant. However, before accepting this interpretation, the adequacy of the fitted model should be checked using suitable diagnostics.

A confidence interval for the acceleration factor is found by exponentiating the confidence limits for the logarithm of the acceleration factor. In this example, the logarithm of the acceleration factor for the treatment effect is the estimated coefficient of *Treat* in the model for the hazard function, multiplied by -1, which is -0.573, and the standard error of this estimate is 0.473. Thus, a 95% confidence interval for the acceleration factor has limits of $\exp\{-0.573 \pm 1.96 \times 0.473\}$, and the required interval is from 0.70 to 4.48. Notice that this interval estimate includes unity, which is consistent with the earlier finding of a non-significant treatment difference.

Finally, in terms of the parameterisation of the model in Section 6.1.1, the fitted hazard function for the ith patient, $i = 1, 2, \ldots, 38$, is given by

$$\hat{h}_i(t) = e^{-\hat{\eta}_i}\hat{h}_0(e^{-\hat{\eta}_i}t),$$

where

$$\hat{\eta}_i = -0.029\, Size_i - 0.293\, Index_i + 0.573\, Treat_i,$$

and from Equation (6.1),

$$\hat{h}_0(t) = \frac{e^{\hat{\theta}}\hat{\kappa}t^{\hat{\kappa}-1}}{1 + e^{\hat{\theta}}t^{\hat{\kappa}}}.$$

The estimated parameters in this form of the estimated baseline hazard function, $\hat{h}_0(t)$, are given by $\hat{\theta} = -22.644$ and $\hat{\kappa} = 2.956$. A graph of this function is shown in Figure 6.8.

This figure indicates that the baseline hazard is increasing over time. Comparison with the baseline hazard function for a fitted Weibull model, also shown in this figure, indicates that under the log-logistic model, the estimated baseline hazard function does not increase quite so rapidly.

6.7* The proportional odds model

In the general proportional odds model, the odds of an individual surviving beyond some time t are expressed as

$$\frac{S_i(t)}{1 - S_i(t)} = e^{\eta_i}\frac{S_0(t)}{1 - S_0(t)}, \tag{6.25}$$

where

$$\eta_i = \beta_1 x_{1i} + \beta_2 x_{2i} + \cdots + \beta_p x_{pi}$$

is a linear combination of the values of p explanatory variables, X_1, $X_2, \ldots,$ X_p, measured on the ith individual, and $S_0(t)$, the baseline survivor function, is the survivor function for an individual whose explanatory variables all take the value zero.

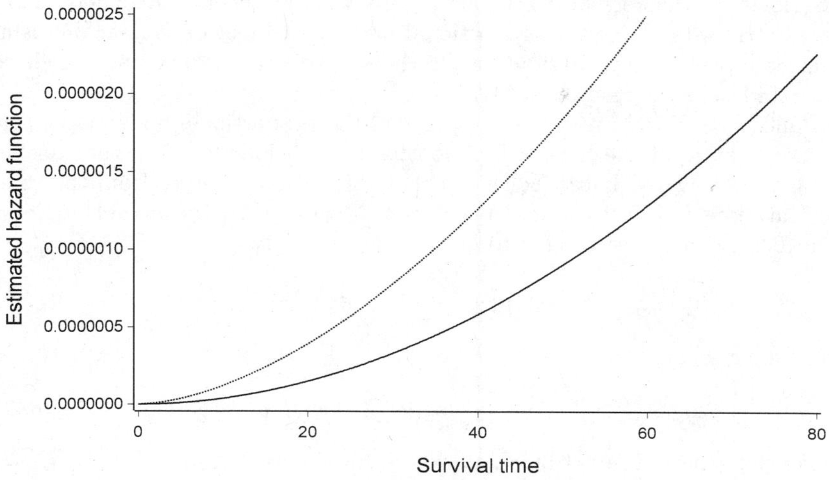

Figure 6.8 *Estimated baseline hazard function for the fitted log-logistic model (—) and a fitted Weibull model (···).*

In this model, the explanatory variables act multiplicatively on the odds of survival beyond t. The logarithm of the ratio of the odds of survival beyond t for the ith individual, relative to an individual for whom the explanatory variables are all equal to zero, is therefore just η_i. The model is therefore a linear model for the log-odds ratio.

Now consider the particular case of a two-group study, in which individuals receive either a standard treatment or new treatment. Let the single indicator variable X take the value zero if an individual is on the standard treatment and unity if on the new. The odds of the ith individual surviving beyond time t is then

$$\frac{S_i(t)}{1 - S_i(t)} = e^{\beta x_i} \frac{S_0(t)}{1 - S_0(t)},$$

where x_i is the value of X for the ith individual, $i = 1, 2, \ldots, n$. Thus, if $S_N(t)$ and $S_S(t)$ are the survivor functions for individuals on the new and standard treatments, respectively,

$$\frac{S_N(t)}{1 - S_N(t)} = e^{\beta} \frac{S_S(t)}{1 - S_S(t)},$$

and the log-odds ratio is simply β. The parameters in the linear component of the model therefore have an immediate interpretation.

As for the proportional hazards model, a non-parametric estimate of the baseline hazard function can be obtained. The model is then fitted by estimating the β-parameters in the linear component of the model, and the baseline survivor function, from the data. A method for accomplishing this has been described by Bennett (1983a), but details will not be included here. Fully parametric versions of the proportional odds model can be derived by using a specific probability distribution for the survival times. One such model is described below in Section 6.7.1.

One particularly important property of the proportional odds model concerns the ratio of the hazard function for the ith individual to the baseline hazard, $h_i(t)/h_0(t)$. It can be shown that this ratio converges from the value $e^{-\eta_i}$ at time $t = 0$, to unity at $t = \infty$. To show this, the model in Equation (6.25) can be rearranged to give

$$S_i(t) = S_0(t)\left\{e^{-\eta_i} + (1 - e^{-\eta_i})S_0(t)\right\}^{-1},$$

and taking logarithms, we get

$$\log S_i(t) = \log S_0(t) - \log\left\{e^{-\eta_i} + (1 - e^{-\eta_i})S_0(t)\right\}. \tag{6.26}$$

Using the general result from Equation (1.5), the hazard function is

$$h_i(t) = -\frac{\mathrm{d}}{\mathrm{d}t}\log S_i(t),$$

and so

$$h_i(t) = h_0(t) - \frac{(1 - e^{-\eta_i})f_0(t)}{e^{-\eta_i} + (1 - e^{-\eta_i})S_0(t)},$$

after differentiating both sides of Equation (6.26) with respect to t, where $f_0(t)$ is the baseline probability density function. After some rearrangement, this equation becomes

$$h_i(t) = h_0(t) - \frac{f_0(t)}{(e^{\eta_i} - 1)^{-1} + S_0(t)}. \tag{6.27}$$

From Equation (1.4), we also have that $h_0(t) = f_0(t)/S_0(t)$ and substituting for $f_0(t)$ in Equation (6.27) gives

$$h_i(t) = h_0(t)\left\{1 - \frac{S_0(t)}{(e^{\eta_i} - 1)^{-1} + S_0(t)}\right\}.$$

Finally, after further rearrangement, the hazard ratio is given by

$$\frac{h_i(t)}{h_0(t)} = \{1 + (e^{\eta_i} - 1)S_0(t)\}^{-1}.$$

As t increases from 0 to ∞, the baseline survivor function decreases monotonically from 1 to 0. When $S_0(t) = 1$, the hazard ratio is $e^{-\eta_i}$ and as t increases to ∞, the hazard ratio converges to unity.

In practical applications, it is common for the hazard functions obtained for patients in two or more groups to converge with time. For example, in a follow-up study of patients in a clinical trial, the effect on survival of the treatment, or the initial stage of disease, may wear off. Similarly, in studies where a group of patients with some disease are being compared with a control group of disease-free individuals, an effective cure of the disease would lead to the survival experience of each group becoming more similar over time. This suggests that the proportional odds model, with its property of convergent hazard functions, might be of considerable value. However, there are two reasons why this general model has not been widely used in practice. The first of these is that computer software is not generally available for fitting a proportional odds model in which the baseline survivor function is of unspecified form. The second is that the model is likely to give similar results to a Cox regression model that includes a time-dependent variable to produce non-proportional hazards. This particular approach to modelling survival data with non-proportional hazards was outlined in Section 4.4.3, and is considered more fully in Chapter 8.

6.7.1 The log-logistic proportional odds model

If survival times for individuals are assumed to have a log-logistic distribution, the baseline survivor function is

$$S_0(t) = \left\{1 + e^{\theta} t^{\kappa}\right\}^{-1},$$

where θ and κ are unknown parameters. The baseline odds of survival beyond time t are then given by

$$\frac{S_0(t)}{1 - S_0(t)} = e^{-\theta} t^{-\kappa}.$$

The odds of the ith individual surviving beyond time t are therefore

$$\frac{S_i(t)}{1 - S_i(t)} = e^{\eta_i - \theta} t^{-\kappa},$$

and so the survival time of the ith individual has a log-logistic distribution with parameters $\theta - \eta_i$ and κ. The log-logistic distribution therefore has the *proportional odds property*, and the distribution is the natural one to use in conjunction with the proportional odds model. In fact, this is the only distribution to share both the accelerated failure time property and the proportional odds property.

This result also means that the estimated β-coefficients in the linear component of the proportional odds model in Equation (6.25) can be obtained by multiplying the α-coefficients in the log-logistic accelerated failure time model of Equation (6.20) by $\hat{\kappa} = \hat{\sigma}^{-1}$, where $\hat{\sigma}$ is the estimated value of the parameter σ. The coefficients of the explanatory variables under the proportional odds model can then be obtained from those under the accelerated failure time model, and vice versa. The results of a survival analysis based on a proportional odds model can therefore be interpreted in terms of an acceleration factor or the ratio of the odds of survival beyond some time, whichever is the more convenient.

As for other models for survival data, the proportional odds model can be fitted using the method of maximum likelihood. Alternative models may then be compared on the basis of the statistic $-2\log\hat{L}$.

In a two-group study, a preliminary examination of the likely suitability of the model can easily be undertaken. The log-odds of the ith individual surviving beyond time t are

$$\log\left\{\frac{S_i(t)}{1-S_i(t)}\right\} = \beta x_i - \theta - \kappa\log t,$$

where x_i is the value of an indicator variable that takes the value zero if an individual is in one group and unity if in the other. The Kaplan-Meier estimate of the survivor function is then obtained for the individuals in each group and the estimated log-odds of survival beyond time t, $\log\left\{\hat{S}_i(t)/[1-\hat{S}_i(t)]\right\}$, are plotted against $\log t$. If the plot shows two parallel straight lines, this would indicate that the log-logistic model was appropriate. If the lines were straight but not parallel, this would suggest that the parameter κ in the model was not the same for each treatment group. Parallel curves in this plot suggest that although the proportional odds assumption is valid, the survival times cannot be taken to have a log-logistic distribution.

Example 6.5 Prognosis for women with breast cancer

In this example to illustrate the use of the proportional odds model, the model is fitted to the data on the survival times of breast cancer patients. In order to assess the likely suitability of the proportional odds model, the Kaplan-Meier estimate of the survivor function for the negatively and positively stained women is computed. For the two groups of women, the log-odds of survival beyond time t are estimated and plotted against $\log t$. The resulting graph is shown in Figure 6.9. The lines are reasonably straight and parallel, and so we go on to use the log-logistic proportional odds model to summarise these data.

The model can be fitted using software for fitting the log-logistic accelerated failure time model. In Example 6.3, this latter model was fitted to the data on the survival of breast cancer patients. The estimated values of κ and θ in the proportional odds model are 1.243 and -6.787, respectively, the same as those in the accelerated failure time model. However, the estimated value of β in the linear component of the proportional odds model is $\hat{\beta} = -1.149\times 1.243 = -1.428$. This is an estimate of the logarithm of the ratio of the odds of a positively stained woman surviving beyond time t, relatively to one who is negatively stained. The corresponding odds ratio is $e^{-1.428} = 0.24$, so that the odds of a woman surviving beyond t are about four times greater if that woman has a negatively stained tumour.

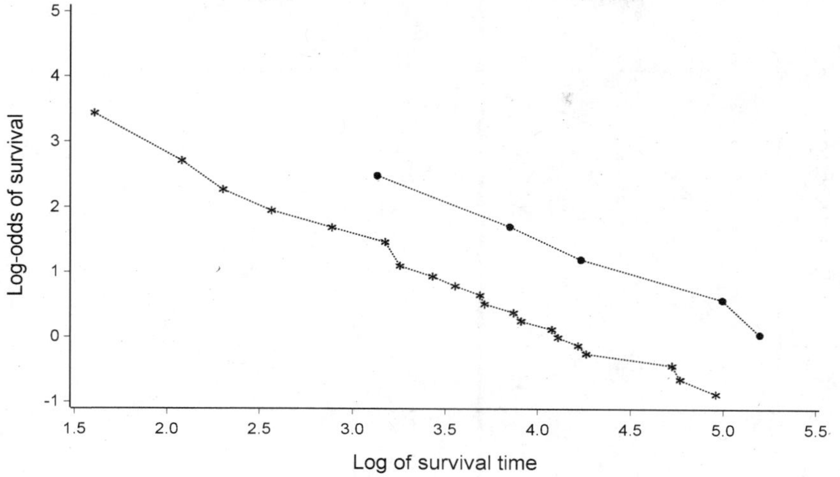

Figure 6.9 *Estimated values of the log-odds of survival beyond t plotted against* $\log t$ *for women with positively stained (*) and negatively stained (•) tumours.*

6.8* Some other distributions for survival data

Although a number of distributions for survival data have already been considered in some detail, there are others that can be useful in specific circumstances. Some of these are mentioned in this section.

When the hazard of death is expected to increase or decrease with time in the short term, and to then become constant, a hazard function that follows a *general exponential curve* or *Mitscherlich curve* may be appropriate. We would then take the hazard function to be

$$h(t) = \theta - \beta e^{-\gamma t},$$

where $\theta > 0$, $\beta > 0$ and $\gamma > 0$. This is essentially a Gompertz hazard function, defined in Section 5.9, with an additional constant. The general shape of this function is depicted in Figure 6.10. This function has a value of $\theta - \beta$ when $t = 0$ and increases to a horizontal asymptote at a hazard of θ. Similarly the function

$$h(t) = \theta + \beta e^{-\gamma t},$$

where $\theta > 0$, $\beta > 0$ and $\gamma > 0$, could be used to model a hazard which decreases from $\theta + \beta$ to a horizontal asymptote at θ.

Using Equation (1.6), the corresponding survivor function can be found, from which the probability density function can be obtained. The probability distribution corresponding to this specification of the hazard function is known as the *Gompertz-Makeham distribution.*

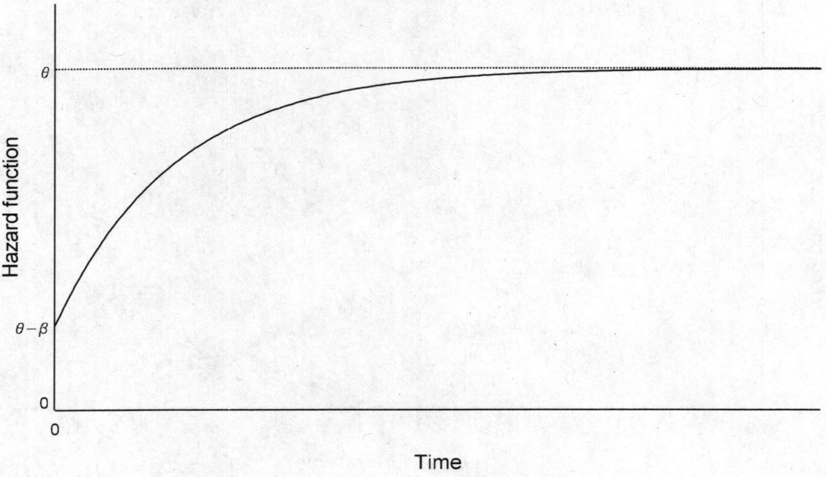

Figure 6.10 *An asymptotic hazard function, where* $h(t) = \theta - \beta e^{-\gamma t}$.

To model a hazard function that decreases and then increases symmetrically about the minimum value, a quadratic hazard function might be suitable. Thus, if

$$h(t) = \theta + \beta t + \gamma t^2,$$

for values of θ, β and γ which give the required shape of hazard and ensure that $h(t) \geqslant 0$, explicit forms for the survivor function and probability density function can be obtained.

Another form of hazard function that decreases to a single minimum and increases thereafter is the 'bathtub' hazard. The model with

$$h(t) = \alpha t + \frac{\beta}{1 + \gamma t}$$

provides a straightforward representation of this form of hazard, and corresponding expressions for the survivor and density functions can be found.

Each of the models described in this section can be fitted by constructing a log-likelihood function, using the result in Expression (5.38) of Chapter 5, and maximising this with respect to the unknown model parameters. In principle, the unknown parameters in the hazard function can also depend on the values of explanatory variables. Non-linear optimisation routines can then be used to maximise the log-likelihood.

6.9* Flexible parametric models

The main advantage of the Cox regression model for survival analysis is often perceived to be the flexibility of the baseline hazard function, since it can accommodate the pattern needed for any particular data set. In contrast, the parametric models described in this chapter lead to baseline hazard functions that depend on a very small number of unknown parameters, and so have a limited ability to capture the underlying form of a baseline hazard. This advantage of the Cox model is often overplayed. Since the baseline hazard function in a Cox model is estimated from the data to give a step-function with jumps at each event time, it can behave very erratically, as illustrated in Example 3.14 of Chapter 3. Also, the estimated survivor function for an individual with given characteristics is constant between event times, so that it may not be possible to estimate the survival rate at a precise time. Moreover, survival rates at times that are beyond the longest event time in a data set cannot be estimated.

Example 6.6 Recurrence-free survival in breast cancer patients
A cohort study of breast cancer in a large number of hospitals was carried out by the German Breast Cancer Study Group to compare three cycles of chemotherapy with six cycles, and also to investigate the effect of additional hormonal treatment consisting of a daily dose of 30 mg of tamoxifen over two years. The patients in the study had primary histologically proven non-metastatic node-positive breast cancer who had been treated with mastectomy. The response variable of interest is recurrence-free survival, which is the time from entry to the study until a recurrence of the cancer or death. Earlier analyses of the data had shown that recurrence-free survival was not affected by the number of cycles of chemotherapy, and so only the factor associated with whether or not a patient received tamoxifen is included in this example. In addition to this treatment factor, data were available on patient age, menopausal status, size and grade of the tumour, number of positive lymph nodes, progesterone and oestrogen receptor status. Further details on the background to the study are given by Schumacher et al. (1994).

The data in this example relate to data from 41 centres and 686 patients with complete data, and were included in Sauerbrei and Royston (1999). The variables in this data set are as follows:

Id:	Patient number
Treat:	Hormonal treatment (0 = no tamoxifen, 1 = tamoxifen)
Age:	Patient age (years)
Men:	Menopausal status (1 = premenopausal, 2 = postmenopausal)
Size:	Tumour size (mm)
Grade:	Tumour grade (1 – 3)
Nodes:	Number of positive lymph nodes
Prog:	Progesterone receptor status (femtomoles)
Oest:	Oestrogen receptor status, (femtomoles)
Time:	Recurrence-free survival time (days)
Status:	Event indicator (0 = censored, 1 = relapse or death)

Data for 20 of the 686 patients in this breast cancer study are shown in Table 6.5.

Table 6.5 *Recurrence-free survival times of 20 breast cancer patients.*

Id	*Treat*	*Age*	*Men*	*Size*	*Grade*	*Nodes*	*Prog*	*Oest*	*Time*	*Status*
1	0	70	2	21	2	3	48	66	1814	1
2	1	56	2	12	2	7	61	77	2018	1
3	1	58	2	35	2	9	52	271	712	1
4	1	59	2	17	2	4	60	29	1807	1
5	0	73	2	35	2	1	26	65	772	1
6	0	32	1	57	3	24	0	13	448	1
7	1	59	2	8	2	2	181	0	2172	0
8	0	65	2	16	2	1	192	25	2161	0
9	0	80	2	39	2	30	0	59	471	1
10	0	66	2	18	2	7	0	3	2014	0
11	1	68	2	40	2	9	16	20	577	1
12	1	71	2	21	2	9	0	0	184	1
13	1	59	2	58	2	1	154	101	1840	0
14	0	50	2	27	3	1	16	12	1842	0
15	1	70	2	22	2	3	113	139	1821	0
16	0	54	2	30	2	1	135	6	1371	1
17	0	39	1	35	1	4	79	28	707	1
18	1	66	2	23	2	1	112	225	1743	0
19	1	69	2	25	1	1	131	196	1781	0
20	0	55	2	65	1	4	312	76	865	1

In analysing these data, we might be interested in the treatment effect after adjusting for other explanatory variables, and in estimating the adjusted hazard functions for the two treatment groups.

It is difficult to discern pattern in the estimated baseline hazard function in a fitted Cox regression model, as the value of the hazard at each event time is determined from the number of events and the number at risk at that time. A smoothed estimate of this function is therefore desirable. One approach to this is to apply a smoothing process to the estimated cumulative baseline hazard, followed by numerical differentiation to give a smooth estimate of the hazard function itself. Although this estimate is useful in a descriptive analysis, it is not straightforward to use the fitted curve to estimate survival rates from the fitted model, nor to validate the fit of such a curve.

A much better approach is to model the underlying baseline hazard parametrical, but allowing this function to have a greater flexibility than that allowed by the fully parametric models in Chapters 5 and 6. A particularly appealing approach was described Royston and Parmar (2002), who showed how the Weibull proportional hazards model and the log-logistic proportional odds model can be extended to provide a flexible parametric modelling procedure.

6.9.1 The Royston and Parmar model

We begin with the Weibull model for the hazard of death at time t, where

$$h_i(t) = \exp(\boldsymbol{\beta}'\boldsymbol{x}_i)h_0(t),$$

in which the baseline hazard function is $h_0(t) = \lambda\gamma t^{\gamma-1}$, λ and γ are unknown parameters that determine the scale and shape of the underlying Weibull distribution, and $\boldsymbol{x}_i$ is the vector of values of p explanatory variables for the ith of n individuals. The corresponding cumulative hazard function is

$$H_i(t) = \int_0^t h_i(u)\,\mathrm{d}u = \exp(\boldsymbol{\beta}'\boldsymbol{x}_i)\lambda t^{\gamma},$$

and so the log-cumulative hazard is

$$\log H_i(t) = \boldsymbol{\beta}'\boldsymbol{x}_i + \log\lambda + \gamma\log t.$$

Now set $\eta_i = \boldsymbol{\beta}'\boldsymbol{x}_i$, and let $\gamma_0 = \log\lambda$, $\gamma_1 = \gamma$ and $y = \log t$, so that the log-cumulative hazard function for the Weibull model can be written

$$\log H_i(t) = \gamma_0 + \gamma_1 y + \eta_i.$$

This formulation shows that the log-cumulative hazard function is linear in $y = \log t$.

The next step is to generalise the linear term in y to a *natural cubic spline* in y. To define this, the range of values of y is divided into a number of intervals, where the boundary between each interval is called a *knot*. In the simplest case, we take the smallest and largest y-values and divide the range into two halves. There would then be two *boundary knots* at the extreme values of y and one *internal knot* between them. A cubic expression in y is then fitted between adjacent knots. For example, suppose that the range of values of y is from $k_{\min}$ to $k_{\max}$, and that one knot is specified at the point where $y = k_1$. A cubic expression in y is then defined for $y \in (k_{\min}, k_1)$ and for $y \in (k_1, k_{\max})$. These two cubic expressions are then constrained to have a smooth join at the internal knot k_1, to give a cubic spline. Finally, a linear term in y is assumed for $y < k_{\min}$ and for $y > k_{\max}$, which leads to a *restricted cubic spline*. This is illustrated in Figure 6.11, which shows a restricted cubic spline with boundary knots at $k_{\min}$ and $k_{\max}$ and an internal knot at k_1.

The algebraic form of a restricted cubic spline in y with one knot is

$$\gamma_0 + \gamma_1 y + \gamma_2 \nu_1(y),$$

where

$$\nu_1(y) = (y - k_1)^3_+ - \lambda_1(y - k_{\min})^3_+ - (1 - \lambda_1)(y - k_{\max})^3_+,$$

with

$$(y - a)^3_+ = \max\{0, (y - a)^3\},$$

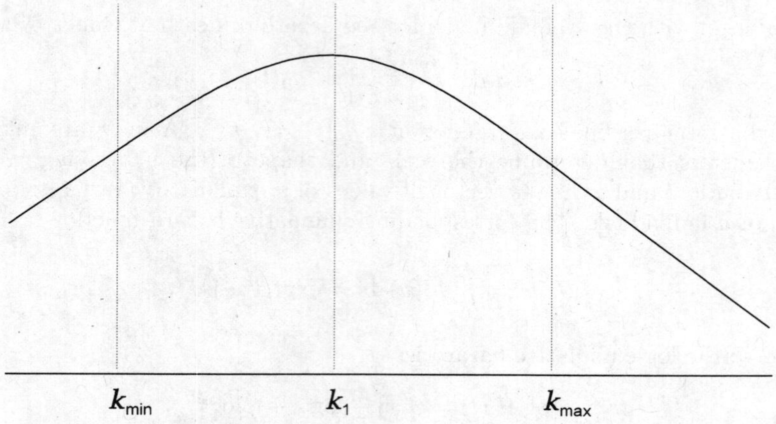

Figure 6.11 *Restricted cubic spline with an internal knot at k_1 and boundary knots at $k_{\min}$ and $k_{\max}$.*

for any value a, and

$$\lambda_1 = \frac{k_{\max} - k_1}{k_{\max} - k_{\min}}.$$

The model for the log-cumulative hazard function then becomes

$$\log H_i(t) = \begin{cases} \gamma_0 + \gamma_1 y + \eta_i, & y < k_{\min}, \\ \gamma_0 + \gamma_1 y - \gamma_2\{\lambda_1 (y - k_{\min})^3\} + \eta_i, & y \in (k_{\min}, k_1), \\ \gamma_0 + \gamma_1 y + \gamma_2\{(y - k_1)^3 - \lambda_1 (y - k_{\min})^3\} + \eta_i, & y \in (k_1, k_{\max}), \\ \gamma_0 + \gamma_1 y + \gamma_2\{(y - k_1)^3 - \lambda_1 (y - k_{\min})^3 & \\ \qquad -(1 - \lambda_1)(y - k_{\max})^3\} + \eta_i, & y > k_{\max}. \end{cases}$$

When $y > k_{\max}$, the expression for $\log H_i(t)$ simplifies to

$$\gamma_0 + \gamma_1 y + \gamma_2 (k_{\max} - k_1)(k_{\min} - k_1)(3y - k_{\min} - k_1 - k_{\max}) + \eta_i,$$

which confirms that $\log H_i(t)$ is a linear function of y for $y < k_{\min}$ and $y > k_{\max}$, and cubic functions of y for values of y between $k_{\min}$ and k_1, and between k_1 and $k_{\max}$.

The flexibility of the parametric model for $\log H_i(t)$ can be increased by increasing the number of internal knots. The greater the number of knots, the more complex the curve. In general, for a model with m internal knots, non-linear terms $\nu_1(y), \nu_2(y), \ldots, \nu_m(y)$ are defined, so that for a model with m knots,

$$\log H_i(t) = \gamma_0 + \gamma_1 y + \gamma_2 \nu_1(y) + \cdots + \gamma_{m+1} \nu_m(y) + \eta_i, \qquad (6.28)$$

where for the jth knot at k_j, $j = 1, 2, \ldots, m$,

$$\nu_j(y) = (y - k_j)_+^3 - \lambda_j(y - k_{\min})_+^3 - (1 - \lambda_j)(y - k_{\max})_+^3, \tag{6.29}$$

and

$$\lambda_j = \frac{k_{\max} - k_j}{k_{\max} - k_{\min}}.$$

The model defined by Equation (6.28) is the Royston and Parmar model.

The extended parametric form of the baseline hazard function means that the survival times no longer have a Weibull distribution under this model, nor any other recognisable distribution, although the model still assumes proportional hazards amongst the explanatory variables. The model in Equation (6.28) can also be expressed in terms of a baseline cumulative hazard function, $H_0(t)$, by writing $H_i(t) = \exp(\eta_i)H_0(t)$, where

$$H_0(t) = \exp\{\gamma_0 + \gamma_1 y + \gamma_2 \nu_1(y) + \cdots + \gamma_{m+1}\nu_m(y)\}. \tag{6.30}$$

The corresponding survivor function is $S_i(t) = \exp\{-H_i(t)\}$, for the ith individual, so that

$$S_i(t) = \exp\{-\exp[\gamma_0 + \gamma_1 y + \gamma_2 \nu_1(y) + \cdots + \gamma_{m+1}\nu_m(y) + \eta_i]\}, \tag{6.31}$$

which can also be expressed as

$$S_i(t) = \{S_0(t)\}^{\exp(\eta_i)},$$

where $S_0(t) = \exp\{-H_0(t)\}$ is the baseline survivor function.

In terms of hazard functions, the model in Equation (6.28) can be expressed as

$$h_i(t) = \frac{\mathrm{d}H_i(t)}{\mathrm{d}t} = \exp(\eta_i)h_0(t). \tag{6.32}$$

In this equation, the baseline hazard function, $h_0(t)$, is found by differentiating $H_0(t)$ in Equation (6.30) with respect to t, which gives

$$h_0(t) = t^{-1}\{\gamma_1 + \gamma_2 \nu_1'(y) + \cdots + \gamma_{m+1}\nu_m'(y)\}H_0(t),$$

where

$$\nu_j'(y) = \begin{cases} 0, & y \leqslant k_{\min}, \\ -3\lambda_j(y - k_{\min})^2, & y \in (k_{\min}, k_j), \\ 3(y - k_j)^2 - 3\lambda_j(y - k_{\min})^2, & y \in (k_j, k_{\max}), \\ 3(y - k_j)^2 - 3\lambda_j(y - k_{\min})^2 - 3(1 - \lambda_j)(y - k_{\max})^2, & y \geqslant k_{\max}, \end{cases}$$

is the first derivative of $\nu_j(y)$ with respect to y, $j = 1, 2, \ldots, m$, and $y = \log t$. This baseline hazard involves $m + 2$ unknown parameters, $\gamma_0, \gamma_1, \ldots, \gamma_{m+1}$, and provides an approximate parametric representation of the non-parametric baseline hazard function in a corresponding Cox regression model.

6.9.2 Number and position of the knots

The position chosen for the knots will affect the form of the parametric model for the cumulative hazard function. Although some authors have proposed using automatic or data driven procedures, Royston and Parmar (2002) caution against this, on the grounds that they can be unduly affected by local features of the data set, and that it is difficult to take account of this when constructing standard errors of parameter estimates. They suggest that the boundary knots are taken at the smallest and largest values of the logarithms of observed event times. Internal knots are then taken to give equal spacing between percentiles of the distribution of the logarithms of the uncensored survival times. Specifically, one internal knot would be placed at the median of the uncensored values of $\log t$, two internal knots would be placed at the 33% and 67% percentiles, three knots would be placed at the quartiles, and so on. Usually, no more than 4 or 5 knots will be needed in practical applications.

To determine the number of knots to be used, we start with zero knots, and fit the standard Weibull parametric model. A model with one internal knot is then fitted, and compared to the model with zero knots, and then a model with two internal knots is then fitted and compared to that with one knot, and so on. As the position of the knots changes as their number is increased, for example from one at the 50th percentile to two at the 33rd and 67th percentiles of the distribution of the uncensored log survival times, models with different numbers of knots are not necessarily nested. This means that the $-2\log\hat{L}$ statistic cannot generally be used to determine whether increasing the number of knots gives a significant improvement in the fit. Instead, the AIC statistic introduced in Section 3.6.1 of Chapter 3, can be used. We will take the AIC statistic to be $-2\log\hat{L} + 2q$, where q is the number of unknown parameters in the fitted model, so that for a model with p β-parameters and m knots, $q = p + m + 2$. Models with the smallest values of this statistic are generally the most suitable, and so the number of knots is increased until the AIC statistic cannot be reduced any further. Models can be compared in a similar manner using the BIC statistic, also defined in Section 3.6.1 of Chapter 3.

Experience in using these parametric models suggests that the number of knots is barely affected by covariate adjustment. This means that any variable selection can be based on standard Weibull or Cox models, and once the explanatory variables for inclusion in the Royston and Parmar model have been determined, the form of the spline function can be found by increasing the number of knots in the parametric model for the adjusted log-cumulative baseline hazard function.

6.9.3 Fitting the model

The model for the log-cumulative hazard function in Equation (6.28), or equivalently, the model for the hazard or survivor functions in Equations (6.31) and (6.32), is fully parametric. This means that the model can be fitted using the method of maximum likelihood. From Equation (5.38) in Section 5.6.1 of Chapter 5, the likelihood function is

$$\prod_{i=1}^{n} \{h_i(t_i)\}^{\delta_i} S_i(t_i),$$

where the survivor and hazard functions for the ith individual at time t_i, $S_i(t_i)$ and $h_i(t_i)$, are given in Equations (6.31) and (6.32), and δ_i is the event indicator. The logarithm of this likelihood function can be maximised using standard optimisation routines, and this leads to fitted survivor and hazard functions that are smooth functions of the survival time t. The fitting process also leads to standard errors of the parameter estimates and functions of them, such as estimates of the hazard and survivor functions at any given time.

Example 6.7 Recurrence-free survival in breast cancer patients
We now return to the data on recurrence-free survival in breast cancer patients, introduced in Example 6.6. As an initial step in the analysis of these data, the suitability of a Weibull model is investigated using a log-cumulative hazard plot, stratified by treatment. Although the presence of additional explanatory variables hinders the interpretation of such a plot for just one factor, the graph shown in Figure 6.12 does not exhibit straight lines for the two treatment groups. The assumption of a Weibull distribution for the survival times is therefore not appropriate. However, the vertical separation of two curves in this plot appears constant suggesting that the proportional hazards assumption for the treatment effect is valid.

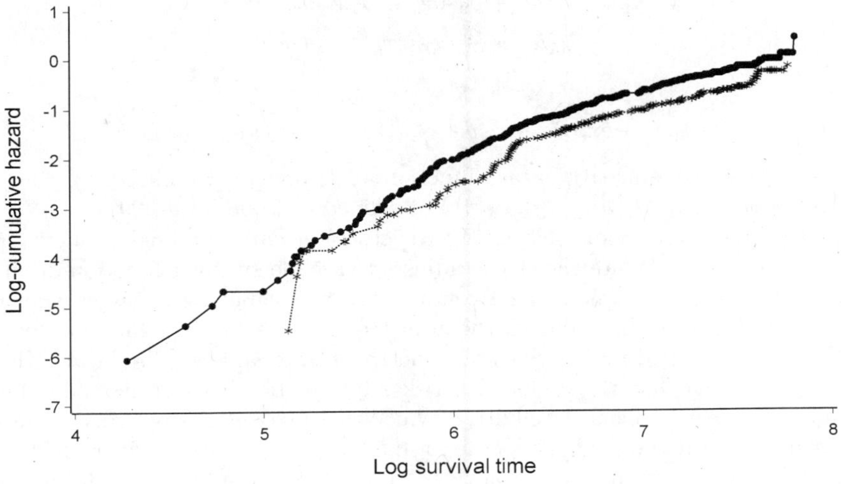

Figure 6.12 *Log-cumulative hazard plot for the women not on tamoxifen (•) and those in the tamoxifen group (∗).*

At this stage, a variable selection process may be used to determine which of the other explanatory factors, *Age*, *Men*, *Size*, *Grade*, *Nodes*, *Prog*, and *Oest*, are needed in the model in addition to *Treat*, but in this example, all of them will be included. Royston and Parmar models with increasing numbers of knots are then fitted. Table 6.6 gives the value of the *AIC* statistic for the models fitted, where the model with zero knots is the standard Weibull model.

Table 6.6 *Values of the AIC statistic for models with up to four knots.*

Number of knots	*AIC*
0	5182.4
1	5147.9
2	5147.1
3	5146.1
4	5148.2

There is a large reduction in the value of the *AIC* statistic on fitting a restricted cubic spline with one internal knot, indicating that this model is a substantial improvement on the standard Weibull model. On adding a second and third knot, the *AIC* statistic is reduced further, but the decrease is much less than that when one knot is added. On adding a fourth internal knot, the *AIC* statistic increases. This analysis shows that the best fitting model has three knots, although this is not a marked improvement on that with just one knot. The fitted model with three knots is most simply expressed in terms of the estimated log-cumulative hazard function for the ith patient, given by

$$\log \hat{H}_i(t) = \exp(\hat{\beta}_1 \, Treat_i + \hat{\beta}_2 Age_i + \hat{\beta}_3 Men_i + \hat{\beta}_4 Size_i + \hat{\beta}_5 \, Grade_i \\ + \hat{\beta}_6 Nodes_i + \hat{\beta}_7 Prog_i + \hat{\beta}_8 \, Oest_i) \hat{H}_0(t),$$

where

$$\hat{H}_0(t) = -\exp\{\hat{\gamma}_0 + \hat{\gamma}_1 y + \hat{\gamma}_2 \nu_1(y) + \hat{\gamma}_3 \nu_2(y) + \hat{\gamma}_4 \nu_3(y)\}$$

is the baseline cumulative hazard function for a model with 3 knots, $y = \log t$ and the functions $\nu_1(y), \nu_2(y), \nu_3(y)$ are defined in Equation (6.29).

A visual summary of the fit of the Royston and Parmar models is shown in Figure 6.13. This figure shows the adjusted baseline survivor function on fitting a Cox regression model that contains the 8 explanatory variables, shown as a step-function. In addition, the adjusted baseline survivor function for a Weibull model, and models with one and three internal knots, is shown. This figure confirms that the underlying risk adjusted baseline survivor function from the Cox model is not well fitted by a Weibull model. A Royston and Parmar model with one knot tracks the estimated Cox baseline survivor function much more closely, and that with three knots gives an improved performance at the longer survival times.

The estimated values of the parameters and their standard errors in the Royston and Parmar model with three knots, are given in Table 6.7. Also

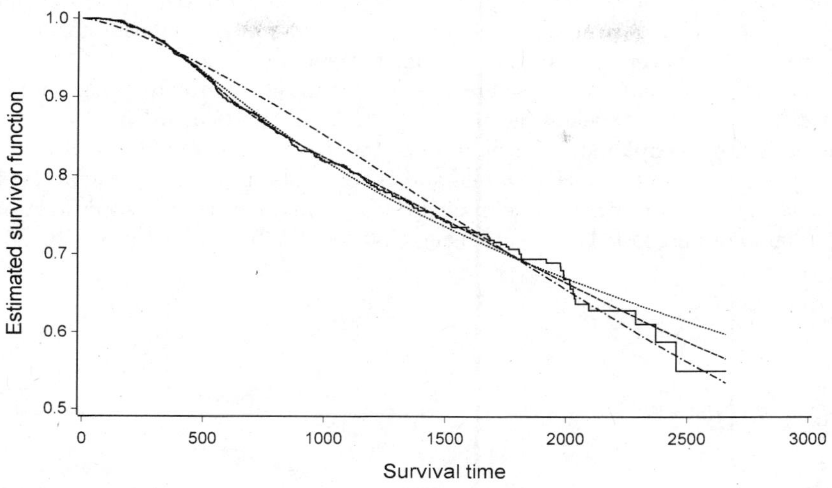

Figure 6.13 *Risk adjusted survivor functions for a fitted Cox regression model (—), Weibull model (-·-) and Royston-Parmar models with 1 (······) and 3 (- - -) knots.*

Table 6.7 *Parameter estimates and their standard errors for a Royston and Parmar model with 3 knots and a Cox regression model.*

Parameter	Royston and Parmar model		Cox regression model	
	Estimate	se (Estimate)	Estimate	se (Estimate)
β_1	−0.3386	0.1290	−0.3372	0.1290
β_2	−0.0096	0.0093	−0.0094	0.0093
β_3	0.2753	0.1831	0.2670	0.1833
β_4	0.0077	0.0040	0.0077	0.0039
β_5	0.2824	0.1059	0.2801	0.1061
β_6	0.0497	0.0074	0.0499	0.0074
β_7	−0.0022	0.0006	−0.0022	0.0006
β_8	0.0002	0.0004	0.0002	0.0004
γ_0	−20.4691	3.2958		
γ_1	2.9762	0.5990		
γ_2	−0.4832	0.5873		
γ_3	1.4232	0.8528		
γ_4	−0.9450	0.4466		

shown in this table are the estimated β-parameters in a fitted Cox model and their standard errors. The estimates and their standard errors for the two models are very similar. The adjusted hazard ratio for a patient on tamoxifen relative to one who is not, is 0.71 under both models, so that the hazard of recurrence of cancer or death is lower for patients on tamoxifen.

The Royston and Parmar model has the advantage of providing a parametric estimate of the baseline hazard. The fitted baseline hazard function, adjusted for the 8 explanatory variables, for the Weibull model and the Royston and Parmar spline models with one and three knots, is shown in Figure 6.14. The Royston and Parmar model indicates that the underlying hazard function is unimodal, and so it is not surprising that the Weibull model is a poor fit.

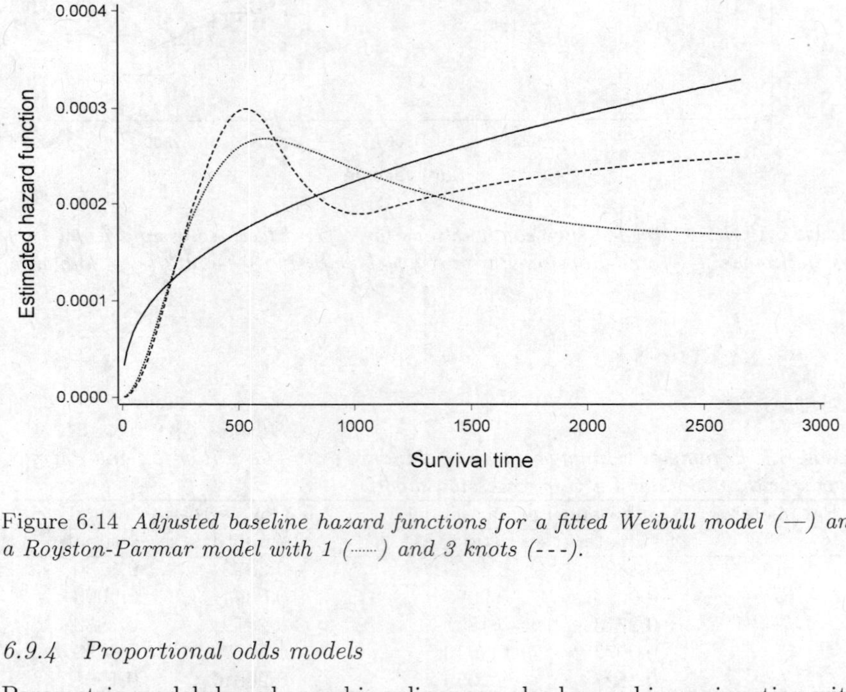

Figure 6.14 *Adjusted baseline hazard functions for a fitted Weibull model (—) and a Royston-Parmar model with 1 (·······) and 3 knots (- - -).*

6.9.4 Proportional odds models

Parametric models based on cubic splines can also be used in conjunction with proportional odds models described in Section 6.7. The general proportional odds model for the odds of survival beyond time t, $S_i(t)/\{1 - S_i(t)\}$, is such that

$$\frac{S_i(t)}{1 - S_i(t)} = e^{\boldsymbol{\beta}'\boldsymbol{x}_i} \frac{S_0(t)}{1 - S_0(t)},$$

where $\boldsymbol{x}_i$ is the vector of values of the explanatory variables for the ith individual and $S_0(t)$ is the baseline survivor function, that is the survivor function for an individual whose explanatory variables all take the value zero. If a log-logistic model with parameters θ, κ is assumed for the survival times, as in

Section 6.7.1, the log odds of survival beyond time t is, from Equation (6.2), $S(t) = \{1 + e^{\theta} t^{\kappa}\}^{-1}$. Taking this to be the baseline survivor function, $S_0(t)$ is then such that

$$\log\left(\frac{S_0(t)}{1 - S_0(t)}\right) = -\theta - \kappa \log t = \gamma_0 + \gamma_1 y,$$

where $\gamma_0 = -\theta$, $\gamma_1 = -\kappa$, and the model is linear in $y = \log t$. Extending this model to incorporate non-linear terms to give a restricted cubic spline with m internal knots, and using the same notation as in Equation (6.28), we get

$$\log\left(\frac{S_0(t)}{1 - S_0(t)}\right) = \gamma_0 + \gamma_1 y + \gamma_2 \nu_1(y) + \cdots + \gamma_{m+1} \nu_m(y),$$

which is analogous to the expression for the cumulative baseline hazard function in Equation (6.30). The proportional odds model that includes spline terms can then be expressed as

$$\log\left(\frac{S_i(t)}{1 - S_i(t)}\right) = \gamma_0 + \gamma_1 y + \gamma_2 \nu_1(y) + \cdots + \gamma_{m+1} \nu_m(y) + \eta_i,$$

where $\eta_i = \boldsymbol{\beta}' \boldsymbol{x}_i$.

This flexible proportional odds model is used in just the same way as the flexible proportional hazards model, and is particularly suited to situations where the hazard function is unimodal. The model can also be expressed in terms of the odds of an event occurring before time t, $\log[F(t)/\{1 - F(t)\}]$, and as this is simply $-\log[S(t)/\{1 - S(t)\}]$, the resulting parameter estimates will only differ in sign.

The model can be fitted using the method of maximum likelihood, as described in Section 6.9.3, and leads to an estimate of the survivor function. Estimates of the corresponding hazard and cumulative hazard functions can then straightforwardly be obtained.

Example 6.8 Recurrence-free survival in breast cancer patients

The unimodal hazard function identified in Example 6.7 suggests that a log-logistic model may be a better fit to the recurrence-free survival times for women with breast cancer. Table 6.8 gives the value of the *AIC* statistic for the model for the log odds of surviving beyond time t that has a flexible baseline survivor function, where the model with zero knots is the standard proportional odds model. As in Example 6.7, the explanatory variables *Age*, *Men*, *Size*, *Grade*, *Nodes*, *Prog* and *Oest* are included in the model, in addition to the treatment factor, *Treat*. Notice that the values of the *AIC* statistic behave somewhat erratically for models with 1, 2 and 3 knots, with the value of the $-2 \log \hat{L}$ statistic increasing slightly on adding a fourth knot. This feature can occur when the models being fitted are barely distinguishable, and since the models being fitted have increasing numbers of knots at different locations, not all the models are nested. In this case, a model for the log odds of surviving

Table 6.8 *Values of the AIC statistic for models with up to four knots.*

Number of knots	AIC
0	5154.0
1	5135.4
2	5135.8
3	5134.1
4	5136.2

beyond time t that contains three knots is the best fit, although the fit of this model is barely distinguishable from the model with just one knot.

For the model with three knots, the estimated parameter associated with the treatment effect is 0.5287. The ratio of the odds of surviving beyond time t for a patient on tamoxifen, relative to one who is not, is $\exp(0.5287) = 1.70$, and so the odds of a patient on tamoxifen surviving beyond any given time are 1.7 times that for a patient who has not received that treatment. This result is entirely consistent with the corresponding hazard ratio for the treatment effect, given in Example 6.7.

6.10* Modelling cure rates

In survival analysis, it is generally assumed that all individuals will eventually experience the end-point of interest, if the follow-up period is long enough. This is certainly the case if the end-point is death from any cause. However, in some studies, a substantial proportion of individuals may not have experienced the end-point before the end of the study. This may be because the treatment has effectively cured the patient. For example, in a cancer trial, interest may centre on a comparison of two treatments, where the end-point is death from a particular type of cancer. If the treatment cures the individual, there will be a number of patients who do not die from the cancer during the course of a relatively long follow-up period. This can lead to a larger proportion of censored observations than is usually encountered, which is sometimes referred to as *heavy censoring*. However, strictly speaking, an individual who does not die during the follow-up period has a censored time, whereas those who are cured cannot die from the disease under study.

Individuals who have been cured, or more generally, those who can no longer experience the event under study, will eventually fail for some reason, but may remain alive throughout a very long time period. In this situation, the survivor function estimated from a group of individuals will tend to level off at a value greater than zero. It may then be assumed that the population consists of a mixture of individuals: those who are susceptible to the end-point, and those who are not. The latter then correspond to the cured individuals, and the proportion with prolonged survival is called the *cured fraction*. Standard methods of survival analysis can then be adapted, so that the probability of cure is modelled simultaneously with the time to the event.

Models for the time to an event can be extended to incorporate a cured fraction, π, the probability of being cured. In a fully parametric model, the survivor function becomes

$$S(t) = (1 - \pi)S_n(t) + \pi, \tag{6.33}$$

where $S_n(t)$ is the survivor function of the non-cured individuals. In Equation (6.33), $S(t)$ is the overall survivor function for a group consisting of cured and non-cured individuals, and the model is termed a *parametric mixture model.* As $t \to \infty$, the survivor function of non-cured individuals tends to zero, and so, from Equation (6.33), $S(t)$ tends to π, the probability of cure. The corresponding hazard function for the whole group is

$$h(t) = -\frac{\mathrm{d}\log S(t)}{\mathrm{d}t} = \frac{f_n(t)}{S_n(t) + \pi/(1-\pi)}, \tag{6.34}$$

where

$$f_n(t) = -\frac{\mathrm{d}}{\mathrm{d}t} S_n(t)$$

is the density function of the non-cured individuals.

If a proportional hazards model can be assumed for the survival time of the non-cured individuals, the hazard of death at time t in such an individual is

$$h_{ni}(t) = \exp(\boldsymbol{\beta}'\boldsymbol{x}_i)h_{n0}(t),$$

where $\boldsymbol{\beta}'\boldsymbol{x}_i = \beta_1 x_{1i} + \beta_2 x_{2i} + \cdots + \beta_p x_{pi}$ is a linear combination of the values of p explanatory variables, $X_1, X_2, \ldots, X_p$, measured on this individual, and $h_{n0}(t)$ is the baseline hazard function of the non-cured individuals. The survivor function for the non-cured individuals is then

$$S_{ni}(t) = [S_{n0}(t)]^{\exp(\boldsymbol{\beta}'\boldsymbol{x}_i)},$$

where $S_{n0}(t) = \exp\{-\int_0^t h_{n0}(u)\,\mathrm{d}u\}$ is their baseline survivor function.

In addition, the probability of being cured may depend on a number of explanatory variables, especially those relating to treatment group, denoted $Z_1, Z_2, \ldots, Z_p$. The dependence of the probability that the ith of n individuals is cured on these variables can then be modelled by taking the logistic transformation of the cured fraction to be a linear combination of their values, $z_{1i}, z_{2i}, \ldots, z_{pi}$. Then,

$$\text{logit}\,(\pi_i) = \log\left(\frac{\pi_i}{1-\pi_i}\right) = \phi_0 + \boldsymbol{\phi}'\boldsymbol{z}_i,$$

for $i = 1, 2, \ldots, n$, where $\boldsymbol{\phi}'\boldsymbol{z}_i = \phi_0 + \phi_1 z_{1i} + \phi_2 z_{2i} + \cdots + \phi_p z_{pi}$ and $\phi_0, \phi_1, \ldots, \phi_p$ are unknown parameters. The cure probability is then

$$\pi_i = \{1 + \exp(-\boldsymbol{\phi}'\boldsymbol{z}_i)\}^{-1}.$$

The same explanatory variables may feature in both the survival model for the non-cured individuals and the model for the probability of cure. Also, in contrast to a survival model, the model for the cure probability will generally include a constant term ϕ_0, which is the logistic transformation of a common cure probability, when there are no other explanatory variables in the model.

Now suppose that the survival times for non-cured individuals can be modelled using a Weibull distribution, with baseline hazard function given by $h_{n0}(t) = \lambda\gamma t^{\gamma-1}$. The hazard function for the non-cured individuals is then

$$h_{ni}(t) = \exp(\boldsymbol{\beta}'\boldsymbol{x}_i)\lambda\gamma t^{\gamma-1}, \tag{6.35}$$

and the corresponding survivor function is

$$S_{ni}(t) = [\exp(-\lambda t^{\gamma})]^{\exp(\boldsymbol{\beta}'\boldsymbol{x}_i)} = \exp\{-e^{\boldsymbol{\beta}'\boldsymbol{x}_i}\lambda t^{\gamma}\}. \tag{6.36}$$

As for other models described in this chapter, the model that incorporates a cured fraction can be fitted using the method of maximum likelihood. Suppose that the data consist of n survival times $t_1, t_2, \ldots, t_n$, and that δ_i is the event indicator for the ith individual so that $\delta_i = 1$ if the ith individual dies and zero otherwise. From Equation (5.38), the likelihood function is

$$L(\boldsymbol{\beta}, \boldsymbol{\phi}, \lambda, \gamma) = \prod_{i=1}^{n} \{h_i(t_i)\}^{\delta_i} S_i(t_i),$$

where $h_i(t_i)$ and $S_i(t_i)$ are found by substituting $h_{ni}(t_i)$ and $S_{ni}(t_i)$ from Equations (6.35) and (6.36) into Equations (6.33) and (6.34).

The corresponding log-likelihood function, $\log L(\boldsymbol{\beta}, \boldsymbol{\phi}, \lambda, \gamma)$ can then be maximised using computer software for numerical optimisation. This process leads to estimates $\hat{\boldsymbol{\beta}}, \hat{\boldsymbol{\phi}}, \hat{\lambda}, \hat{\gamma}$ of the unknown parameters and their standard errors. In addition, models with different explanatory variables in either the model for the probability of cure or the survival models for non-cured individuals, can be compared using the values of the statistic $-2\log L(\hat{\boldsymbol{\beta}}, \hat{\boldsymbol{\phi}}, \hat{\lambda}, \hat{\gamma})$ in the usual way.

A number of extensions to this model are possible. For example, an accelerated failure time model can be used instead of a proportional hazards model for the non-cured individuals. A Royston and Parmar model can also be used to provide a more flexible model for the baseline hazard function in the non-cured individuals.

6.11* Effect of covariate adjustment

We conclude this chapter with an illustration of an important feature that can be encountered when developing parametric models for survival data. In linear regression analysis, one effect of adding covariates to a model is to reduce the residual mean square, and hence increase the precision of estimates based on the model, such as a treatment effect. The estimated treatment effect, adjusted for explanatory variables, will then have a smaller standard error than the unadjusted effect. In modelling survival data, the inclusion of relevant explanatory variables often has a negligible effect on standard errors of parameter estimates. Indeed, the standard error of an estimated treatment effect, for example, may even be larger after adjusting for covariates. Essentially, this is because the treatment effect does not have the same interpretation in models with and without covariates, a point made by Ford, Norrie and Ahmadi (1995). Nevertheless, it is important to include relevant explanatory variables in the model, and to check that the fitted model is appropriate, in order to ensure that a proper estimate of the treatment effect is obtained.

To illustrate this in a little more detail, suppose that t_i is the observed value of the random variable T_i, that is associated with the survival time of the ith of n individuals, $i = 1, 2, \ldots, n$. We will consider the situation where there are two treatment groups, with $n/2$ individuals in each group, and where there is a further explanatory variable whose values are available for each individual. The two explanatory variables will be labelled X_1, X_2, where X_1 refers to the treatment effect, and takes the value 0 or 1. The values of X_1, X_2 for the ith individual will be denoted x_{1i}, x_{2i}, respectively, and we will write $z_{ji} = x_{ji} - \bar{x}_j$, for $j = 1, 2$, where $\bar{x}_j$ is the sample mean of the values of the explanatory variable X_j. A proportional hazards model will be adopted for the dependence of the hazard of death at time t, for the ith individual, on the values z_{1i}, z_{2i}, in which the baseline hazard is a constant value, λ. Consequently, the hazard function can be expressed in the form

$$h_i(t) = \lambda \exp(\beta_1 z_{1i} + \beta_2 z_{2i}), \tag{6.37}$$

and under this model, the survival times are exponentially distributed, with means $\{\lambda \exp(\beta_1 z_{1i} + \beta_2 z_{2i})\}^{-1}$. Using results given in Section 6.5.1, this model may also be expressed in accelerated failure time form as

$$\log T_i = \mu - \beta_1 z_{1i} - \beta_2 z_{2i} + \epsilon_i, \tag{6.38}$$

where $\mu = -\log \lambda$ and ϵ_i has a Gumbel distribution, that is $\log \epsilon_i$ has a unit exponential distribution. The model represented in Equations (6.37) or (6.38) will be referred to as Model (1).

Using the results for maximum likelihood estimation given in Appendix A, it can be shown that the approximate variance of the estimated treatment effect, $\hat{\beta}_1$, in Model (1), is

$$\text{var}\,(\hat{\beta}_1) = \frac{1}{[1 - \{\text{corr}\,(z_1, z_2)\}^2] \sum_{i=1}^{n} z_{1i}^2},$$

where $\text{corr}\,(z_1, z_2)$ is the sample correlation between the values z_{1i} and z_{2i}. Since z_{1i} is either -0.5 or 0.5, and there are equal numbers of individuals in each group, $\sum_{i=1}^{n} z_{1i}^2 = n/4$, and so

$$\text{var}\,(\hat{\beta}_1) = \frac{4}{n[1 - \{\text{corr}\,(z_1, z_2)\}^2]}. \tag{6.39}$$

Now consider the model that only includes the variable associated with the treatment effect, X_1, so that

$$h_i(t) = \lambda \exp(\beta_1 z_{1i}), \tag{6.40}$$

or equivalently,

$$\log T_i = \mu - \beta_1 z_{1i} + \epsilon_i, \tag{6.41}$$

where again $\log \epsilon_i$ has a unit exponential distribution. The model described by Equations (6.40) or (6.41) will be referred to as Model (2). In this model, the approximate variance of $\hat{\beta}_1$ is given by $\text{var}\,(\hat{\beta}_1) = 4n^{-1}$. Since the term $1 - \{\,\text{corr}\,(z_1, z_2)\}^2$ in Equation (6.39) is always less than or equal to unity, the variance of $\hat{\beta}_1$ in Model (1) is at least equal to that of Model (2). The addition of the explanatory variable X_2 to Model (1) cannot therefore decrease the variance of the estimated treatment effect.

The reason for this is that Model (1) and Model (2) cannot both be valid for the same data set. If Model (1) is correct, and Model (2) is actually fitted, the residual term in Equation (6.41) is not ϵ_i but $\epsilon_i - \beta_2 z_{2i}$. Similarly, if Model (2) is correct, but Model (1) is actually fitted, we cannot assume that the logarithm of ϵ_i in Equation (6.38) has a unit exponential distribution. Moreover, the parameter β_1 is now estimated less precisely because a redundant parameter, β_2, is included in the model.

More detailed analytic and simulation studies are given in the paper by Ford et al. (1995), which confirm the general point that the inclusion of explanatory variables in models for survival data cannot be expected to increase the precision of an estimated treatment effect.

6.12 Further reading

The properties of random variables that have probability distributions such as the logistic, lognormal and gamma, are presented in Johnson and Kotz (1994). Chhikara and Folks (1989) give a detailed study of the inverse Gaussian distribution.

A description of the log-linear model for survival data is contained in many of the major textbooks on survival analysis; see in particular Cox and Oakes (1984), Kalbfleisch and Prentice (2002), Klein and Moeschberger (2005) or Lawless (2002).

Cox and Oakes (1984) show that the Weibull distribution is the only one to have both the proportional hazards property and the accelerated failure time property. They also demonstrate that the log-logistic distribution is the only one that shares the accelerated failure time property and the proportional odds property.

A non-parametric version of the accelerated failure time model, which does not require the specification of a probability distribution for the survival data, has been introduced by Wei (1992). This paper, and the published discussion, Fisher (1992), includes comments on whether the accelerated failure time model should be used more widely in the analysis of survival data.

The application of the accelerated failure time and proportional odds models to the analysis of reliability data is described by Crowder et al. (1991). The general proportional odds model for survival data was introduced by Bennett (1983a), and Bennett (1983b) describes the log-logistic proportional odds model. The model has been further developed by Yang and Prentice (1999).

The piecewise exponential model, mentioned in Section 6.3.1, in which hazards are constant over particular time intervals, was introduced by Breslow (1974). Breslow also points out that the Cox regression model is equivalent to a piecewise exponential model with constant hazards between each death time. The piecewise exponential model and the use of the normal, lognormal, logistic and log-logistic distributions for modelling survival times are described in Aitkin et al. (1989).

Use of the quadratic hazard function was discussed by Gaver and Acar (1979) and the bathtub hazard function was proposed by Hjorth (1980).

A more general way of modelling survival data is to use a general family of distributions for survival times, which includes the Weibull and log-logistic as special cases. The choice between alternative distributions can then be made within a likelihood framework. In particular, the exponential, Weibull, log-logistic, lognormal and gamma distributions are special cases of the generalised F-distribution described by Kalbfleisch and Prentice (2002). However, this methodology will only tend to be informative in the analysis of data sets in which the number of death times is relatively large.

Estimators of the hazard function based on kernel smoothing are described by Ramlau-Hansen (1983) and in the text of Klein and Moeschberger (2005). The use of cubic splines in regression models was described by Durrleman and Simon (1989). The flexible parametric model for survival analysis was introduced by Royston and Parmar (2002), and a comprehensive account of the model, and its implementation in Stata, is given by Royston and Lambert (2011). Parametric mixture models that incorporate cured fractions, and their extension to semi-parametric models, have been described by a number of authors, including Farewell (1982), Kuk and Chen (1992), Taylor (1995), Sy and Taylor (2000) and Peng and Dear (2000).

Chapter 7

Model checking in parametric models

Diagnostic procedures for the assessment of model adequacy are as important in parametric modelling as they are when the Cox regression model is used in the analysis of survival data. Procedures based on residuals are particularly relevant, and so we begin this chapter by defining residuals for parametric models, some of which stem from those developed for the Cox model, described in Chapter 4. This is followed by a summary of graphical procedures for assessing the suitability of models fitted to data that are assumed to have a Weibull, log-logistic or lognormal distribution. Other ways of examining the fit of a parametric regression model are then considered, along with methods for the detection of influential observations. We conclude with a summary of how the assumption of proportional hazards can be examined after fitting the Weibull proportional hazards model.

7.1 Residuals for parametric models

Suppose that T_i is the random variable associated with the survival time of the ith individual, $i = 1, 2, \ldots, n$, and that $x_{1i}, x_{2i}, \ldots, x_{pi}$ are the values of p explanatory variables, $X_1, X_2, \ldots, X_p$, for this individual. Assuming an accelerated failure time model for T_i, we have that

$$\log T_i = \mu + \alpha_1 x_{1i} + \alpha_2 x_{2i} + \cdots + \alpha_p x_{pi} + \sigma\epsilon_i,$$

where ϵ_i is a random variable with a probability distribution that depends on the distribution adopted for T_i, and μ, σ and α_j, $j = 1, 2, \ldots, p$, are unknown parameters. If the observed survival time of the ith individual is censored, the corresponding residual will also be censored, complicating the interpretation of these quantities.

7.1.1 Standardised residuals

A natural form of residual to adopt in accelerated failure time modelling is the *standardised residual* defined by

$$r_{Si} = \{\log t_i - \hat{\mu} - \hat{\alpha}_1 x_{1i} - \hat{\alpha}_2 x_{2i} - \cdots - \hat{\alpha}_p x_{pi}\} / \hat{\sigma}, \qquad (7.1)$$

where t_i is the observed survival time of the ith individual, and $\hat{\mu}$, $\hat{\sigma}$, $\hat{\alpha}_j$, $j = 1, 2, \ldots, p$, are the estimated parameters in the fitted accelerated failure time model. This residual has the appearance of a quantity of the form 'observation − fitted value', and would be expected to have the same distribution as that of ϵ_i in the accelerated failure time model, if the model were correct. For example, if a Weibull distribution is adopted for T_i, the r_{Si} would be expected to behave as if they were a possibly censored sample from a Gumbel distribution, if the fitted model is correct. The estimated survivor function of the residuals would then be similar to the survivor function of ϵ_i, that is, $S_{\epsilon_i}(\epsilon)$. Using the general result in Section 4.1.1 of Chapter 4, $-\log S_{\epsilon_i}(\epsilon)$ has a unit exponential distribution, and so it follows that $-\log S_{\epsilon_i}(r_{Si})$ will have an approximate unit exponential distribution, if the fitted model is appropriate. This provides the basis for a diagnostic plot that may be used in the assessment of model adequacy, described in Section 7.2.4.

7.1.2 *Cox-Snell residuals*

The Cox-Snell residuals that were defined for the Cox regression model in Section 4.1.1 of Chapter 4 are essentially the estimated values of the cumulative hazard function for the ith observation, at the corresponding event time, t_i. Residuals that have a similar form may also be used in assessing the adequacy of parametric models. The main difference is that now the survivor and hazard functions are parametric functions that depend on the distribution adopted for the survival times. In particular, the estimated survivor function for the ith individual, on fitting an accelerated failure time model, from Equation (6.12), is given by

$$\hat{S}_i(t) = S_{\epsilon_i}\left(\frac{\log t - \hat{\mu} - \hat{\alpha}_1 x_{1i} - \hat{\alpha}_2 x_{2i} - \cdots - \hat{\alpha}_p x_{pi}}{\hat{\sigma}}\right), \tag{7.2}$$

where $S_{\epsilon_i}(\epsilon)$ is the survivor function of ϵ_i in the accelerated failure time model, $\hat{\alpha}_j$ is the estimated coefficient of x_{ji}, $j = 1, 2, \ldots, p$, and $\hat{\mu}$, $\hat{\sigma}$ are the estimated values of μ and σ. The form of $S_{\epsilon_i}(\epsilon)$ for some commonly used distributions for T_i was summarised in Table 6.2 of Chapter 6.

The Cox-Snell residuals for a parametric model are defined by

$$r_{Ci} = \hat{H}_i(t_i) = -\log \hat{S}_i(t_i), \tag{7.3}$$

where $\hat{H}_i(t_i)$ is the estimated cumulative hazard function, and $\hat{S}_i(t_i)$ is the estimated survivor function in Equation (7.2), evaluated at t_i. As in the context of the Cox regression model, these residuals can be taken to have a unit exponential distribution when the correct model has been fitted, with censored observations leading to censored residuals; see Section 4.1.1 for details.

The Cox-Snell residuals in Equation (7.3) are very closely related to the standardised residuals in Equation (7.1), since from Equation (7.2), we see that $r_{Ci} = -\log S_{\epsilon_i}(r_{Si})$. Assessment of whether the standardised residuals have a particular distribution is therefore equivalent to assessing whether the corresponding Cox-Snell residuals have a unit exponential distribution.

7.1.3 *Martingale residuals*

The martingale residuals provide a measure of the difference between the observed number of deaths in the interval $(0, t_i)$, which is either 0 or 1, and the number predicted by the model. Observations with unusually large martingale residuals are not well fitted by the model. The analogue of the martingale residual, defined for the Cox regression model in Equation (4.6) of Chapter 4, is such that

$$r_{Mi} = \delta_i - r_{Ci}, \tag{7.4}$$

where δ_i is the event indicator for the ith observation, so that δ_i is unity if that observation is an event and zero if censored, and now r_{Ci} is the Cox-Snell residual given in Equation (7.3). For reasons given in Section 7.1.5, the martingale residuals for a parametric accelerated failure time model sum to zero, but are not symmetrically distributed about zero. Strictly speaking, it is no longer appropriate to refer to these residuals as martingale residuals since the derivation of them, based on martingale methods, does not carry over to the accelerated failure time model. However, for semantic convenience, we will continue to refer to the quantities in Equation (7.4) as martingale residuals.

7.1.4 *Deviance residuals*

The deviance residuals, which were first presented in Equation (4.7) of Chapter 4, can be regarded as an attempt to make the martingale residuals symmetrically distributed about zero, and are defined by

$$r_{Di} = \text{sgn}(r_{Mi}) \left[-2 \left\{r_{Mi} + \delta_i \log(\delta_i - r_{Mi})\right\}\right]^{\frac{1}{2}}. \tag{7.5}$$

It is important to note that these quantities are not components of the deviance for the fitted parametric model, but nonetheless it will be convenient to continue to refer to them as deviance residuals.

7.1.5* *Score residuals*

Score residuals, which parallel the score residuals, or Schoenfeld residuals, used in connection with the Cox regression model, can be defined for any parametric model. The score residuals are the components of the derivatives of the log-likelihood function, with respect to the unknown parameters, μ, σ and α_j, $j = 1, 2, \ldots, p$, and evaluated at the maximum likelihood estimates of these parameters, $\hat{\mu}$, $\hat{\sigma}$ and $\hat{\alpha}_j$. From Equation (6.24) of Chapter 6, the log-likelihood function for n observations is

$$\log L(\boldsymbol{\alpha}, \mu, \sigma) = \sum_{i=1}^{n} \left\{-\delta_i \log(\sigma t_i) + \delta_i \log f_{\epsilon_i}(z_i) + (1 - \delta_i) \log S_{\epsilon_i}(z_i)\right\},$$

where $z_i = (\log t_i - \mu - \alpha_1 x_{1i} - \alpha_2 x_{2i} - \cdots - \alpha_p x_{pi})/\sigma$, $f_{\epsilon_i}(\epsilon)$ and $S_{\epsilon_i}(\epsilon)$ are the density and survivor functions of ϵ_i, and δ_i is the event indicator.

Differentiating this log-likelihood function with respect to the parameters μ, σ, and α_j, for $j = 1, 2, \ldots, p$, gives the following derivatives:

$$\frac{\partial \log L}{\partial \mu} = \sigma^{-1} \sum_{i=1}^{n} g(z_i),$$

$$\frac{\partial \log L}{\partial \sigma} = \sigma^{-1} \sum_{i=1}^{n} \{z_i g(z_i) - \delta_i\},$$

$$\frac{\partial \log L}{\partial \alpha_j} = \sigma^{-1} \sum_{i=1}^{n} x_{ji} g(z_i),$$

where the function $g(z_i)$ is given by

$$g(z_i) = \frac{(1-\delta_i) f_{\epsilon_i}(z_i)}{S_{\epsilon_i}(z_i)} - \frac{\delta_i f'_{\epsilon_i}(z_i)}{f_{\epsilon_i}(z_i)},$$

and $f'_{\epsilon_i}(z_i)$ is the derivative of $f_{\epsilon_i}(z_i)$ with respect to z_i.

The ith component of each derivative, evaluated at the maximum likelihood estimates of the unknown parameters, is then the score residual for the corresponding term. Consequently, from the definition of the standardised residual in Equation (7.1), the ith score residual for μ is

$$\hat{\sigma}^{-1} g(r_{Si}),$$

that for the scale parameter, σ, is

$$\hat{\sigma}^{-1} \{r_{Si}\, g(r_{Si}) - \delta_i\},$$

and that for the jth explanatory variable in the model, X_j, is

$$r_{Uji} = \hat{\sigma}^{-1} x_{ji}\, g(r_{Si}).$$

Of these, the score residuals for X_j are the most important, and as in Section 4.1.6 are denoted r_{Uji}. Specific expressions for these residuals are given in the sequel for some particular parametric models. Because the sums of score residuals are the derivatives of the log-likelihood function at its maximum, these residuals must sum to zero.

7.2 Residuals for particular parametric models

In this section, the form of the residuals for parametric models based on Weibull, log-logistic and lognormal distributions for the survival times are described.

7.2.1 Weibull distribution

The residuals described in Section 7.1 may be used in conjunction with either the proportional hazards or the accelerated failure time representations of the Weibull model. We begin with the proportional hazards model described in Chapter 5, according to which the hazard of death at time t for the ith individual is

$$h_i(t) = \exp(\beta_1 x_{1i} + \beta_2 x_{2i} + \cdots + \beta_p x_{pi}) h_0(t),$$

where $h_0(t) = \lambda\gamma t^{\gamma-1}$ is the baseline hazard function. The corresponding estimate of the cumulative hazard function is

$$\hat{H}_i(t) = \exp(\hat{\beta}_1 x_{1i} + \hat{\beta}_2 x_{2i} + \cdots + \hat{\beta}_p x_{pi}) \hat{\lambda} t^{\hat{\gamma}}$$

which are the Cox-Snell residuals, as defined in Equation (7.3).

In the accelerated failure time form of the model, ϵ_i has a Gumbel distribution, with survivor function

$$S_{\epsilon_i}(\epsilon) = \exp(-e^{\epsilon}). \tag{7.6}$$

The standardised residuals are then as given in Equation (7.1), and if an appropriate model has been fitted, these will be expected to behave as a possibly censored sample from a Gumbel distribution. This is equivalent to assessing whether the Cox-Snell residuals, defined below, have a unit exponential distribution.

The Cox-Snell residuals, $r_{Ci} = -\log S_{\epsilon_i}(r_{Si})$, are, from Equation (7.6), simply the exponentiated standardised residuals, that is $r_{Ci} = \exp(r_{Si})$. These residuals lead immediately to the martingale and deviance residuals for the Weibull model, using Equations (7.4) and (7.5).

The score residuals for the Weibull model are found from the general results in Section 7.1.5. In particular, the ith score residual for the jth explanatory variable in the model, X_j, is

$$r_{Uji} = \hat{\sigma}^{-1} x_{ji} \left(e^{r_{Si}} - \delta_i\right),$$

where r_{Si} is the ith standardised residual and δ_i the event indicator. We also note that the ith score residual for μ is $\hat{\sigma}^{-1}(e^{r_{Si}} - \delta_i)$, which is $\hat{\sigma}^{-1}(r_{Ci} - \delta_i)$. Since these score residuals sum to zero, it follows that the sum of the martingale residuals, defined in Equation (7.4), must be zero in the Weibull model.

7.2.2 Log-logistic distribution

In the log-logistic accelerated failure time model, the random variable ϵ_i has a logistic distribution with survivor function

$$S_{\epsilon_i}(\epsilon) = \left(1 + e^{\epsilon}\right)^{-1}.$$

Accordingly, the standardised residuals, obtained from Equation (7.1), should behave as a sample from a logistic distribution, if the fitted model is correct. Equivalently, the Cox-Snell residuals for the log-logistic accelerated failure time model are given by

$$r_{Ci} = -\log S_{\epsilon_i}(r_{Si}),$$

that is,

$$r_{Ci} = \log\{1 + \exp(r_{Si})\},$$

where r_{Si} is the ith standardised residual. The score residuals are found from the general results in Section 7.1.5, and we find that the ith score residual for the jth explanatory variable in the model is

$$r_{Uji} = \hat{\sigma}^{-1} x_{ji} \left\{ \frac{\exp(r_{Si}) - \delta_i}{1 + \exp(r_{Si})} \right\}.$$

7.2.3 *Lognormal distribution*

If the survival times are assumed to have a lognormal distribution, then ϵ_i in the log-linear formulation of the accelerated failure time model is normally distributed. The estimated survivor function for the ith individual, from Equation (6.23), is

$$\hat{S}_i(t) = 1 - \Phi\left(\frac{\log t - \hat{\mu} - \hat{\alpha}_1 x_{1i} - \hat{\alpha}_2 x_{2i} - \cdots - \hat{\alpha}_p x_{pi}}{\hat{\sigma}} \right),$$

and so the Cox-Snell residuals become

$$r_{Ci} = -\log\{1 - \Phi(r_{Si})\},$$

where, as usual, r_{Si} is the ith standardised residual in Equation (7.1). Again the martingale and deviance residuals are obtained from these, and the score residuals are obtained from the results in Section 7.1.5. Specifically, the ith score residual for X_j, is

$$r_{Uji} = \hat{\sigma}^{-1} \left\{ \frac{(1 - \delta_i) f_{\epsilon_i}(r_{Si})}{1 - \Phi(r_{Si})} + \delta_i r_{Si} \right\},$$

where $f_{\epsilon_i}(r_{Si})$ is the standard normal density function at r_{Si}, and $\Phi(r_{Si})$ is the corresponding distribution function.

7.2.4 *Analysis of residuals*

In the analysis of residuals after fitting a parametric model to survival data, one of the most useful plots is based on comparing the distribution of the Cox-Snell residuals with the unit exponential distribution. As noted in Section 7.1.1, this is equivalent to comparing the distribution of the standardised residuals to that of the random variable ϵ_i in the log-linear form of the accelerated failure time model. This comparison is made using a cumulative hazard, or log-cumulative hazard, plot of the residuals, as shown in Section 4.2.1 of Chapter 4, where the use of this plot in connection with residuals after fitting the Cox regression model was described. In summary, the Kaplan-Meier estimate of the survivor function of the Cox-Snell residuals, denoted $\hat{S}(r_{Ci})$, is obtained, and $-\log \hat{S}(r_{Ci})$ is plotted against r_{Ci}. A straight line with unit slope and zero intercept will suggest that the fitted model is appropriate. Alternatively, a log-cumulative hazard plot of the residuals, obtained by plotting $\log\{-\log \hat{S}(r_{Ci})\}$ against $\log r_{Ci}$, will also give a straight line with unit slope and passing through the origin, if the fitted survival model is satisfactory.

In Section 4.2.1, substantial criticisms were levied against the use of this plot. However, these criticisms do not have as much force for residuals derived from parametric models. The reason for this is that the non-parametric estimate of the baseline cumulative hazard function, used in the Cox regression model, is now replaced by an estimate of a parametric function. This function usually depends on just two parameters, μ and σ, and so fewer parameters are being estimated when an accelerated failure time model is fitted to survival data. The Cox-Snell residuals for a parametric model are therefore much more likely to be approximated by a unit exponential distribution, when the correct model has been fitted.

Other residual plots that are useful include index plots of martingale or deviance residuals, which can be used to identify observations not well fitted by the model. A plot of martingale or deviance residuals against the survival times, the rank order of the times, or explanatory variables, shows whether there are particular times, or particular values of explanatory variables, for which the model is not a good fit. Plots of martingale or deviance residuals against the estimated acceleration factor, $\exp(-\hat{\boldsymbol{\alpha}}'\boldsymbol{x}_i)$, or simply the estimated linear component of the accelerated failure time model, $\hat{\boldsymbol{\alpha}}'\boldsymbol{x}_i$, also provide information about the relationship between the residuals and the likely survival time of an individual. Those with large values of the estimated acceleration factor will tend to have shorter survival times. Index plots of score residuals, or plots of these residuals against the survival times, or the rank order of the survival times, might be examined in a more comprehensive assessment of model adequacy.

Example 7.1 Chemotherapy in ovarian cancer patients

In Example 5.10 of Chapter 5, data on the survival times of patients with ovarian cancer were presented. The data were analysed using a Weibull proportional hazards model, and the model chosen contained variables corresponding to the age of the woman, *Age*, and the treatment group to which the woman was assigned, *Treat*. In the accelerated failure time representation of the model, the estimated survivor function for the ith woman is

$$\hat{S}_i(t) = S_{\epsilon_i}\left(\frac{\log t - \hat{\mu} - \hat{\alpha}_1\, Age_i - \hat{\alpha}_2\, Treat_i}{\hat{\sigma}}\right),$$

where $S_{\epsilon_i}(\epsilon) = \exp(-e^{\epsilon})$, so that

$$\hat{S}_i(t) = \exp\left\{ -\exp\left(\frac{\log t - 10.4254 + 0.0790\, Age_i - 0.5615\, Treat_i}{0.5489} \right) \right\}.$$

The standardised residuals are the values of

$$r_{Si} = (\log t_i - 10.4254 + 0.0790\, Age_i - 0.5615\, Treat_i)/0.5489,$$

for $i = 1, 2, \ldots, 26$, and these are given in Table 7.1. Also given are the values of the Cox Snell residuals, which for the Weibull model, are such that $r_{Ci} = \exp(r_{Si})$.

Table 7.1 *Values of the standardised and Cox-Snell residuals for 26 ovarian cancer patients.*

Patient	r_{Si}	r_{Ci}	Patient	r_{Si}	r_{Ci}
1	−1.320	0.267	14	−1.782	0.168
2	−1.892	0.151	15	−0.193	0.825
3	−2.228	0.108	16	−1.587	0.204
4	−2.404	0.090	17	−0.917	0.400
5	−3.270	0.038	18	−1.771	0.170
6	−0.444	0.642	19	−1.530	0.217
7	−1.082	0.339	20	−2.220	0.109
8	−0.729	0.482	21	−0.724	0.485
9	0.407	1.503	22	−1.799	0.165
10	0.817	2.264	23	0.429	1.535
11	−1.321	0.267	24	−0.837	0.433
12	−0.607	0.545	25	−1.287	0.276
13	−1.796	0.166	26	−1.886	0.152

A cumulative hazard plot of the Cox-Snell residuals is given in Figure 7.1. In this figure, the plotted points lie on a line that has an intercept and slope close to zero and unity, respectively. However, there is some evidence of a systematic deviation from the straight line, giving some cause for concern about the adequacy of the fitted model.

Plots of the martingale and deviance residuals against the rank order of the survival times are shown in Figures 7.2 and 7.3, respectively. Both of these plots show a slight tendency for observations with longer survival times to have smaller residuals, but these are also the observations that are censored.

The graphs in Figure 7.4 show the score residuals for the two variables in the model, *Age* and *Treat*, plotted against the rank order of the survival times. The plot of the score residuals for *Age* shows that there are three observations with relatively large residuals. These correspond to patients 14, 4 and 26 in the original data set given in Table 5.6. However, there does not appear to be anything unusual about these observations. The score residual for *Treat* for patient 26 is also somewhat larger than the others. This points to the fact that the model is not a good fit to the data from patients 14, 4 and 26.

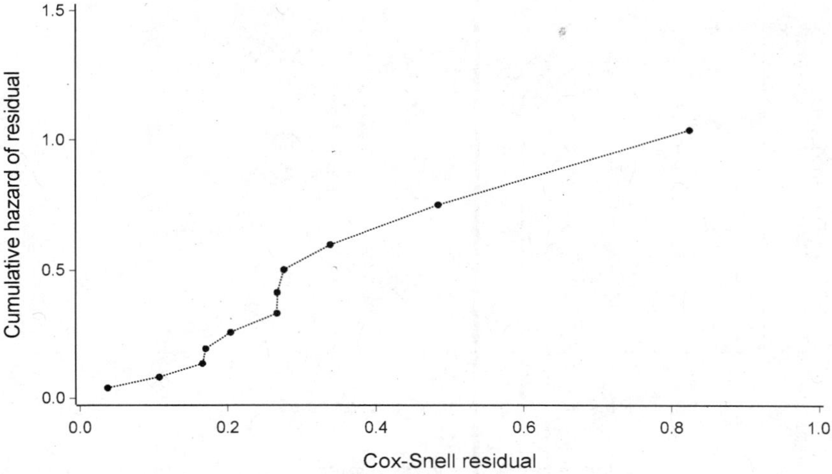

Figure 7.1 *Cumulative hazard plot of the Cox-Snell residuals.*

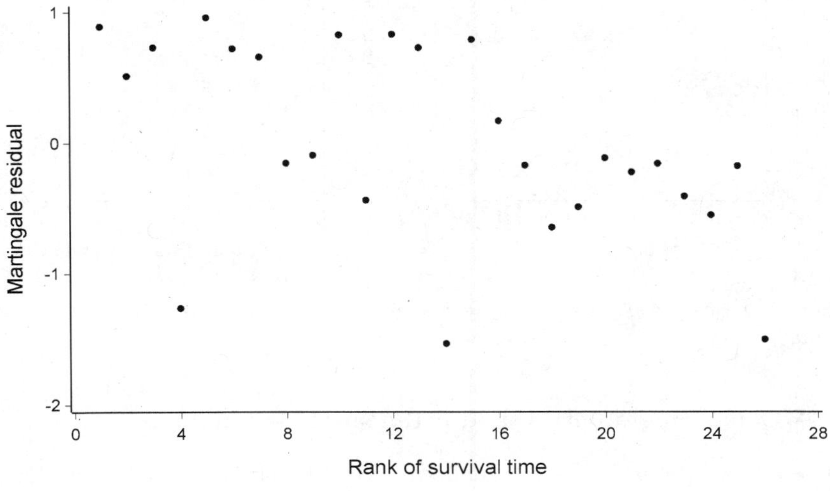

Figure 7.2 *Plot of the martingale residuals against rank order of survival time.*

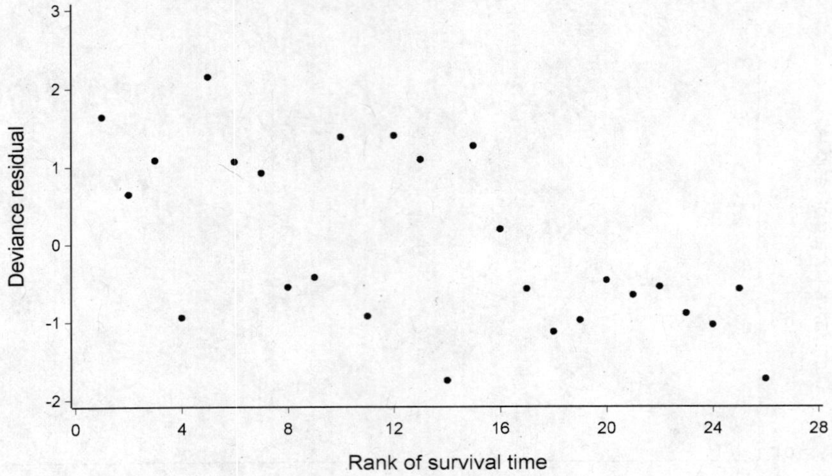

Figure 7.3 *Plot of the deviance residuals against rank order of survival time.*

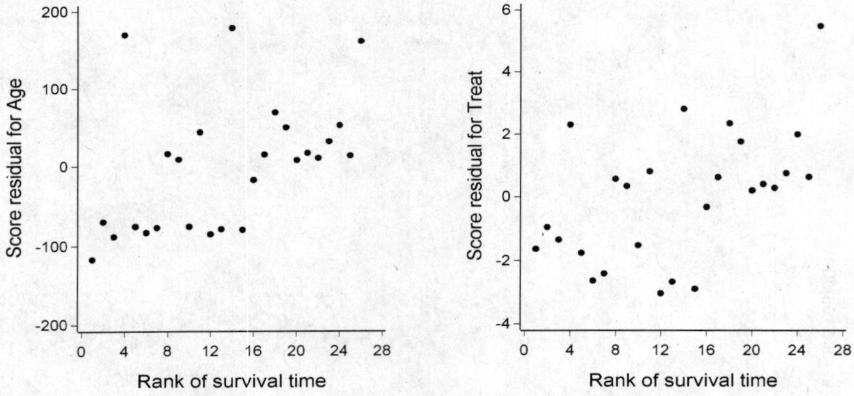

Figure 7.4 *Score residuals plotted against rank order of survival time for Age and Treat.*

7.3 Comparing observed and fitted survivor functions

In parametric modelling, the estimated survivor function is a continuous function of the survival time, t, and so this function can be plotted for particular values of the explanatory variables included in the model. When there is just a single sample of survival data, with no explanatory variables, the fitted survivor function can be compared directly with the Kaplan-Meier estimate of the survivor function, described in Section 2.1.2 of Chapter 2. If the fitted survivor function is close to the Kaplan-Meier estimate, which is a step-function, the fitted model is an appropriate summary of the data. Similarly, suppose that the model incorporates one or two factors that classify individuals according to treatment group, or provide a cross-classification of treatment group and gender. For each group of individuals defined by the combinations of levels of the factors in the model, the fitted survivor function can then be compared with the corresponding Kaplan-Meier estimate of the survivor function.

In situations where the values of a number of explanatory variables are recorded, groups of individuals are formed from the values of the estimated linear component of the fitted model. For the ith individual, whose values of the explanatory variables in the model are $\boldsymbol{x}_i$, this is just the risk score in a proportional hazards model, $\hat{\boldsymbol{\beta}}'\boldsymbol{x}_i$, or the value of $\hat{\boldsymbol{\alpha}}'\boldsymbol{x}_i$ in an accelerated failure time model. The following discussion is based on the risk score, where large positive values correspond to a greater hazard, but it could equally well be based on the linear component of an accelerated failure time model, or the value of the acceleration factor.

The values of the risk score for each individual are arranged in increasing order, and these values are used to divide the individuals into a number of groups. For example, if three groups were used, there would be individuals with low, medium and high values of the risk score. The actual number of groups formed in this way will depend on the size of the database. For larger databases, five or even seven groups might be constructed. In particular, with five groups, there would be 20% of the individuals in each group; those with the lowest and highest values of the risk score would be at low and high risk, respectively, while the middle 20% would be of medium risk.

The next step is to compare the observed and fitted survivor functions in each of the groups. Suppose that $\hat{S}_{ij}(t)$ is the model-based estimate of the survivor function for the ith individual in the jth group. The average fitted survivor function is then obtained for each group, or just the groups with the smallest, middle and highest risk scores, from

$$\bar{S}_j(t) = \frac{1}{n_j} \sum_{i=1}^{n_j} \hat{S}_{ij}(t),$$

where n_j is the number of observations in the jth group. The value of $\bar{S}_j(t)$ would be obtained for a range of t values, so that a plot of the values of $\bar{S}_j(t)$ against t, for each value of j, yields a smooth curve. The corresponding observed survivor function for a particular group is the Kaplan-Meier estimate of the survivor function for the individuals in that group. Superimposing these two sets of estimates gives a visual representation of the agreement between the observed and fitted survivor functions. This procedure is analogous to that described in Section 3.11.1 for the Cox regression model.

Using this approach, it is often easier to detect departures from the fitted model, than from plots based on residuals. However, the procedure can be criticised for using the same fitted model to define the groups, and to obtain the estimated survivor function for each group. If the database is sufficiently large, the survivor function could be estimated from half of the data, and the fit of the model evaluated on the remaining half. Also, since the method is based on the values of the risk score, no account is taken of differences between individuals who have different sets of values of the explanatory variables, but just happen to have the same value of the risk score.

Example 7.2 Chemotherapy in ovarian cancer patients
In this example, we examine the fit of a Weibull proportional hazards model to the data on the survival times of 26 women, following treatment for ovarian cancer. A Weibull model that contains the variables *Age* and *Treat* is fitted, as in Example 5.10, so that the fitted survivor function for the ith individual is

$$\hat{S}_i(t) = \exp\left\{-e^{\hat{\eta}_i}\hat{\lambda}t^{\hat{\gamma}}\right\}, \tag{7.7}$$

where $\hat{\eta}_i = 0.144\, Age_i - 1.023\, Treat_i$ is the risk score, $i = 1, 2, \ldots, 26$. This is equivalent to the accelerated failure time representation of the model, used in Example 7.1. The values of $\hat{\eta}_i$ are then arranged in ascending order and divided into three groups, as shown in Table 7.2.

Table 7.2 *Values of the risk score, with the patient number in parentheses, for three groups of ovarian cancer patients.*

Group	Risk score				
1 (low risk)	4.29 (14)	4.45 (2)	4.59 (20)	5.15 (22)	5.17 (5)
	5.17 (19)	5.31 (17)	5.59 (4)	5.59 (12)	
2 (medium risk)	5.87 (16)	6.02 (13)	6.16 (8)	6.18 (18)	6.31 (26)
	6.45 (6)	6.45 (9)	6.45 (11)	7.03 (25)	
3 (high risk)	7.04 (15)	7.04 (24)	7.17 (7)	8.19 (23)	
	8.48 (1)	9.34 (3)	9.63 (10)	9.63 (21)	

The next step is to obtain the average survivor function for each group by averaging the values of the estimated survivor function, in Equation (7.7), for the patients in the three groups. This is done for $t = 0, 1, \ldots, 1230$, and the three average survivor functions are shown in Figure 7.5. The Kaplan-Meier estimate of the survivor function for the individuals in each of the three groups shown in Table 7.2 is then calculated, and this is also shown in Figure 7.5.

From this plot, we see that the model is a good fit to the patients in the high-risk group. For those in the middle group, the agreement between the observed and fitted survivor functions is not that good, as the fitted model leads to estimates of the survivor function that are a little too high. In fact, the patients in this group have the largest values of the martingale residuals, which also indicates that the death times of these individuals are not adequately summarised by the fitted model. There is only one death among the individuals in the low-risk group, and so little can be said about the fit of the model to this set of patients.

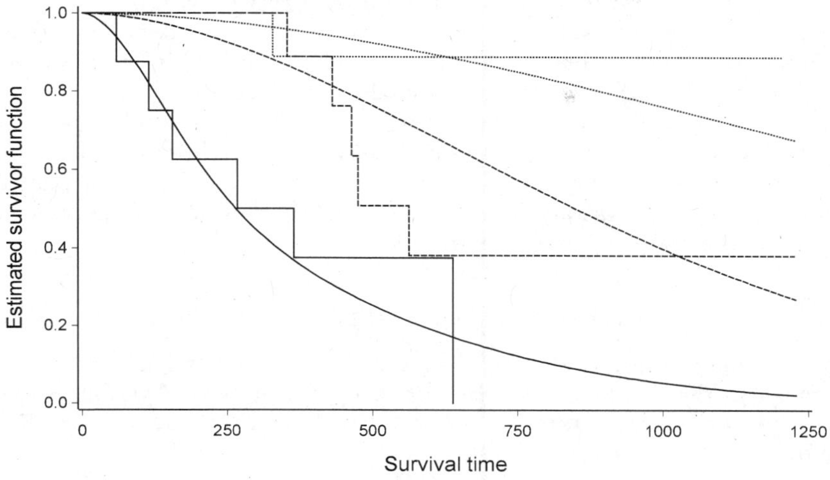

Figure 7.5 *Plot of the observed and fitted survivor functions for patients of low (⋯⋯), medium (- - -) and high (—) risk. The observed survivor function is the step-function.*

7.4 Identification of influential observations

As when fitting the Cox regression model, it will be important to identify observations that exert an undue influence on particular parameter estimates, or on the complete set of parameter estimates. These two aspects of influence are considered in turn in this section.

A number of influence diagnostics for the Weibull proportional hazards model have been proposed by Hall, Rogers and Pregibon (1982), derived from the accelerated failure time representation of the model. However, they may also be used with other parametric models. These diagnostics are computed from the estimates of all $p + 2$ parameters in the model, and their variance-covariance matrix. For convenience, the vector of $p + 2$ parameters will be denoted by $\boldsymbol{\theta}$, so that $\boldsymbol{\theta}' = (\mu, \alpha_1, \alpha_2, \ldots, \alpha_p, \sigma)$. The vector $\hat{\boldsymbol{\theta}}'$ will be used to denote the corresponding vector of estimates of the parameters.

7.4.1 Influence of observations on a parameter estimate*

An approximation to the change in the estimated value of θ_j, the jth component of the vector $\boldsymbol{\theta}$, on omitting the ith observation, $\Delta_i\hat{\theta}_j$, is the jth component of the $(p + 2) \times 1$ vector

$$\text{var}\,(\hat{\boldsymbol{\theta}})\boldsymbol{u}_i. \tag{7.8}$$

In Expression (7.8), $\text{var}\,(\hat{\boldsymbol{\theta}})$ is the estimated variance-covariance matrix of the parameters in $\boldsymbol{\theta}$, and $\boldsymbol{u}_i$ is the $(p + 2) \times 1$ vector of values of the first partial derivatives of the log-likelihood for the ith observation, with respect to the $p+2$ parameters in $\boldsymbol{\theta}$, evaluated at $\hat{\boldsymbol{\theta}}$. The vector $\boldsymbol{u}_i$ is therefore the vector of values of the score residuals for the ith observation, defined in Section 7.1.5.

The quantities $\Delta_i\hat{\alpha}_j$ are components 2 to $p-1$ of the vector in Expression (7.8), which we will continue to refer to as delta-betas rather than as delta-alphas. These values may be standardised through division by the standard error of $\hat{\alpha}_j$, leading to standardised delta-betas. Index plots or plots of the standardised or unstandardised values of $\Delta_i\hat{\alpha}_j$ provide informative summaries of this aspect of influence.

7.4.2 Influence of observations on the set of parameter estimates*

Two summary measures of the influence of the ith observation on the set of parameters that make up the vector $\boldsymbol{\theta}$ have been proposed by Hall, Rogers and Pregibon (1982). These are the statistics F_i and C_i. The quantity F_i is given by

$$F_i = \frac{\boldsymbol{u}_i'\boldsymbol{R}^{-1}\boldsymbol{u}_i}{(p+2)\{1-\boldsymbol{u}_i'\boldsymbol{R}^{-1}\boldsymbol{u}_i\}}, \tag{7.9}$$

where the $(p+2)\times(p+2)$ matrix $\boldsymbol{R}$ is the cross-product matrix of score residuals, that is, $\boldsymbol{R}=\sum_{i=1}^{n}\boldsymbol{u}_i\boldsymbol{u}_i'$. Equivalently, $\boldsymbol{R}=\boldsymbol{U}'\boldsymbol{U}$, where $\boldsymbol{U}$ is the $n\times(p+2)$ matrix whose ith row is the transpose of the vector of score residuals, $\boldsymbol{u}_i'$. An alternative measure of the influence of the ith observation on the set of parameter estimates is the statistic

$$C_i = \frac{\boldsymbol{u}_i'\operatorname{var}(\hat{\boldsymbol{\theta}})\boldsymbol{u}_i}{\{1-\boldsymbol{u}_i'\operatorname{var}(\hat{\boldsymbol{\theta}})\boldsymbol{u}_i\}^2}. \tag{7.10}$$

The statistics F_i and C_i will typically have values that are quite different from each other. However, in each case a relatively large value of the statistic will indicate that the corresponding observation is influential. Exactly how such observations influence the estimates would need to be investigated by omitting that observation from the data set and refitting the model.

Example 7.3 Chemotherapy in ovarian cancer patients
We now go on to investigate whether there are any influential observations in the data on the survival times following chemotherapy treatment for ovarian cancer. The unstandardised delta-betas for *Age* and *Treat*, plotted against the rank order of the survival times, are shown in Figures 7.6 and 7.7.

In Figure 7.6, two observations have relatively large values of the delta-beta for *Age*. These occur for patients 4 and 5 in the original data set. Both women have short survival times, and in addition one is relatively old at 74 years and the other relatively young at 43 years. The delta-betas for *Treat* displayed in Figure 7.7 show no unusual features.

We next investigate the influence of each observation on the set of parameter estimates. The values of F_i and C_i, defined in Equations (7.9) and (7.10),

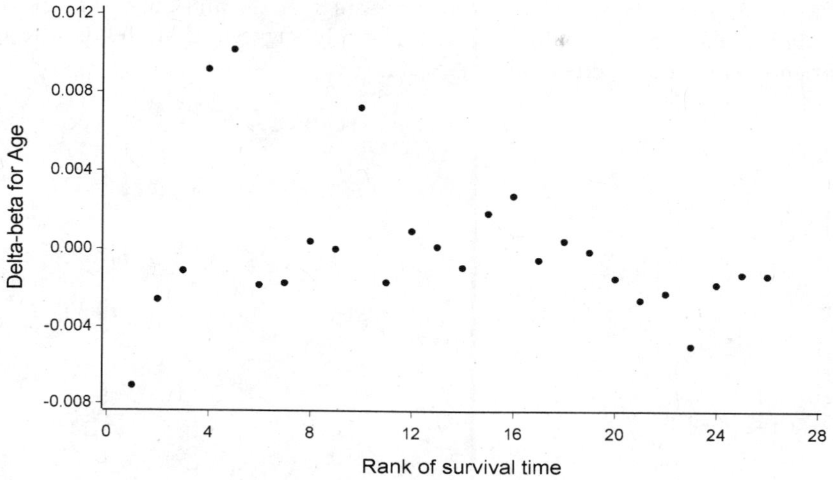

Figure 7.6 *Plot of the delta-betas for Age against rank order of survival time.*

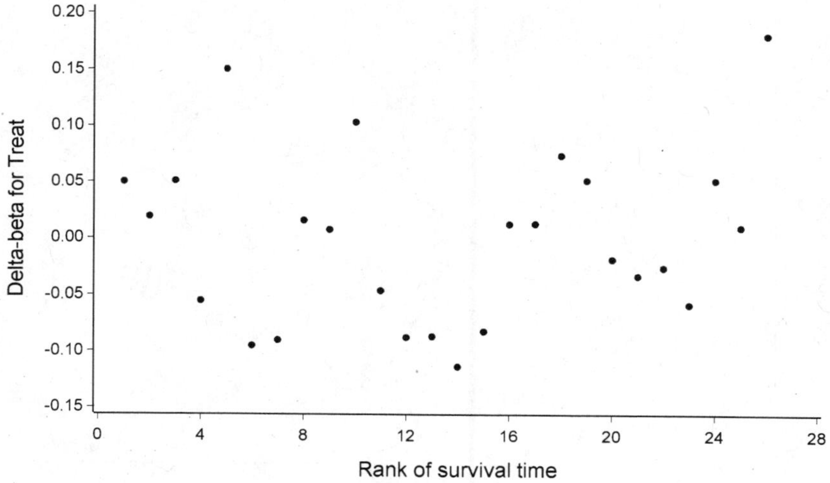

Figure 7.7 *Plot of the delta-betas for Treat against rank order of survival time.*

are plotted against the rank order of the survival times in Figures 7.8 and 7.9. Figure 7.8 clearly shows that the observation corresponding to patient 5 is influential, and that the influence of patients 1, 4, 14 and 26 should be investigated in greater detail. Figure 7.9 strongly suggests that the data from patients 5 and 26 is influential.

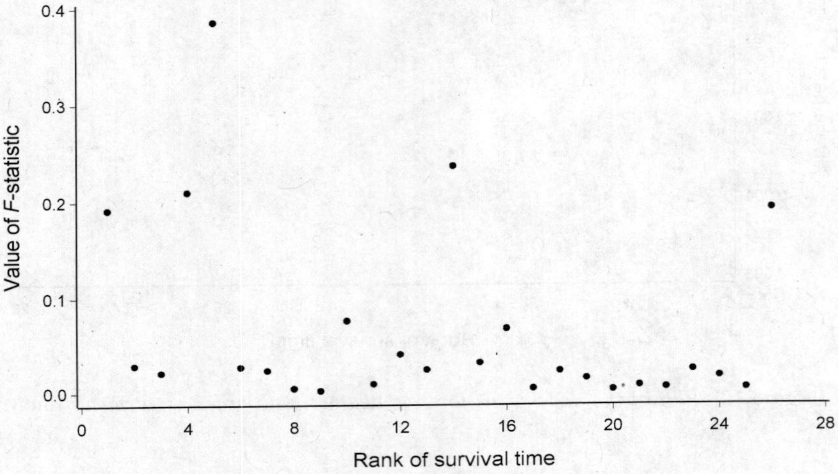

Figure 7.8 *Plot of the F-statistic against rank order of survival time.*

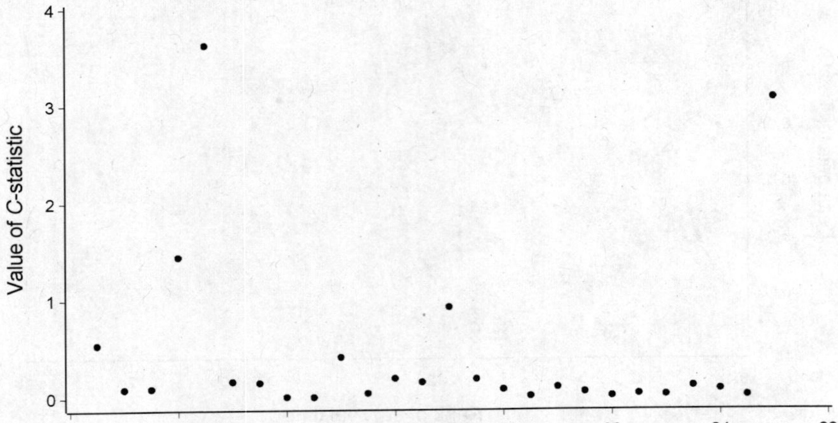

Figure 7.9 *Plot of the C-statistic against rank order of survival time.*

The linear component of the fitted hazard function in the model fitted to all 26 patients is

$$0.144\, Age_i - 1.023\, Treat_i,$$

while that on omitting each of observations 1, 4, 5, 14 and 26 in turn is as follows:

Omitting patient number 1:	$0.142\, Age_i - 1.016\, Treat_i$
Omitting patient number 4:	$0.175\, Age_i - 1.190\, Treat_i$
Omitting patient number 5:	$0.177\, Age_i - 0.710\, Treat_i$
Omitting patient number 14:	$0.149\, Age_i - 1.318\, Treat_i$
Omitting patient number 26:	$0.159\, Age_i - 0.697\, Treat_i$

These results show that the effect of omitting the data from patient 1 on the parameter estimates is small. When the data from patient 4 are omitted, the estimated coefficient of *Age* is most affected, whereas when the data from patient 14 are omitted, the coefficient of *Treat* is changed the most. On leaving out the data from patients 5 and 26, both estimates are considerably affected.

The hazard ratio for a patient on the combined treatment (*Treat* = 2), relative to one on the single treatment (*Treat* = 1), is estimated by $e^{-1.023} = 0.36$, when the model is fitted to all 26 patients. When the observations from patients 1, 4, 5, 14 and 26 are omitted in turn, the estimated age-adjusted hazard ratios are 0.36, 0.30, 0.49, 0.27 and 0.50, respectively. The data from patients 5 and 26 clearly have the greatest effect on the estimated hazard ratio; in each case the estimate is increased, and the magnitude of the treatment effect is diminished. Omission of the data from patients 4 or 14 decreases the estimated hazard ratio, thereby increasing the estimated treatment difference.

7.5 Testing proportional hazards in the Weibull model

The Weibull model is most commonly used as a parametric proportional hazards model, and so it will be important to test that the proportional hazards assumption is tenable. In Section 4.4.3 of Chapter 4, it was shown how a time-dependent variable can be used in testing proportionality of hazards in the Cox regression model. Parametric models containing time-dependent variables are more complicated, and because software for fitting such models is not widely available, further details on this approach will not be given here.

In the Weibull model, the assumption of proportional hazards across a number of groups, g, say, corresponds to the assumption that the shape parameter γ in the baseline hazard function is the same in each group. One way of testing this assumption is to fit a separate Weibull model to each of the g groups, where the linear component of the model is the same in each case. The models fitted to the data from each group will then have different shape parameters as well as different scale parameters. The values of the statistic $-2\log\hat{L}$ for each of these g separate models are then summed to give a value of $-2\log\hat{L}$ for a model that has different shape parameter for each group. Denote this by $-2\log\hat{L}_1$. We then combine the g sets of data and fit a Weibull proportional hazards model that includes the factor associated with the group effects and interactions between this factor and other terms in the model. This model then corresponds to there being a common shape parameter for each group. The inclusion of group effects in the model leads to there being different scale parameters for each group. The value of $-2\log\hat{L}$ for this model, $-2\log\hat{L}_0$, say, is then compared with $-2\log\hat{L}_1$. The difference between the values of these two statistics is the change in $-2\log\hat{L}$ due to constraining the Weibull shape parameters to be equal, and can be compared with a chi-squared distribution on $g-1$ degrees of freedom. If the difference is not significant, the assumption of proportional hazards is justified.

Example 7.4 Chemotherapy in ovarian cancer patients
Data from the study of survival following treatment for ovarian cancer, given in Example 5.10 of Chapter 5, are now used to illustrate the procedure for testing the assumption that the Weibull shape parameter is the same for the patients in each of the two treatment groups. The first step is to fit a Weibull proportional hazards model that contains *Age* alone to the data from the women in each treatment group. When such a model is fitted to the data from those on the single chemotherapy treatment, the value of the statistic $-2\log\hat{L}$ is 22.851, while that for the women on the combined treatment is 16.757. The sum of the two values of $-2\log\hat{L}$ is 39.608, which is the value of the statistic for a Weibull model with different shape parameters for the two treatment groups, and different coefficients of *Age* for each group. For the model with different age effects for each treatment group, a treatment effect, and common shape parameter, the value of $-2\log\hat{L}$ is 39.708. The change in $-2\log\hat{L}$ on constraining the shape parameters to be equal is therefore 0.10, which is not significant when compared with a chi-squared distribution on one degree of freedom. The two shape parameters may therefore be taken to be equal.

Some alternatives to the proportional hazards model are described in Chapter 6, and further comments on how to deal with situations in which the hazards are not proportional are given in Chapter 11.

7.6 Further reading

There have been relatively few publications on model checking in parametric survival models, compared to the literature on model checking in the Cox regression model. Residuals and influence measures for the Weibull proportional hazards model are described by Hall, Rogers and Pregibon (1982). Hollander and Proschan (1979) show how to assess whether a sample of censored observations is drawn from a particular probability distribution. Weissfeld and Schneider (1994) describe and illustrate a number of residuals that can be used in conjunction with parametric models for survival data. Cohen and Barnett (1995) describe how the interpretation of cumulative hazard plots of residuals can be helped by the use of simulated envelopes for the plots. Influence diagnostics for use in parametric survival modelling are given by Weissfeld and Schneider (1990) and Escobar and Meeker (1992). A SAS macro for evaluating influence diagnostics for the Weibull proportional hazards model is described by Escobar and Meeker (1988). These papers involve arguments based on local influence, a topic that is explored in general terms by Cook (1986), and reviewed in Rancel and Sierra (2001). A method for testing the assumptions of proportional hazards and accelerated failure times against a general model for the hazard function is presented by Ciampi and Etezadi-Amoli (1985). An interesting application of parametric modelling, based on data on times to reoffending by prisoners released on parole, which incorporates elements of model checking, is given by Copas and Heydari (1997).

Chapter 8

Time-dependent variables

When explanatory variables are incorporated in a model for survival data, the values taken by such variables are those recorded at the time origin of the study. For example, consider the study to compare two treatments for prostatic cancer first described in Example 1.4 of Chapter 1. Here, the age of a patient, serum haemoglobin level, size of the tumour, value of the Gleason index, and of course the treatment group, were all recorded at the time when a patient was entered into the study. The impact of these variables on the hazard of death is then evaluated.

In many studies that generate survival data, individuals are monitored for the duration of the study. During this period, the values of certain explanatory variables may be recorded on a regular basis. Thus, in the example on prostatic cancer, the size of the tumour and other variables, may be recorded at frequent intervals. If account can be taken of the values of explanatory variables as they evolve, a more satisfactory model for the hazard of death at any given time would be obtained. For example, in connection with the prostatic cancer study, more recent values of the size of the tumour may provide a better indication of future life expectancy than the value at the time origin.

Variables whose values change over time are known as *time-dependent variables*, and in this chapter we see how such variables can be incorporated in models used in the analysis of survival data.

8.1 Types of time-dependent variables

It is useful to consider two types of variables that change over time, which may be referred to as *internal variables* and *external variables*.

Internal variables relate to a particular individual in a study, and can only be measured while a patient is alive. Such data arises when repeated measurements of certain characteristics are made on a patient over time, and examples include measures of lung function such as vital capacity and peak flow rate, white blood cell count, systolic blood pressure and serum cholesterol level. Variables that describe changes in the status of a patient are also of this type. For example, following a bone marrow transplant, a patient may be susceptible to the development of graft versus host disease. A binary explanatory variable, that reflects whether the patient is suffering from this life-threatening side effect at any given time, is a further example of an internal variable. In each case, such variables reflect the condition of the patient and their values may well be associated with the survival time of the patient.

On the other hand, external variables are time-dependent variables that do not necessarily require the survival of a patient for their existence. One type of external variable is a variable that changes in such a way that its value will be known in advance at any future time. The most obvious example is the age of a patient, in that once the age at the time origin is known, that patient's age at any future time will be known exactly. However, there are other examples, such as the dose of a drug that is to be varied in a predetermined manner during the course of a study, or planned changes to the type of immunosuppressant to be used following organ transplantation. Another type of external variable is one that exists totally independently of any particular individual, such as the level of atmospheric sulphur dioxide, or air temperature. Changes in the values of such quantities may well have an effect on the lifetime of individuals, as in studies concerning the management of patients with certain types of respiratory disease.

Time-dependent variables also arise in situations where the coefficient of a time-constant explanatory variable is a function of time. In Section 3.9 of Chapter 3, it was explained that the coefficient of an explanatory variable in the Cox proportional hazards model is a log-hazard ratio, and so under this model, the hazard ratio is constant over time. If this ratio were in fact a function of time, then the coefficient of the explanatory variable that varies with time is referred to as a *time-varying coefficient*. In this case, the log-hazard ratio is not constant and so we no longer have a proportional hazards model. More formally, suppose that the coefficient of an explanatory variable, X, is a linear function of time, t, so that we may write the term as $\beta t X$. This means that the corresponding log-hazard ratio is a linear function of time. This was precisely the sort of term introduced into the model in order to test the assumption of proportional hazards in Section 4.4.3 of Chapter 4. This term can also be written as $\beta X(t)$, where $X(t) = Xt$ is a time-dependent variable. In general, suppose that a model includes the explanatory variable, X, with a time-varying coefficient of the form $\beta(t)$. The corresponding term in the model would be $\beta(t)X$, which can be expressed as $\beta X(t)$. In other words, a term that involves a time-varying coefficient can be expressed as a time-dependent variable with a constant coefficient. However, if $\beta(t)$ is a non-linear function of one or more unknown parameters, for example $\beta_0 \exp(\beta_1 t)$, the term is not so easily fitted in a model.

All these different types of time-dependent variables can be introduced into the Cox regression model, in the manner described in the following section.

8.2 A model with time-dependent variables

According to the Cox proportional hazards model described in Chapter 3, the hazard of death at time t for the ith of n individuals in a study can be written in the form

$$h_i(t) = \exp\left\{\sum_{j=1}^{p} \beta_j x_{ji}\right\} h_0(t),$$

where x_{ji} is the baseline value of the jth explanatory variable, X_j, $j = 1, 2, \ldots$, p, for the ith individual, $i = 1, 2, \ldots, n$, and $h_0(t)$ is the baseline hazard function. Generalising this model to the situation in which some or all of the explanatory variables are time-dependent, we write $x_{ji}(t)$ for the value of the jth explanatory variable at time t, in the ith individual. The Cox regression model then becomes

$$h_i(t) = \exp\left\{\sum_{j=1}^{p} \beta_j x_{ji}(t)\right\} h_0(t). \tag{8.1}$$

In this model, the baseline hazard function, $h_0(t)$, is interpreted as the hazard function for an individual for whom all the variables are zero at the time origin, and remain at this same value through time.

Since the values of the variables $x_{ji}(t)$ in the model given in Equation (8.1) depend on the time t, the relative hazard $h_i(t)/h_0(t)$ is also time-dependent. This means that the hazard of death at time t is no longer proportional to the baseline hazard, and the model is no longer a proportional hazards model.

To provide an interpretation of the β-parameters in this model, consider the ratio of the hazard functions at time t for two individuals, the rth and sth, say. This is given by

$$\frac{h_r(t)}{h_s(t)} = \exp\left[\beta_1\{x_{r1}(t) - x_{s1}(t)\} + \cdots + \beta_p\{x_{rp}(t) - x_{sp}(t)\}\right].$$

The coefficient β_j, $j = 1, 2, \ldots, p$, can therefore be interpreted as the log-hazard ratio for two individuals whose value of the jth explanatory variable at a given time t differ by one unit, with the two individuals having the same values of all the other $p - 1$ variables at that time.

8.2.1 Fitting the Cox model*

When the Cox regression model is extended to incorporate time-dependent variables, the partial log-likelihood function, from Equation (3.6) in Chapter 3, can be generalised to

$$\sum_{i=1}^{n} \delta_i \left\{\sum_{j=1}^{p} \beta_j x_{ji}(t_i) - \log \sum_{l \in R(t_i)} \exp\left(\sum_{j=1}^{p} \beta_j x_{jl}(t_i)\right)\right\}, \tag{8.2}$$

in which $R(t_i)$ is the risk set at time t_i, the death time of the ith individual in the study, $i = 1, 2, \ldots, n$, and δ_i is an event indicator that is zero if the survival time of the ith individual is censored and unity otherwise. This expression can then be maximised to give estimates of the β-parameters.

In order to use Equation (8.1) in this maximisation process, the values of each of the variables in the model must be known at each death time for all individuals in the risk set at time t_i. This is no problem for external variables whose values are preordained, but it may be a problem for external variables that exist independently of the individuals in a study, and certainly for internal variables.

To illustrate the problem, consider a trial of two maintenance therapies for patients who have suffered a myocardial infarct. The serum cholesterol level of such patients may well be measured at the time when a patient is admitted to the study, and at regular intervals of time thereafter. This variable is then a time-dependent variable, and will be denoted $X(t)$. It is then plausible that the hazard of death for any particular patient, the ith, say, at time t, $h_i(t)$, is more likely to be influenced by the value of the explanatory variable $X(t)$ at time t, than its value at the time origin, where $t = 0$.

Now suppose that the ith individual dies at time t_i and that there are two other individuals, labelled r and s, in the risk set at time t_i. We further suppose that individual r dies at time t_r, where $t_r > t_i$, and that the survival time of individual s, t_s, is censored at some time after t_r. The situation is illustrated graphically in Figure 8.1. In this figure, the vertical dotted lines refer to points in patient time when the value of $X(t)$ is measured.

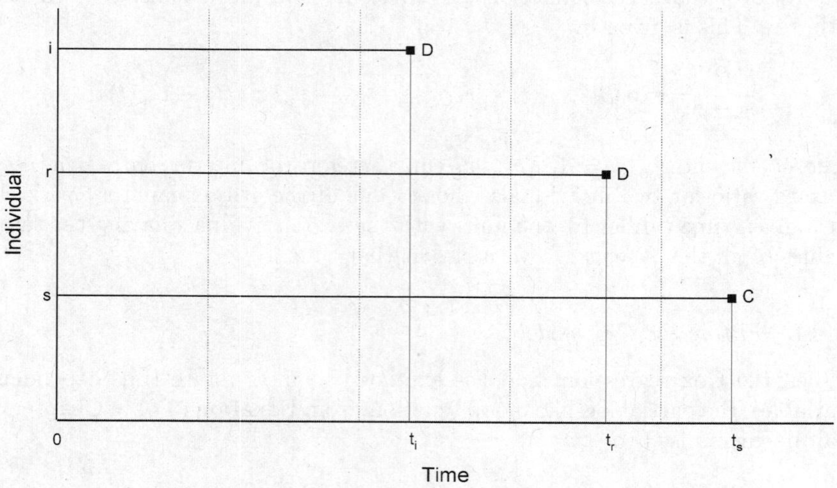

Figure 8.1 *Survival times of three patients in patient time.*

If individuals r and s are the only two in the risk set at time t_i, and X is the only explanatory variable that is measured, the contribution of the ith individual to the log-likelihood function in Expression (8.2) will be

$$\beta x_i(t_i) - \log \sum_l \exp\{\beta x_l(t_i)\},$$

where $x_i(t_i)$ is the value of $X(t)$ for the ith individual at their death time, t_i, and l in the summation takes the values i, r, and s. This expression is therefore equal to

$$\beta x_i(t_i) - \log \left\{ e^{\beta x_i(t_i)} + e^{\beta x_r(t_i)} + e^{\beta x_s(t_i)} \right\}.$$

This shows that the value of the time-dependent variable $X(t)$ is needed at the death time of the ith individual, and at time t_i for individuals r and s. In addition, the value of the variable $X(t)$ will be needed for individuals r and s at t_r, the death time of individual r.

For terms in a model that are explicit functions of time, such as interactions between time and a variable or factor measured at baseline, there is no difficulty in obtaining the values of the time-dependent variables at any time for any individual. Indeed, it is usually straightforward to incorporate such variables in the Cox model when using statistical software that has facilities for dealing with time-dependent variables. For other variables, such as serum cholesterol level, the values of the time-dependent variable at times other than that at which it was measured has to be approximated. There are then several possibilities.

One option is to use the last recorded value of the variable before the time at which the value of the variable is needed. When the variable has been recorded for an individual before and after the time when the value is required, the value closest to that time might be used. Another possibility is to use linear interpolation between consecutive values of the variable. Figure 8.2 illustrates these approximations.

In this figure, the continuous curve depicts the actual value of a time-dependent variable at any time, and the dotted vertical lines signify times when the variable is actually measured. If the value of the variable is required at time t in this figure, we could use either the value at P, the last recorded value of the variable, the value at R, the value closest to t, or the value at Q, the linearly interpolated value between P and R.

Linear interpolation is clearly not an option when a time-dependent variable is a categorical variable. In addition, some categorical variables may be such that individuals can only progress through the levels of the variable in a particular direction. For example, the performance status of an individual may only be expected to deteriorate, so that the value of this categorical variable might only change from 'good' to 'fair' and from 'fair' to 'poor'. As another example, following a biopsy, a variable associated with the occurrence of a tumour will take one of two values, corresponding to absence and presence. It might then be very unlikely for the status to change from 'present' to 'absent' in consecutive biopsies.

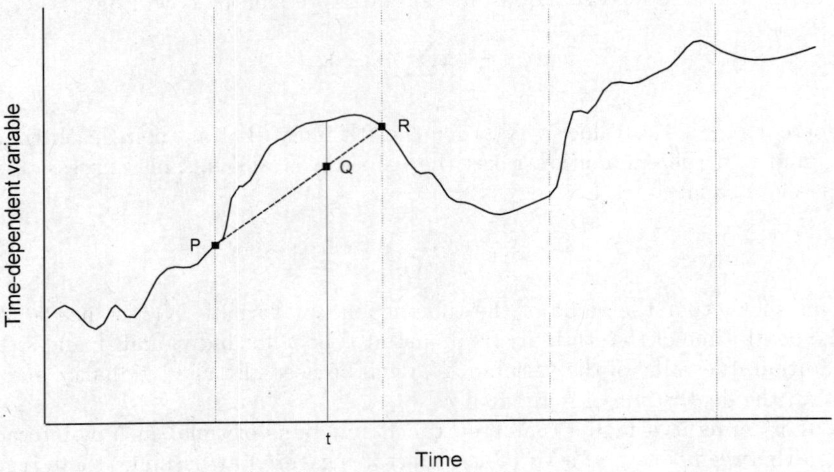

Figure 8.2 *Computation of the value of a time-dependent variable at intermediate times.*

Anomalous changes in the values of time-dependent variables can be detected by plotting the values of the variable against time for each patient. This may then lead on to a certain amount of data editing. For example, consider the plot in Figure 8.3, which shows the biopsy result, absent or present, for a particular patient at a number of time points. In this diagram, at least one of the observations made at times t_A and t_B must be incorrect. The observation at t_A might then be changed to 'absent' or that at t_B to 'present'.

If inferences of interest turn out to be sensitive to the method of interpolation used, extreme caution must be exercised when interpreting the results. Indeed, this feature could indicate that the value of the time-dependent variable is subject to measurement error, substantial inherent variation or perhaps the values have not been recorded sufficiently regularly.

8.2.2 Estimation of baseline hazard and survivor functions*

After a Cox regression model that includes time-dependent variables has been fitted, the baseline hazard function, $h_0(t)$ and the corresponding baseline survivor function, $S_0(t)$, can be estimated. This involves an adaptation of the results given in Section 3.10 of Chapter 3 to cope with the additional complication of time-dependent variables, in which the values of the explanatory variables need to be updated with their time-specific values. In particular, the Nelson-Aalen estimate of the baseline cumulative hazard function, given in

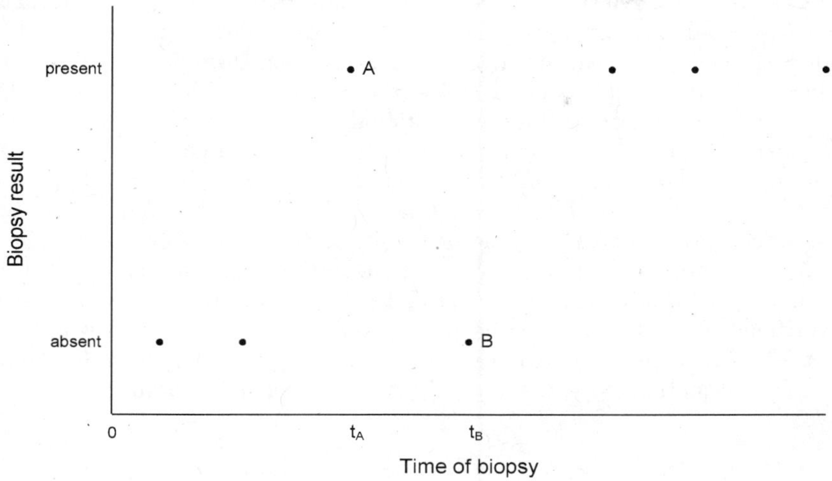

Figure 8.3 *Values of a time-dependent categorical variable.*

Equation (3.28), becomes

$$\tilde{H}_0(t) = -\log \tilde{S}_0(t) = \sum_{j=1}^{k} \frac{d_j}{\sum_{l \in R(t_{(j)})} \exp\{\hat{\boldsymbol{\beta}}' \boldsymbol{x}_l(t)\}}, \tag{8.3}$$

for $t_{(k)} \leqslant t < t_{(k+1)}$, $k = 1, 2, \ldots, r-1$, where $\boldsymbol{x}_l(t)$ is the vector of values of the explanatory variables for the lth individual at time t, and d_j is the number of events at the jth ordered event time, $t_{(j)}$, $j = 1, 2, \ldots, r$. Similar modifications can be made to the other results in Section 3.10. With this modification, computation of the summation over the risk set is much more complicated, since for every event time, $t_{(j)}$, $j = 1, 2, \ldots, r$, the value of each time-dependent variable, for all individuals in the risk set, is needed at that event time.

Having obtained an estimate of the cumulative hazard function, the corresponding baseline hazard function can be estimated using Equation (3.30), and an estimate of the baseline survivor function is $\tilde{S}_0(t) = \exp\{-\tilde{H}_0(t)\}$.

The survivor function for a particular individual is much more difficult to estimate. This is because the result that $S_i(t)$ can be expressed as a power of the baseline survivor function, $S_0(t)$, given in Equation (3.25) of Chapter 3, no longer holds. Instead, the survivor function for the ith individual is obtained from the integrated hazard function, which, from Equation (1.7) in Chapter 1, is given by

$$S_i(t) = \exp\left\{-\int_0^t \exp\left(\sum_{j=1}^{p} \beta_j x_{ji}(u)\right) h_0(u)\,\mathrm{d}u\right\}. \tag{8.4}$$

This survivor function therefore depends not only on the baseline hazard function $h_0(t)$, but also on the values of the time-dependent variables over the interval from 0 to t. The survivor function may therefore depend on future values of the time-dependent variables in the model, which will generally be unknown. However, approximate conditional probabilities of surviving a certain time interval can be found from the probability that an individual survives over an interval of time, from t to $t+h$, say, conditional on being alive at time t. This probability is $\mathrm{P}(T_i \geqslant t+h \mid T_i \geqslant t)$, where T_i is the random variable associated with the survival time of the ith individual. Using the standard result for conditional probability, given in Section 3.3.1 of Chapter 3, this probability becomes $\mathrm{P}(T_i \geqslant t+h)/\mathrm{P}(T_i \geqslant t)$, which is the ratio of the survivor functions at times $t+h$ and t, that is, $S_i(t+h)/S_i(t)$. We now assume that any time-dependent variable remains constant through this interval, so that from Equation (8.4), the approximate conditional probability is

$$\begin{aligned} P_i(t, t+h) &= \frac{\exp\left\{-\exp\left(\sum_{j=1}^{p} \beta_j x_{ji}(t)\right) \int_0^{t+h} h_0(u)\,\mathrm{d}u\right\}}{\exp\left\{-\exp\left(\sum_{j=1}^{p} \beta_j x_{ji}(t)\right) \int_0^{t} h_0(u)\,\mathrm{d}u\right\}}, \\ &= \exp\left[-\{H_0(t+h) - H_0(t)\}\exp\left(\sum_{j=1}^{p} \beta_j x_{ji}(t)\right)\right], \end{aligned}$$

where $H_0(t)$ is the baseline cumulative hazard function. An estimate of this approximate conditional probability of surviving through the interval $(t, t+h)$ is then

$$\tilde{P}_i(t,\, t+h) = \exp\left[-\left\{\tilde{H}_0(t+h) - \tilde{H}_0(t)\right\}\exp\left(\sum_{j=1}^{p} \hat{\beta}_j x_{ji}(t)\right)\right], \qquad (8.5)$$

where $\tilde{H}_0(t)$ is the estimated baseline cumulative hazard function obtained on fitting the Cox regression model with p possibly time-dependent variables with values $x_{ji}(t)$, $j = 1, 2, \ldots, p$, for the ith individual, $i = 1, 2, \ldots, n$, and $\hat{\beta}_j$ is the estimated coefficient of the jth time-dependent variable. This result was given by Altman and De Stavola (1994).

Corresponding estimates of the conditional probability of an event in the interval $(t, t+h)$ are $1 - \tilde{P}_i(t, t+h)$, and these quantities can be used to obtain an estimate of the expected number of events in each of a number of successive intervals of width h. Comparing these values with the observed number of events in these intervals leads to an informal assessment of model adequacy.

8.3 Model comparison and validation

Models for survival data that include time-dependent variables can be compared in the same manner as Cox proportional hazards models, using the procedure described in Section 3.5 of Chapter 3. In particular, the model-fitting process leads to a maximised partial likelihood function, from which the value of the statistic $-2\log\hat{L}$ can be obtained. Changes in the value of this statistic between alternative nested models may then be compared to percentage points of the chi-squared distribution, with degrees of freedom equal to the difference in the number of β-parameters being fitted. For this reason, the model-building strategies discussed in Chapter 3 apply equally in situations where there are time-dependent variables.

8.3.1 *Comparison of treatments*

In order to examine the magnitude of a treatment effect after taking account of variables that change over time, the value of $-2\log\hat{L}$ for a model that contains the time-dependent variables and any other prognostic factors is compared with that for the model that contains the treatment term, in addition to these other variables. But in this analysis, if no treatment effect is revealed, one explanation could be that the time-dependent variable has *masked* the treatment difference.

To fix ideas, consider the example of a study to compare two cytotoxic drugs in the treatment of patients with leukaemia. Here, a patient's survival time may well depend on subsequent values of that patient's white blood cell count. If the effect of the treatment is to increase white blood cell count, no treatment difference will be identified after including white blood cell count as a time-dependent variable in the model. On the other hand, the treatment effect may appear in the absence of this variable. An interpretation of this is that the time-dependent variable has accounted for the treatment difference, and so provides an explanation as to how the treatment has been effective.

In any event, much useful information will be gained from a comparison of the results of an analysis that incorporates time-dependent variables with an analysis that uses baseline values alone.

8.3.2 *Assessing model adequacy*

After fitting a model that includes time-dependent variables, a number of the techniques for evaluating the adequacy of the model, described in Chapter 4, can be implemented. In particular, an overall martingale residual can be computed for each subject, from an adaptation of the result in Equation (4.6). The martingale residual for the ith subject is now

$$r_{Mi} = \delta_i - \exp\{\hat{\boldsymbol{\beta}}'\boldsymbol{x}_i(t_i)\}\tilde{H}_0(t_i),$$

where $\boldsymbol{x}_i(t_i)$ is the vector of values of explanatory variables for the ith individual, which may be time-dependent, evaluated at t_i, the event time of that individual. Also, $\hat{\boldsymbol{\beta}}$ is the vector of coefficients, δ_i is the event indicator that takes the value unity if t_i is an event and zero otherwise, and $\tilde{H}_0(t_i)$ is the estimated baseline cumulative hazard function at t_i, obtained from Equation (8.3). The deviance residuals may also be computed from the martingale residuals, using Equation (4.7) of Chapter 4.

The plots described in Section 4.2.2 of Chapter 4 will often be helpful. In particular, an index plot of the martingale residuals will enable outlying observations to be identified. However, diagnostic plots for assessing the functional form of covariates, described in Section 4.2.3, turn out to be not so useful when a time-dependent variable is being studied. This is because there will then be a number of values of the time-dependent covariate for any one individual, and it is not clear what the martingale residuals for the null model should be plotted against.

For detecting influential values, the delta-betas, introduced in Section 4.3.1 of Chapter 4, provide a helpful means of investigating the effect of each observation on individual parameter estimates. Changes in the value of the $-2 \log \hat{L}$ statistic, on omitting each observation in turn, can give valuable information about the effect of each observation on the set of parameter estimates.

8.4 Some applications of time-dependent variables

One application of time-dependent variables is in connection with evaluating the assumption of proportional hazards. This was discussed in detail in Section 4.4.3 of Chapter 4. In this application, a variable formed from the product of an explanatory variable, X, and time, t, is added to the linear part of the Cox model, and the null hypothesis that the coefficient of Xt is zero is tested. If this estimated coefficient is found to be significantly different from zero, there is evidence that the assumption of proportional hazards is not valid.

In many circumstances, the waiting time from the occurrence of some catastrophic event until a patient receives treatment may be strongly associated with the patient's survival. For example, in a study of factors affecting the survival of patients who have had a myocardial infarct, the time from the infarct to when the patient arrives in hospital may be crucial. Some patients may die before receiving treatment, while those who arrive at the hospital soon after their infarct will tend to have a more favourable prognosis than those for whom treatment is delayed. It will be important to take account of this aspect of the data when assessing the effects of other explanatory variables on the survival times of these patients.

In a similar example, Crowley and Hu (1977) show how a time-dependent variable can be used in organ transplantation studies. Here, one feature of interest is the effect of a transplant on the patient's survival time. Suppose that in a study on the effectiveness of a particular type of organ transplant, a patient is judged to be suitable for a transplant at some time t_0. They then wait some period of time until a suitable donor organ is found, and if the patient survives this period, they receive a transplant at time t_1.

In studies of this type, the survival times of patients who have received a transplant cannot be compared with those who have not had a transplant in the usual way. The reason for this is that in order to receive a transplant, a patient must survive the waiting time to transplant. Consequently, the group who survive to the time of transplant is not directly comparable with the group who receive no such transplant. Similarly, it is not possible to compare the times that the patients who receive a transplant survive after the transplant with the survival times of the group not receiving a transplant. Here, the time origin would be different for the two groups, and so they are not comparable at the time origin. This means that it is not possible to identify a time origin from which standard methods for survival analysis can be used.

The solution to this problem is to introduce a time-dependent variable $X_1(t)$, which takes the value zero if a patient has not received a transplant at time t, and unity otherwise. Adopting a Cox regression model, the hazard of death for the ith individual at time t is then

$$h_i(t) = \exp\{\eta_i + \beta_1 x_{1i}(t)\}h_0(t),$$

where η_i is a linear combination of the explanatory variables that are not time-dependent, whose values have been recorded at the time origin for the ith individual, and $x_{1i}(t)$ is the value of X_1 for that individual at time t.

Under this model, the hazard function is $\exp(\eta_i)h_0(t)$ for patients who do not receive a transplant before time t, and $\exp\{\eta_i + \beta_1\}h_0(t)$ thereafter. The effect of a transplant on the patient's survival experience is then reflected in β_1. In particular, for two patients who have the same values of other explanatory variables in a model, e^{β_1} is the hazard of death at time t for the patient who receives a transplant before time t, relative to the hazard at that time for the patient who does not. Values of $-2\log\hat{L}$ can be compared after fitting the models with and without the time-dependent variable X_1. A significant difference in these values means that the transplant has an effect on survival.

In a refinement to this model, Cox and Oakes (1984) suggested that the term $\beta_1 x_{1i}(t)$ be replaced by $\beta_1 + \beta_2 \exp\{-\beta_3(t - t_1)\}$ for patients receiving a transplant at time t_1. In this model, the effect of the transplant is to increase the hazard to some value $\exp(\eta_i + \beta_1 + \beta_2)h_0(t)$ immediately after the transplant, when $t = t_1$, and to then decrease exponentially to $\exp(\eta_i + \beta_1)h_0(t)$, which is less than the initial hazard $\exp(\eta_i)h_0(t)$ if $\beta_1 < 0$. See Figure 8.4, which shows graphically the behaviour of the hazard ratio, $h_i(t)/h_0(t)$, for a transplant patient for whom η_i is the linear component of the model. Although this is an attractive model, it does have the disadvantage that specialist software is required to fit it.

In situations where a particular explanatory variable is changing rapidly, new variables that reflect such changes may be defined. The dependence of the hazard on the values of such variables can then be explored. For example, in an oncological study, the percentage increase in the size of a tumour over a period of time might be a more suitable prognostic variable than either the size of the tumour at the time origin, or the time-dependent version of that variable. If this route is followed, the computational burden of fitting time-dependent variables can be avoided.

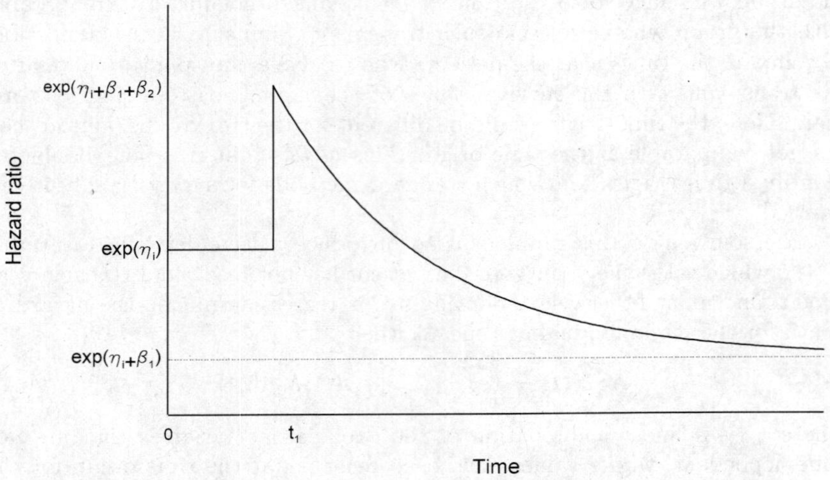

Figure 8.4 *The hazard ratio* $\exp\{\eta_i + \beta_1 + \beta_2 e^{-\beta_3(t-t_1)}\}$, $t > t_1$, *for individual i who receives a transplant at* t_1.

8.5 Three examples

In this section, three examples of survival analyses that involve time-dependent variables are given. In the first, data from a study concerning the use of bone marrow transplantation in the treatment of leukaemia is used to illustrate how a variable that is associated with the state of a patient, and whose value changes over the follow-up period, can be included in a model. In the second example, data from Example 5.10 of Chapter 5 on the comparison of two chemotherapy treatments for ovarian cancer are analysed to explore whether there is an interaction between age and survival time. The third example is designed to illustrate how information on a time-varying explanatory variate recorded during the follow-up period can be incorporated in a model for survival times. Studies in which the values of certain explanatory variables are recorded regularly throughout the follow-up period of each patient generate large sets of data. For this reason, artificial data from a small number of individuals will be used in Example 8.3 to illustrate the methodology.

Example 8.1 Bone marrow transplantation in the treatment of leukaemia
Patients suffering from acute forms of leukaemia often receive a bone marrow transplant. This provides the recipient with a new set of parent blood-forming cells, known as stem cells, which in turn produce a supply of healthy red and white blood cells. Klein and Moeschberger (2005) describe a multicentre study of factors that affect the prognosis for leukaemia patients treated in this manner. This study involved patients suffering from acute lymphoblastic leukaemia (ALL) and acute myelocytic leukaemia (AML), with those suffering

from AML being further divided into low-risk and high-risk, according to their status at the time of transplantation. The survival time from the date of the transfusion is available for each patient, together with the values of a number of explanatory variables concerning the characteristics of the donor and recipient, and adverse events that occurred during the recovery process. Before the bone marrow transplant, patients were treated with a combination of cyclophosphamide and busulfan, in order to destroy all abnormal blood cells. The time taken for the blood platelets to return to a normal level is then an important variable in terms of the prognosis for a patient, and so the values of this variable were also recorded.

This example is based on the data from just one hospital, St. Vincent in Sydney, Australia. The observed survival time of each patient was recorded in days, together with the values of an event indicator which is unity if a patient died, and zero if the patient was still alive at the end of the study period. The prognostic variables to be used in this example concern the disease group, the ages of the patient and the bone marrow donor, an indicator variable that denotes whether the platelet count returned to a normal level of 40×10^9 per litre, and the time taken to return to this value. Two patients, numbers 7 and 21, died before the platelet count had returned to normal, and so for these patients, no value is given for the time to return to a normal platelet count. The variables recorded are therefore as follows:

Time: Survival time in days
Status: Event indicator (0 = censored, 1 = event)
Group: Disease group (1 = ALL, 2 = low-risk AML,
3 = high-risk AML)
Page: Age of patient
Dage: Age of donor
Precovery: Platelet recovery indicator (0 = no, 1 = yes)
Ptime: Time in days to return of platelets to normal level (if $P = 1$)

The database used in this example is given in Table 8.1.

The aim of the analysis of these data is to examine whether there are any differences between the survival times of patients in the three disease groups, after adjusting for prognostic variables. In order to investigate the effect of the time taken for platelets to return to their normal level on patient survival, a time-dependent variable, $Plate(t)$, is defined. This variable takes the value zero at times t when the platelets have not returned to normal levels, and then switches to unity once a normal level has been achieved. Formally,

$$Plate(t) = \begin{cases} 0 & \text{if } t < \text{time at which platelets returned to normal,} \\ 1 & \text{if } t \geqslant \text{time at which platelets returned to normal,} \end{cases}$$

so that $Plate(t) = 0$ for all t when a patient dies before platelet recovery.

We first fit a Cox proportional hazards model that contains the variables associated with the age of the patient and donor, *Page* and *Dage*. When either

Table 8.1 *Survival times of patients following bone marrow transplantation.*

Patient	*Time*	*Status*	*Group*	*Page*	*Dage*	*Precovery*	*Ptime*
1	1199	0	1	24	40	1	29
2	1111	0	1	19	28	1	22
3	530	0	1	17	28	1	34
4	1279	1	1	17	20	1	22
5	110	1	1	28	25	1	49
6	243	1	1	37	38	1	23
7	86	1	1	17	26	0	
8	466	1	1	15	18	1	100
9	262	1	1	29	32	1	59
10	1850	0	2	37	36	1	9
11	1843	0	2	34	32	1	19
12	1535	0	2	35	32	1	21
13	1447	0	2	33	28	1	24
14	1384	0	2	21	18	1	19
15	222	1	2	28	30	1	52
16	1356	0	2	33	22	1	14
17	1136	0	3	47	27	1	15
18	845	0	3	40	39	1	20
19	392	1	3	43	50	1	24
20	63	1	3	44	37	1	16
21	97	1	3	48	56	0	
22	153	1	3	31	25	1	59
23	363	1	3	52	48	1	19

of these variables is added on their own or in the presence of the other, there is no significant reduction in the value of the $-2\log\hat{L}$ statistic.

The time-dependent variable $Plate(t)$ is now added to the null model. The value of $-2\log\hat{L}$ is reduced from 67.13 to 62.21, a reduction of 4.92 on 1 d.f., which is significant at the 5% level ($P = 0.026$). This suggests that time to platelet recovery does affect survival. After allowing for the effects of this variable, there is still no evidence that the hazard of death is dependent on the age of the patient or donor.

The estimated coefficient of $Plate(t)$ in the model that contains this variable alone is -2.696, and the fact that this is negative indicates that there is a greater hazard of death at any given time for a patient whose platelets are not at a normal level. The hazard ratio at any given time is $\exp(-2.696) = 0.067$, and so a patient whose platelets have recovered to normal at a given time has about one-fifteenth the risk of death at that time. However, a 95% confidence interval for the corresponding true hazard ratio is $(0.006, 0.751)$, which shows that the point estimate of the relative risk is really quite imprecise.

To quantify the effect of disease group on survival, the change in $-2\log\hat{L}$ when the factor *Group* is added to the model that contains the time-dependent variable *Plate*(t) is 6.49 on 2 d.f., which is significant at the 5% level ($P = 0.039$). The parameter estimates associated with disease group show that the hazard of death is much greater for those suffering from ALL and those in the high-risk group of AML sufferers. The hazard ratios for an ALL patient relative to a low-risk AML patient is 7.97 and that for a high-risk AML patient relative to a low-risk one is 11.77.

For the model that contains the factor *Group* and the time-dependent variable *Plate*(t), the estimated baseline cumulative hazard and survivor functions are given in Table 8.2. These have been obtained using the estimate of the baseline cumulative hazard function given in Equation (8.3).

Table 8.2 *Estimated baseline cumulative hazard, $\tilde{H}_0(t)$, baseline survivor function, $\tilde{S}_0(t)$, and survivor function for an ALL patient with Plate$(t) = 1$, $\tilde{S}_1(t)$.*

Time, t	$\tilde{H}_0(t)$	$\tilde{S}_0(t)$	$\tilde{S}_1(t)$
0	0.0000	1.0000	1.0000
63	0.1953	0.8226	0.9810
86	0.3962	0.6728	0.9618
97	0.6477	0.5232	0.9383
110	1.2733	0.2799	0.8823
153	1.9399	0.1437	0.8264
222	2.6779	0.0687	0.7685
243	3.4226	0.0326	0.7143
262	4.2262	0.0146	0.6600
363	5.0987	0.0061	0.6057
392	6.0978	0.0022	0.5491
466	7.2663	0.0007	0.4895
1279	13.0700	0.0000	0.2766

In this table, $\tilde{H}_0(t)$ and $\tilde{S}_0(t)$ are the estimated cumulative hazard and survivor functions for an individual with AML and for whom the platelet recovery indicator, *Plate*(t), remains at zero throughout the study. Also given in this table are the values of the estimated survivor function for an individual with ALL, but for whom *Plate*$(t) = 1$ for all values of t, denoted $\tilde{S}_1(t)$. Since the value of *Plate*(t) is zero for each patient at the start of the study, and for most patients this changes to unity at some later point in time, these two estimated survivor functions illustrate the effect of platelet recovery at any specific time. For example, the probability of an ALL patient surviving beyond 97 days is only 0.52 if their platelets have not recovered to a normal level by this time. On the other hand, if such a patient has experienced platelet recovery by this time, they would have an estimated survival probability of 0.94. The estimated survivor function for an ALL patient whose platelet recovery status changes at some time t_0 from 0 to 1 can also be obtained from Table 8.2, since this will be $\tilde{S}_0(t)$ for $t \leqslant t_0$ and $\tilde{S}_1(t)$ for $t > t_0$. Estimates of the survivor function may also be obtained for individuals in the other disease groups.

In this illustration, the data from two patients who died before their platelet count had reached a normal level have a substantial impact on inferences about the effect of platelet recovery. If patients 7 and 21 are omitted from the database, the time-dependent variable is no longer significant when added to the null model ($P = 0.755$). The conclusion about the effect of platelet recovery time on survival is therefore dramatically influenced by the data for these two patients.

Example 8.2 Chemotherapy in ovarian cancer patients

Consider again the data on patient survival following diagnosis of ovarian cancer, given in Example 5.10 of Chapter 5. When a Cox proportional hazards model that contains the variables *Age*, the age of a patient at the time origin, and *Treat*, the treatment group, is fitted to the data on the survival times of patients with ovarian cancer, the estimated hazard function for the ith of 26 patients in the study is

$$\hat{h}_i(t) = \exp\{0.147\, Age_i - 0.796\, Treat_i\} h_0(t).$$

The value of the $-2 \log \hat{L}$ statistic for this model is 54.148.

We now fit a model that contains *Age* and *Treat*, and a term corresponding to an interaction between age and survival time. This interaction will be modelled by including the time-dependent variable *Tage*, whose values are formed from the product of *Age* and the survival time t, that is, $Tage = Age \times t$. Since the values of *Tage* are dependent upon t, this time-dependent variable cannot be fitted in the same manner as *Age* and *Treat*. When *Tage* is added to the model, the fitted hazard function becomes

$$\hat{h}_i(t) = \exp\{0.216\, Age_i - 0.664\, Treat_i - 0.0002\, Age_i\, t\} h_0(t).$$

Under this model, the hazard of death at t for a patient of a given age on the combined treatment ($Treat = 2$), relative to one of the same age on the single treatment ($Treat = 1$), is $\exp(-0.664) = 0.52$, which is not very different from the value of 0.45 found using the model that does not contain the variable *Tage*. However, the log-hazard ratio for a patient aged a_2 years, relative to one aged a_1 years, is

$$0.216(a_2 - a_1) - 0.0002(a_2 - a_1)t$$

at time t. This model therefore allows the log-hazard ratio for *Age* to be linearly dependent on survival time.

The value of $-2 \log \hat{L}$ for the model that contains *Age*, *Treat* and *Tage* is 53.613. The change in $-2 \log \hat{L}$ on adding the variable *Tage* to a model that contains *Age* and *Treat* is therefore 0.53, which is not significant ($P = 0.465$). We therefore conclude that the time-dependent variable *Tage* is not in fact needed in the model.

Example 8.3 Data from a cirrhosis study
Although the data to be used in this example are artificial, it is useful to provide a background against which these data can be considered. Suppose therefore that 12 patients have been recruited to a study on the treatment of cirrhosis of the liver. The patients are randomised to receive either a placebo or a new treatment that will be referred to as Liverol. Six patients are allocated to Liverol and six to the placebo. At the time when the patient is entered into the study, the age and baseline value of the patient's bilirubin level are recorded. The natural logarithm of the bilirubin value (in μmol/l) will be used in this analysis, and the variables measured are summarised below:

Time:	Survival time of the patient in days
Status:	Event indicator (0 = censored, 1 = uncensored)
Treat:	Treatment group (0 = placebo, 1 = Liverol)
Age:	Age of the patient in years
Lbr:	Logarithm of bilirubin level

The values of these variables are given in Table 8.3.

Table 8.3 *Survival times of 12 patients in a study on cirrhosis of the liver.*

Patient	*Time*	*Status*	*Treat*	*Age*	*Lbr*
1	281	1	0	46	3.2
2	604	0	0	57	3.1
3	457	1	0	56	2.2
4	384	1	0	65	3.9
5	341	0	0	73	2.8
6	842	1	0	64	2.4
7	1514	1	1	69	2.4
8	182	0	1	62	2.4
9	1121	1	1	71	2.5
10	1411	0	1	69	2.3
11	814	1	1	77	3.8
12	1071	1	1	58	3.1

Patients are supposed to return to the clinic three, six and twelve months after the commencement of treatment, and yearly thereafter. On these occasions, the bilirubin level is again measured and recorded. Data are therefore available on how the bilirubin level changes in each patient throughout the duration of the study. Table 8.4 gives the values of the logarithm of the bilirubin value at each time in the follow-up period for each patient.

In taking log(bilirubin) to be a time-dependent variable, the value of the variate is that recorded at the most recent follow-up visit, for each patient. In this calculation, the change to a new value will be assumed to take place immediately after the reading was taken, so that patient 1, for example, is assumed to have a log(bilirubin) value of 3.2 for any time t when $t \leqslant 47$,

Table 8.4 *Follow-up times and* log*(bilirubin) values for the 12 patients in the cirrhosis study.*

Patient	Follow-up time	Log(bilirubin)
1	47	3.8
	184	4.9
	251	5.0
2	94	2.9
	187	3.1
	321	3.2
3	61	2.8
	97	2.9
	142	3.2
	359	3.4
	440	3.8
4	92	4.7
	194	4.9
	372	5.4
5	87	2.6
	192	2.9
	341	3.4
6	94	2.3
	197	2.8
	384	3.5
	795	3.9
7	74	2.9
	202	3.0
	346	3.0
	917	3.9
	1411	5.1
8	90	2.5
	182	2.9
9	101	2.5
	410	2.7
	774	2.8
	1043	3.4
10	182	2.2
	847	2.8
	1051	3.3
	1347	4.9
11	167	3.9
	498	4.3
12	108	2.8
	187	3.4
	362	3.9
	694	3.8

3.8 for $47 < t \leqslant 184$, 4.9 for $184 < t \leqslant 251$, and 5.0 for $251 < t \leqslant 281$. The values of *Lbr* for a given individual then follow a step-function in which the values are assumed constant between any two adjacent time points.

The data are first analysed using the baseline log(bilirubin) value alone. A Cox proportional hazards model is used, and the values of $-2 \log \hat{L}$ on fitting particular models are as shown in Table 8.5.

Table 8.5 *Values of* $-2 \log \hat{L}$ *for models without a time-dependent variable.*

Terms in model	$-2 \log \hat{L}$
null model	25.121
Age	22.135
Lbr	21.662
Age, Lbr	18.475

Both *Age* and *Lbr* appear to be needed in the model, although the evidence for including *Age* as well as *Lbr* is not very strong. When *Treat* is added to the model that contains *Age* and *Lbr*, the reduction in the value of $-2 \log \hat{L}$ is 5.182 on 1 d.f. This is significant at the 5% level ($P = 0.023$). The coefficient of *Treat* is -3.052, indicating that the drug Liverol is effective in reducing the hazard of death. Indeed, other things being equal, Liverol reduces the hazard of death by a factor of 0.047.

We now analyse these data, taking the log(bilirubin) values to be time-dependent. Let *Lbrt* be the time-dependent variate formed from the values of log(bilirubin). The values of $-2 \log \hat{L}$ on fitting Cox regression models to the data are then given in Table 8.6.

Table 8.6 *Values of* $-2 \log \hat{L}$ *for models with a time-dependent variable.*

Terms in model	$-2 \log \hat{L}$
null model	25.121
Age	22.135
Lbrt	12.050
Age, Lbrt	11.145

It is clear from this table that the hazard function depends on the time-dependent variable *Lbrt*, and that after allowing for this, the effect of *Age* is slight. We therefore add the treatment effect *Treat* to the model that contains *Lbrt* alone. The effect of this is that $-2 \log \hat{L}$ is reduced from 12.050 to 10.676, a reduction of 1.374 on 1 d.f. This reduction is not significant ($P = 0.241$) leading to the conclusion that after taking account of the dependence of the hazard of death on the evolution of the log(bilirubin) values, no treatment effect is discernible.

The estimated hazard function for the ith individual is given by

$$\hat{h}_i(t) = \exp\{3.605\, Lbr_i(t) - 1.479\, Treat_i\} h_0(t),$$

where $Lbr_i(t)$ is the value of log(bilirubin) for this patient at time t. The estimated ratio of the hazard of death at time t for two individuals on the same treatment who have values of *Lbr* that differ by 0.1 units at t is $e^{0.3605} = 1.43$. This means that the individual whose log(bilirubin) value is 0.1 units greater has close to a 50% increase in the hazard of death at time t.

One possible explanation for the difference between the results of these two analyses is that the effect of the treatment is to change the values of the bilirubin level, so that after changes in these values over time have been allowed for, no treatment effect is visible.

The baseline cumulative hazard function may now be estimated for the model that contains the time-dependent variable *Lbrt* and *Treat*. The estimated values of this function are tabulated in Table 8.7.

Table 8.7 *Estimated baseline cumulative hazard function, $\tilde{H}_0(t)$, for the cirrhosis study.*

Follow-up time (t)	$\tilde{H}_0(t)$
0	0.000
281	0.009×10^{-6}
384	0.012×10^{-6}
457	0.541×10^{-6}
814	0.908×10^{-6}
842	1.577×10^{-6}
1071	3.318×10^{-6}
1121	6.007×10^{-6}
1514	6.053×10^{-6}

This table shows that the cumulative hazard function is increasing in a non-linear fashion, which indicates that the baseline hazard is not constant, but increases with time. The corresponding baseline survivor function could be obtained from this estimate. However, a model with $Lbrt = 0$ for all t is not at all easy to interpret, and so the estimated survivor function is obtained for an individual for whom $Lbrt = 3$. This function is shown in Figure 8.5, for a patient in either treatment group. This figure clearly shows that patients on placebo have a much poorer prognosis than those on Liverol.

Finally, we illustrate how estimates of the conditional probabilities of survival from time t to time $t + 360$ days can be obtained, using the result given in Equation (8.5). Using the values of the time-dependent variable given in Tables 8.3 and 8.4, the values of $\sum_{j=1}^{p} \hat{\beta}_j x_{ji}(t)$, the prognostic index at time t for the ith patient, $i = 1, 2, \ldots, 12$, can be calculated for $t = 0$, 360, 720, 1080, and 1440. For this calculation, the log(bilirubin) value at one of these times is taken to be the value recorded at the immediately preceding follow-up time. Table 8.7 is then used to obtain the values of $\tilde{H}_0(t + 360) - \tilde{H}_0(t)$, and then

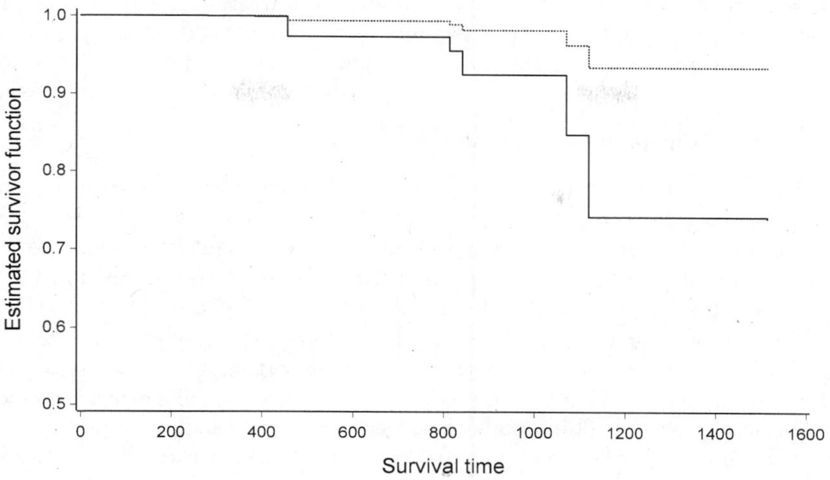

Figure 8.5 *Estimated survivor function for a patient with Lbr = 3, for all t, who is on placebo (—) or Liverol (·······).*

$\tilde{P}_i(t, t+360)$ is obtained from Equation (8.5). The full set of results will not be given here, but as an example, the estimated approximate conditional probabilities of surviving through consecutive intervals of 360 days, for patients 1 and 7, are shown in Table 8.8.

Table 8.8 *Approximate conditional survival probabilities for patients 1 and 7.*

Time interval	$\tilde{P}_1(t, t+h)$	$\tilde{P}_7(t, t+h)$
0–	0.999	1.000
360–	0.000	0.994
720–	0.000	0.969
1080–	0.000	0.457
1440–	0.045	0.364

Note that because these estimates are survival probabilities conditional on being alive at the start of an interval, they are not necessarily decreasing functions of time. These estimates again show that patients on Liverol have a greater probability of surviving for a period of one year, if they are alive at the start of that year, than patients on the placebo. Finally, the values of $1 - \tilde{P}_i(t, t+h)$ are approximate estimates of the probability of death within each interval, conditional on a patient being alive at the start. Summing these estimates over all 12 patients leads to the values 0.02, 2.46, 5.64, 6.53, 3.16, for each of the five intervals, respectively. These can be compared to the observed numbers of deaths in each interval, which are 1, 2, 3, 1 and 1, respectively.

There is therefore a tendency for the model to overestimate the numbers of deaths, but because of the small size of the data set, this does not provide a very reliable assessment of the predictive power of the model.

8.6 Counting process format

Models that include time-dependent variables can be fitted by maximising the partial log-likelihood function in Equation (8.2). This can be accomplished using software that enables the value of any time-dependent variable to be determined at different event times in the data set, as explained in Section 8.2.1, and this approach was used in the examples of Section 8.5.

Time-dependent variables may also be included in a model by expressing the data in *counting process format.* This involves setting intervals of time over which the values of all explanatory variables are constant. The event indicator is then set to zero for all intervals except the final interval. The upper limit of the final interval is the event time, or censoring time, of the individual, and the value of the event indicator is set to unity if there is an event at the end of that interval, and zero otherwise. Variables associated with the lower and upper limits of each time interval, *Start* and *Stop*, say, are then used to specify survival experience, and the variable *Status* denotes whether or not an event has occurred at each stop time. The survival data are then represented by a trio of values (*Start*, *Stop*, *Status*) for each interval, and this format of data is called the *counting process* or *(start, stop, status) format.* Many software packages for survival analysis can process data expressed in this general form. Further details on the counting process format, and its application to other areas of survival analysis, are given in Section 13.1.3 of Chapter 13.

Example 8.4 Data from a cirrhosis study
To illustrate the counting process form of survival data, consider again the data from Example 8.3. For patient 1, the data for whom were given in Table 8.4, the log(bilirubin) value was 3.2 when measured at baseline, 3.8 from day 47, 4.9 from day 184 and 5.0 from day 251. This patient died on day 281, and so the value of the event indicator is 0 until the end of the final interval. The values of the explanatory variables *Status*, *Treat*, *Age* and the time-dependent variable *Lbrt* in the intervals $(0, 47]$, $(47, 184]$, $(184, 251]$ and $(251, 281]$, are then as shown in Table 8.9. In this notation for the time intervals, $(a, b]$ denotes the interval for a time t, where $a < t \leqslant b$.

Table 8.9 *Data for the first patient in the cirrhosis study in the counting process format.*

Time interval	*Start*	*Stop*	*Status*	*Treat*	*Age*	*Lbrt*
$(0, 47]$	0	47	0	0	46	3.2
$(47, 184]$	47	184	0	0	46	3.8
$(184, 251]$	184	251	0	0	46	4.9
$(251, 281]$	251	281	1	0	46	5.0

The database now has four lines of data for Patient 1, and we proceed in a similar manner for the data from the remaining patients. A Cox regression model with the variables *Age*, *Treat* and the time-dependent variable *Lbrt* is then fitted to the extended data set, which leads to the same results as those given in Example 8.3.

8.7 Further reading

The possibility of incorporating time-dependent variables in a proportional hazards model was raised by Cox (1972). The appropriate partial likelihood function was given in his paper, and discussed in greater detail in Cox (1975). Kalbfleisch and Prentice (2002) include a detailed account of the construction of the partial likelihood function. The classification of time-dependent variables outlined in Section 8.1 is due to Prentice and Kalbfleisch (1979), who amplify on this in Kalbfleisch and Prentice (2002). Andersen (1992) reviews the uses of time-dependent variables in survival analysis and includes an example on which the hypothetical study of Example 8.3 is loosely based.

A number of practical problems encountered in the analysis of survival data with time-dependent variables are discussed by Altman and De Stavola (1994), who include a review of software available at that time. A comprehensive analysis of data on primary biliary cirrhosis, which includes an assessment of conditional survival probabilities is also provided. See Christensen et al. (1986) for a further illustration. Klein and Moeschberger (2005) give the full data set on survival following bone marrow transplantation, part of which was used in Example 8.1, and use this in a number of detailed illustrative examples.

The model described in Section 8.4 in connection with organ transplantation was presented by Crowley and Hu (1977) and Cox and Oakes (1984) in an analysis of the 'Stanford heart transplant data'. This famous data set is given in Crowley and Hu (1977) and an update is provided by Cox and Oakes (1984). See also Aitkin, Laird and Francis (1983) and the ensuing discussion.

Relatively little work has been done on incorporating time-dependent variables in a fully parametric model for survival data. However, Petersen (1986) shows how a parametric model with time-dependent variables can be fitted. The Royston and Parmar model, described in Section 6.9 of Chapter 6, can be extended to include time-dependent variables by adding an interaction between potential time-dependent variables and the spline variables, $\nu_1(y), \nu_2(y), \ldots$, in the baseline cumulative hazard function of Equation (6.30) of Chapter 6.

Joint models for longitudinal and survival data that describe underlying relationships between measurements made on an individual at multiple times and the time to an event, are also relevant in this context. Recent review papers include Tsiatis and Davidian (2004), Tseng, Hsieh and Wang (2005), McCrink, Marshall and Cairns (2013) and the text of Rizopoulis (2012).

Chapter 9

Interval-censored survival data

In many studies where the response variable is a survival time, the exact time of the event of interest will not be known. Instead, the event will be known to have occurred during a particular interval of time. Data in this form are known as *grouped* or *interval-censored* survival data.

Interval-censored data commonly arise in studies where there is a non-lethal end-point, such as the recurrence of a disease or condition. However, most survival analyses are based on interval-censored data, in the sense that the survival times are often taken as the nearest day, week or month. In this chapter, some methods for analysing interval-censored data will be described and illustrated. Models in which specific assumptions are made about the form of the underlying hazard function are considered in Sections 9.1 to 9.4, and fully parametric models are discussed in Section 9.5.

9.1 Modelling interval-censored survival data

In this chapter, a number of methods for the analysis of interval-censored survival data will be discussed in the context of a study on disease recurrence. In the management of patients who have been cured of ulcers, carcinomas or other recurrent conditions, the patients are usually provided with medication to maintain their recovery. These patients are subsequently examined at regular intervals in order to detect whether a recurrence has occurred. Naturally, some patients may experience symptoms of a recurrence and be subsequently diagnosed as having had a recurrence at a time other than one of the scheduled screening times.

Now suppose that the study is designed to compare two maintenance therapies, a new and a standard treatment, say, and that a number of explanatory variables are recorded for each individual when they are recruited to the study. The vector $\boldsymbol{x}_i$ will be used to denote the set of values of p explanatory variables, $X_1, X_2, \ldots, X_p$, for the ith individual in the study. The first of these variables, X_1, will be taken to be an indicator variable corresponding to the treatment group, where $X_1 = 0$ if an individual is on the standard treatment and $X_1 = 1$ if on the new treatment.

Clearly, one way of analysing such data is to ignore the interval censoring. A survival analysis is then carried out on the times of a detected recurrence.

However, the data set used in this analysis will be based on a mixture of recurrences detected at scheduled screening times, known as *screen-detected recurrences* and recurrences diagnosed following the occurrence of symptoms or *interval-detected recurrences*. This leads to a difficulty in interpreting the results of the analysis.

To illustrate the problem, consider a study to compare two treatments for suppressing the recurrence of an ulcer, a new and a standard treatment, say. Also suppose that both treatments have exactly the same effect on the recurrence time, but that the new treatment suppresses symptoms. The recurrence of an ulcer in a patient on the new treatment will then tend to be detected later than that in a patient on the standard treatment. Therefore, interval-detected recurrences will be identified sooner in a patient on the standard treatment. The interval-detected recurrence times will then be shorter for this group of patients, indicating an apparent advantage of the new treatment over the standard.

If the time interval between successive screenings is short, relative to the average time to recurrence, there will be few interval-detected recurrences. Standard methods for survival analysis may then be used.

Example 9.1 Recurrence of an ulcer

In a double-blind clinical trial to compare treatments for the inhibition of relapse after primary therapy has healed an ulcer, patients are randomised to receive one or other of two treatments, labelled A and B. Regular visits to a clinic were arranged for the patients, and endoscopies were performed 6 months and 12 months after randomisation. A positive endoscopy result indicates that an ulcer has recurred in the time since the last negative result. Information is therefore obtained on whether or not an ulcer has recurred in the interval from 0 to 6 months or in the interval from 6 to 12 months. Additionally, some patients presented at the clinic between scheduled visits, suffering from symptoms of recurrence. These patients had endoscopies at these times in order to detect if a recurrence had in fact occurred.

At entry to the trial, the age of each person, in years, and the duration of verified disease (1 = less than five years, 2 = greater than or equal to five years) was recorded, in addition to the treatment group (A or B). There are two variables associated with ulcer detection in the data set, namely the time of the last visit, in months, and the result of the endoscopy (1 = no ulcer detected, 2 = ulcer detected). Those with times other than 6 or 12 months had presented with symptoms between scheduled visits.

The study itself was multinational and the full set of data is given in Whitehead (1989). In this example, only the data from Belgium will be used, and the relevant data are given in Table 9.1.

Once an ulcer is detected by endoscopy, a patient is treated for this and is then no longer in the study. There were some patients who either did not have an endoscopy six months after trial entry, or who dropped out after a negative unscheduled endoscopy in the first six months. These patients have

Table 9.1 *Data on the recurrence of an ulcer following treatment for the primary disease.*

Patient	Age	Duration	Treatment	Time of last visit	Result
1	48	2	*B*	7	2
2	73	1	*B*	12	1
3	54	1	*B*	12	1
4	58	2	*B*	12	1
5	56	1	*A*	12	1
6	49	2	*A*	12	1
7	71	1	*B*	12	1
8	41	1	*A*	12	1
9	23	1	*B*	12	1
10	37	1	*B*	5	2
11	38	1	*B*	12	1
12	76	2	*B*	12	1
13	38	2	*A*	12	1
14	27	1	*A*	6	2
15	47	1	*B*	6	2
16	54	1	*A*	6	1
17	38	1	*B*	10	2
18	27	2	*B*	7	2
19	58	2	*A*	12	1
20	75	1	*B*	12	1
21	25	1	*A*	12	1
22	58	1	*A*	12	1
23	63	1	*B*	12	1
24	41	1	*A*	12	1
25	47	1	*B*	12	1
26	58	1	*A*	3	2
27	74	2	*A*	2	2
28	75	2	*A*	6	1
29	72	1	*A*	12	1
30	59	1	*B*	12	2
31	52	1	*B*	12	1
32	75	1	*B*	12	2
33	76	1	*A*	12	1
34	34	2	*A*	6	1
35	36	1	*B*	12	1
36	59	1	*B*	12	1
37	44	1	*A*	12	2
38	28	2	*B*	12	1
39	62	1	*B*	12	1
40	23	1	*A*	12	1
41	49	1	*B*	12	1
42	61	1	*A*	12	1
43	33	2	*B*	12	1

been omitted from the data set on the grounds that there is no information about whether an ulcer has recurred in the first six months of the study. This means that those patients in Table 9.1 whose last visit was greater than 6 months after randomisation would have had a negative endoscopy at 6 months.

In modelling the data from this study, duration of disease is denoted by an indicator variable *Dur*, which is zero when the duration is less than 5 years and unity otherwise. The treatment effect is denoted by a variable *Treat*, which takes the value zero if an individual is on treatment A and unity if on treatment B. The patient's age is reflected in the continuous variate *Age*.

We first analyse the recurrence times in Table 9.1 ignoring the interval censoring. The recurrence times of those patients who have not had a detected recurrence by the time of their last visit are taken to be censored, and a Cox regression model is fitted.

Table 9.2 *Values of $-2\log\hat{L}$ on fitting a Cox regression model to data on the time to recurrence of an ulcer.*

Variables in model	$-2\log\hat{L}$
None	79.189
Dur	79.157
Age	78.885
Age + *Dur*	78.872
Age + *Dur* + *Treat*	78.747
Treat	79.097

From the values of the $-2\log\hat{L}$ statistic for different models, given in Table 9.2, it is clear that neither age nor duration of disease are important prognostic factors. Moreover, the reduction in $-2\log\hat{L}$ on adding the treatment effect to the model, adjusted or unadjusted for the prognostic factors, is nowhere near significant.

The estimated coefficient of *Treat* in the model that contains *Treat* alone is 0.189, and the standard error of this estimate is 0.627. The estimated hazard of a recurrence under treatment B (*Treat* $= 1$), relative to that under treatment A (*Treat* $= 0$), is therefore $\exp(0.189) = 1.21$. The standard error of the estimated hazard ratio is found using Equation (3.13) in Chapter 3, and is 0.758. The fact that the estimated hazard ratio is greater than unity gives a slight indication that treatment A is superior to treatment B, but not significantly so.

9.2 Modelling the recurrence probability in the follow-up period

Suppose that patients are followed up to time t_s, at which time the last scheduled screening test is carried out. Information on whether or not a recurrence was detected at any time up to and including the last screen is then recorded. Let $p_i(t_s)$ be the probability of a recurrence up to time t_s for the ith patient,

$i = 1, 2, \ldots, n$, with vector of explanatory variables $\boldsymbol{x}_i$. We now adopt a Cox proportional hazards model, according to which the hazard of a recurrence at t_s, for the ith patient, is given by

$$h_i(t_s) = \exp(\eta_i)h_0(t_s),$$

where $\eta_i = \boldsymbol{\beta}'\boldsymbol{x}_i = \beta_1 x_{1i} + \beta_2 x_{2i} + \cdots + \beta_p x_{pi}$ is the risk score, and $h_0(t_s)$ is the baseline hazard function at t_s.

The probability that the ith individual experiences a recurrence after time t_s is the survivor function $S_i(t_s)$, so that $S_i(t_s) = 1 - p_i(t_s)$. Now, from Equation (3.25) in Section 3.10 of Chapter 3,

$$S_i(t_s) = \{S_0(t_s)\}^{\exp(\eta_i)}, \tag{9.1}$$

where $S_0(t_s)$ is the value of the survivor function at t_s for an individual on the standard treatment for whom all the other explanatory variables are zero. The probability of a recurrence up to time t_s under this model is therefore

$$p_i(t_s) = 1 - \{S_0(t_s)\}^{\exp(\eta_i)},$$

and so

$$\log[-\log\{1 - p_i(t_s)\}] = \eta_i + \log\{-\log S_0(t_s)\}.$$

Writing $\beta_0 = \log\{-\log S_0(t_s)\}$, the model can be expressed as

$$\log[-\log\{1 - p_i(t_s)\}] = \beta_0 + \beta_1 x_{1i} + \beta_2 x_{2i} + \cdots + \beta_p x_{pi}. \tag{9.2}$$

This is a linear model for the complementary log-log transformation of the probability of a recurrence up to time t_s. The model can be fitted to data on a binary response variable that takes the value zero for those individuals in the study who have not experienced a recurrence before t_s, the time of the last screen, and unity otherwise.

As in modelling survival data, models fitted to data on a binary response variable can be compared on the basis of the statistic $-2\log\hat{L}$. Here, $\hat{L}$ is the maximised likelihood of the binary data, and $-2\log\hat{L}$ is generally known as the *deviance*. Differences in the deviance for two nested models have an asymptotic chi-squared distribution, and so models fitted to binary data can be compared in the same manner as the models used in survival analysis.

When the model in Equation (9.2) is fitted to the observed data, the estimate of the constant, $\hat{\beta}_0$, is an estimate of $\log\{-\log S_0(t_s)\}$, from which an estimate of the baseline survivor function at t_s can be obtained. Also, the ratio of the hazard of a recurrence for an individual on the new treatment, relative to one on the standard, is $\exp(\beta_1)$. This can be estimated by $\exp(\hat{\beta}_1)$, where $\hat{\beta}_1$ is the parameter estimate corresponding to X_1, the indicator variable that corresponds to the treatment group. Values of the hazard ratio less than unity suggest that the risk of a recurrence at any time is smaller under the new treatment than under the standard. A confidence interval for the hazard ratio may be obtained from the standard error of $\hat{\beta}_1$ in the usual manner.

This method of estimating the hazard ratio from interval-censored survival data is not particularly efficient, since data on the times that a recurrence is detected are not utilised. However, the method is appropriate when interest simply centres on the risk of a recurrence in a specific time period. It is also the method that would be adopted in modelling quantities such as the probability of a relapse in the first year of treatment, or the probability of no recurrence in a five-year period after trial entry.

Example 9.2 Recurrence of an ulcer
We now model the probability of an ulcer recurring in the 12 months following recruitment to the study described in Example 9.1. Of the 43 patients in the data set, 11 of them had experienced a recurrence in this 12-month period, namely patients 1, 10, 14, 15, 17, 18, 26, 27, 30, 32 and 37. A binary response variable is now defined, which takes the value unity if a patient has experienced a recurrence and zero otherwise. A model in which the complementary log-log transformation of the recurrence probability is related to age, duration of disease and treatment group is then fitted to the binary observations.

Table 9.3 gives the deviances on fitting complementary log-log models with different terms to the binary response variable. All the models fitted include a constant term.

Table 9.3 *Deviances on fitting complementary log-log models to data on the recurrence of an ulcer in 12 months.*

Variables in model	Deviance	d.f.
Constant	48.902	42
Dur	48.899	41
Age	48.573	41
Treat	48.531	41
Dur + *Age*	48.565	40
Dur + *Treat*	48.531	40
Age + *Treat*	48.175	40
Dur + *Age* + *Treat*	48.172	39
Dur + *Age* + *Treat* + *Treat* × *Age*	47.944	38
Dur + *Age* + *Treat* + *Treat* × *Dur*	48.062	38

In this example, the effects of age, duration of disease and treatment group have been modelled using the variates *Age*, *Dur*, and *Treat*, defined in Example 9.1. However, factors corresponding to duration and treatment could have been used in conjunction with packages that allow factors to be included directly. This would not make any difference to the deviances in Table 9.3, but it may have an effect on the interpretation of the parameter estimates. See Sections 3.2 and 3.9 for fuller details.

It is clear from Table 9.3 that no variable reduces the deviance by a significant amount. For example, the change in the deviance on adding *Treat* to the model that only contains a constant is 0.371, which is certainly not significant when compared to percentage points of the chi-squared distribution on 1 d.f.

Approximately the same change in deviance is found when *Treat* is added to the model that contains *Age* and *Dur*, showing that the treatment effect is of a similar magnitude after allowing for these two variables. Moreover, there is no evidence whatsoever of an interaction between treatment and the variables *Age* and *Dur*.

On fitting a model that contains *Treat* alone, the estimated coefficient of *Treat* is 0.378, with a standard error of 0.629. Thus, the ratio of the hazard of a recurrence before 12 months in a patient on treatment B (*Treat* = 1), relative to that for a patient on treatment A (*Treat* = 0), is $\exp(0.378) = 1.46$. The risk of a recurrence in the year following randomisation is thus greater under treatment B than it is under treatment A, but not significantly so. This hazard ratio is not too different from the value of 1.21 obtained in Example 9.1. The standard error of the estimated hazard ratio, again found using Equation (3.13) in Chapter 3, is 0.918, which is also very similar to that found in Example 9.1.

A 95% confidence interval for the log-hazard ratio has limits of $0.378 \pm 1.96 \times 0.629$, and so the corresponding interval estimate for the hazard ratio itself is $(0.43, 5.01)$. Notice that this interval includes unity, a result which was foreshadowed by the non-significant treatment effect.

The estimated constant term in this fitted model is -1.442. This is an estimate of $\log\{-\log S_0(12)\}$, the survivor function at 12 months for a patient on treatment A. The estimated probability of a recurrence after 12 months for a patient on treatment A is therefore $\exp(-e^{-1.442}) = 0.79$. The corresponding value for a patient on treatment B is $0.79^{\exp(0.378)} = 0.71$. The probabilities of a recurrence in the first 12 months are therefore 0.21 for a patient on treatment A, and 0.29 for a patient on treatment B. This again shows that patients on treatment B have a slightly higher probability of the recurrence of an ulcer in the year following randomisation.

9.3* Modelling the recurrence probability at different times

In this section, a method for analysing interval-censored survival data is described, which takes account of whether or not a recurrence is detected at different examination times.

Suppose that patients enter a study at time 0 and are followed up to time t_k. During the course of this follow-up period, the individuals are screened on a regular basis in order to detect a recurrence of the disease or condition under study. Denote the examination times by $t_1, t_2, \ldots, t_k$, which are such that $t_1 < t_2 < \cdots < t_k$. Further, let t_0 denote the time origin, so that $t_0 = 0$ and let $t_{k+1} = \infty$.

For each individual, information will be recorded on whether or not a recurrence has occurred at times $t_1, t_2, \ldots, t_k$. It can then be determined whether a given individual has experienced a recurrence in the jth time interval from t_{j-1} to t_j. Thus, a patient who has a recurrence detected at time t_j has an actual recurrence time of t, where $t_{j-1} \leqslant t < t_j$, $j = 1, 2, \ldots, k$. Note that the study will not provide any information about whether a recurrence occurs after the final screening time, t_k.

Now let p_{ij} be the probability of a recurrence being detected in the ith patient, $i = 1, 2, \ldots, n$, at time t_j, so that p_{ij} is the probability that patient i experiences a recurrence in the jth time interval, $j = 1, 2, \ldots, k$. Also let π_{ij} be the probability that the ith of n patients is found to be free of the disease at time t_{j-1} and has a recurrence in the jth time interval, $j = 1, 2, \ldots, k$. This is therefore the conditional probability of a recurrence in the jth interval, given that the recurrence occurs after t_{j-1}. Using T_i to denote the random variable associated with the recurrence time of the ith individual, we therefore have

$$p_{ij} = \mathrm{P}(t_{j-1} \leqslant T_i < t_j),$$

and

$$\pi_{ij} = \mathrm{P}(t_{j-1} \leqslant T_i < t_j \mid T_i \geqslant t_{j-1}),$$

for $j = 1, 2, \ldots, k$.

We now consider individuals who have not had a detected recurrence by the last examination time, t_k. For these individuals, we define T_i to be the random variable associated with the time to either a recurrence or death, and the corresponding probability of a recurrence or death in the interval from time t_k is given by

$$p_{i,k+1} = \mathrm{P}(T_i \geqslant t_k) = 1 - \sum_{j=1}^{k} p_{ij}.$$

Also, the corresponding conditional probability of a recurrence or death in the interval (t_k, ∞) is

$$\pi_{i,k+1} = \mathrm{P}(T_i \geqslant t_k \mid T_i \geqslant t_k) = 1.$$

It then follows that

$$p_{ij} = (1 - \pi_{i1})(1 - \pi_{i2}) \cdots (1 - \pi_{i,j-1})\pi_{ij}, \tag{9.3}$$

for $j = 2, 3, \ldots, k + 1$, with $p_{i1} = \pi_{i1}$.

Now let r_{ij} be unity if the ith patient has a recurrence detected in the interval from t_{j-1} to t_j, $j = 1, 2, \ldots, k+1$, and zero if no recurrence is detected in that interval, with $r_{i,k+1} = 1$. Also let s_{ij} be unity if a patient has a detected recurrence after t_j, and zero otherwise. Then,

$$s_{ij} = r_{i,j+1} + r_{i,j+2} + \cdots + r_{i,k+1},$$

for $j = 1, 2, \ldots, k$.

The sample likelihood of the $n(k + 1)$ values r_{ij} is

$$\prod_{i=1}^{n} \prod_{j=1}^{k+1} p_{ij}^{r_{ij}},$$

and on substituting for p_{ij} from Equation (9.3), the likelihood function becomes

$$\prod_{i=1}^{n}\prod_{j=1}^{k+1}\{(1-\pi_{i1})\cdots(1-\pi_{i,j-1})\pi_{ij}\}^{r_{ij}}.$$

This function can be written as

$$\prod_{i=1}^{n}\pi_{i1}^{r_{i1}}\{(1-\pi_{i1})\pi_{i2}\}^{r_{i2}}\cdots\{(1-\pi_{i1})\cdots(1-\pi_{ik})\pi_{i,k+1}\}^{r_{i,k+1}},$$

which reduces to

$$\prod_{i=1}^{n}\pi_{i,k+1}^{r_{i,k+1}}\prod_{j=1}^{k}\pi_{ij}^{r_{ij}}(1-\pi_{ij})^{s_{ij}}. \tag{9.4}$$

However, $\pi_{i,k+1} = 1$, and so the likelihood function in Equation (9.4) becomes

$$\prod_{i=1}^{n}\prod_{j=1}^{k}\pi_{ij}^{r_{ij}}(1-\pi_{ij})^{s_{ij}}. \tag{9.5}$$

This is the likelihood function for nk observations r_{ij} from a binomial distribution with response probability π_{ij}, and where the binomial denominator is $r_{ij} + s_{ij}$. This denominator is equal to unity when a patient is at risk of having a detected recurrence after time t_j, and zero otherwise. In fact, the denominator is zero when both r_{ij} and s_{ij} are equal to zero, and the likelihood function in Expression (9.5) is unaffected by observations for which $r_{ij} + s_{ij} = 0$. Data records for which the binomial denominator is zero are therefore uninformative, and so they can be omitted from the data set. If there are m observations remaining after these deletions, so that $m \leqslant nk$, the likelihood function in Expression (9.5) is that of m observations from binomial distributions with parameters 1 and π_{ij}, in other words, m observations from a *Bernoulli distribution*.

The next step is to note that for the ith patient,

$$1-\pi_{ij} = \mathrm{P}(T_i \geqslant t_j \mid T_i \geqslant t_{j-1}),$$

so that

$$1-\pi_{ij} = \frac{S_i(t_j)}{S_i(t_{j-1})}.$$

Adopting a proportional hazards model for the recurrence times, the hazard of a recurrence being detected at time t_j in the ith individual can be expressed as

$$h_i(t_j) = \exp(\eta_i)h_0(t_j),$$

where $h_0(t_j)$ is the baseline hazard at t_j, and η_i is the risk score for the ith individual. Notice that this assumption means that the hazards need only be proportional at the scheduled screening times t_j, and not at intermediate times. This is less restrictive than the usual proportional hazards assumption, which requires that hazards be proportional at every time.

Using the result in Equation (9.1),

$$1 - \pi_{ij} = \left\{ \frac{S_0(t_j)}{S_0(t_{j-1})} \right\}^{\exp(\eta_i)},$$

and on taking logarithms we find that

$$\log(1 - \pi_{ij}) = \exp(\eta_i) \log \{S_0(t_j)/S_0(t_{j-1})\}.$$

Consequently,

$$\begin{aligned} \log\{-\log(1 - \pi_{ij})\} &= \eta_i + \log\left[-\log\{S_0(t_j)/S_0(t_{j-1})\}\right] \\ &= \eta_i + \gamma_j, \end{aligned}$$

say. This is a linear model for the complementary log-log transformation of π_{ij}, in which the parameters γ_j, $j = 1, 2, \ldots, k$, are associated with the k time intervals. The model can be fitted using standard methods for modelling binary data.

In modelling the probability of a recurrence in the jth time interval for the ith patient, π_{ij}, the data are the values r_{ij}. Data records for which both r_{ij} and s_{ij} are equal to zero are omitted, and so the binomial denominator is unity for each remaining observation. The parameters γ_j are incorporated in the model by fitting terms corresponding to a k-level factor associated with the period of observation, or by including suitable indicator variables as described in Section 3.2. Note that a constant term is not included in the model. The estimates of the β-coefficients in η_i, obtained on fitting this model, can again be interpreted as log-hazard ratios. Also, estimates of the γ_j can be used to obtain estimates of the π_{ij}. This process is illustrated in Example 9.3 below.

Example 9.3 Recurrence of an ulcer

The data on the time to detection of an ulcer recurrence, given in Example 9.1, are now analysed using the method described above. To prepare the data set for analysis using this approach, the two additional variables, *Period* and R, are introduced. The first of these, *Period*, is used to signify the period, and the variable is given the value unity for each observation. The second variable, R, contains the values r_{i1}, $i = 1, 2, \ldots, 43$, and so R is equal to unity if an ulcer is detected in the first period and zero otherwise. For these data, patients 10, 14, 15, 26 and 27 experienced a recurrence in the interval from 0 to 6 months, and so the value of R is unity for these five individuals and zero for the remaining 38.

We then add a second block of data to this set. This block is a duplication of the records for the patients who have not had a recurrence at the six-month mark and for whom the last visit is made after 6 months. There are 38 patients who have not had a recurrence at six months, but three of these, patients 16,

28 and 34, took no further part in the study. The second block of data therefore contains 35 records. The variable *Period* now takes the value 2 for these 35 observations, since they correspond to the second time period. The variable R contains the values r_{i2} for this second block of data. Therefore, R takes the value unity for patients 1, 17, 18, 30, 32 and 37 and zero otherwise, since these are the only six patients who have a detectable recurrence at 12 months.

The combined set of data has $43 + 35 = 78$ rows, and includes the variable *Period*, which defines the period in which an endoscopy is performed ($1 =$ 0–6 months, $2 =$ 6–12 months), and the variable R, which defines the endoscopy result ($0 =$ negative, $1 =$ positive). The value of s_{ij} is unity for all records except those for which $r_{ij} = 1$, when it is zero. The binomial denominators $r_{ij} + s_{ij}$ are therefore equal to unity for each patient, since every patient in the extended data set is at risk of a detectable recurrence. Instead of giving a full listing of the modified data set, the records for the combinations of patient and period, for the first 18 patients, are shown in Table 9.4.

The dependence of the complementary log-log transformation of the probabilities π_{ij} on certain explanatory variables can now be investigated by fitting models to the binary response variable R. Each model includes a two-level factor, *Period*, associated with the period, but no constant term. The term in the model that corresponds to the period effect is γ_j, $j = 1, 2$. The deviances for the models fitted are summarised in Table 9.5.

From this table we see that the effect of adding either *Age* or *Dur* to the model that contains *Period* alone is to reduce the deviance by less than 0.3. There is therefore no evidence that the age of a person or the duration of disease are associated with a recurrence. Adding *Treat* to the model that contains *Period* alone, the reduction in deviance is 0.10 on 1 d.f. This leads us to conclude that there is no significant difference between the two treatments. The treatment effect, after adjusting for the variables *Age* and *Dur*, is of a similar magnitude.

To check whether there are interactions between treatment and the two prognostic factors, we look at the effect of adding the terms *Treat* × *Age* and *Treat* × *Dur* to that model that contains *Period*, *Age* and *Dur*. From Table 9.5, the resulting change in deviance is very small, and so there is no evidence of any such interactions.

In summary, the modelling process shows that π_{ij}, the probability that the ith patient has a recurrence in the jth period, does not depend on the patient's age or the duration of the disease, and, more importantly, does not depend on the treatment group.

To further quantify the treatment effect, consider the model that includes both *Treat* and *Period*. The equation of the fitted model can be written as

$$\log\{-\log(1 - \hat{\pi}_{ij})\} = \hat{\gamma}_j + \hat{\beta}\ Treat_i, \tag{9.6}$$

where γ_j is the effect of the jth period, $j = 1, 2$, and $Treat_i$ is the value of the indicator variable *Treat*, for the ith individual. This variable is zero if that patient is on treatment A and unity otherwise.

Table 9.4 *Modified data on the recurrence of an ulcer in two periods, for the first 18 patients.*

Patient	Age	Duration	Treat-ment	Time of last visit	Result	Period	R
1	48	2	B	7	2	1	0
1	48	2	B	7	2	2	1
2	73	1	B	12	1	1	0
2	73	1	B	12	1	2	0
3	54	1	B	12	1	1	0
3	54	1	B	12	1	2	0
4	58	2	B	12	1	1	0
4	58	2	B	12	1	2	0
5	56	1	A	12	1	1	0
5	56	1	A	12	1	2	0
6	49	2	A	12	1	1	0
6	49	2	A	12	1	2	0
7	71	1	B	12	1	1	0
7	71	1	B	12	1	2	0
8	41	1	A	12	1	1	0
8	41	1	A	12	1	2	0
9	23	1	B	12	1	1	0
9	23	1	B	12	1	2	0
10	37	1	B	5	2	1	1
11	38	1	B	12	1	1	0
11	38	1	B	12	1	2	0
12	76	2	B	12	1	1	0
12	76	2	B	12	1	2	0
13	38	2	A	12	1	1	0
13	38	2	A	12	1	2	0
14	27	1	A	6	2	1	1
15	47	1	B	6	2	1	1
16	54	1	A	6	1	1	0
17	38	1	B	10	2	1	0
17	38	1	B	10	2	2	1
18	27	2	B	7	2	1	0
18	27	2	B	7	2	2	1

The estimated coefficient of *Treat* in this model is 0.195 and the standard error of this estimate is 0.626. The hazard of a recurrence on treatment B at any given time, relative to that on treatment A, is $\exp(0.195) = 1.21$. Since this exceeds unity, there is the suggestion that the risk of recurrence is less on treatment A than on treatment B, but the evidence for this is not statistically significant. The standard error of the estimated hazard ratio is 0.757. For comparison, from Example 9.2, the estimated hazard ratio at 12 months was found to be 1.46, with a standard error of 0.918. These values are very similar to those obtained in this example. Moreover, the results of analyses

Table 9.5 *Deviances on fitting complementary log-log models that do not include a constant to the variable R.*

Terms fitted in model	Deviance	d.f.
Period	62.982	76
Period + Age	62.685	75
Period + Dur	62.979	75
Period + Age + Dur	62.685	74
Period + Age + Dur + Treat	62.566	73
Period + Age + Dur + Treat + Treat × Age	62.278	72
Period + Age + Dur + Treat + Treat × Dur	62.552	72
Period + Treat	62.884	75

that accommodate interval censoring are comparable to those found in Example 9.1, in which the Cox proportional hazards model was used without taking account of the fact that the data are interval-censored.

The model in Equation (9.6) can be used to provide estimates of the π_{ij}. The estimates of the period effects in this model are $\hat{\gamma}_1 = -2.206$, $\hat{\gamma}_2 = -1.794$, and so the estimated probability of a recurrence in the first period, for a patient on treatment A, denoted $\hat{\pi}_{A1}$, is given by

$$\log\{-\log(1 - \hat{\pi}_{A1})\} = \hat{\gamma}_1 + \hat{\beta} \times 0 = -2.206,$$

and from this, $\hat{\pi}_{A1} = 0.104$. Other fitted probabilities can be calculated in a similar manner, and the results of these calculations are shown in Table 9.6. The corresponding observed proportions of individuals with a recurrence for each combination of treatment and period are also displayed. The agreement between the observed and fitted probabilities is good, which indicates that the model is a good fit.

Table 9.6 *Fitted and observed probabilities of an ulcer recurring in the two time periods.*

Period	Treatment A		Treatment B	
	Fitted	Observed	Fitted	Observed
(0, 6)	0.104	0.158	0.125	0.083
(6, 12)	0.153	0.077	0.183	0.227

If desired, probabilities of a recurrence in either period 1 or period 2 could also be estimated. The probability that a patient on treatment A has a recurrence in either period 1 or period 2 is

$$\text{P}\{\text{recurrence in } (0, 6)\} + \text{P}\{\text{recurrence in } (6, 12) \text{ and no recurrence in } (0, 6)\}.$$

The joint probability of a recurrence in $(6, 12)$ and no recurrence in $(0, 6)$ can be expressed as

$$\text{P}\{\text{recurrence in } (6, 12) \mid \text{no recurrence in } (0, 6)\} \times \text{P}\{\text{no recurrence in } (0, 6)\},$$

and so the required probability is estimated by

$$\hat{\pi}_{A1} + \hat{\pi}_{A2}(1 - \hat{\pi}_{A1}) = 0.104 + 0.153 \times 0.896 = 0.241.$$

Similarly, that for treatment B is

$$\hat{\pi}_{B1} + \hat{\pi}_{B2}(1 - \hat{\pi}_{B1}) = 0.125 + 0.183 \times 0.875 = 0.285.$$

This again indicates the superiority of treatment A, but there is insufficient data for this effect to be declared significant.

9.4* Arbitrarily interval-censored survival data

The methods of analysis described in the previous sections may be adopted when different individuals have the same observation times. In this section, we consider a more general form of interval censoring, where the observation times differ between individuals. Then, each individual may have a different time interval in which the event of interest has occurred, and data in this form are referred to as *arbitrarily interval-censored data.* A method for analysing such data, assuming proportional hazards, which is based on a non-linear model for binary data, proposed by Farrington (1996), is now developed.

9.4.1 Modelling arbitrarily interval-censored data

Suppose that the event time for the ith of n individuals is observed to occur in the interval $(a_i, b_i]$, where the use of different types of bracket indicates that the actual event time is greater than a_i, but less than or equal to b_i. In other words, the event has not occurred by time a_i, but has occurred by time b_i, where the values of a_i and b_i may well be different for each individual in the study. We will further suppose that the values of a number of explanatory variables have also been recorded for each individual in the study.

When the values of both a_i and b_i are observed for an individual, the interval-censored observation is said to be *confined.* If the event time for an individual is left-censored at time b_i, so that the event is only known to have occurred some time before b_i, then $a_i = 0$. Similarly, if the event time is right-censored at time a_i, so that the event is only known to have occurred after time a_i, the upper limit of the interval, b_i, is effectively infinite.

The survivor function for the ith individual will be denoted by $S_i(t)$, so that the probability of an event occurring in the interval $(a_i, b_i]$ is $S_i(a_i) - S_i(b_i)$. The likelihood function for the n observations is then

$$\prod_{i=1}^{n} \{S_i(a_i) - S_i(b_i)\}. \tag{9.7}$$

Now suppose that the n observations consist of l left-censored observations, r right-censored observations, and c observations that are confined, so that

$n = l + r + c$. For the purpose of this exposition, we will assume that the data have been arranged in such a way that the first l observations are left-censored ($a_i = 0$), the next r are right-censored ($b_i = \infty$), and the remaining c observations are confined ($0 < a_i < b_i < \infty$). Since $S_i(0) = 1$ and $S_i(\infty) = 0$, the contributions of a left- and right-censored observation to the likelihood function will be $1 - S_i(b_i)$ and $S_i(a_i)$, respectively. Consequently, from Equation (9.7), the overall likelihood function can be written as

$$\prod_{i=1}^{l}\{1 - S_i(b_i)\} \prod_{i=l+1}^{l+r} S_i(a_i) \prod_{i=l+r+1}^{n} \{S_i(a_i) - S_i(b_i)\},$$

and a re-expression of the final product in this function gives

$$\prod_{i=1}^{l}\{1 - S_i(b_i)\} \prod_{i=l+1}^{l+r} S_i(a_i) \prod_{i=l+r+1}^{n} S_i(a_i)\{1 - S_i(b_i)/S_i(a_i)\}. \tag{9.8}$$

We now show that this likelihood is equivalent to that for a corresponding set of $n + c$ independent binary observations, $y_1, y_2, \ldots, y_{n+c}$, where the ith is assumed to be an observation from a Bernoulli distribution with response probability p_i, $i = 1, 2, \ldots, n+c$. The likelihood function for this set of binary data is then

$$\prod_{i=1}^{n+c} p_i^{y_i}(1 - p_i)^{1-y_i}, \tag{9.9}$$

where y_i takes the value 0 or 1, for $i = 1, 2, \ldots, n + c$.

To see the relationship between the response probabilities, p_i, in Expression (9.9), and the values of the survivor function in Expression (9.8), consider first the left-censored observations. Suppose that each of these l observations contributes a binary observation with $y_i = 1$ and $p_i = 1 - S_i(b_i)$, $i = 1, 2, \ldots, l$. The contribution of these l observations to Expression (9.9) is then

$$\prod_{i=1}^{l} p_i = \prod_{i=1}^{l}\{1 - S_i(b_i)\},$$

which is the first term in Expression (9.8). For a right-censored observation, we take $y_i = 0$ and $p_i = 1 - S_i(a_i)$ in Expression (9.9), and the contribution to the likelihood function in Expression (9.9) from r such observations is

$$\prod_{i=l+1}^{l+r} (1 - p_i) = \prod_{i=l+1}^{l+r} S_i(a_i),$$

and this is the second term in Expression (9.8). The situation is a little more complicated for an observation that is confined to the interval $(a_i, b_i]$, since two binary observations are needed to give the required component of Expression (9.8). One of these is taken to have $y_i = 0$, $p_i = 1 - S_i(a_i)$, while the other is such that $y_{c+i} = 1, p_{c+i} = 1-\{S_i(b_i)/S_i(a_i)\}$, for $i = l+r+1, l+r+2, \ldots, n$. Combining these two terms leads to a component of the likelihood in Expression (9.9) of the form

$$\prod_{i=l+r+1}^{n} (1-p_i)p_{c+i},$$

which corresponds to

$$\prod_{i=l+r+1}^{n} S_i(a_i)\{1 - S_i(b_i)/S_i(a_i)\}$$

in Expression (9.8).

This shows that by suitably defining a set of $n+c$ binary observations, with response probabilities expressed in terms of the survivor functions for the three possible forms of interval-censored observation, the likelihood function in Expression (9.9) is equivalent to that in Expression (9.8). Accordingly, maximisation of the log-likelihood function for $n+c$ binary observations is equivalent to maximising the log-likelihood for the interval-censored data.

9.4.2 Proportional hazards model for the survivor function

The next step in the development of a procedure for modelling arbitrarily interval-censored survival data is to construct expressions for the survivor functions that make up the likelihood function in Expression (9.8). A proportional hazards model will be assumed, so that from Equation (9.1),

$$S_i(t) = S_0(t)^{\exp(\boldsymbol{\beta}'\boldsymbol{x}_i)}, \tag{9.10}$$

where $S_0(t)$ is the baseline survivor function and $\boldsymbol{x}_i$ is the vector of values of p explanatory variables for the ith individual, $i = 1, 2, \ldots, n$, with coefficients that make up the vector $\boldsymbol{\beta}$.

The baseline survivor function will be modelled as a step-function, where the steps occur at the k ordered censoring times, $t_{(1)}, t_{(2)}, \ldots, t_{(k)}$, where $0 < t_{(1)} < t_{(2)} < \cdots < t_{(k)}$, which are a subset of the times at which observations are interval-censored. This means that the $t_{(j)}$, $j = 1, 2, \ldots, k$, are a subset of the values of a_i and b_i, $i = 1, 2, \ldots, n$. Exactly how these times are chosen will be described later in Section 9.4.3.

We now define

$$\theta_j = \log \frac{S_0(t_{(j-1)})}{S_0(t_{(j)})},$$

where $t_{(0)} = 0$, so that $\theta_j \geqslant 0$, and at times $t_{(j)}$, we have

$$S_0(t_{(j)}) = e^{-\theta_j} S_0(t_{(j-1)}), \tag{9.11}$$

for $j = 1, 2, \ldots, k$.

Since the first step in the baseline survivor function occurs at $t_{(1)}$, $S_0(t) = 1$ for $0 \leqslant t < t_{(1)}$. From time $t_{(1)}$, the baseline survivor function, using Equation (9.11), has the value $S_0(t_{(1)}) = \exp(-\theta_1)S_0(t_{(0)})$, which, since $t_{(0)} = 0$, means that $S_0(t) = \exp(-\theta_1)$, for $t_{(1)} \leqslant t < t_{(2)}$. Similarly, from time $t_{(2)}$, the survivor function is $\exp(-\theta_2)S_0(t_{(1)})$, that is $S_0(t) = \exp\{-(\theta_1 + \theta_2)\}$, $t_{(2)} \leqslant t < t_{(3)}$, and so on, until $S_0(t) = \exp\{-(\theta_1 + \theta_2 + \cdots + \theta_k)\}$, $t \geqslant t_{(k)}$. Consequently,

$$S_0(t) = \exp\left(-\sum_{r=1}^{j} \theta_r\right), \tag{9.12}$$

for $t_{(j)} \leqslant t < t_{(j+1)}$, and so the baseline survivor function, at any time t_i, is given by

$$S_0(t_i) = \exp\left(-\sum_{j=1}^{k} \theta_j\, d_{ij}\right), \tag{9.13}$$

where

$$d_{ij} = \begin{cases} 1 & \text{if } t_{(j)} \leqslant t_i, \\ 0 & \text{if } t_{(j)} > t_i, \end{cases}$$

for $j = 1, 2, \ldots, k$. The quantities d_{ij} will be taken to be the values of k indicator variables, $D_1, D_2, \ldots, D_k$, for the ith observation in the augmented data set. Note that the values of the D_j, $j = 1, 2, \ldots, k$, will differ at each observation time, t_i.

Combining the results in Equations (9.10) and (9.13), the survivor function for the ith individual, at times a_i, b_i, can now be obtained. In particular,

$$S_i(a_i) = S_0(a_i)^{\exp(\boldsymbol{\beta}'\boldsymbol{x}_i)} = \left\{\exp\left(-\sum\nolimits_{j=1}^{k} \theta_j\, d_{ij}\right)\right\}^{\exp(\boldsymbol{\beta}'\boldsymbol{x}_i)},$$

which can be expressed in the form

$$S_i(a_i) = \exp\left\{-\exp(\boldsymbol{\beta}'\boldsymbol{x}_i)\sum\nolimits_{j=1}^{k} \theta_j\, d_{ij}\right\},$$

where $d_{ij} = 1$ if $t_{(j)} \leqslant a_i$, and $d_{ij} = 0$, otherwise. An expression for $S_i(b_i)$ can be obtained in a similar way, leading to

$$S_i(b_i) = \exp\left\{-\exp(\boldsymbol{\beta}'\boldsymbol{x}_i)\sum\nolimits_{j=1}^{k} \theta_j\, d_{ij}\right\},$$

where $d_{ij} = 1$ if $t_{(j)} \leqslant b_i$, and $d_{ij} = 0$, otherwise.

From these expressions for $S_i(a_i)$ and $S_i(b_i)$, the response probabilities, p_i, used in Expression (9.9), can be expressed in terms of the unknown parameters $\theta_1, \theta_2, \ldots, \theta_k$, and the unknown coefficients of the p explanatory variables in the model, $\beta_1, \beta_2, \ldots, \beta_p$. As in Section 9.4.1, for a left-censored observation, $p_i = 1 - S_i(b_i)$, and for a right-censored observation, $p_i = 1 - S_i(a_i)$. In the case of a confined observation, $p_i = 1 - S_i(a_i)$ for one of the two binary observations. For the other,

$$\begin{aligned} p_{c+i} &= 1 - S_i(b_i)/S_i(a_i), \\ &= 1 - \frac{\exp\left\{-\exp(\boldsymbol{\beta}'\boldsymbol{x}_i)\sum_{j=1}^{k}\theta_j\, d_{1ij}\right\}}{\exp\left\{-\exp(\boldsymbol{\beta}'\boldsymbol{x}_i)\sum_{j=1}^{k}\theta_j\, d_{2ij}\right\}}, \end{aligned}$$

where the values d_{1ij} in the numerator are equal to unity if $t_{(j)} \leqslant b_i$, and zero otherwise, and the values d_{2ij} in the denominator are equal to unity if $t_{(j)} \leqslant a_i$, and zero otherwise. Consequently, the θ-terms in the numerator for which $t_{(j)} \leqslant a_i$ cancel with those in the denominator, and this leaves

$$p_{c+i} = 1 - \exp\left\{-\exp(\boldsymbol{\beta}'\boldsymbol{x}_i)\sum_{j=1}^{k}\theta_j\, d_{ij}\right\},$$

where here $d_{ij} = 1$ if $a_i < t_{(j)} \leqslant b_i$.

It then follows that in each case, the response probability can be expressed in the form

$$p_i = 1 - \exp\left\{-\exp(\boldsymbol{\beta}'\boldsymbol{x}_i)\sum_{j=1}^{k}\theta_j\, d_{ij}\right\}, \tag{9.14}$$

where

$$d_{ij} = \begin{cases} 1 & \text{if } t_{(j)} \text{ is in the interval } A_i, \\ 0 & \text{otherwise,} \end{cases}$$

for $j = 1, 2, \ldots, k$, and the intervals A_i are as shown in Table 9.7.

Table 9.7 *Definition of intervals, A_i, used for constructing indicator variables.*

Type of observation	Value of y_i	Interval, A_i
Left-censored	1	$(0, b_i]$, $i = 1, 2, \ldots, l$
Right-censored	0	$(0, a_i]$, $i = l+1, l+2, \ldots, l+r$
Confined	0	$(0, a_i]$, $i = l+r+1, l+r+2, \ldots, n$
	1	$(a_{i-c}, b_{i-c}]$, $i = n+1, n+2, \ldots, n+c$

This leads to a non-linear model for a set of binary response variables, with values y_i, and corresponding response probabilities p_i, found from Equation (9.14), for $i = 1, 2, \ldots, n+c$. The model contains $k+p$ unknown parameters, namely $\theta_1, \theta_2, \ldots, \theta_k$ and $\beta_1, \beta_2, \ldots, \beta_p$. This model is known as a *generalised non-linear model*, since it is not possible to express a simple function of p_i as a linear combination of the unknown parameters, except in the case where there are no explanatory variables in the model. The model can be fitted using computer software for generalised non-linear modelling. Note that in the fitting process, the θ-parameters should be constrained to be non-negative.

After fitting a model, the value of the statistic $-2\log\hat{L}$ can be found, and this may be used to compare alternative models in the usual manner. The general procedure is to fit the k terms involving the θ-parameters, and to then examine the effect of adding and subtracting the explanatory variables in the data set.

Once an appropriate model has been found, the baseline survivor function in Equation (9.12) is estimated using

$$\hat{S}_0(t) = \exp\left(-\sum_{r=1}^{j}\hat{\theta}_r\right), \tag{9.15}$$

for $t_{(j)} \leqslant t < t_{(j+1)}$, $j = 1, 2, \ldots, k$, where $t_{(k+1)} = \infty$, and $\hat{\theta}_j$ is the estimated value of θ_j. The estimated survivor function for the ith individual follows from

$$\begin{aligned}\hat{S}_i(t) &= \hat{S}_0(t)^{\exp(\hat{\boldsymbol{\beta}}'\boldsymbol{x}_i)}\\ &= \exp\left\{-\exp(\hat{\boldsymbol{\beta}}'\boldsymbol{x}_i)\sum\nolimits_{r=1}^{j}\hat{\theta}_r\right\},\end{aligned} \tag{9.16}$$

for $i = 1, 2, \ldots, n$, where $\hat{\boldsymbol{\beta}}$ is the vector of estimated coefficients of the explanatory variables. Furthermore, the estimates of the β-parameters are interpretable as log-hazard ratios, in the usual manner, and their standard errors, produced during the fitting process, can be used to obtain confidence limits.

9.4.3 Choice of the step times

We have seen that the baseline survivor function is assumed to have steps at times $t_{(j)}$, $j = 1, 2, \ldots, k$, which are a subset of the observed censoring times, a_i and b_i, $i = 1, 2, \ldots, n$. It might be considered to be desirable for the $t_{(j)}$ to be formed from all distinct censoring times, that is all the unique values of a_i and b_i. However, this will generally lead to the introduction of far too many θ-parameters in the non-linear model. Instead, a subset of the available times is chosen.

Each interval used in the binary data model, and denoted by A_i in the preceding section, must include at least one of the times $t_{(j)}$. If this is the case, at least one of the values of d_{ij} in Equation (9.14) will be equal to unity and hence the term $\sum_{j=1}^{k}\theta_j\, d_{ij}$ will be greater than zero. Suppose that the interval A_i is $(u_i, v_i]$. This requirement is then achieved by taking $t_{(1)}$ to be the smallest of the values of v_i, $t_{(2)}$ to be the smallest v_i such that $u_i \geqslant t_{(1)}$, $t_{(3)}$ to be the smallest v_i such that $u_i \geqslant t_{(2)}$, and so on, until $t_{(k)}$ is the smallest value of v_i such that $u_i \geqslant t_{(k-1)}$.

Once this subset of k times has been identified, the model can be fitted. Models containing explanatory variables are fitted, and for each model the estimates of the k θ-parameters and the relevant β-parameters are found. The fitting process will lead to a value of the $-2\log\hat{L}$ statistic, and these values can be compared for models with the same number of θ-parameters, but different explanatory variables, in the usual way.

Sometimes, it may be desirable to increase the number of steps in the estimated baseline hazard function, by the addition of some of the remaining censoring times. This entails adding a new θ-parameter for each additional time point. One way of doing this is to fit the minimal set of censoring times, and to then add each additional time point in turn, for the full set of explanatory variables. The time that leads to the biggest reduction in the value of $-2\log\hat{L}$ is then added to the minimal set. All remaining times are then added one by one, and again that which reduces $-2\log\hat{L}$ the most is added to the set. This process may be continued until the reduction on adding an additional θ-parameter ceases to be significant at some chosen level, and so long as all the estimated θ-parameters remain positive.

It is important to note that this modelling procedure is only valid if the set of possible censoring times is finite, that is, it does not increase with the number of observations. Otherwise, the number of θ's increases indefinitely and asymptotic results used in comparing models will no longer be valid.

This procedure for modelling arbitrarily interval-censored data is now illustrated.

Example 9.4 Occurrence of breast retraction

In the treatment of early breast cancer, a tumourectomy, followed by radiation therapy, may be used as an alternative to mastectomy. Chemotherapy may also be used in conjunction with the radiotherapy in order to enhance its effect, but there is evidence that this adjuvant chemotherapy increases the effect of the radiation on normal tissue. This in turn leads to breast retraction, which has a negative impact on the appearance of the breast. In a retrospective study to assess the effect of this type of treatment on breast cosmesis, 46 women who had been treated with radiotherapy alone were compared with 48 who had received a combination of radiotherapy and chemotherapy. Patients were observed every 4 to 6 months, but less frequently as their recovery progressed. On these occasions, the cosmetic effect of the treatment was monitored, with the extent of breast retraction being measured on a four-point scale: none, minimal, moderate, severe. The event of interest was the time in months to the first appearance of moderate or severe retraction. The exact time of occurrence of breast retraction will be unknown, and the only information available will concern whether or not retraction is identified when a patient visits the clinic. Moreover, since the visit times were not the same for each patient, and a number of patients failed to keep appointments, the data are regarded as arbitrarily interval-censored. The data obtained in this study were included in Finkelstein and Wolfe (1985), and are given in Table 9.8.

In this data set, there are five patients for whom breast retraction had occurred before the first visit. For each of these patients, the start of the interval is set to zero, that is $a_i = 0$, and the observed times are left-censored, so that $l = 5$. There are 38 patients who had not experienced retraction by

Table 9.8 *Data on the time in months to breast retraction in patients with breast cancer.*

Radiotherapy			Radiotherapy and Chemotherapy		
(45, ∗]	(25, 37]	(37, ∗]	(8, 12]	(0, 5]	(30, 34]
(6, 10]	(46, ∗]	(0, 5]	(0, 22]	(5, 8]	(13, ∗]
(0, 7]	(26, 40]	(18, ∗]	(24, 31]	(12, 20]	(10, 17]
(46, ∗]	(46, ∗]	(24, ∗]	(17, 27]	(11, ∗]	(8, 21]
(46, ∗]	(27, 34]	(36, ∗]	(17, 23]	(33, 40]	(4, 9]
(7, 16]	(36, 44]	(5, 11]	(24, 30]	(31, ∗]	(11, ∗]
(17, ∗]	(46, ∗]	(19, 35]	(16, 24]	(13, 39]	(14, 19]
(7, 14]	(36, 48]	(17, 25]	(13, ∗]	(19, 32]	(4, 8]
(37, 44]	(37, ∗]	(24, ∗]	(11, 13]	(34, ∗]	(34, ∗]
(0, 8]	(40, ∗]	(32, ∗]	(16, 20]	(13, ∗]	(30, 36]
(4, 11]	(17, 25]	(33, ∗]	(18, 25]	(16, 24]	(18, 24]
(15, ∗]	(46, ∗]	(19, 26]	(17, 26]	(35, ∗]	(16, 60]
(11, 15]	(11, 18]	(37, ∗]	(32, ∗]	(15, 22]	(35, 39]
(22, ∗]	(38, ∗]	(34, ∗]	(23, ∗]	(11, 17]	(21, ∗]
(46, ∗]	(5, 12]	(36, ∗]	(44, 48]	(22, 32]	(11, 20]
(46, ∗]			(14, 17]	(10, 35]	(48, ∗]

their final visit. For these patients, the upper limit of the time interval is shown as an asterisk (∗) in Table 9.8. The observations for these patients are therefore right-censored and so $r = 38$. The remaining $c = 51$ patients experience breast retraction within confined time intervals, and the total number of observations is $n = l + c + r = 94$.

The first step in fitting a model to these arbitrarily interval-censored data is to expand the data set by adding a further 51 lines of data, repeating that for the patients whose intervals are confined, so that the revised database has $n + c = 145$ observations. The values, y_i, of the binary response variable, Y, are then added. These are such that $Y = 1$ for a left-censored observation, and $Y = 0$ for a right-censored observation. For confined observations, where the data are duplicated, one of the pairs of observations has $Y = 0$ and the other $Y = 1$. The treatment effect will be represented by the value of a variable labelled *Treat*, which will be zero for a patient on radiotherapy and unity for a patient on radiotherapy and chemotherapy. For illustration, the values of the binary response variable, Y, are shown for the first three patient treated with radiotherapy alone, in Table 9.9.

Table 9.9 *Augmented data set for the first three patients on radiotherapy.*

Patient	A	B	U	V	*Treat*	Y
1	45	∗	0	45	0	0
2	6	10	0	6	0	0
2	6	10	6	10	0	1
3	0	7	0	7	0	1

In this table, the variables A and B refer to the times of the start and end of each interval, and so their values are a_i, b_i and the variables U and V contain the values of u_i, v_i that form the limits of the intervals, A_i, in the binary data model.

We now determine the time points, $t_{(j)}$, that are to be used in calculating the baseline survivor function, using the procedure described in Section 9.4.3. The first of these is the smallest of the values v_i, which form the variable V in the data set. This is found for the observation $(0, 4]$, for which $V = 4$, so that $t_{(1)} = 4$. The smallest value of V for which $U \geqslant 4$ occurs for the observation $(4, 8]$, and so $t_{(2)} = 8$. Next, the smallest value of V with $U \geqslant 8$ occurs for the observation $(8, 12]$, giving $t_{(3)} = 12$. There are six other times found in this way, namely 17, 23, 30, 34, 39 and 48, and so the minimal subset of times has $k = 9$ in this example.

Variables with values d_{ij}, that correspond to each of the k censoring times, $t_{(j)}$, are now added to the database that has 145 records. Since $k = 9$ in this case, nine variables, $D_1, D_2, \ldots, D_9$, are introduced, where the values of D_j, $j = 1, 2, \ldots, 9$, are d_{ij}, for $i = 1, 2, \ldots, 145$. These values are such that $d_{ij} = 1$ if $u_i < t_{(j)} \leqslant v_i$, and zero otherwise, and so they can straightforwardly be obtained from the variables U and V in Table 9.9. The values of $D_1, D_2, \ldots, D_9$, for the three patients included in Table 9.9, are shown in Table 9.10.

Table 9.10 *Database for binary data analysis, for the first three patients on radiotherapy.*

Patient	*Treat*	Y	D_1	D_2	D_3	D_4	D_5	D_6	D_7	D_8	D_9
1	0	0	1	1	1	1	1	1	1	1	0
2	0	0	1	0	0	0	0	0	0	0	0
2	0	1	0	1	0	0	0	0	0	0	0
3	0	1	1	0	0	0	0	0	0	0	0

We now have the database to which a non-linear model for the binary response data in Y is fitted. The model is such that we take Y to have a Bernoulli distribution with response probability as given in Equation (9.14), that is a binomial distribution with parameters $1, p_i$. Here, the SAS procedure `proc nlmixed` has been used to fit the non-linear model to the binary data.

On fitting the null model, that is the model that contains all 9 D-variables, but not the treatment effect, the value of the statistic $-2 \log \hat{L}$ is 285.417. On adding *Treat* to the model, the value of $-2 \log \hat{L}$ is reduced to 276.983. This reduction of 8.43 on 1 d.f. is significant at the 1% level ($P = 0.0037$), and so we conclude that the interval-censored data do provide strong evidence of a treatment effect. The estimated coefficient of *Treat* is 0.8212, with a standard error of 0.2881. The corresponding hazard ratio for a patient on the combination of radiotherapy and chemotherapy, relative to a patient on radiotherapy alone, is exp(0.8212) = 2.27. The interpretation of this is that patients on the combined treatment have just over twice the risk of breast retraction, compared to patients on radiotherapy. A 95% confidence interval for the corresponding true hazard ratio has limits $\exp(0.8212 \pm 1.96 \times 0.2881)$, which leads to the interval $(1.29, 4.00)$.

The minimal subset of times at which the estimated baseline survivor function is estimated can be enlarged by adding additional censoring times from the data set. However, there are no additional times that lead to a significant reduction in the value of the $-2 \log \hat{L}$ statistic, with the estimated θ-parameters remaining positive.

The estimated values of the coefficients of the D-variables are the values $\hat{\theta}_j$, for $j = 1, 2, \ldots, 9$, and these can be used to provide an estimate of the survivor function for the two treatment groups. Equation (9.15) gives the form of the estimated baseline survivor function, which is the estimated survivor function for the patients on radiotherapy alone. The corresponding estimate for the patients who receive adjuvant chemotherapy is obtained using Equation (9.16), and is just $\{\hat{S}_0(t_{(j)})\}^{\exp(\hat{\beta})}$, with $\hat{\beta} = 0.8212$. On fitting the model that contains the treatment effect and the 9 D-variables, the estimated values of θ_j, for $j = 1, 2, \ldots, 9$, are 0.0223, 0.0603, 0.0524, 0.0989, 0.1620, 0.0743, 0.1098, 0.2633 and 0.4713, respectively. From these values, the baseline survivor function, at the times $t_{(j)}$, $j = 1, 2, \ldots, 9$, can be estimated, and this estimate is given as $\hat{S}_0(t_{(j)})$ in Table 9.11. Also given in this table is the estimated survivor function for patients on the combined treatment, denoted $\hat{S}_1(t_{(j)})$.

Table 9.11 *Estimated survivor functions for a patient on radiotherapy alone, $\hat{S}_0(t)$, and adjuvant chemotherapy, $\hat{S}_1(t)$.*

Time interval	$\hat{S}_0(t)$	$\hat{S}_1(t)$
0–	1.000	1.000
4–	0.978	0.951
8–	0.921	0.829
12–	0.874	0.736
17–	0.791	0.588
23–	0.673	0.407
30–	0.625	0.343
34–	0.560	0.268
39–	0.430	0.147
48–	0.269	0.050

The survivor functions for the two groups of patients are shown in Figure 9.1. From the estimated survivor functions, the median time to breast retraction for patients on radiotherapy is estimated to be 39 months, while that for patients who received adjuvant chemotherapy is 23 months. More precise estimates of these median times could be obtained if a greater number of censoring times were used in the analysis.

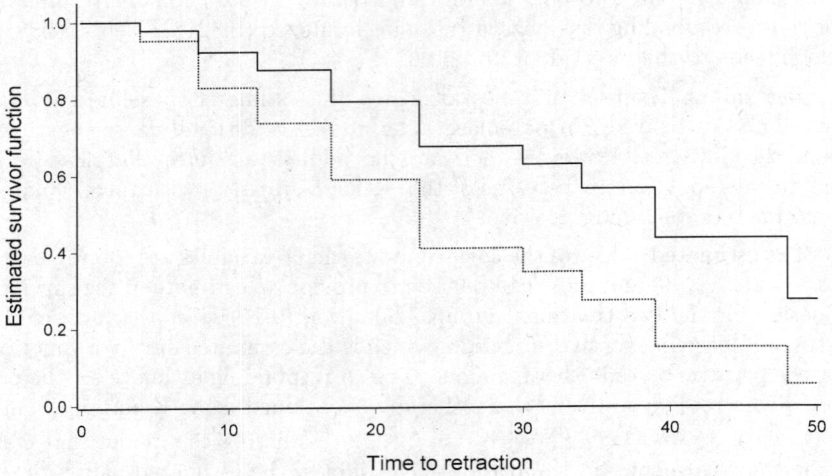

Figure 9.1 *Estimated survivor functions for a patient on radiotherapy (—) and the combination of radiotherapy and chemotherapy (······).*

9.5 Parametric models for interval-censored data

The methods for modelling interval-censored data that have been described in previous sections are based on the Cox proportional hazards model. In fact, it is much more straightforward to model such data assuming a parametric model for the survival times. In Section 9.4, the likelihood function for n arbitrarily interval-censored observations consisting of l that are left-censored at time a_i, r that are right-censored at b_i, and c that are confined to the interval (a_i, b_i), was given as

$$\prod_{i=1}^{l}\{1 - S_i(b_i)\} \prod_{i=l+1}^{l+r} S_i(a_i) \prod_{i=l+r+1}^{n} \{S_i(a_i) - S_i(b_i)\}. \tag{9.17}$$

If a parametric model for the survival times is assumed, then $S_i(t)$ has a fully parametric form. For example, if the survival times have a Weibull distribution with scale parameter λ and shape parameter γ, from Equation (5.37) in Section 5.6 of Chapter 5, the survivor function for the ith individual is

$$S_i(t) = \exp\left\{-\exp(\boldsymbol{\beta}'\boldsymbol{x}_i)\lambda t^{\gamma}\right\},$$

where $\boldsymbol{x}_i$ is the vector of values of explanatory variables for that individual, with coefficients $\boldsymbol{\beta}$. Alternatively, the accelerated failure time form of the survivor function, given in Equation (6.16) of Section 6.5 of Chapter 6, may be used. The Weibull survivor function leads to expressions for the survivor functions in Expression (9.17), for any values of a_i and b_i. The corresponding log-likelihood function can then be maximised with respect to the parameters λ, γ and the β's. No new principles are involved. The same procedure can be adopted for any other parametric model described in Chapter 6.

In some situations, the database may be a combination of censored and uncensored observations. The likelihood function in Expression (9.17) may then be further extended to allow for the uncensored observations. This is achieved by including an additional factor of the form $\prod_i f(t_i)$, which is the product of the density functions at the event times, over the uncensored observations. A number of software packages include facilities for the parametric modelling of interval-censored data.

Example 9.5 Occurrence of breast retraction
The interval-censored data on the times to breast retraction in women being treated for breast cancer, given in Example 9.4, are now used to illustrate parametric modelling for interval-censored data.

If a common Weibull distribution is assumed for the data in both treatment groups, the value of $-2\log\hat{L}$ is 297.585. If the treatment effect is added to this model, and the assumption of proportional hazards is made, so that the shape parameter is constant, the value of $-2\log\hat{L}$ reduces to 286.642. This reduction of 10.943 on 1 d.f. is highly significant ($P = 0.001$). Comparing this with the results of the analysis in Example 9.4, we find that the significance of the treatment effect is a little greater under the assumed Weibull model. Furthermore, the estimated hazard ratio for a patient on radiotherapy with adjuvant chemotherapy, relative to a patient on radiotherapy alone, is 2.50, and a corresponding 95% confidence interval is $(1.44, 4.35)$. These values do not differ much from those found in Example 9.4.

9.6 Discussion

In many situations, the method for analysing interval-censored survival data that has been presented in Section 9.4, or the fully parametric approach of Section 9.5, will be the most appropriate. Even when studies are designed to be such that the examination times are the same for each patient in the study, missed, postponed or cancelled appointments may lead to observation times that do differ across the patients. In this case, and for studies where this is a natural feature, methods for handling arbitrarily interval-censored data will be required.

When the observation times are the same for each patient, the method for analysing interval-censored data that has been presented in Section 9.3 will generally be the most suitable. However, this approach is not optimal, since recurrences detected between scheduled examinations, that is, interval-detected recurrences, are only counted at the next examination time. If the intervals between successive examination times are not too large, the difference between the results of an analysis based on the model in Section 9.3, and one that uses the actual times of interval-detected recurrences, will be negligible.

In fact, if the number of intervals is not too small, and the time between successive examinations not too large, the results will not be too different from an analysis that assumes the recurrence times to be continuous, outlined in Section 9.1.

As mentioned earlier, the model described in Section 9.3 only requires hazards to be proportional at scheduled screening times. This means that the model is useful when the hazards are not necessarily proportional between screening times. Furthermore, the model could be relevant in situations where although actual survival times are available, the hazards can only be taken to be proportional at specific times. On the other hand, the method for analysing arbitrarily interval-censored data in Section 9.4, requires hazards to be proportional at each of the times used in constructing the baseline survivor function, which is more restrictive. Further comments on methods for analysing survival data where hazards are non-proportional are included in Chapter 11.

9.7 Further reading

Much of Sections 9.1 to 9.3 of this chapter are based on the summary of methods for processing interval-censored survival data given by Whitehead (1989). The approach described in Section 9.3 is based on Prentice and Gloeckler (1978). A method for fitting the proportional hazards model to interval-censored data was proposed by Finkelstein (1986), but the method for modelling arbitrarily interval-censored data in Section 9.4 is due to Farrington (1996), who also develops additive and multiplicative models for such data.

A number of approaches to the analysis of interval-censored data involve the analysis of binary observations. Collett (2003) describes a model-based approach to the analysis of binary data. Other books that include material on the analysis of binary data include Hosmer and Lemeshow (2000), Dobson (2001) and Morgan (1992).

The use of the complementary log-log transformation in the analysis of interval-censored data was described by Thompson (1981). Becker and Melbye (1991) show how a log-linear model can be used to obtain an estimate of the survivor function from interval-censored data, assuming a constant hazard in each interval.

There are a number of other approaches to the analysis of interval-censored data, some of which are described in the tutorial provided by Lindsey and Ryan (1998). Lindsey (1998) reviews the use of parametric models for the analysis of interval-censored data. Pan (2000) suggests using multiple imputation, based on the approximate Bayesian bootstrap, to impute values for censored observations. Farrington (2000) provides a comprehensive account of diagnostic methods for use with proportional hazards models for interval-censored data.

Chapter 10

Frailty models

In modelling survival data, we attempt to explain observed variation in times to events such as death by differences in the values of certain explanatory variables that have been recorded for each individual in a study. However, even after allowing for the effects of such variables, there will still be variation in their observed survival times. Some individuals may have a greater hazard of death than others, and are therefore likely to die sooner. They may be described as being more *frail*, and variation in survival times can be explained by variability in this *frailty effect* across individuals.

Situations where the survival times amongst groups of individuals in a study are not independent are frequently encountered. The survival times of individuals within the same group will then tend to be more similar than they would be for individuals from different groups. This effect can then be modelled by assuming that the individuals within a group share the same frailty. Since the frailty is common to all individuals within a group, a degree of dependence between the survival times of individuals within the group is introduced. Consequently, models with *shared frailty* can be used in modelling survival data where some association between the event times is anticipated, as in studies involving groups of individuals that share a common feature, or when an individual experiences repeated times to an event. Such models are described in this chapter.

10.1 Introduction to frailty

Variation in survival times is almost always found amongst individuals in a study. Even when a number of individuals share the same values of demographic variables such as age and gender, or the same values of other explanatory variables that have been measured, their survival times will generally be different. These differences may be explained by the fact that certain variables that influence survival were not measured, or that an individual's survival time depends on variables that it was not possible to measure. There may be many such variables and our knowledge of these may be limited to the extent that we simply do not know what the variables are that might explain this variability.

To illustrate, consider the survival times of patients who have been diagnosed with a life-threatening cancer. Patient survival time following diagnosis will depend on many factors, including the type of cancer and stage of the tumour, characteristics of the patient such as their age, weight and lifestyle, and the manner in which the cancer is treated. A group of patients who have the same values of each measured explanatory variable may nevertheless be observed to have different survival times. This variation or *heterogeneity* between individuals may arise because some individuals are not as strong as others in ways that cannot be summarised in terms of a relatively small number of known variables. Indeed, we can never aspire to know what all the factors are that may have an effect on the survival of cancer patients, let alone be able to measure them, but we can take account of them in a modelling process.

Variation between the survival times of a group of individuals can be described in terms of some individuals being more frail than others. Those who have higher values of a frailty term tend to die sooner than those who are less frail. However, the extent of an individual's frailty cannot be measured directly; if it could, we might attempt to include it in a model for survival times. Instead, we only observe the impact that the frailty effects have on the observable survival times.

10.1.1 Random effects

In the models described in earlier chapters, the effects corresponding to factors of interest have always been assumed to be fixed. The possible values of a *fixed effect* do not vary, and they are assumed to be measured without error. For example, the factor associated with gender has two distinct levels, male and female, that will not change from study to study, and it will often be of interest to summarise outcome differences between the two genders. On the other hand, a *random effect* is assumed to have levels drawn from a population of possible values, where the actual levels are representative of that population. As an example, in a multicentre clinical trial, the centres adopted might be considered to be drawn from a larger number of possible centres. We would then model centre variation using a random effect, and there would be little interest in comparing outcomes between particular centres.

Random effects are assumed to be observations on a random variable that has some underlying probability distribution, with the variance of this distribution used to summarise the extent of differences in their values. Such effects typically have many possible values and it is unrealistic to represent differences between them using fixed effects, as this would introduce a large number of unknown parameters into a model. By taking them to be random effects, there is just one parameter to estimate, namely the variance of their assumed underlying distribution.

10.1.2 Individual frailty

Since the unknown frailty values attributed to individuals in a study are essentially drawn from a large number of possible values, we take frailty to be a random effect. In situations where the variance of the underlying distribution of random effects is small, the frailty effects will not differ much and the effect on inferences will be negligible. However, if the frailty variance is large, the observed survival times of individuals may differ markedly, even after allowing for the effects of other potential explanatory variables.

In the presence of frailty, individuals who are more frail will tend to die earlier. This means that at any point in time when the survival times of a sample of individuals are observed, those who are still alive will be less frail than the corresponding population from which the sample has been drawn. Since frailty is acting as a *selection effect*, there are consequences for what can actually be observed. For example, if each individual has a constant hazard of death, and frailty effects are present, the more frail individuals will die earlier, while those who are less frail will survive longer. The observed hazard function may therefore appear to decline over time. As an illustration of this, consider a group of individuals who have experienced a non-fatal heart attack. For such individuals, the hazard of death is generally observed to decline with time, and there are two possible reasons for this. First, the individuals may simply adjust to any damage to the heart that has been caused by the heart attack, so that the underlying hazard of death does decline. Alternatively, the hazard of death may be constant, but the observed decrease in the hazard may be due to frailty; higher risk individuals die earlier, so that at any time, the individuals who remain alive are those that are less frail. Data on the survival times cannot be used to distinguish between these two possible explanations for the apparent decline in the hazard of death. By the same token, when allowance is made for frailty effects, estimated hazard ratios and their associated standard errors may be quite different from the values obtained when frailty effects are ignored. This feature will be illustrated in Section 10.3.

10.1.3 Shared frailty

Models that take account of individual levels of frailty can be used to assess how the values of unmeasured variables may affect survival. However, the notion of frailty is more widely used in situations where a number of individuals share something in common. In a multicentre study, for example, the survival experience of individuals from the same centre may be more similar than that for individuals from different centres. This could be because of different clinical teams in the different centres, or different nursing practices across the centres. Similarly, in an animal experiment, animals from the same litter will be more alike than animals from different litters, because of genetic and environmental influences. Their survival times will therefore be correlated, and one way of modelling this association between survival times is to assume that all the individuals within a group share the same frailty. In paired organ studies involving eyes, ears or kidneys, where the time to some event is recorded on each organ within the pair, frailty might be included in a model to allow for any association between the pairs of observed event times. Shared frailty models therefore provide a method for modelling survival data when the survival times are not independent.

Some studies lead to repeated or recurrent event times within an individual. Examples of this type of situation include studies on the times between successive adverse events, such as migraine or nausea, the times to the failure of tooth fillings in an individual, and times to the failure of transplanted kidneys in patients that receive more than one transplant. Here again, the event times within an individual may not be independent, and to model this we can assume that the frailty is the same for each of these event times. The concept of a shared frailty can therefore be extended to situations where there are repeated events within an individual.

10.2 Modelling individual frailty

Variation between the survival times of individuals can be modelled by supposing that each person has his or her own value of a frailty. This frailty term is assumed to act multiplicatively on the hazard of death of an individual. Those with a frailty greater than unity will have increased hazard, while those who have a frailty less than unity will have a reduced hazard of the event occurring.

Consider a proportional hazards model for the hazard of an event occurring at some time t, in an individual with a hazard function that depends on the values of p explanatory variables $X_1, X_2, \ldots, X_p$, and on some unknown baseline hazard function $h_0(t)$. The hazard function for the ith of n individuals is then

$$h_i(t) = \exp(\boldsymbol{\beta}'\boldsymbol{x}_i)h_0(t), \qquad (10.1)$$

where $\boldsymbol{x}_i$ is the vector of values of the explanatory variables for the ith individual, and $\boldsymbol{\beta}$ is the vector of their unknown coefficients $\beta_1, \beta_2, \ldots, \beta_p$. The baseline hazard $h_0(t)$ may be unspecified as in the Cox regression model (Chapter 3) or a parametric function of t, such as a Weibull model (Chapters 5, 6).

We now introduce a multiplicative frailty term, z_i, and write

$$h_i(t) = z_i \exp(\boldsymbol{\beta}'\boldsymbol{x}_i)h_0(t). \qquad (10.2)$$

The frailty term z_i cannot be negative, and the greater the frailty, the greater is the hazard of the event occurring. A value of $z_i = 1$ brings us back to the standard model of Equation (10.1), corresponding to the situation where there are no frailty effects. Values of z_i between 0 and 1 correspond to situations where the hazard is less than that in the underlying proportional hazards model, and occur when individuals have increased fortitude. Differences in the values of the z_i across the sample of n individuals will then represent variation in the hazard of death at any given time due to frailty effects.

It is generally more convenient to work with an alternative representation of the frailty effect, obtained by setting $z_i = \exp(u_i)$. The model in Equation (10.2) can then be written

$$h_i(t) = \exp(\boldsymbol{\beta}'\boldsymbol{x}_i + u_i)h_0(t). \qquad (10.3)$$

In this model, $u_i = \log z_i$ is a *random effect* in the linear component of the proportional hazards model. Note that whereas a frailty z_i cannot be negative, u_i can take any value, positive or negative, and $u_i = 0$ corresponds to the case where $z_i = 1$ and there is no frailty. In Equation (10.3), the linear component of the proportional hazards model has been extended to include a random effect, and this part of the model for survival times is now akin to mixed models used in other areas of general and generalised linear modelling.

The u_i in Equation (10.3) are regarded as the observed values, or *realisations*, of n independent and identically distributed random variables U_i, $i = 1, 2, \ldots, n$, where each random variable, U_i, is assumed to have a common probability distribution. So although the individual frailties across a group of individuals may all be different, they are drawn from the same underlying probability distribution.

Example 10.1 Prognosis for women with breast cancer

The data in Example 1.2 of Chapter 1 on the survival times of two groups of women, with tumours that were negatively or positively stained, shows that there is variability in the survival times of the women within each group. In the negatively stained group, actual survival times range from 23 to beyond 224 months, while in the positively stained group, they range from 5 to over 225 months. To summarise these data, a Weibull proportional hazards model containing a factor associated with positive or negative staining is fitted, as in Example 5.6. The estimated baseline hazard function is $\hat{h}_0(t) = \hat{\lambda}\hat{\gamma}t^{\hat{\gamma}-1}$, where $\hat{\lambda} = 0.00414$ and $\hat{\gamma} = 0.937$. The corresponding estimated survivor function for the ith woman, $i = 1, 2, \ldots, 45$, is given by

$$\hat{S}_i(t) = \exp\{-\exp(\hat{\beta}x_i)\hat{\lambda}t^{\hat{\gamma}}\},$$

using Equation (5.37) of Chapter 5, where $x_i = 0$ for a woman with negative staining and $x_i = 1$ for one with positive staining, and $\hat{\beta} = 0.934$. The corresponding hazard ratio for a woman with a positively stained tumour, relative to one whose tumour is negatively stained, is 2.545, with a 95% confidence interval of (0.93, 6.98). The fitted Weibull survivor functions are shown in Figure 10.1, superimposed on the Kaplan-Meier estimate of the survivor functions. The Weibull model does not appear to be a very good fit to the survival times of women with positively stained tumours.

In this figure, the data have been summarised in just two curves. However, the introduction of frailty would lead to separate estimated survivor functions for each woman, and we will return to this in Example 10.2.

10.2.1 Frailty distributions*

In the model of Equation (10.3), it is common to assume that the random variables U_i, $i = 1, 2, \ldots, n$, that are associated with the random effects, have a normal distribution with zero mean and common variance σ_u^2. If

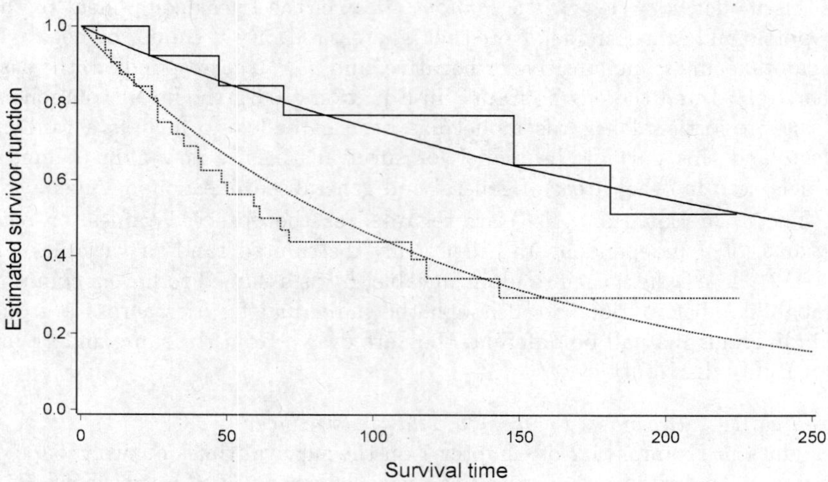

Figure 10.1 *Observed and fitted Weibull survivor functions for women with positive (⋯⋯) and negative (—) staining.*

$U_i \sim N(0, \sigma_u^2)$, then $Z_i = \exp(U_i)$ has a lognormal distribution. This distribution was introduced in Section 6.1.2 of Chapter 6. Since $z_i = 1$ in the model of Equation (10.2) corresponds to the situation where there is no frailty, it is desirable for the frailty distribution to be centred on unity. By taking the random frailty effects, U_i, to be distributed about a mean of zero, the corresponding distribution of Z_i has a median of unity. However, the expected value of Z_i, which is

$$\mathrm{E}\,(Z_i) = \exp(\sigma_u^2/2), \tag{10.4}$$

will be different from 1.0, and the variance of Z_i is given by

$$\mathrm{var}\,(Z_i) = \exp(\sigma_u^2)\{\exp(\sigma_u^2) - 1\}. \tag{10.5}$$

The results in Equations (10.4) and (10.5) show how the mean and variance of a lognormal frailty distribution can be found from the variance, σ_u^2, of the corresponding normally distributed random effect. An alternative approach is to take U_i to have a normal distribution with mean $-\sigma_u^2/2$ and variance σ_u^2. Although Z_i would then have a mean of unity, this formulation is not widely used in practice.

A distribution that is very similar to the lognormal distribution is the gamma distribution, described in Section 6.1.3, and so this is an alternative distribution for the frailty random variable, Z_i. This frailty distribution is sometimes more convenient to work with than the lognormal model, and can be used to investigate some of the consequences of introducing a frailty effect, which we do in Section 10.3.

If we take Z_i to have a gamma distribution with both unknown parameters equal to θ, and density

$$f(z_i) = \frac{\theta^\theta z_i^{\theta-1} e^{-\theta z_i}}{\Gamma(\theta)}, \quad \theta \geqslant 0,$$

for $z_i > 0$, so that $Z_i \sim \Gamma(\theta, \theta)$, this frailty distribution has a mean of unity and a variance of $1/\theta$. The larger the value of θ, the smaller the frailty variance, and as $\theta \to \infty$, the frailty variance tends to zero, corresponding to the case where the z_i are all equal to unity and there is no frailty. The corresponding distribution of $U_i = \exp(Z_i)$ has density

$$f(u_i) = \frac{\theta^\theta e^{\theta u_i} \exp(-\theta e^{u_i})}{\Gamma(\theta)}, \quad \theta \geqslant 0, \tag{10.6}$$

for $-\infty < u_i < \infty$, and U_i is said to have an *exp-gamma distribution.* This distribution is also referred to as the log-gamma distribution, but this nomenclature is inconsistent with the definition of a lognormal distribution. The modal value of U_i is zero, but the distribution is asymmetric and the mean and variance of U_i are expressed in terms of *digamma* and *trigamma functions.* Specifically,

$$\mathrm{E}\,(U_i) = \Psi(\theta) - \log\theta, \tag{10.7}$$

where the digamma function, $\Psi(\theta)$, can be obtained from the series expansion

$$\Psi(\theta) = -\lambda + \sum_{j=0}^{\infty} \frac{\theta - 1}{(1+j)(\theta+j)},$$

and here, $\lambda = 0.577216$ is Euler's constant. Also, the variance of U_i is the derivative of $\Psi(\theta)$, written $\Psi'(\theta)$, and known as the trigamma function. This function can also be obtained using a series expansion, and

$$\mathrm{var}\,(U_i) = \Psi'(\theta) = \sum_{j=0}^{\infty} \frac{1}{(\theta+j)^2}. \tag{10.8}$$

The digamma and trigamma functions are available as standard functions in many statistical software packages.

The lognormal and gamma distributions for frailty, and the corresponding normal and exp-gamma distributions for the random effects, will be compared later in Example 10.3.

10.2.2 Observable survivor and hazard functions*

The survivor function for the ith individual, from Equations (1.6) and (1.7) in Chapter 1, is

$$S_i(t) = \exp\left\{-\int_0^t h_i(t)\,\mathrm{d}t\right\},$$

where $h_i(t)$ is given in Equation (10.2). Therefore

$$S_i(t) = \exp\{-z_i e^{\boldsymbol{\beta}'\boldsymbol{x}_i} H_0(t)\}, \tag{10.9}$$

where $H_0(t)$ is the baseline cumulative hazard function. This is the survivor function for the ith individual conditional on the frailty z_i, and is termed a *conditional model* for the survival times.

The individual frailties z_i cannot be observed directly, and so what we observe is the effect that they have on the overall survivor function for the group of individuals. The observable survivor function is therefore the individual functions averaged over all possible values of z_i, that is the expected value of $S_i(t)$ with respect to the frailty distribution. If the corresponding random variables Z_i had a discrete distribution, where only a few specific values of the frailty were possible, we would obtain this expectation by summing the products of the possible values of $S_i(t)$ for the different z_i values and the probability that Z_i was equal to z_i. However, we generally assume a continuous distribution for the Z_i, and in this situation, the survivor function that is observed is found by integrating $S_i(t)$ in Equation (10.9) with respect to the distribution of Z_i. The resulting survivor function is

$$S_i^*(t) = \int_0^\infty S_i(t) f(z_i)\,\mathrm{d}z_i = \int_0^\infty \exp\{-z_i e^{\boldsymbol{\beta}'\boldsymbol{x}_i} H_0(t)\} f(z_i)\,\mathrm{d}z_i, \tag{10.10}$$

where $f(z_i)$ is the density function of the frailty distribution. The quantity $S_i^*(t)$ is the *unconditional* or *observable survivor function*, and Equation (10.10) defines an *unconditional model* for the survival times.

Once $S_i^*(t)$ has been obtained for a particular model, the corresponding *observable hazard function*, $h_i^*(t)$, can be found using the relationship in Equation (1.5) of Chapter 1, so that

$$h^*(t) = -\frac{\mathrm{d}}{\mathrm{dt}}\{\log S^*(t)\}. \tag{10.11}$$

In general the integral in Equation (10.10) has to be evaluated numerically, but as we shall see in the following section, this can be accomplished analytically in the special case of gamma frailty effects.

10.3 The gamma frailty distribution

The gamma distribution is often used to model frailty effects as it leads to a closed form representation of the observable survivor and hazard functions, as shown in this section.

Suppose that each individual in a study has a distinct frailty value, z_i, and that these are observations on independent and identically distributed random variables Z_i, $i = 1, 2, \ldots, n$, where $Z_i \sim \Gamma(\theta, \theta)$. Now, from Equation (10.10), the observable survivor function is

$$S_i^*(t) = \int_0^\infty S_i(t) f(z_i)\,\mathrm{d}z_i,$$

so that

$$S_i^*(t) = \int_0^\infty \exp\{-z_i e^{\boldsymbol{\beta}'\boldsymbol{x}_i} H_0(t)\} \frac{\theta^\theta z_i^{\theta-1} e^{-\theta z_i}}{\Gamma(\theta)} \, \mathrm{d}z_i,$$

and on some rearrangement, this becomes

$$\frac{\theta^\theta [\theta + e^{\boldsymbol{\beta}'\boldsymbol{x}_i} H_0(t)]^{-\theta}}{\Gamma(\theta)} \int_0^\infty y_i^{\theta-1} e^{-y_i} \, \mathrm{d}y_i,$$

where $y_i = \{\theta + e^{\boldsymbol{\beta}'\boldsymbol{x}_i} H_0(t)\} z_i$. Then, from the definition of a gamma function,

$$\int_0^\infty y_i^{\theta-1} e^{-y_i} \, \mathrm{d}y_i = \Gamma(\theta),$$

and so

$$S_i^*(t) = \{1 + \theta^{-1} e^{\boldsymbol{\beta}'\boldsymbol{x}_i} H_0(t)\}^{-\theta}. \tag{10.12}$$

Equation (10.11) leads to the observable hazard function, given by

$$h_i^*(t) = \frac{e^{\boldsymbol{\beta}'\boldsymbol{x}_i} h_0(t)}{1 + \theta^{-1} e^{\boldsymbol{\beta}'\boldsymbol{x}_i} H_0(t)}. \tag{10.13}$$

In the next section, some of the consequences of introducing a frailty effect are illustrated.

10.3.1 Impact of frailty on an observable hazard function

To illustrate the effect that a frailty term has on the hazard function, we will take the frailty random variable Z_i to have a $\Gamma(\theta, \theta)$ distribution. Suppose that the baseline hazard function $h_0(t)$ is a constant, λ, and that we are fitting a model to a single sample of survival times so that there are no covariates. Using Equation (10.13), the observable hazard function is then

$$h^*(t) = \frac{\theta\lambda}{\theta + \lambda t},$$

which declines non-linearly from the value λ when $t = 0$ to zero. The presence of frailty effects therefore provides an alternative explanation for a decreasing hazard function. Specifically, the overall hazard of an event might actually be constant, but heterogeneity between the survival times of the individuals in the study will mean that a decline in hazard is observed.

Similar features are found if we assume that the underlying baseline hazard is dependent upon time. In the case where the underlying baseline hazard is Weibull, with $h_0(t) = \lambda\gamma t^{\gamma-1}$, and where there are no covariates,

$$h^*(t) = \frac{\theta\lambda\gamma t^{\gamma-1}}{\theta + \lambda t^\gamma}.$$

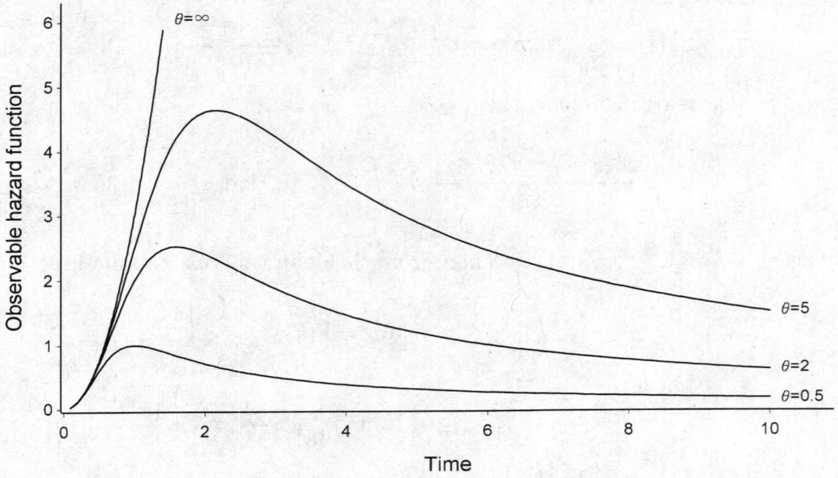

Figure 10.2 *Observable hazard function for Weibull baseline hazards with* $h_0(t) = 3t^2$ *and gamma frailty distributions with* $\theta = 0.5, 2, 5$ *and* ∞.

A plot of $h^*(t)$ against t for a Weibull hazard with $\lambda = 1$, $\gamma = 3$ and various values of θ is shown in Figure 10.2.

One limitation of a Weibull baseline hazard function, noted in Section 5.1.2 of Chapter 5, is that it is monotonic. However, as we can see in Figure 10.2, when there is a degree of frailty present, we may observe unimodal hazard functions. Consequently, an observed unimodal hazard may be the result of frailty effects, rather than the intrinsic behaviour of the underlying baseline hazard.

10.3.2 Impact of frailty on an observable hazard ratio

Suppose that the hazard function for the ith individual is

$$h_i(t) = z_i \exp(\beta x_i) h_0(t),$$

where x_i is the value of a binary covariate X that takes values 0, 1 and z_i is a realisation of a $\Gamma(\theta, \theta)$ random variable. The corresponding observable hazard function is

$$h_i^*(t) = \frac{e^{\beta x_i} h_0(t)}{1 + \theta^{-1} e^{\beta x_i} H_0(t)},$$

from Equation (10.13), and the observable hazard ratio for $X = 1$ relative to $X = 0$ is

$$\psi^*(t) = \frac{1 + \theta^{-1} H_0(t)}{1 + \theta^{-1} e^{\beta} H_0(t)} e^{\beta}. \tag{10.14}$$

This hazard ratio is no longer constant but a function of time t, and so proportional hazards no longer pertains. For example, in the particular case where the underlying baseline hazard is assumed to be a constant λ, $H_0(t) = \lambda t$ and the hazard ratio becomes

$$\frac{1 + \theta^{-1}\lambda t}{1 + \theta^{-1}e^{\beta}\lambda t} e^{\beta},$$

a non-linear function of t.

To illustrate the dependence of the observable hazard ratio on time, Figure 10.3 shows the hazard ratio $\psi^*(t)$ for a Weibull baseline hazard with $\lambda = 1$, $\gamma = 3$, $\psi = e^{\beta} = 3$ and various values of θ.

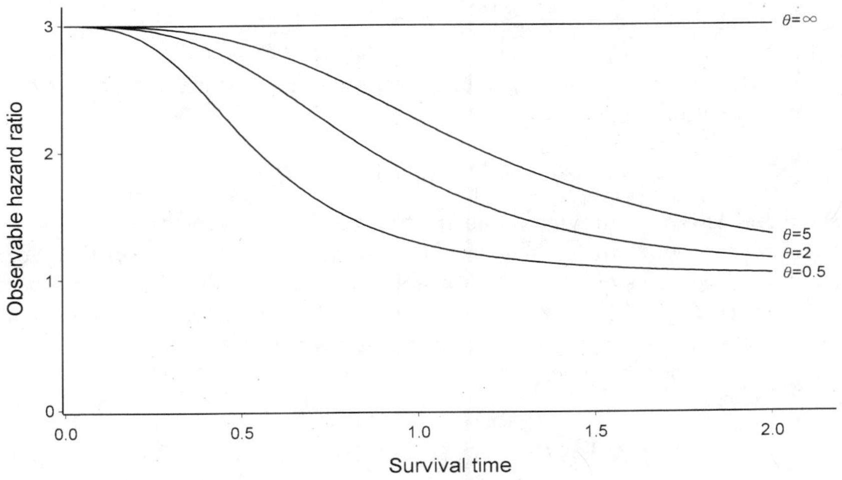

Figure 10.3 *Observable hazard ratio for Weibull baseline hazard with* $h_0(t) = 3t^2$, $\beta = \log 3$, *and gamma frailty distributions with* $\theta = 0.5, 2, 5$ *and* ∞.

The hazard ratio has a constant value of 3 when there is no frailty, that is when $\theta = \infty$, but when the frailty variance exceeds zero, the observable hazard ratio declines over time. This dependence of the hazard ratio on time could be used to account for any observed non-proportionality in the hazards.

These results show that the inclusion of a random effect in a Weibull proportional hazards regression model can lead to hazards not being proportional, and to a non-monotonic hazard function. Although this has been illustrated using a Weibull model with gamma frailty, the conclusions drawn apply more generally. This means that models that include random effects provide an alternative way of modelling data where the hazard function is unimodal, or where the hazards are not proportional.

10.4 Fitting parametric frailty models

Fitting the model in Equation (10.3) entails estimating the values of the coefficients of the explanatory variables, the variance of frailty distribution and the baseline hazard function. Models in which $h_0(t)$ is fully specified, such as the Weibull proportional hazards model or an accelerated failure time model, can be fitted using the method of maximum likelihood. Denote the observed survival data by the pairs (t_i, δ_i), $i = 1, 2, \ldots, n$, where t_i is the survival time and δ_i is an event indicator, which takes the value zero for a censored observation and unity for an event. If the random effects u_i in Equation (10.3) had known values, the likelihood function would be

$$\prod_{i=1}^{n} \{h_i(t_i)\}^{\delta_i} S_i(t_i), \tag{10.15}$$

as in Equation (5.10) of Chapter 5. In this expression, the hazard function for the ith of n individuals is given in Equation (10.3) and the corresponding survivor function is

$$S_i(t_i) = \exp\{-\exp(\boldsymbol{\beta}'\boldsymbol{x}_i + u_i)H_0(t_i)\}, \tag{10.16}$$

where $H_0(t_i)$ is the cumulative hazard function evaluated at time t_i.

However, the u_i are not known, but are independent and identically distributed realisations of a random variable that has a probability distribution with density $f(u_i)$. In this situation, we integrate the likelihood contributions over possible values of the random effects, so that from Equation (10.15), the likelihood function becomes

$$\prod_{i=1}^{n} \int_0^{\infty} \{h_i(t_i)\}^{\delta_i} S_i(t_i) f(u_i)\, \mathrm{d}u_i, \tag{10.17}$$

or equivalently, when working with the frailty terms z_i,

$$\prod_{i=1}^{n} \int_0^{\infty} \{h_i(t_i)\}^{\delta_i} S_i(t_i) f(z_i)\, \mathrm{d}z_i. \tag{10.18}$$

Numerical methods are generally needed to maximise this function, or its logarithm.

Once the unknown parameters in a fully parametric model have been estimated, it is possible to obtain estimates of the random effects. To do this, we use a version of Bayes' theorem, according to which the probability of an event A, conditional on an event B, is given by

$$\mathrm{P}(A \mid B) = \frac{P(B \mid A)P(A)}{P(B)}. \tag{10.19}$$

We now write $L(t_i \,|\, u_i)$ for the likelihood of the ith event time t_i when the random effect u_i is regarded as fixed, which from combining Equation (10.16) with Expression (10.15), is

$$L(t_i \,|\, u_i) = \{\exp(\boldsymbol{\beta}'\boldsymbol{x}_i + u_i)h_0(t_i)\}^{\delta_i} \exp\{-\exp(\boldsymbol{\beta}'\boldsymbol{x}_i + u_i)H_0(t_i)\}.$$

This can be interpreted as the probability of t_i conditional on the random effect u_i. Next, the probability of a particular value of the random effect is the density function $f(u_i)$. Using Equation (10.19), the probability of u_i conditional on t_i can be expressed as

$$\pi(u_i \,|\, t_i) = \frac{L(t_i \,|\, u_i)f(u_i)}{P(t_i)}, \qquad (10.20)$$

where $P(t_i)$ is the marginal probability of the data, obtained by integrating $L(t_i \,|\, u_i)f(u_i)$ with respect to u_i. This ensures that $\pi(u_i \,|\, t_i)$ integrates to 1, and so defines a proper probability density function. The mean or mode of the distribution of the random variable associated with the ith random effect, U_i, conditional on the data, $\pi(u_i \,|\, t_i)$, can then be obtained. Finally, substituting estimates of the unknown β-coefficients and the variance of the frailty distribution, we get an estimate of the mean or modal value of the distribution of U_i, $\hat{u}_i$, say, which can be regarded as an estimate of the random effect. Because of the link to Bayes' theorem in Equation (10.19), $\pi(u_i \,|\, t_i)$ is referred to as the *posterior density* of U_i, and the estimates $\hat{u}_i$ are termed *empirical Bayes estimates.* In a similar way, the posterior variance of U_i can be obtained from $\pi(u_i \,|\, t_i)$, which leads to the standard error of $\hat{u}_i$. Corresponding estimates of the frailty effects and their standard errors are obtained from $\hat{z}_i = \exp(\hat{u}_i)$.

Once frailty effects have been estimated, Equations (10.9) or (10.16) can be used to obtain fully parametric estimates of the survivor function. The median survival time for a particular individual can then be found from the expression

$$\left\{\frac{\log 2}{\hat{\lambda}\exp(\hat{\boldsymbol{\beta}}'\boldsymbol{x}_i + \hat{u}_i)}\right\}^{1/\hat{\gamma}}, \qquad (10.21)$$

which is a straightforward adaptation of the result in Equation (5.42) of Chapter 5.

Parametric survival models with frailty are most easily fitted when the frailty effects have a gamma distribution, and so the fitting process for this particular model is described in the following section.

10.4.1 Gamma frailty*

When the frailty random variable, Z_i, is assumed to have a gamma distribution, a closed form can be obtained for the integrated likelihood in Equation (10.18). To show this, on substituting for the hazard function, survivor function and density of Z_i into Equation (10.18), the likelihood function is

$$\prod_{i=1}^{n}\int_0^{\infty}\{z_i e^{\boldsymbol{\beta}'\boldsymbol{x}_i} h_0(t_i)\}^{\delta_i}\ \exp\{-z_i e^{\boldsymbol{\beta}'\boldsymbol{x}_i} H_0(t_i)\}\ \frac{\theta^{\theta} z_i^{\theta-1} e^{-\theta z_i}}{\Gamma(\theta)}\,\mathrm{d}z_i.$$

Collecting terms in z_i, this becomes

$$\prod_{i=1}^{n}\frac{\theta^{\theta}}{\Gamma(\theta)}\{e^{\boldsymbol{\beta}'\boldsymbol{x}_i} h_0(t_i)\}^{\delta_i}\int_0^{\infty} z_i^{\theta+\delta_i-1}\exp\{-[\theta+e^{\boldsymbol{\beta}'\boldsymbol{x}_i} H_0(t_i)]z_i\}\,\mathrm{d}z_i.$$

Next, the density of a gamma random variable Y with parameters r and θ is

$$f(y)=\frac{\theta^{r} y^{r-1} e^{-\theta y}}{\Gamma(r)}, \tag{10.22}$$

and so

$$\int_0^{\infty} y^{r-1} e^{-\theta y}\,\mathrm{d}y=\frac{\Gamma(r)}{\theta^{r}},$$

from which

$$\int_0^{\infty} z_i^{\theta+\delta_i-1}\exp\{-[\theta+e^{\boldsymbol{\beta}'\boldsymbol{x}_i} H_0(t_i)]z_i\}\,\mathrm{d}z_i=\frac{\Gamma(\theta+\delta_i)}{\{\theta+e^{\boldsymbol{\beta}'\boldsymbol{x}_i} H_0(t_i)\}^{\theta+\delta_i}}.$$

Consequently, the likelihood function becomes

$$\prod_{i=1}^{n}\frac{\theta^{\theta}}{\Gamma(\theta)}\{e^{\boldsymbol{\beta}'\boldsymbol{x}_i} h_0(t_i)\}^{\delta_i}\frac{\Gamma(\theta+\delta_i)}{\{\theta+e^{\boldsymbol{\beta}'\boldsymbol{x}_i} H_0(t_i)\}^{\theta+\delta_i}}.$$

The corresponding log-likelihood function is

$$\sum_{i=1}^{n}\{\theta\log\theta-\log\Gamma(\theta)+\log\Gamma(\theta+\delta_i)+\delta_i[\boldsymbol{\beta}'\boldsymbol{x}_i+\log h_0(t_i)]\}$$
$$-\sum_{i=1}^{n}(\theta+\delta_i)\log\{\theta+e^{\boldsymbol{\beta}'\boldsymbol{x}_i} H_0(t_i)\}, \tag{10.23}$$

and now that no integration is involved, standard numerical methods can be used to maximise this function with respect to θ, the βs and the parameters in the baseline hazard function, to give the maximum likelihood estimates. Standard errors of these estimates are found from the corresponding information matrix; see Appendix A. The estimated variance of the random effects can then be found by using the maximum likelihood estimate of θ, $\hat{\theta}$, in Equation (10.8).

To obtain estimates of the frailty effects when they are assumed to have a gamma distribution, it is more convenient to work with the z_i rather than the corresponding random effects u_i. Writing $L(t_i \mid z_i)$ for the likelihood of t_i

when the frailty z_i is regarded as fixed, the numerator of Equation (10.20) is then $L(t_i \mid z_i)f(z_i)$, which is

$$[z_i e^{\boldsymbol{\beta}'\boldsymbol{x}_i} h_0(t_i)]^{\delta_i} \exp\{-z_i e^{\boldsymbol{\beta}'\boldsymbol{x}_i} H_0(t_i)\} \frac{\theta^\theta z_i^{\theta-1} e^{-\theta z_i}}{\Gamma(\theta)}.$$

Ignoring terms that do not involve z_i, the posterior density of Z_i, $\pi(z_i \mid t_i)$, is proportional to

$$z_i^{\theta+\delta_i-1} \exp\{-[\theta + e^{\boldsymbol{\beta}'\boldsymbol{x}_i} H_0(t_i)]z_i\}.$$

From the general form of a two-parameter gamma density function, shown in Equation (10.22), it follows that the posterior distribution of Z_i is a gamma distribution with parameters $\theta + \delta_i$ and $\theta + e^{\boldsymbol{\beta}'\boldsymbol{x}_i} H_0(t_i)$. Then since the expected value of a gamma random variable with parameters r, θ is r/θ, the expectation of Z_i given the data, is

$$\mathrm{E}\,(Z_i \mid t_i) = \frac{\theta + \delta_i}{\theta + e^{\boldsymbol{\beta}'\boldsymbol{x}_i} H_0(t_i)}.$$

From this, an estimate of the frailty effect for the ith individual is

$$\hat{z}_i = \frac{\hat{\theta} + \delta_i}{\hat{\theta} + e^{\hat{\boldsymbol{\beta}}'\boldsymbol{x}_i} \hat{H}_0(t_i)},$$

where $\hat{H}_0(t)$ is the estimated baseline cumulative hazard function. Similarly, the variance of a gamma random variable is r/θ^2 and so

$$\mathrm{var}\,(Z_i \mid t_i) = \frac{\theta + \delta_i}{\{\theta + e^{\boldsymbol{\beta}'\boldsymbol{x}_i} H_0(t_i)\}^2}.$$

The estimated variance of Z_i reduces to $\hat{z}_i^2/(\hat{\theta} + \delta_i)$ and so the standard error of $\hat{z}_i$ is given by

$$\mathrm{se}\,(\hat{z}_i) = \frac{\hat{z}_i}{\sqrt{(\hat{\theta} + \delta_i)}}.$$

Interval estimates for the frailty terms can then be found, and the ratio of $\hat{z}_i$ to its standard error can be compared to percentage points of a standard normal distribution to give a P-value for a test of the hypothesis that the ith frailty effect is zero. However, the results of a series of unplanned hypothesis tests about frailty effects must be adjusted to allow for repeated significance testing, for example by using the Bonferroni correction. With this correction, the P-value for the frailty terms of n individuals are each divided by n before interpreting the significance levels.

As this analysis shows, working with gamma frailties is mathematically straightforward and leads to closed form estimates of many useful quantities. In other situations, numerical methods are needed to evaluate the summary statistics of the conditional distribution of the frailty given the data.

Example 10.2 Prognosis for women with breast cancer
When a frailty term with a gamma distribution is included in a Weibull model for the survival times of women with negatively and positively stained tumours, outlined in Example 10.1, the resulting hazard function is $h_i(t) = z_i \exp(\beta x_i)\lambda\gamma t^{\gamma-1}$, and the corresponding fitted survivor function is

$$\hat{S}_i(t) = \exp\{-\hat{z}_i \exp(\hat{\beta} x_i)\hat{\lambda} t^{\hat{\gamma}}\}.$$

The variance of the underlying gamma distribution for the frailty is $\hat{\theta}^{-1} = 3.40$, and estimates of the frailty effects follow from the method outlined in this section.

In the presence of frailty, $\hat{\beta} = 2.298$, and the hazard ratio for a positively stained woman relatively to one who is negatively stained is 9.95. However, the 95% confidence interval for this estimate ranges from 0.86 to 115.54, reflecting the much greater uncertainty about the staining effect when account is taken of frailty. It is also important to note that the estimated hazard ratio is conditional on frailty, and so refers to a woman with a specific frailty value. The revised estimates of λ and γ are 0.00008 and 1.9091, respectively, and the individual frailty values are shown in Table 10.1, alongside the observed survival times. Note that women with the shortest survival times have the largest estimated frailty effects.

Table 10.1 *Survival times of women with tumours that were negatively or positively stained and corresponding gamma frailties.*

Negative staining		Positive staining			
Survival time	Frailty	Survival time	Frailty	Survival time	Frality
23	3.954	5	4.147	68	0.444
47	3.050	8	3.827	71	0.412
69	2.290	10	3.579	76*	0.083
70*	0.514	13	3.192	105*	0.047
71*	0.507	18	2.581	107*	0.045
100*	0.348	24	1.981	109*	0.044
101*	0.344	26	1.816	113	0.179
148	0.888	26	1.816	116*	0.039
181	0.646	31	1.472	118	0.166
198*	0.127	35	1.254	143	0.116
208*	0.117	40	1.038	154*	0.023
212*	0.113	41	1.001	162*	0.021
224*	0.103	48	0.788	188*	0.016
		50	0.739	212*	0.013
		59	0.564	217*	0.012
		61	0.534	225*	0.011

* Censored survival times.

The individual estimates of the survivor functions are shown in Figure 10.4. This figure illustrates the extent of variation in the estimated survivor functions that stems from the frailty effect, and shows that there is some separation

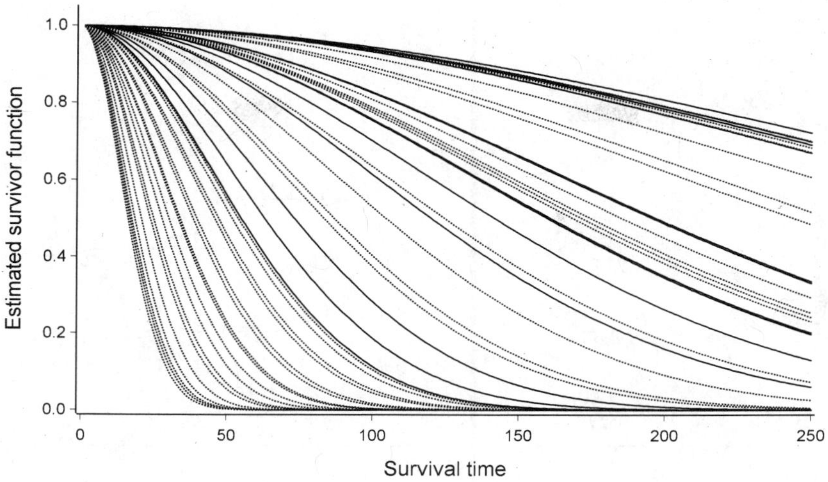

Figure 10.4 *Fitted Weibull survivor functions for women with positive (⋯⋯) and negative (—) staining.*

in the estimates for those women whose tumours were positively or negatively stained.

The median survival times, found using Equation (10.21), vary from 55 to 372 months for women in the negatively stained group, and from 16 to 355 months for those in the positively stained group. Of the 32 women with positively stained tumours, 18 have estimated median survival times that are less than any of those in the negatively stained group. This confirms that once allowance is made for frailty effects, differences between survival times in the two groups of women are not as pronounced.

The observable survivor function under this model, from Equation (10.12), can be estimated by $\{1 + \hat{\theta}^{-1}\hat{H}_0(t)\}^{-\hat{\theta}}$ for a woman with a negatively stained tumour and $\{1 + \hat{\theta}^{-1}e^{\hat{\beta}}\hat{H}_0(t)\}^{-\hat{\theta}}$ for one with a positively stained tumour. These functions are shown in Figure 10.5, superimposed on the corresponding Kaplan-Meier estimate of the survivor functions. Comparing this with Figure 10.1, we see that once allowance is made for frailty, the Weibull model is a much better fit to the observed survival times. This figure also provides a visual confirmation of the suitability of the fitted model.

The observable, or unconditional, hazard ratio, for a woman with a positively stained tumour relative to one whose tumour was negatively stained, derived from Equation (10.14), is given in Figure 10.6. This figure shows how the observable hazard ratio varies over time; the hazard is much greater at earlier times, but declines quite rapidly. This is due to the selection effect of frailty, whereby women who are more frail die sooner. There are also many

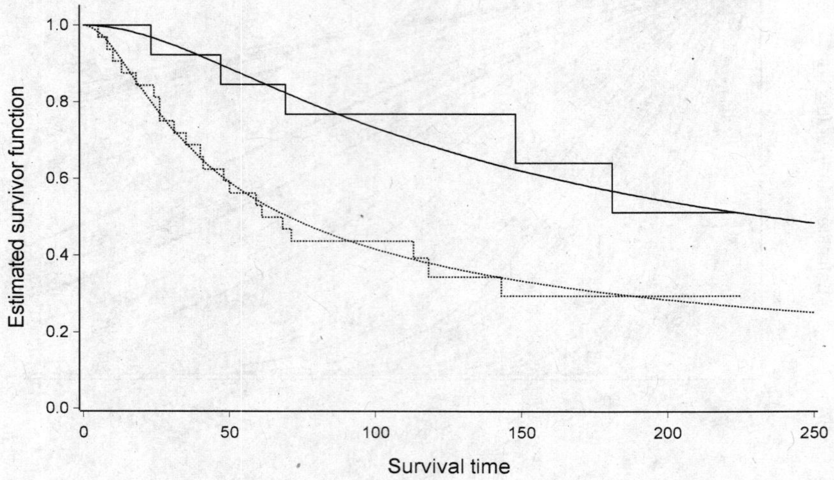

Figure 10.5 *Fitted survivor functions for the Weibull gamma frailty model, with the corresponding observed survivor functions, for women with positive (⋯⋯) and negative (—) staining.*

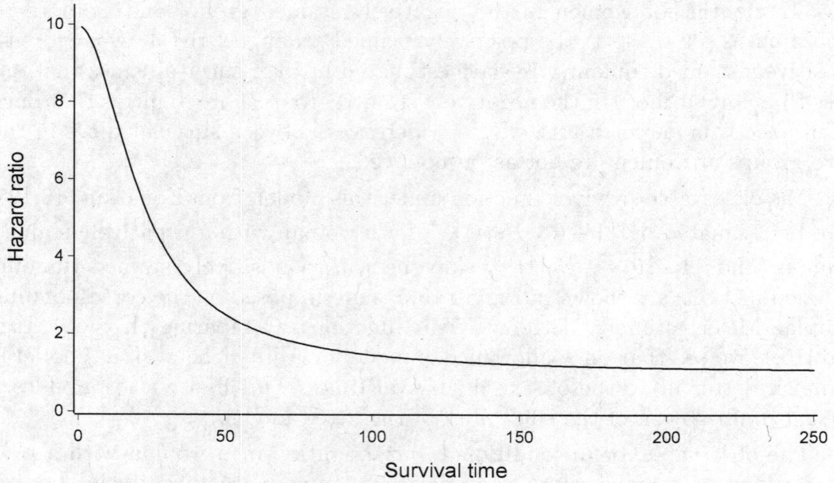

Figure 10.6 *Ratio of the hazard of death for a women with a positively stained tumour relative to one whose tumour is negatively stained.*

more early deaths in the positively stained group, which is why the observed hazard ratio varies in this way.

10.5 Fitting semi-parametric frailty models

When no underlying parametric form is assumed for the baseline hazard function, as in the Cox regression model, the procedure for fitting a frailty model described in the previous section can no longer be used. This is because the likelihood function in Expression (10.15) is no longer fully specified. The approach that is now most widely implemented in standard software packages involves maximising the sum of the partial log-likelihood for the Cox model that includes the random effects, $\log L_p(\boldsymbol{\beta}, \boldsymbol{u})$, and the log-likelihood of the random effects. This log-likelihood function is

$$\log L_p(\boldsymbol{\beta}, \boldsymbol{u}) + \sum_{i=1}^{n} \log f(u_i), \qquad (10.24)$$

where $\boldsymbol{\beta}$ is the vector of coefficients of p explanatory variables in a Cox regression model, and $\boldsymbol{u}$ is the vector of random effects for the n individuals. The partial log-likelihood is found by replacing $\boldsymbol{\beta}'\boldsymbol{x}_i$ in Equation (3.6) of Chapter 3 by $\boldsymbol{\beta}'\boldsymbol{x}_i + u_i$, to give

$$\log L_p(\boldsymbol{\beta}, \boldsymbol{u}) = \sum_{i=1}^{n} \delta_i \left\{ \boldsymbol{\beta}'\boldsymbol{x}_i + u_i - \log \sum_{l \in R(t_i)} \exp(\boldsymbol{\beta}'\boldsymbol{x}_l + u_l) \right\},$$

where δ_i is the event indicator and $R(t_i)$ is the set of patients at risk of death at time t_i. The random effects, u_i, are the observed values of frailty random variables, $U_i = \exp(Z_i)$, where Z_i is usually taken to have either a lognormal or a gamma distribution.

10.5.1 Lognormal frailty effects*

When frailty effects are assumed to be lognormally distributed, the random effects, u_i, in Expression (10.24), are realisations of an $N(0, \sigma_u^2)$ random variable, with density

$$f(u_i) = \frac{1}{\sigma_u \sqrt{(2\pi)}} \exp\left(-\frac{u_i^2}{2\sigma_u^2}\right).$$

The log-likelihood function in Expression (10.24) is then

$$\log L_p(\boldsymbol{\beta}, \boldsymbol{u}) - n \log\{\sigma_u \sqrt{(2\pi)}\} - \frac{1}{2\sigma_u^2} \sum_{i=1}^{n} u_i^2. \qquad (10.25)$$

Since this log-likelihood is only used to estimate the p components of $\boldsymbol{\beta}$ and the n components of $\boldsymbol{u}$, the term involving σ_u^2 alone can be omitted to give

$$\log L_{pen}(\boldsymbol{\beta}, \boldsymbol{u}, \sigma_u^2) = \log L_p(\boldsymbol{\beta}, \boldsymbol{u}) - \frac{1}{2\sigma_u^2} \sum_{i=1}^{n} u_i^2. \qquad (10.26)$$

This is known as a *penalised partial log-likelihood*, since the effect of the second term is to assign penalties to the partial log-likelihood function when the u_i have more extreme values, that is values that are further from their expected value of zero. The σ_u^2 term in Equation (10.26) essentially controls the relative importance of the two components of this log-likelihood function.

The maximisation process proceeds iteratively by starting with a provisional estimate of σ_u^2 and finding the estimates of the βs and the us that maximise $\log L_{pen}(\boldsymbol{\beta}, \boldsymbol{u}, \sigma_u^2)$. Next, a *marginal log-likelihood*, $\log L_m(\boldsymbol{\beta}, \sigma_u^2)$, is obtained by integrating the log-likelihood in Expression (10.25) over the random effects u_i. Ripatti and Palmgren (2000) show that, at estimates $\hat{\boldsymbol{\beta}}$ of $\boldsymbol{\beta}$, this is well-approximated by

$$\log L_m(\sigma_u^2) = \log L_{pen}(\hat{\boldsymbol{\beta}}, \hat{\boldsymbol{u}}, \sigma_u^2) - \frac{1}{2}\log(\sigma_u^{2n}) - \frac{1}{2}\log|\boldsymbol{I}_u|, \tag{10.27}$$

where $\boldsymbol{I}_u$ is the $n \times n$ observed information matrix for the random effects, formed from the negative second partial derivatives of $\log L_{pen}(\boldsymbol{\beta}, \boldsymbol{u}, \sigma_u^2)$ with respect to the u_i, $i = 1, 2, \ldots, n$, evaluated at $\hat{\boldsymbol{\beta}}, \hat{\boldsymbol{u}}$, and $|\boldsymbol{I}_u|$ is the determinant of that matrix. Using the estimates of the βs, the marginal log-likelihood in Equation (10.27) is then maximised with respect to σ_u^2 to give a revised estimate of σ_u^2. This process is repeated until the difference between two successive estimates of σ_u^2 is sufficiently small.

Estimates of the random effects, $\hat{u}_i$, and hence the frailty terms $\hat{z}_i = \exp(\hat{u}_i)$, are also obtained from this iterative process. Moreover, the maximum likelihood estimate of the variance of the random effect is given by

$$\hat{\sigma}_u^2 = n^{-1}\left\{\sum_{i=1}^{n} \hat{u}_i^2 + \text{trace}\,(\boldsymbol{I}_u^{-1})\right\},$$

where $\text{trace}\,(\boldsymbol{I}_u^{-1})$ is the sum of the diagonal elements of the inverse of $\boldsymbol{I}_u$. The standard error of this estimate is

$$\text{se}\,(\hat{\sigma}_u^2) = \surd(2\hat{\sigma}_u^2)\left[n + \frac{1}{\hat{\sigma}_u^4}\,\text{trace}\,(\boldsymbol{I}_u^{-1}\boldsymbol{I}_u^{-1}) - 2\frac{1}{\hat{\sigma}_u^2}\,\text{trace}\,(\boldsymbol{I}_u^{-1})\right]^{-1/2}.$$

Maximum likelihood estimates of variances tend to be biased, and instead estimates based on the method of *restricted maximum likelihood (REML)* estimation are preferred. For example, in the case of estimating the variance of a single sample of observations, $x_1, x_2, \ldots, x_n$, from a normal distribution, the maximum likelihood estimate of the variance is the biased estimate $n^{-1}\sum_i(x_i - \bar{x})^2$ whereas the corresponding REML estimate turns out to be the usual unbiased estimate $(n-1)^{-1}\sum_i(x_i - \bar{x})^2$.

REML estimates are obtained from a likelihood function that is independent of $\boldsymbol{\beta}$, and the REML estimate of the variance of the random frailty term is

$$\tilde{\sigma}_u^2 = n^{-1}\left\{\sum_{i=1}^{n} \tilde{u}_i^2 + \text{trace}\,(\tilde{\boldsymbol{V}}_u)\right\},$$

where $\tilde{\boldsymbol{V}}_u$ is the estimated variance-covariance matrix of the REML estimates of the u_i, $\tilde{u}_i$. The trace of this matrix is just the sum of the estimated variances of the $\tilde{u}_i$. This is the preferred estimate of the variance of a normally distributed random frailty effect. The standard error of $\tilde{\sigma}_u^2$ can be found from

$$\text{se}\,(\tilde{\sigma}_u^2) = \sqrt{(2\tilde{\sigma}_u^2)} \left[n + \frac{1}{\tilde{\sigma}_u^4} \text{trace}\,(\tilde{\boldsymbol{V}}_u \tilde{\boldsymbol{V}}_u) - 2\frac{1}{\tilde{\sigma}_u^2} \text{trace}\,(\tilde{\boldsymbol{V}}_u) \right]^{-1/2}.$$

Both $\tilde{\sigma}_u^2$ and its standard error generally feature in the output of software packages that have the facility for fitting Cox regression models with lognormal frailty.

For fully parametric frailty models, the cumulative baseline hazard function and the corresponding survivor function can be estimated using the maximum likelihood estimates of the unknown parameters. However, in semi-parametric frailty models, estimates of the baseline hazard and cumulative hazard cannot be extended to take account of the frailty terms, and so estimated survivor functions cannot easily be obtained.

10.5.2 Gamma frailty effects*

When the random variable associated with frailty effects is assumed to have a gamma distribution with unit mean and variance $1/\theta$, the corresponding random effects, u_i, have an exp-gamma distribution, introduced in Section 10.2.1. Using the density function in Equation (10.6), the log-likelihood function in Expression (10.24) is now

$$\log L_p(\boldsymbol{\beta}, \boldsymbol{u}) + n\theta \log \theta - n \log \Gamma(\theta) - \sum_{i=1}^{n} \{\theta e^{u_i} - \theta u_i\}.$$

This log-likelihood function will be used to estimate the components of $\boldsymbol{\beta}$ and $\boldsymbol{u}$, and so terms involving θ alone can be omitted to give the penalised partial log-likelihood function

$$\log L_{pen}(\boldsymbol{\beta}, \boldsymbol{u}, \theta) = \log L_p(\boldsymbol{\beta}, \boldsymbol{u}) - \theta \sum_{i=1}^{n} \{e^{u_i} - u_i\}, \qquad (10.28)$$

in which $\theta \sum_{i=1}^{n} \{e^{u_i} - u_i\}$ is the penalty term.

To obtain estimates of $\boldsymbol{\beta}$, $\boldsymbol{u}$ and θ, estimates of $\boldsymbol{\beta}$ and $\boldsymbol{u}$ are first taken to be the values that maximise Equation (10.28) for a given value of θ. The marginal log-likelihood for θ, at estimates $\hat{\boldsymbol{\beta}}$ and $\hat{\boldsymbol{u}}$ of $\boldsymbol{\beta}$ and $\boldsymbol{u}$, is then used to obtain a revised estimate of θ. This has been shown by Therneau and Grambsch (2000) to be given by

$$\begin{aligned} \log L_m(\theta) = {} & \log L_{pen}(\hat{\boldsymbol{\beta}}, \hat{\boldsymbol{u}}, \theta) + n\theta(1 + \log \theta) \\ & - \sum_{i=1}^{n} \left\{ (\theta + \delta_i) \log(\theta + \delta_i) - \log \left[\frac{\Gamma(\theta + \delta_i)}{\Gamma(\theta)} \right] \right\}, \end{aligned} \qquad (10.29)$$

where δ_i is the event indicator for the ith individual. Maximising $\log L_m(\theta)$ in Equation (10.29) with respect to θ, leads to $\hat{\theta}$. This estimate is then used with Equation (10.28) to obtain updated estimates of $\boldsymbol{\beta}$ and $\boldsymbol{u}$, and so on until the process converges. No closed form estimate of θ, nor its standard error, is available.

As the frailty variance, $1/\theta$, tends to zero, the marginal log-likelihood in Equation (10.29) becomes

$$\log L_p(\hat{\boldsymbol{\beta}}) - \sum_{i=1}^{n} \delta_i,$$

where $\log L_p(\hat{\boldsymbol{\beta}})$ is the maximised partial log-likelihood for the Cox regression model when there is no frailty. By taking the marginal log-likelihood to be $\log L_m(\theta) + \sum_{i=1}^{n} \delta_i$, the maximised marginal log-likelihood in the presence of frailty is then directly comparable to that for the model with no frailty. This is helpful in comparing models, as we will see in Section 10.6.

10.6 Comparing models with frailty

In many cases, frailty acts as a nuisance term in the model. While it is important to take account of its effects, the main interest is in determining which explanatory variables are needed in a model, and obtaining estimates of their effects, in the presence of frailty. The methods described in Section 5.7 of Chapter 5, based on the change in the $-2\log\hat{L}$ statistic, can be used to compare parametric models that incorporate frailty. Model selection strategies for determining which factors to include in a parametric model in the presence of frailty can then be straightforwardly implemented. The fitted models can subsequently be used to draw inferences about their effects, allowing for frailty.

The situation is more complicated for the Cox regression model. This is because a penalised likelihood does not behave in the same way as the usual likelihood or partial likelihood functions, since it contains unobservable frailty effects. Instead, the maximised marginal log-likelihood statistic is used, which is $\log L_m(\hat{\sigma}_u^2)$ or $\log L_m(\hat{\theta})$ for lognormal and gamma frailties, respectively. This statistic is generally given in computer output from fitting Cox regression models that include frailty. Differences in the values of $-2\log L_m(\hat{\sigma}_u^2)$ or $-2\log L_m(\hat{\theta})$, or $-2\log\hat{L}_m$ for short, can be compared with percentage points of a χ^2 distribution in the usual manner. In the case of lognormal frailty effects, the marginal likelihood based on the maximum likelihood estimates of the βs is used, rather than that based on the REML estimates.

10.6.1 *Testing for the presence of frailty*

In parametric models, the hypothesis of no frailty effects can be evaluated by comparing $-2\log\hat{L}$ values for models with and without frailty effects, for a given set of covariates, with percentage points of a chi-squared distribution on one degree of freedom, χ_1^2. However, some care is needed as the standard asymptotic theory that underpins the result that differences in $-2\log\hat{L}$ values have a chi-squared distribution, is no longer valid. Essentially this is because the hypothesis of no frailty effect corresponds to testing the hypothesis that the variance of the frailty term is zero, and this is the smallest possible value that the variance can take. Tests based on changes in $-2\log\hat{L}$ then tend to be conservative, and the resulting P-value for a difference will be larger than it should be. In this situation, the difference in $-2\log\hat{L}$ values, when frailty is added, can be compared informally to percentage points of a χ_1^2 distribution. If the observed difference is relatively large or small, conclusions about the degree of frailty will be clear.

For a more precise determination of the significance of the frailty effect, we can use the result that the asymptotic distribution of the change in $-2\log\hat{L}$, when a frailty term is added to a fully parametric model, is an equally weighted mixture of a χ_0^2 and χ_1^2 distributions, written $0.5(\chi_0^2+\chi_1^2)$. A χ_0^2 distribution has a point mass at zero, and so if the random variable W has a $0.5(\chi_0^2+\chi_1^2)$ distribution, $\text{P}(W=0)=0.5$ and $\text{P}(W>w)=0.5\text{P}(\chi_1^2>w)$ for $w>0$. Consequently, to apply this result, the P-value for testing the hypothesis that the frailty variance is zero is just half of that obtained from using a χ_1^2 distribution.

In borderline cases, other methods may be needed, such as *bootstrapping*. This procedure can be used to obtain an interval estimate of the variance of a frailty term. Briefly, bootstrapping involves resampling the data *with replacement* to give a new sample of n survival times. The survival model that includes a frailty term is then fitted to this sample, and the variance of the random effect is then estimated. This is repeated a large number of times. The 2.5% and 97.5% percentiles of the distribution of the bootstrap variance estimates then define a 95 per cent interval estimate for the variance.

In the case of the Cox regression model, fitted using the method of penalised partial log-likelihood outlined in Section 10.5, the significance of a frailty term is assessed using the $-2\log\hat{L}_m$ statistic formed from the maximised marginal log-likelihood. For lognormal frailty effects, the maximised marginal log-likelihood for the model with frailty, obtained from maximum likelihood estimation and not REML, can be compared directly with the maximised partial log-likelihood for the corresponding Cox regression model without frailty. A similar process is used when gamma frailty effects are assumed, but here the total number of events, $\sum_{i=1}^{n}\delta_i$, has to be added to the maximised marginal log-likelihood, as explained in Section 10.5.2. As with parametric modelling, this test procedure is only approximate, and bootstrapping may be required for a more reliable assessment of the magnitude of the frailty effect.

Example 10.3 Survival of patients registered for a lung transplant

The likely survival time of a patient from when they are assessed as needing an organ transplant is of great interest to patients and clinicians alike. In a study to quantify this survival time and to identify factors associated with survival from listing for a lung transplant, data were obtained on the UK patients who were registered for a transplant in 2004. Survival times were measured from the date of registration until death, regardless of all intervening treatments, including transplantation. Survival was censored at the date of removal from the list, the last known follow-up date, or at 30 April 2012 for patients still alive. In addition, the age at registration, gender, body mass index and primary disease were recorded, where primary disease was categorised as fibrosis, chronic obstructive pulmonary disease (COPD), suppurative disease and other. There are 196 patients in the data set, of whom 123 died during the study period. Data for the first 20 patients are shown in Table 10.2.

Table 10.2 *Survival times of 20 patients from listing for a lung transplant.*

Patient	Survival time	Status	Age	Gender	BMI	Disease
1	2324	1	59	1	29.6	COPD
2	108	1	28	1	22.6	Suppurative
3	2939	0	55	1	32.1	Fibrosis
4	1258	0	62	1	30.0	Fibrosis
5	2904	0	51	1	30.4	Fibrosis
6	444	1	59	1	26.9	Fibrosis
7	158	1	55	2	24.6	COPD
8	1686	1	53	2	26.8	COPD
9	142	1	47	1	32.2	Fibrosis
10	1624	1	53	2	15.7	COPD
11	16	1	62	1	26.4	Fibrosis
12	2929	0	50	1	29.0	COPD
13	1290	1	55	2	17.1	COPD
14	2854	0	47	1	20.0	Other
15	237	1	23	1	15.9	Suppurative
16	136	1	65	1	16.0	COPD
17	2212	1	24	2	19.5	Suppurative
18	371	1	54	1	28.9	Fibrosis
19	683	1	24	2	20.2	Suppurative
20	290	1	53	1	25.2	Fibrosis

We first fit a Weibull proportional hazards model that contains age, gender, body mass index and primary disease. The value of the $-2\log\hat{L}$ statistic for this model is 2043.73. A lognormal frailty term is now introduced, by adding a normally distributed random effect to the linear component of the model, and maximising the likelihood function in Expression (10.17). The Weibull model with lognormal frailty has a $-2\log\hat{L}$ value of 2026.85, and the change in $-2\log\hat{L}$ on adding the random effect is 16.88. Comparing this reduction with percentage points of a χ_1^2 distribution, the frailty effect is highly significant, with a P-value of less than 0.001. This means that there is substantial heterogeneity between the survival times of the patients in this study, after allowing for the effects of the four explanatory variables. A less conservative estimate of the significance of the frailty effect is found by referring the change in $-2\log\hat{L}$ to a $0.5(\chi_0^2+\chi_1^2)$ distribution, equivalent to halving the P-value from a comparison with a χ_1^2 distribution, and it is then even more significant. The variance of the normal random effect corresponding to the lognormal frailty is $\hat{\sigma}_u^2 = 2.254$. Using Equations (10.4) and (10.5), the mean and variance of the lognormal frailty effect are 3.09 and 81.20, respectively.

We next fit a Weibull model that contains age, gender, body mass index and primary disease, together with a gamma frailty effect. This model is fitted by maximising the log-likelihood function in Expression (10.23), from which the gamma frailty effect has variance $\hat{\theta}^{-1} = 3.015$. The corresponding variance of the random effect is calculated from Equation (10.8), and is 10.19. The Weibull model with gamma frailty has a $-2\log\hat{L}$ value of 2023.69, and so addition of the frailty term leads to a reduction in the value of the $-2\log\hat{L}$ statistic of 20.04. This change is highly significant ($P < 0.001$), and greater than that when a lognormal frailty is introduced.

In this example, the variance of the two distributions for the frailty term, and the corresponding distributions of the random effect, are quite different. To explore this in more detail, Figures 10.7 and 10.8 show the fitted normal and exp-gamma probability density functions for the random variable U, and the corresponding fitted lognormal and gamma probability density functions for the frailty random variable, Z.

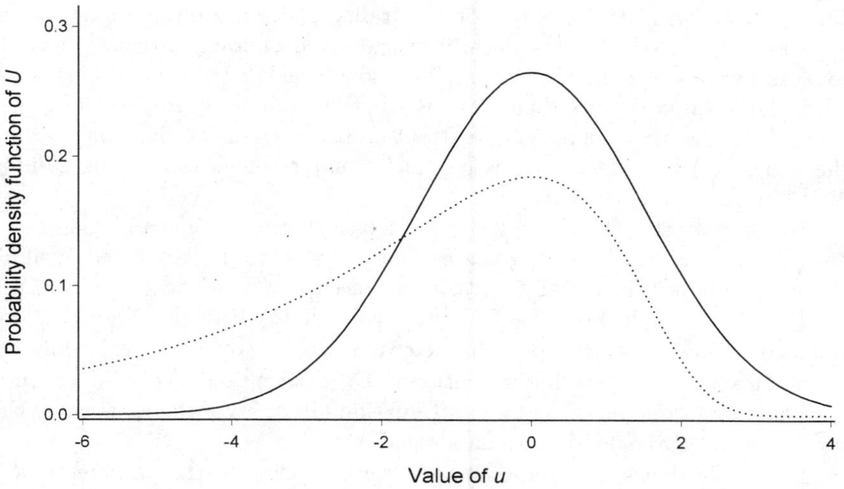

Figure 10.7 *Fitted probability density functions for the normal (—) and exp-gamma (·······) random effects.*

Figure 10.7 shows the asymmetry in the exp-gamma distribution of the random effect, and although the mode is zero, the mean, from Equation (10.7), is −2.05. This explains the disparity in the estimated variances of the normal

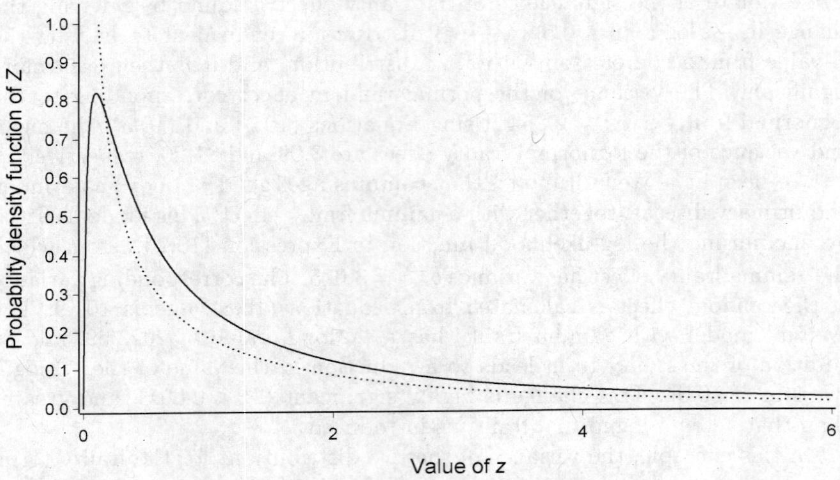

Figure 10.8 *Fitted probability density functions for the lognormal (—) and gamma (……) frailty effects.*

and exp-gamma distributions for the random effect. Figure 10.8 shows that the estimated density functions of the frailty effect are quite similar when z_i exceeds 0.2. However, the density of the fitted gamma distribution tends to ∞ as z_i tends to zero, whereas the fitted lognormal distribution is unimodal. Also, the mean of the fitted gamma distribution is unity, whereas from Equation (10.4), the fitted lognormal distribution has a mean of 3.09, which is why the lognormal frailty variance is so much greater than that for the gamma distribution.

To compare the parameter estimates for the various terms and their standard errors, Table 10.3 shows the estimates for the different fitted Weibull models, including the estimated variances of the random effects, u_i, and the frailty effects, z_i, denoted $\widehat{\text{var}}\,(u_i)$ and $\widehat{\text{var}}\,(z_i)$, respectively. Note that for a normal random effect, the estimated variance is $\widehat{\text{var}}\,(u_i) = \hat{\sigma}_u^2$, while for gamma frailty, $\widehat{\text{var}}\,(z_i) = 1/\hat{\theta}$. Equation (10.5) is then used to obtain the variance of a lognormal frailty term and Equation (10.8) gives the variance of the random effect corresponding to gamma frailty.

This table shows that there is a general tendency for the parameter estimates to be further from zero when a frailty term is added, and the standard errors are also larger. However, inferences about the impact of the factors on patient survival from listing are not much affected by the inclusion of a frailty term, and there is little difference in the results obtained when either a lognormal or gamma frailty effect is included. The only factor to have any effect on patient survival is primary disease, with the hazard of death in patients with COPD being less than that for patients with other diseases. Also, on the basis

Table 10.3 *Parameter estimates (standard error) in fitted Weibull models.*

Term	No frailty	Lognormal frailty	Gamma frailty
Age	0.015 (0.012)	0.014 (0.018)	0.003 (0.020)
Gender: Male	0.080 (0.198)	0.226 (0.325)	0.433 (0.412)
BMI	−0.024 (0.024)	−0.029 (0.039)	−0.014 (0.049)
Disease: COPD	−0.675 (0.377)	−0.960 (0.597)	−1.008 (0.694)
Disease: Fibrosis	0.363 (0.344)	0.887 (0.575)	1.382 (0.724)
Disease: Other	−0.254 (0.391)	−0.231 (0.623)	−0.076 (0.768)
Weibull shape ($\hat{\gamma}$)	0.663 (0.051)	1.040 (0.141)	1.304 (0.231)
Weibull scale ($\hat{\lambda}$)	0.0061 (0.0042)	0.0004 (0.0005)	0.0003 (0.0004)
$\widehat{\text{var}}\,(u_i)$	–	2.254	10.186
$\widehat{\text{var}}\,(z_i)$	–	81.197	3.015
$-2\log\hat{L}$	2043.73	2026.85	2023.69

of the $-2\log\hat{L}$ statistic, the model with gamma frailty might be preferred to that with lognormal frailty.

To avoid making specific assumptions about the form of the underlying baseline hazard function, we fit a Cox regression model that contains age, gender, body mass index and primary disease, and that also includes a lognormal or gamma frailty term. These models are fitted by maximising the penalised log-likelihood functions in Equations (10.26) and (10.28), respectively. To test the hypothesis that all frailty effects are zero in the presence of the four explanatory variables, we compare the value of the $-2\log\hat{L}$ statistic for the fitted Cox model, which is 1159.101, with values of the maximised marginal log-likelihood statistic, $-2\log\hat{L}_m$, for Cox models with frailty.

When a lognormal frailty term is added, the value of the maximised marginal log-likelihood statistic, $-2\log L_m(\hat{\sigma}_u^2)$ from Equation (10.27), is 1157.477, and this leads to a change in the value of the $-2\log\hat{L}_m$ statistic of 1.62, which is not significant ($P = 0.203$).

On fitting models with gamma frailty, the value of the $\log L_m(\hat{\theta})$ statistic from Equation (10.29) is −699.653, and adding the observed number of deaths, 123, to this and multiplying by −2, gives 1153.306. This can be compared with the value of $-2\log\hat{L}$ for the Cox regression model that contains the same explanatory variables, but no frailty effects, 1159.101. The reduction in the value of this test statistic is 5.80, which is significant when compared to percentage points of a χ^2 distribution on 1 d.f. ($P = 0.016$). This now shows a significant frailty effect after allowing for survival differences due to primary disease and the other factors.

The variances of the normal and exp-gamma random effects are smaller in the Cox model than in the corresponding Weibull model, and the frailty effect is less significant. This suggests that the fitted Cox regression model explains more of the variation in survival times from listing for a transplant than a Weibull model.

To compare the parameter estimates for the various terms in a Cox regression model and their standard errors, Table 10.4 shows the estimates for the different models fitted, and the estimated variances of the random effects, $\widehat{\text{var}}\,(u_i)$ and frailty effects, $\widehat{\text{var}}\,(z_i)$. For lognormal frailty, REML estimates are given. Equations (10.5) and (10.8) have again been used to estimate the variance of the frailty effects for lognormal frailty and the variance of the random effects for gamma frailty.

Table 10.4 *Parameter estimates (standard error) in fitted Cox models.*

Term	No frailty	Lognormal frailty	Gamma frailty
Age	0.013 (0.012)	0.012 (0.015)	0.006 (0.018)
Gender: Male	0.078 (0.198)	0.146 (0.267)	0.305 (0.352)
BMI	−0.023 (0.024)	−0.028 (0.032)	−0.024 (0.042)
Disease: COPD	−0.621 (0.371)	−0.754 (0.482)	−0.887 (0.598)
Disease: Fibrosis	0.377 (0.340)	0.704 (0.459)	1.225 (0.607)
Disease: Other	−0.218 (0.386)	−0.185 (0.512)	−0.089 (0.659)
$\widehat{\text{var}}\,(u_i)$	–	1.223	2.147
$\widehat{\text{var}}\,(z_i)$	–	8.149	5.572
$-2\log\hat{L}_m$	1159.10	1157.48	1153.31

As with the Weibull model, some parameter estimates are larger when a frailty term is added and the standard errors are larger, but the parameter estimates in Tables 10.3 and 10.4 are broadly similar. As for the Weibull model, the gamma frailty model leads to the smallest value of the $-2\log\hat{L}$ statistic and is a better fit to the data.

Estimates of frailty effects can be obtained using the approach outlined in Section 10.4. For example, from estimates of the frailty terms, $\hat{z}_i$, for the Cox model with lognormal frailty, there are 7 patients with values of $\hat{z}_i$ greater than 3, namely patients 11, 36, 69, 70, 87, 113 and 163. The survival times of these patients are 16, 21, 3, 4, 38, 22 and 35 days respectively, and so the patients with largest frailty are those whose survival is shortest, as expected.

10.7 The shared frailty model

Models that seek to explain heterogeneity in the survival times of individuals can provide improved estimates of the effects of covariates, or help to explain features such as non-proportional hazards. However, frailty models are particularly useful in modelling situations where there is some characteristic whose values are shared by groups of individuals. Some examples of potential areas of application were given in Section 10.1.3.

To formulate a shared frailty model for survival data, suppose that there are g groups of individuals with n_i individuals in the ith group, $i = 1, 2, \ldots, g$. For the proportional hazards model, the hazard of death at time t for the jth individual, $j = 1, 2, \ldots, n_i$, in the ith group, is then

$$h_{ij}(t) = z_i \exp(\boldsymbol{\beta}'\boldsymbol{x}_{ij})h_0(t), \tag{10.30}$$

where $\boldsymbol{x}_{ij}$ is a vector of values of p explanatory variables for the jth individual in the ith group, $\boldsymbol{\beta}$ is the vector of their coefficients, $h_0(t)$ is the baseline hazard function, and the z_i are frailty effects that are common for all n_i individuals within the ith group. The hazard function in Equation (10.30) can also be written in the form

$$h_{ij}(t) = \exp(\boldsymbol{\beta}'\boldsymbol{x}_{ij} + u_i)h_0(t),$$

where $u_i = \log(z_i)$, and are assumed to be realisations of g random variables $U_1, U_2, \ldots, U_g$. The distribution assumed for U_i is taken to have zero mean, and the normal distribution is a common choice.

The form of the baseline hazard may be fully specified as in a Weibull model, or unspecified as in the Cox model. The general parametric accelerated failure time model that incorporates a shared frailty component is, from Equation (6.8) in Chapter 6, of the form

$$h_{ij}(t) = e^{-\eta_{ij}} h_0(t/e^{\eta_{ij}}),$$

where $\eta_{ij} = \boldsymbol{\alpha}'\boldsymbol{x}_{ij} + u_i$. Equivalently, extending Equation (6.9), this model can be expressed in log-linear form as

$$\log T_{ij} = \mu + \boldsymbol{\alpha}'\boldsymbol{x}_{ij} + u_i + \sigma\epsilon_{ij},$$

where T_{ij} is the random variable associated with the survival time of the jth individual in the ith group, μ and σ are intercept and scale parameters, and ϵ_{ij} has some specified probability distribution.

10.7.1 Fitting the shared frailty model*

Suppose that the survival times for the jth individual in the ith group are denoted t_{ij}, for $j = 1, 2, \ldots, n_i$ and $i = 1, 2, \ldots, g$, and write δ_{ij} for the corresponding event indicator, which is unity if t_{ij} is an event time and zero otherwise. Also, let $S_{ij}(t)$ and $h_{ij}(t)$ be the survivor and hazard functions for the jth individual in the ith group. For a fully parametric model, the likelihood function for the observations in the ith group, when the frailty terms are known, is

$$L_i(\boldsymbol{\beta}) = \prod_{j=1}^{n_i} h_{ij}(t_{ij})^{\delta_{ij}} S_{ij}(t_{ij}).$$

As in Section 10.4, we next integrate this likelihood over the u_i to give

$$\int_0^\infty L_i(\boldsymbol{\beta}) f(u_i)\,\mathrm{d}u_i,$$

where $f(u_i)$ is the probability density function of U_i. Over the g groups, the likelihood function is

$$L(\boldsymbol{\beta}) = \prod_{i=1}^{g} \int_0^\infty L_i(\boldsymbol{\beta}) f(u_i)\,\mathrm{d}u_i.$$

As in the case of individual frailty effects, the integration can only be carried out analytically if the frailty effects have a $\Gamma(\theta, \theta)$ distribution. In this case, the likelihood function for the ith group is

$$\prod_{j=1}^{n_i} \left\{ e^{\boldsymbol{\beta}' \boldsymbol{x}_{ij}} h_0(t_{ij}) \right\}^{\delta_{ij}} \frac{\theta^{\theta} \Gamma(\theta + d_i)}{\Gamma(\theta) \{\theta + \sum_j \exp(\boldsymbol{\beta}' \boldsymbol{x}_{ij}) H_0(t_{ij})\}^{\theta + d_i}},$$

where $d_i = \sum_i \delta_{ij}$ is the number of deaths in the ith group. The corresponding log-likelihood over the g groups is

$$\begin{aligned} \log L(\boldsymbol{\beta}) = & \sum_{i=1}^{g} \{\log \Gamma(\theta + d_i) - \log \Gamma(\theta) - d_i \log \theta\} \\ & - \sum_{i=1}^{g} (\theta + d_i) \log \left[1 + \theta^{-1} \sum_{j=1}^{n_i} \exp(\boldsymbol{\beta}' \boldsymbol{x}_{ij}) H_0(t_{ij}) \right] \\ & + \sum_{i=1}^{g} \sum_{j=1}^{n_i} \delta_{ij} \left[\boldsymbol{\beta}' \boldsymbol{x}_{ij} + \log h_0(t_{ij}) \right], \end{aligned}$$

which can be maximised to give estimates of θ, the parameters in the baseline hazard function, and the βs.

Once this model has been fitted, estimates of the frailty effects, $\hat{z}_i$, can be obtained in the same manner as described in Section 10.4, and we find that

$$\hat{z}_i = \frac{\hat{\theta} + d_i}{\hat{\theta} + \sum_{j=1}^{n_i} \exp(\hat{\boldsymbol{\beta}}' \boldsymbol{x}_{ij}) \hat{H}_0(t_{ij})},$$

with standard error $\hat{z}_i / (\hat{\theta} + d_i)$.

Cox regression models with frailty can again be fitted using penalised partial log-likelihood methods, as in Section 10.5. To adapt the formulae given in that section to the case of shared frailty models, the event indicator δ_i is replaced by d_i, the number of deaths in the ith of g groups, and summations over $i = 1$ to n are replaced by summations over $i = 1$ to g.

10.7.2 Comparing shared frailty models

Again, the results given in Section 10.6 apply equally to shared frailty models. In particular, fully parametric models that include a shared frailty term can be compared using the $-2 \log \hat{L}$ statistic. To test for frailty, the change in the value of the $-2 \log \hat{L}$ statistic on adding frailty effects can be formally compared with percentage points of a $0.5(\chi_0^2 + \chi_1^2)$ distribution, as in Section 10.6.1.

For the Cox model with shared frailty that is fitted using penalised partial log-likelihood methods, the marginal log-likelihood statistics, $-2 \log L_m(\hat{\sigma}_u^2)$ and $-2 \log L_m(\hat{\theta})$, can be used to compare models with lognormal or gamma frailties, respectively. These statistics can also be compared to the value of $-2 \log \hat{L}$ for the Cox regression model without frailty, to assess the extent of frailty effects. However, the limitations of this approach, outlined in Section 10.6.1, also apply here. Note that in the case of gamma frailty, the quantity $\sum_{i=1}^{g} d_i$ needs to be added to $\log L_m(\hat{\theta})$ to ensure comparability with the maximised partial log-likelihood in the absence of frailty, as for univariate frailty.

Estimates of the random effects can be found using the method described in Section 10.4. Such estimates are particularly useful when the frailty term represents centres in a multicentre study, since the rank order of the estimated centre effects provides information about the merits of the different centres in terms of patient survival. But here, the estimated coefficients of the explanatory variables in the model are interpreted as conditional on the shared frailty. This means that hazard ratios relate to a comparison of effects in individuals within the same group. Estimates of the random effects also lead to estimates of the survivor function for individuals with given characteristics, and median survival times can easily be obtained. No new principles are involved.

We conclude with an example that illustrates some of these features.

Example 10.4 Survival following kidney transplantation

Deceased organ donors generally donate both kidneys which are subsequently transplanted into two different recipients, often by different transplant centres. In modelling short-term graft and patient survival, account needs to be taken of a number of factors associated with the recipient, and factors associated with the transplant procedure itself. This illustration is based on the outcomes of all kidney transplants carried out in a particular year, using donors who are deceased following circulatory death. The outcome variable is transplant survival, defined as the earlier of graft failure or death with a functioning graft. Of the many explanatory factors that were recorded, patient age (years), diabetes status (0 = absent, 1 = present) and the cold ischaemic time (CIT), the time in hours between retrieval of the kidney from the donor and transplantation into the recipient, are used in this example.

In addition to these recipient and transplant factors, donor factors may also have an impact on the outcome of the transplant. Although many factors related to the donor are routinely recorded, it is difficult to take account of everything. Moreover, the survival times of the patients who receive the two kidneys from the same donor may be expected to be more highly correlated than the times for recipients of kidneys from different donors. One way of taking account of donor factors, while allowing for association between the outcomes when organs from the same donor are used, is to include the donor as a shared frailty effect. The frailty term is then the same in models for the survival times of two recipients of kidneys from the same donor.

In this study there were 434 transplants using organs from 270 deceased donors. Of these, 106 gave one kidney and 164 donated both kidneys. Data for the 22 recipients of kidneys from the first 15 donors in the year are shown in Table 10.5.

Table 10.5 *Survival times of 20 patients following kidney transplantation.*

Patient	Donor	Survival time	Status	Age	Diabetes	CIT
1	1	1436	0	61	0	14.5
2	2	1442	0	30	0	7.2
3	3	310	1	62	0	14.3
4	4	1059	1	62	0	10.6
5	5	236	1	50	0	18.7
6	6	1372	0	65	0	19.3
7	6	382	1	71	0	12.2
8	7	736	1	46	0	13.6
9	7	1453	0	66	0	13.9
10	8	1122	0	53	0	18.0
11	8	1010	0	42	0	13.8
12	9	1403	0	44	0	12.9
13	10	1449	0	67	0	13.9
14	11	843	1	34	0	16.6
15	12	1446	0	32	0	10.3
16	12	1397	0	51	0	19.0
17	13	1301	0	75	0	12.5
18	13	1442	0	47	0	11.3
19	14	1445	0	69	0	18.8
20	14	1445	0	53	0	23.2
21	15	1445	0	46	0	15.5
22	15	1445	0	49	0	17.2

On fitting a Weibull model containing cold ischaemic time, and the age and diabetic status of the recipient, the value of the $-2 \log \hat{L}$ statistic is 1352.24. To take account of donor effects, a lognormal shared frailty effect is added, and the $-2 \log \hat{L}$ statistic decreases slightly to 1351.60. This reduction of 0.64 on 1 d.f. is not significant ($P = 0.42$) when compared to a χ_1^2 distribution, and remains non-significant ($P = 0.21$) compared to the percentage points of the $0.5(\chi_0^2 + \chi_1^2)$ distribution.

When a lognormal frailty is added to a Cox regression model that contains the same explanatory variables, the maximised marginal log-likelihood, multiplied by -2, is 831.469, whereas for the corresponding Cox regression model without frailty, $-2 \log \hat{L} = 831.868$. Again, the reduction on adding a frailty effect is not significant. Very similar results are obtained when donor effects are modelled using a shared gamma frailty term, and we conclude that there is no reason to include donor effects in the model. The estimated coefficients of the three explanatory variables are very similar under a Cox and Weibull model, and are hardly affected by including random donor effects. We conclude that taking proper account of the donor effects has not materially affected inferences about the effect of explanatory factors on short-term survival of these transplant recipients.

10.8* Some other aspects of frailty modelling

A number of other issues that arise in connection with frailty modelling are discussed briefly in this section.

10.8.1 Model checking

The techniques for model checking described in Chapters 4 and 7 may reveal outlying observations, influential values and inadequacies in the functional form of covariates. In addition, an informal way of assessing the adequacy of a parametric model with gamma frailty is to compare the observed survivor function with the observable function derived from a frailty model, as in Example 10.2. In more complex problems, the baseline survivor function estimated from fitting a Cox model with the same explanatory variables as the frailty model, can be compared to the observable survivor function for an individual with all explanatory variables set to zero. For other choices of frailty distribution the observable survivor function can only be determined numerically, and so this approach is not so useful.

In frailty modelling, the validity of the chosen frailty distribution may also be critically examined. Two particular distributional models have been described in this chapter, the gamma and lognormal distributions, but there are a number of other possibilities. Which of these frailty distributions is chosen is often guided by mathematical convenience and the availability of statistical software. One approach to discriminating between alternative frailty distributions is to consider a general family that includes specific distributions as special cases. The *power variance function (PVF) distribution* is widely used in this context. This distribution has a density function that is a function of three parameters, α, δ and θ, and whose mean and variance are given by

$$\mathrm{E}\,(Z) = \delta\theta^{\alpha-1}, \qquad \mathrm{var}\,(Z) = \delta(1-\alpha)\theta^{\alpha-2},$$

for $\theta \geqslant 0$, $0 < \alpha \leqslant 1$, $\delta > 0$. Setting $\delta = \theta^{1-\alpha}$ gives a distribution with unit mean and variance $(1-\alpha)/\theta$. When $\alpha = 0$ the distribution reduces to a gamma density with variance θ^{-1} and when $\alpha = 0.5$ to an inverse Gaussian distribution. Tests of hypotheses about the value of α can then inform model choice.

Another approach to model checking is to assess the sensitivity of key model-based inferences to the specific choice of frailty model. Comparing hazard ratios from a fully parametric models with those from a Cox regression model that has the same frailty distribution can also be valuable.

10.8.2 Correlated frailty models

An important extension of shared frailty models is to the situation where the frailties of individuals within a group are not identical as in the shared frailty model, but are merely correlated. Such models are particularly relevant when interest centres on the association between event times, as might be the case when studying event times of paired organs, or amongst twins for example. In the bivariate frailty case, correlated frailty can be modelled by extending the model in Equation (10.30) to have a separate frailty for each member of the pair. Then, in the ith pair, the hazard function is

$$h_{ij}(t) = z_{ij} \exp(\boldsymbol{\beta}'\boldsymbol{x}_{ij})h_0(t),$$

for $j = 1, 2$, and a bivariate distribution is adopted for the corresponding frailty random variables (Z_{i1}, Z_{i2}). In the case of lognormal frailties, a bivariate normal distribution could be assumed for the corresponding random effects $U_{ij} = \log(Z_{ij})$ in the linear component of the model, with $\text{corr}\,(U_{i1}, U_{i2}) = \rho$. This correlation need not be the same for each group. The extent of this correlation can then be evaluated. Such models may be fitted using likelihood or penalised likelihood methods, but can also be fitted using Monte Carlo Markov Chain (MCMC) methods.

10.8.3 Dependence measures

When a shared frailty model is being used to account for association between the event times of individuals within a group, a large frailty variance corresponds to a high degree of dependence between the times. In this sense, the frailty variance is a measure of dependence, and the extent of this dependence can be compared in alternative models. For example, on adding certain covariates, the frailty effect may diminish and so a reduction in the frailty variance would indicate that the revised model has been successful in reducing unexplained variation.

Other measures of dependence in parametric models can be based on correlation. In the special case of gamma frailty distributions, Kendall's coefficient of rank correlation, τ, is a useful measure of association between a pair of survival times. Kendall's τ is simply related to the frailty variance θ^{-1}, and is found from $\tau = (1 + 2\theta)^{-1}$. The advantage of this is that it yields a summary statistic of dependence in the range $(0, 1)$.

10.8.4 Numerical problems in model fitting

Frailty models are generally fitted using a combination of numerical integration and optimisation. For this reason, it is important to specify suitable initial values for the unknown parameters. These are best obtained from fitting the corresponding model without frailty, and using a small value for the initial frailty variance. Even then, numerical procedures can lead to computational problems in the fitting process, and instability in the resulting estimates. This is particularly the case when the parameters being estimated have very different scales. For instance, in Example 10.3, estimates of the Weibull shape parameter, λ, are much smaller than estimates of the other parameters, leading to convergence problems. Such difficulties can often be overcome by rescaling certain parameters, in this case by working with $\lambda' = 10000\lambda$, or by reparameterising the model. Variance parameters such as σ_u^2 in a normal random effect may be recoded by estimating $\omega = \log \sigma_u^2$, and writing $\exp(\omega)$ in place of σ_u^2 in the model. If changes such as these are not successful, some changes may be needed to the settings used in the numerical integration process, or the criteria that define convergence of the optimisation process.

10.9 Further reading

Hougaard (2000) includes an extensive discussion of frailty models, and a number of illustrative examples. More recently, the books of Wienke (2011) and Duchateau and Janssen (2008) both give thorough accounts of frailty modelling. General review papers include those of Aalen (1994), Aalen (1998), and Hougaard (1995). General texts on mixed models include Brown and Prescott (2000), Demidenko (2013), West, Welch and Galecki (2007) and Stroup (2013). Texts that include accounts of restricted maximum likelihood estimation (REML) include those of McCulloch, Searle and Neuhaus (2008) and Searle, Casella and McCulloch (2006)

McGilchrist and Aisbett (1991) describe how a Cox model with normal random effects can be fitted and illustrate this with a much discussed example on times to the recurrence of infection following insertion of a catheter in patients on dialysis. Their approach is generalised in Ripatti and Palmgren (2000) who show how random frailty effects that have a multivariate distribution can be fitted using penalised partial log-likelihood methods. Therneau and Grambsch (2000) include a chapter on frailty models and describe how penalised partial log-likelihood methods can be used to fit Cox models with frailty and to test hypotheses about parameters in the fitted models; see also Therneau, Grambsch and Pankratz (2003). An alternative fitting method is based on the expectation-maximization (EM) algorithm, described by Klein (1992) and Klein and Moeschberger (2005).

Instead of comparing Cox regression models with frailty using the maximised marginal log-likelihood, Wald tests can be used. This approach has been described by Therneau and Grambsch (2000), and uses the notion of generalised degrees of freedom, described by Gray (1992). The result that the change in $-2\log\hat{L}$ on adding a frailty effect to a parametric model has an asymptotic $0.5(\chi_0^2 + \chi_1^2)$ distribution was given in Claeskens, Nguti and Janssen (2008).

Lambert et al. (2004) and Nelson et al. (2006) show how the probability integral transformation can be used to fit parametric accelerated failure time models with non-normal random frailty effects. This allows other distributions to be adopted when using computer software designed for fitting models with normal random effects.

There has been relatively little published on methods for checking the adequacy of frailty models, with most emphasis on testing the validity of a gamma frailty. One of the first papers to develop a test for the assumption of a gamma frailty distribution was Shih and Louis (1995), and a goodness of fit test for use with bivariate survival data was given by Shih (1998). Some extensions are described by Glidden (1999). More recently a formal goodness of fit test is given in Geerdens, Claeskens and Janssen (2013), who also briefly review other work in this area.

Chapter 11

Non-proportional hazards and institutional comparisons

Proportional hazards models are widely used in modelling survival data in medical research and other application areas. This assumption of proportionality means that the effect of an explanatory variable or factor on the hazard of an event occurring does not depend on time. This can be quite a strong assumption, and situations frequently arise where this assumption is untenable. Although models that do not assume proportional hazards have been described in earlier chapters, some additional methods are described in this chapter. A particularly important application of non-proportional hazards modelling is the comparison of survival rates between institutions, and so methods that can be used in this context are also described.

11.1 Non-proportional hazards

Models that do not require the assumption of proportional hazards include the accelerated failure time model and the proportional odds model introduced in Chapter 6, and the Cox regression model that includes a time-dependent variable, described in Chapter 8. But often we are faced with a situation where the assumption of proportional hazards cannot be made, and yet none of the above models is satisfactory.

As an illustration, consider a study to compare a surgical procedure with chemotherapy in the treatment of a particular form of cancer. Suppose that the survivor functions under the two treatments are as shown in Figure 11.1, where the time-scale is in years. Clearly the hazards are non-proportional. Death at an early stage may be experienced by patients on the surgical treatment, as a result of patients not being able to withstand the surgery or complications arising from it. In the longer term, patients who have recovered from the surgery have a better prognosis. A similar situation arises when an aggressive form of chemotherapy is compared to a standard. Here also, a long-term advantage to the aggressive treatment may be at the expense of short-term excess mortality.

One approach, which is useful in the analysis of data arising from situations such as these, is to define the end-point of the study to be survival beyond

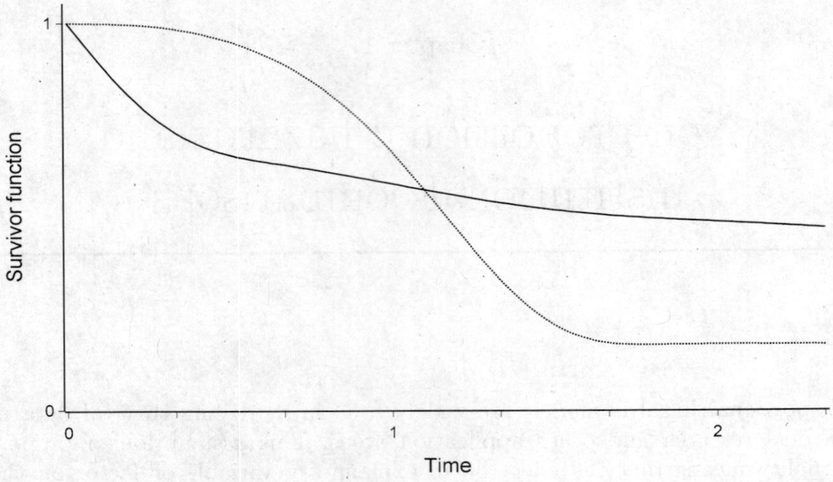

Figure 11.1 *Long-term advantage of surgery (—) over chemotherapy (⋯⋯).*

some particular time. For example, in the study leading to the survivor functions illustrated in Figure 11.1, the treatment difference is roughly constant after two years. The dependence of the probability of survival beyond two years on prognostic variables and treatment might therefore be modelled. This approach was discussed in connection with the analysis of interval-censored survival data in Section 9.2. As shown in that section, there are advantages in using a linear model for the complementary log-log transformation of the survival probability. In particular, the coefficients of the explanatory variables in the linear component of the model can be interpreted as logarithms of hazard ratios. The disadvantages of this approach are that all patients must be followed until the point in time when the survival rates are to be analysed, and that the death data cannot be used until this time. Moreover, faith in the long-term benefits of one or other of the two treatments will be needed to ensure that the trial is not stopped early because of excess mortality in one treatment group.

Strictly speaking, an analysis based on the survival probability at a particular time is only valid when that time is specified at the outset of the study, which may be difficult to do. If the data are used to suggest end-points such as the probability of survival beyond two years, some caution will be needed in interpreting the results of a significance test.

In the study that leads to the survivor functions shown in Figure 11.1, it is clear that an analysis of the two-year survival rate will be appropriate. Now consider a study to compare the use of chemotherapy in addition to surgery with surgery alone, in which the survivor functions are as shown in Figure 11.2. Here, the short-term benefit of the chemotherapy may certainly be

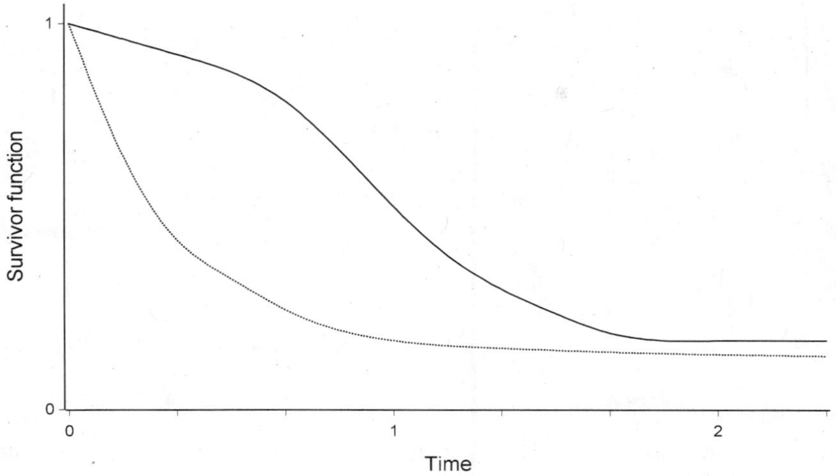

Figure 11.2 *Short-term advantage of chemotherapy and surgery (—) over surgery alone (·······).*

worthwhile, but an analysis of the two-year survival rates will fail to establish a treatment difference. The fact that the difference between the two survival rates is not constant makes it difficult to use an analysis based on survival rates at a given time. However, it might be reasonable to assume that the hazards are proportional over the first year of the study, and to carry out a survival analysis at that time.

11.2 Stratified proportional hazards models

A situation that sometimes occurs is that hazards are not proportional on an overall basis, but that they are proportional in different subgroups of the data. For example, consider a situation in which a new drug is being compared with a standard in the treatment of a particular disease. If the study involves two participating centres, it is possible that in each centre the new treatment halves the hazard of death, but that the hazard functions for the standard drug differ between centres. Then, the hazards between centres for individuals on a given drug are not proportional. This situation is illustrated in Figure 11.3.

In problems of this kind, it may be assumed that patients in each of the subgroups, or *strata*, have a different baseline hazard function, but that all other explanatory variables satisfy the proportional hazards assumption within each stratum. Suppose that the patients in the jth stratum have a baseline hazard function $h_{0j}(t)$, for $j = 1, 2, \dots, g$, where g is the number of strata. The effect of explanatory variables on the hazard function can then be represented by a proportional hazards model for $h_{ij}(t)$, the hazard function for the ith

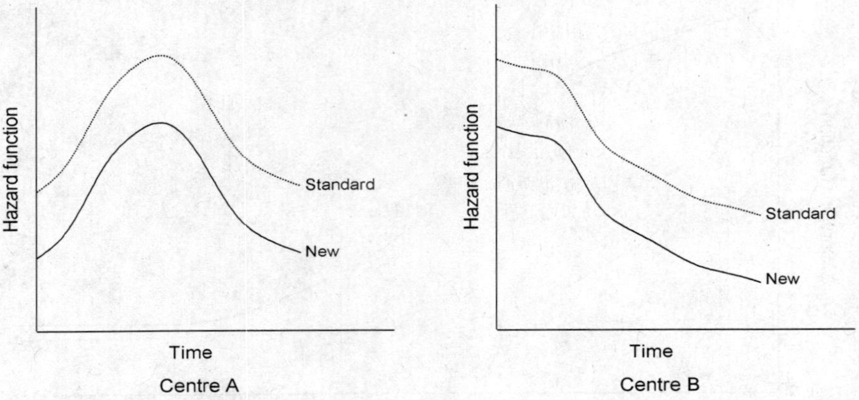

Figure 11.3 *Hazard functions for individuals on a new drug (—) and a standard drug (······) in two centres.*

individual in the jth stratum, where $i = 1, 2, \ldots, n_j$, say, and n_j is the number of individuals in the jth stratum. We then have the *stratified proportional hazards model*, according to which

$$h_{ij}(t) = \exp(\boldsymbol{\beta}'\boldsymbol{x}_{ij})h_{0j}(t),$$

where $\boldsymbol{x}_{ij}$ is the vector of values of p explanatory variables, $X_1, X_2, \ldots, X_p$, recorded on the ith individual in the jth stratum. This model was introduced in connection with the risk adjusted survivor function, described in Section 3.11.1 of Chapter 3.

As an example of this model, consider the particular case where there are two treatments being compared in each of g centres, and no other explanatory variables. Let x_{ij} be the value of an indicator variable X, which is zero if the ith patient in the jth centre is on the standard treatment and unity if on the new treatment. The hazard function for this individual is then

$$h_{ij}(t) = e^{\beta x_{ij}}h_{0j}(t).$$

On fitting this model, the estimated value of β is the log-hazard ratio for a patient on the new treatment, relative to one on the standard, in each centre.

This model for stratified proportional hazards is easily fitted using standard software packages for survival analysis, and nested models can be compared using the $-2\log\hat{L}$ statistic. Apart from the fact that the stratifying variable cannot be included in the linear part of the model, no new principles are involved. When two or more groups of survival data are being compared, the stratified proportional hazards model is in fact equivalent to the stratified log-rank test described in Section 2.8 of Chapter 2.

11.2.1 Non-proportional hazards between treatments

If there are non-proportional hazards between two treatments, misleading inferences can result from ignoring this phenomenon. To illustrate this point, suppose that the hazard function for two groups of individuals, on a new and standard treatment, are as shown in Figure 11.4 (i). If a proportional hazards model were fitted, the resulting fitted hazard functions are likely to be as shown in Figure 11.4 (ii). Incorrect conclusions would then be drawn about the relative merit of the two treatments.

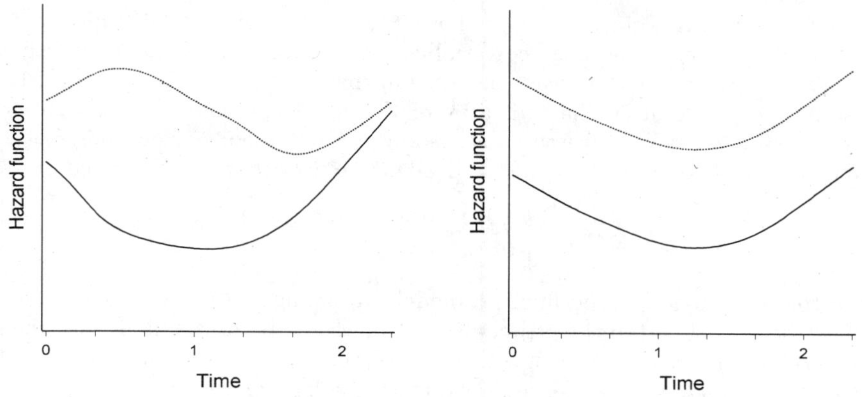

Figure 11.4 *(i) Non-proportional hazards and (ii) the result of fitting a proportional hazards model for individuals on a new treatment (—) and a standard treatment (·······).*

Non-proportional hazards between treatments can be modelled by assuming proportional hazards in a series of consecutive time intervals. This is achieved using a *piecewise Cox model*, which is analogous to the piecewise exponential model introduced in Chapter 6. To illustrate the use of the model, suppose that the time period over which the hazard functions in Figure 11.4 are given is divided into three intervals, namely $(0, t_1]$, $(t_1, t_2]$ and $(t_2, t_3]$. Within each of these intervals, hazards might be assumed to be proportional.

Now let X be an indicator variable associated with the two treatments, where $X = 0$ if an individual is on the standard treatment and $X = 1$ if an individual is on the new treatment. The piecewise Cox regression model can then be fitted by defining two time-dependent variables, $X_2(t)$ and $X_3(t)$, say, which are as follows:

$$X_2(t) = \begin{cases} 1 \text{ if } t \in (t_1, t_2] \text{ and } X = 1, \\ 0 \text{ otherwise;} \end{cases}$$

$$X_3(t) = \begin{cases} 1 \text{ if } t \in (t_2, t_3] \text{ and } X = 1, \\ 0 \text{ otherwise.} \end{cases}$$

In the absence of other explanatory variables, the model for the hazard function for the ith individual at time t can be written as

$$h_i(t) = \exp\{\beta_1 x_i + \beta_2 x_{2i}(t) + \beta_3 x_{3i}(t)\} h_0(t), \tag{11.1}$$

where x_i is the value of X for the ith individual, and $x_{2i}(t)$ and $x_{3i}(t)$ are the values of the two time-dependent variables for the ith individual at t. Under this model, the log-hazard ratio for an individual on the new treatment, relative to one on the standard, is then β_1 for $t \in (0, t_1]$, $\beta_1 + \beta_2$ for $t \in (t_1, t_2]$ and $\beta_1 + \beta_3$ for $t \in (t_2, t_3]$. This model can be fitted in the manner described in Chapter 8.

The model in Equation (11.1) allows the assumption of proportional hazards to be tested by adding the variables $x_{2i}(t)$ and $x_{3i}(t)$ to the model that contains x_i alone. A significant decrease in the value of the $-2 \log \hat{L}$ statistic would indicate that the hazard ratio for the new treatment ($X = 1$) relative to the standard ($X = 0$) was not constant. An equivalent formulation of the model in Equation (11.1) is obtained by defining $x_{1i}(t)$ to be the value of

$$X_1(t) = \begin{cases} 1 & \text{if } t \in (0, t_1] \text{ and } X = 1, \\ 0 & \text{otherwise,} \end{cases}$$

for the ith individual, and fitting a model containing $x_{1i}(t)$, $x_{2i}(t)$ and $x_{3i}(t)$. The coefficients of the three time-dependent variables in this model are then the log-hazard ratios for the new treatment relative to the standard in each of the three intervals. Confidence intervals for the hazard ratio can be obtained directly from this version of the model.

Example 11.1 Survival times of patients with gastric cancer
In a randomised controlled trial carried out by the Gastrointestinal Tumor Study Group, 90 patients with locally advanced gastric carcinoma were recruited. They were randomised to receive chemotherapy alone consisting of a combination of 5-fluorouracil and 1-(2-chloroethyl)-3-(4-methylcyclohexyl)-1-nitrosoureamethyl (methyl CCNU), or a combination of the same chemotherapy treatment with external radiotherapy of 5000 rad. Patients were followed up for over eight years, and the outcome of interest is the number of days from randomisation to death from gastric cancer. The data, as reported by Stablein and Koutrouvelis (1985), are shown in Table 11.1.

Kaplan-Meier estimates of the survivor functions for the patients in each treatment group are shown in Figure 11.5. This figure shows that over the first two years, patients on the combined chemotherapy and radiotherapy treatment have lower survival rates than those on chemotherapy alone. However, in the longer term, the combined therapy is more advantageous. The two lines in the log-cumulative hazard plot in Figure 11.6 are not parallel, again confirming that the treatment effect varies over time. If this aspect of the data had been ignored, and a Cox regression model fitted, the estimated hazard ratio for the combined treatment, relative to the chemotherapy treatment alone, would have been 1.11, and the P-value for the change in the $-2 \log \hat{L}$ statistic

Table 11.1 *Survival times of gastric cancer patients.*

Chemotherapy alone			Chemotherapy and Radiotherapy		
1	383	748	17	185	542
63	383	778	42	193	567
105	388	786	44	195	577
129	394	797	48	197	580
182	408	955	60	208	795
216	460	968	72	234	855
250	489	1000	74	235	1366
262	499	1245	95	254	1577
301	523	1271	103	307	2060
301	524	1420	108	315	2412*
342	535	1551	122	401	2486*
354	562	1694	144	445	2796*
356	569	2363	167	464	2802*
358	675	2754*	170	484	2934*
380	676	2950*	183	528	2988*

* Censored survival times.

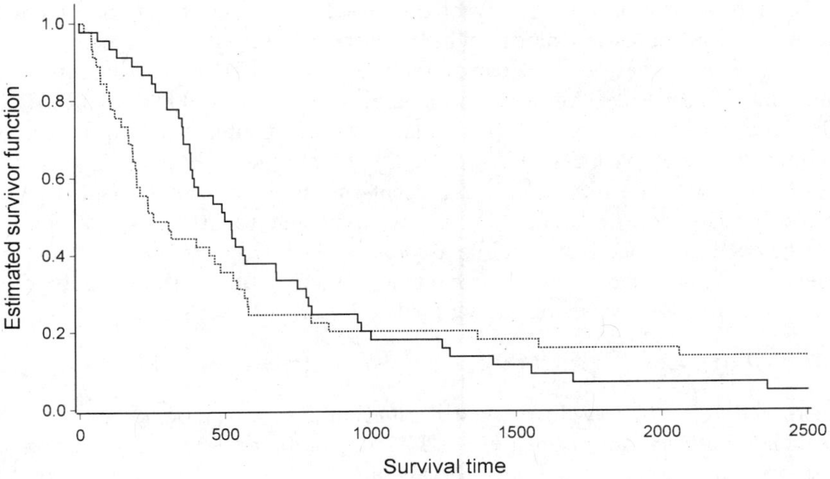

Figure 11.5 *Estimates of the survivor functions for gastric cancer patients on chemotherapy alone (—) or a combination of chemotherapy and radiotherapy (·······).*

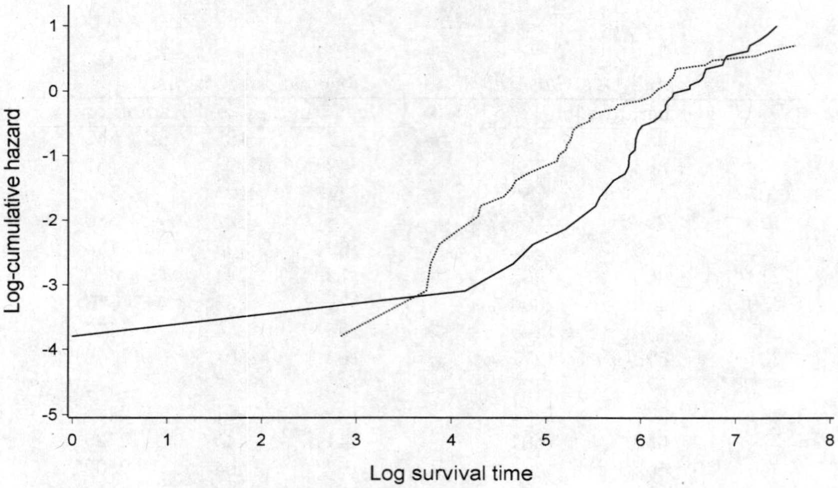

Figure 11.6 *Log-cumulative hazard plot for gastric cancer patients on chemotherapy alone (—) or a combination of chemotherapy and radiotherapy (·······).*

on adding the treatment effect to a null model is 0.64. We would then have concluded there was no evidence of a treatment effect, but since the hazards of death on the two treatments are not proportional, this analysis is incorrect.

A more appropriate summary of the treatment effect is obtained using a piecewise Cox regression model, where the treatment effect is assumed constant in each of a number of separate intervals, but differs across the intervals. Four time intervals will be used in this analysis, namely 1–360, 361–720, 721–1080 and 1081– days. A time-dependent treatment effect is then set up by defining four variables, $X_1(t), X_2(t), X_3(t), X_4(t)$, where $X_j(t) = 1$ when t is within the jth time interval for a patient on the combined treatment, and zero otherwise, for $j = 1, 2, 3, 4$. This is equivalent to fitting an interaction between a time-dependent variable associated with the four intervals and the treatments effect. If $x_{ji}(t)$ is the value of the jth variable for the ith individual at time t, the Cox regression model for the hazard of death at time t is

$$h_i(t) = \exp\{\beta_1 x_{1i}(t) + \beta_2 x_{2i}(t) + \beta_3 x_{3i}(t) + \beta_4 x_{4i}(t)\}\, h_0(t),$$

where $h_0(t)$ is the baseline hazard function. In this model, the four β-coefficients are the log-hazard ratios for the combined treatment relative to chemotherapy alone in the four intervals, and $h_0(t)$ is the hazard function for a patient on the chemotherapy treatment.

On fitting all four time-dependent variables, the value of $-2\log\hat{L}$ is 602.372. For the model in which a treatment effect alone is fitted, on the assumption of proportional hazards, the hazard of death for the ith patient at time t is $h_i(t) = \exp(\beta x_i)h_0(t)$, where x_i is the value of a variable X

for the ith patient, where $X = 0$ for a patient on the chemotherapy treatment and $X = 1$ for a patient on the combined treatment. On fitting this model, $-2\log\hat{L} = 614.946$. The two models are nested and the difference in their $-2\log\hat{L}$ values provides a test of proportional hazards. This difference of 12.57 on 3 d.f. is highly significant, $P = 0.005$, confirming that there is clear evidence of non-proportionality in the hazard ratio for the treatment effect. On fitting the four time-dependent variables, the hazard ratios and 95% confidence intervals are as shown in Table 11.2.

Table 11.2 *Hazard ratios and their corresponding 95% confidence limits on fitting a piecewise Cox regression model.*

Time interval	Hazard ratio	95% confidence limits
1–360	2.40	(1.25, 4.64)
361–720	0.78	(0.34, 1.76)
721–1080	0.33	(0.07, 1.60)
1081–	0.31	(0.08, 1.24)

This table summarises how the treatment effect varies over the four time intervals. In the first year, patients on the combined treatment have over twice the risk of death at any time, compared to those on the chemotherapy treatment alone. In subsequent years, patients on the combined treatment have a reduced hazard of death, although the three interval estimates all include unity, suggesting that these hazard ratios are not significantly different from 1.

11.3* Restricted mean survival

When hazards are not proportional, the hazard ratio is not an appropriate summary of the effect of a covariate or a treatment effect. This is because the hazard ratio is time-dependent, and so a single estimate of this ratio may be misleading. An alternative summary measure, that has the advantage of being straightforward to interpret, is the mean survival time to some predetermined time point, called the *restricted mean survival time*.

To define the restricted mean survival time, suppose that T is a random variable associated with a survival time. The restricted mean survival time to t_0, $\mu(t_0)$, is then the expected value of the minimum of T and t_0 over the follow-up period, so that $\mu(t_0) = \mathrm{E}\,(\min\{T, t_0\})$.

Now,

$$\mathrm{E}\,(\min\{T, t_0\}) = \mathrm{E}\,(T; T \leqslant t_0) + t_0\,\mathrm{P}(T > t_0),$$

and

$$\mathrm{E}\,(T; T \leqslant t_0) = \int_0^{t_0} u f(u)\,\mathrm{d}u,$$

when T has a parametric distribution with density $f(t)$. Integrating by parts,

$$\int_0^{t_0} u f(u)\,\mathrm{d}u = uF(u)\big|_0^{t_0} - \int_0^{t_0} F(u)\,\mathrm{d}u = t_0F(t_0) - \int_0^{t_0} F(u)\,\mathrm{d}u,$$

and in terms of the survivor function, $S(t) = 1 - F(t)$,

$$\int_0^{t_0} uf(u)\,du = t_0\{1 - S(t_0)\} - \int_0^{t_0} \{1 - S(u)\}\,du,$$

so that

$$\int_0^{t_0} uf(u)\,du = \int_0^{t_0} S(u)\,du - t_0 S(t_0).$$

Finally, since $t_0 \mathrm{P}(T > t_0) = t_0 S(t_0)$,

$$\mathrm{E}\left(\min\{T, t_0\}\right) = \int_0^{t_0} S(u)\,du.$$

The restricted mean survival time is therefore the area under the estimated survivor function to t_0, and is an easily understood summary statistic. For example, if time is measured in months, $\mu(24)$ is the average number of months survived over a 24-month period, and so is the two-year life expectancy. This statistic can also be used to summarise the effect of a treatment parameter or other explanatory variables on life expectancy over a defined period of time.

The restricted mean survival can be determined from the Kaplan-Meier estimate of the survivor function. For example, the estimated restricted mean at the rth ordered event time, $t_{(r)}$, is

$$\hat{\mu}(t_{(r)}) = \sum_{j=1}^{r} \hat{S}(t_{(j)})(t_{(j)} - t_{(j-1)}),$$

where $\hat{S}(t_{(j)})$ is the Kaplan-Meier estimate of the survivor function at the jth event time, $t_{(j)}$, and $t_{(0)}$ is defined to be zero. The standard error of this estimate is given by

$$\left(\sum_{j=1}^{r-1} A_j^2 / \{n_j \hat{S}(t_{(j)})\} \right)^{\frac{1}{2}},$$

where

$$A_j = \sum_{i=j}^{r-1} \hat{S}(t_{(i)})(t_{(i+1)} - t_{(i)}).$$

A minor modification to these results is needed when an estimate of restricted survival is required at a time that is not actually an event time.

When there are two groups of survival times, as in a clinical trial to compare two treatments, and non-proportional hazards is anticipated or found, the restricted mean survival time can be determined from the area under the Kaplan-Meier estimates of the two survivor functions. The difference in the estimated restricted mean survival to a given time can then be used as an unadjusted summary measure of the overall treatment effect.

More generally, consider the situation where there is non-proportional hazards between two treatment groups and where information on the values of other explanatory variables is available. Here, parametric models with different underlying hazards could be used, such as a Weibull model with a different shape parameter for each treatment group. The survivor functions under such a model are fully parameterised, and so the restricted mean survival time can be estimated by integrating the fitted survivor function, analytically or numerically.

A greater degree of flexibility in modelling the underlying baseline hazard function is achieved by using the *Royston and Parmar model* described in Section 6.9 of Chapter 6. By adding interaction terms between the treatment factor and the cubic spline functions that define the baseline hazard, different underlying hazard functions for each treatment group can be fitted. Again, the restricted mean survival time can subsequently be obtained by integrating the fitted survivor functions.

11.3.1 Use of pseudo-values

A versatile, and straightforward way of modelling the dependence of the restricted mean survival on explanatory variables is based on *pseudo-values*. These values are formed from the differences between an estimate of some quantity obtained from a complete set of n individuals, and that obtained on omitting the ith, for $i = 1, 2, \ldots, n$. Standard regression models are then used to model the dependence of the pseudo-values on explanatory variables.

To obtain the pseudo-values for the restricted mean, the Kaplan-Meier estimate of the survivor function for the complete set of survival times is first determined, from which the restricted mean survival at some value t_0 is obtained, $\hat{\mu}(t_0)$, say. Then, each observation is omitted in turn, and the restricted mean survival is estimated from the reduced data set, to give $\hat{\mu}_{(-i)}(t_0)$, for $i = 1, 2, \ldots, n$. The ith pseudo-value is then

$$z_i = n\hat{\mu}(t_0) - (n-1)\hat{\mu}_{(-i)}(t_0), \tag{11.2}$$

for $i = 1, 2, \ldots, n$. This measures the contribution made by the ith individual to the estimated restricted mean survival time at t_0, and is defined irrespective of whether or not the observed survival time for that individual is censored.

The ith pseudo-value, z_i, is then assumed to be the observed value of a random variable Z_i, and a generalised linear model may then be used to model the dependence of the expected value of Z_i on treatment factors and explanatory variables. A natural choice would be to assume that Z_i is normally distributed, with a log-linear model for its mean, $\text{E}(Z_i)$. Then, $\log \text{E}(Z_i) = \beta_0 + \boldsymbol{\beta}'\boldsymbol{x}_i$, where β_0 is a constant and $\boldsymbol{x}_i$ is the vector of values of explanatory variables for the ith individual. A linear regression model for $\text{E}(Z_i)$ will often give similar results.

In practical applications, the value to use for t_0 has to be determined in advance of the analysis. When the occurrence of an event over a particular time period is of interest, this time period will determine the value of t_0. For example, if the average time survived over a one-year period following the diagnosis of a particular form of cancer is of interest, t_0 would be 365 days. In other cases, t_0 will be usually be taken to be close to the longest observed event time in the data set.

Example 11.2 Survival times of patients with gastric cancer
An alternative analysis of the data on survival times of patients suffering from gastric cancer, given in Example 11.1, is based on the restricted mean. The restricted mean survival will be calculated at 5 years, obtained as the area under the Kaplan-Meier estimate of the survivor function for patients in each treatment group up to $t = 1826$ days. This is found to be 661.31 (se = 74.45) for patients on the single treatment and 571.89 (se = 94.04) for those on the combined treatment. This means that over a five-year period, patients are expected to survive for 1.8 years on average when on chemotherapy alone, and 1.6 years when on the combined treatment. The 95% confidence intervals for the restricted mean survival time to 1826 days are (515.39, 807.23) and (387.57, 756.21), respectively, for the two treatment groups. As there is a substantial overlap between these intervals, there is no evidence that the restricted mean survival time differs between the two groups.

We next illustrate the use of pseudo-values in analysing these data. First, the Kaplan-Meier estimate of the survivor function for the complete data set is obtained, and from this the estimated restricted mean to 1826 days is 616.60 days. This is an overall estimate of the average patient survival time over this time period. Each of the 90 observations is then omitted in turn, and the Kaplan-Meier estimate recalculated from each set of 89 observations. The restricted mean to 1826 days is then estimated for each of these 90 sets of data, and Equation (11.2) is then used to obtain the 90 pseudo-values. These represent the contribution of each observation to the overall estimate of the five-year restricted mean.

For the data in Table 11.1, the pseudo-values are equal to the observed survival times for patients that die before 1826 days, while for the 10 patients that survive beyond that time, the pseudo-values are all equal to 1826. This pattern in the pseudo-values is due to the censored survival times being the longest observed follow-up times in the data set.

The next step is to model the dependence of the pseudo-values on the treatment effect. This can be done using a log-linear model for the expected value of the ith pseudo-observation, $\text{E}\,(Z_i)$, $i = 1, 2, \ldots, n$, where $\log \text{E}\,(Z_i) = \beta_0 + \beta_1 x_i$, and $x_i = 0$ if the ith patient is on the chemotherapy treatment alone and $x_i = 1$ otherwise. On adding the treatment effect to the log-linear model, the deviance is reduced from 28591297 on 89 d.f. to 28411380 on 88 d.f., and so the F-ratio for testing whether there is a treatment effect is $(28591297 - 28411380)/\{28411380/88\} = 0.56$, which is not significant as an F-statistic on 1, 88 d.f. ($P = 0.46$). Much the same result is obtained using a linear model for $\text{E}(Z_i)$, which is equivalent to using a two-sample t-test to compare the means of the pseudo-values in each treatment group. Patient survival over 1826 days is therefore unaffected by the addition of radiotherapy to the chemotherapy treatment.

In summary, the data in Table 11.1 indicate that there is a longer-term benefit for patients on the combination of chemotherapy and radiotherapy, so long as they survive the first 18 months or so where there is an increased risk of death on this treatment. However, over the five-year follow-up period, on average there is no survival benefit from being on the combined treatment.

11.4 Institutional comparisons

The need for accountability in the health service has led to the introduction of a range of performance indicators that measure the quality of care provided by different institutions. One of the key measures is the risk adjusted mortality rate, which summarises the mortality experienced by patients in different healthcare institutions in a way that takes account of differences in the characteristics of patients being treated. Statistics such as these provide a means of comparing institutional performance on an equal footing. Analogous measures can be defined for survival rates, recovery rates and infection rates, and the methods that are described in this section apply equally to comparisons between other types of organisation, such as schools, universities and providers of financial services. In this section, we describe and illustrate how point and interval estimates for a *risk adjusted failure rate*, $RAFR$, can be obtained from survival data.

The $RAFR$ is an estimate of

$$\frac{\text{Observed failure rate}}{\text{Expected failure rate}} \times \text{Overall failure rate}, \tag{11.3}$$

at a given time, where the observed failure rate is obtained from the Kaplan-Meier estimate of the survivor function for a specific institution at a given time, and the overall failure rate at that time is estimated from the survivor function fitted to the data across all institutions, ignoring differences between them. The expected failure rate for an institution can be estimated from the risk adjusted survivor function, defined in Section 3.11 of Chapter 3, which is the average of the estimated survivor functions for individuals within an institution, at a given time, based on a risk adjustment model. Estimates of each failure rate at a specified time are obtained by subtracting the corresponding value of the estimated survivor function from unity. Once the $RAFR$ has been obtained, the analogous *risk adjusted survival rate*, or $RASR$, can simply be found from $RASR = 1 - RAFR$.

Example 11.3 Comparisons between kidney transplant centres

The methods of this section will be illustrated using data on the transplant survival rates experienced by recipients of organs from deceased donors in eight kidney transplant centres in the UK, in the three-year period from January

2009 to December 2011. There are a number of factors that may affect the centre specific survival rates, and in this illustration, account is taken of donor age, an indicator of whether the donor is deceased following brain death (DBD donor) or circulatory death (DCD donor), recipient age at transplant, diabetic status of the recipient (absent, present) and the elapsed time between retrieval of the kidney from the donor and transplantation into the recipient, known as the cold ischaemic time. Also recorded is the transplant survival time, defined to be the earlier of graft failure and patient death, and an event indicator that is zero if the patient was alive with a functioning graft at the last known date of follow-up, or December 2012 at the latest. The variables are summarised below.

Patient:	Patient identifier
Centre:	Transplant centre $(1, 2, \ldots, 8)$
Tsurv:	Transplant survival time (days)
Tcens:	Event indicator (0 = censored, 1 = transplant failure)
Dage:	Donor age (years)
Dtype:	Donor type (0 = DBD, 1 = DCD)
Rage:	Recipient age (years)
Diab:	Diabetic status (0 = absent, 1 = present)
CIT:	Cold ischaemic time (hours)

There are 1439 patients in the data set, and data for the first 30 patients transplanted in the time period are shown in Table 11.3. The transplanted kidney did not function in patient 7, and so $Tsurv = 0$ for this patient.

Of particular interest is the transplant failure rate at one year, and so the eight transplant centres will be compared using this metric. We first obtain the unadjusted Kaplan-Meier estimate of the survivor function across all 1439 patients, from which the overall one-year failure rate is $1 - 0.904 = 0.096$. The centre-specific one-year failure rates are similarly obtained from the Kaplan-Meier estimate of the survivor function for patients in each centre. Next, the risk adjusted survival rate in each centre is calculated using the method described in Section 3.11.1 of Chapter 3. A Cox regression model that contains the variables *Dage*, *Dtype*, *Rage*, *Diab*, and *CIT*, is fitted to the data, from which the estimated survivor function for the ith patient in the jth centre is

$$\hat{S}_{ij}(t) = \{\hat{S}_0(t)\}^{\exp(\hat{\eta}_{ij})}, \tag{11.4}$$

where

$$\hat{\eta}_{ij} = 0.023\, Dage_{ij} + 0.191\, Dtype_{ij} + 0.002\, Rage_{ij} - 0.133\, Diab_{ij} + 0.016\, CIT_{ij},$$

and $\hat{S}_0(t)$ is the estimated baseline survivor function. The average survivor function at time t in the jth centre, $j = 1, 2, \ldots, 8$, is

$$\hat{S}_j(t) = \frac{1}{n_j} \sum_{i=1}^{n_j} \hat{S}_{ij}(t),$$

Table 11.3 *Transplant survival times of 30 kidney recipients.*

Patient	*Centre*	*Tsurv*	*Tcens*	*Dage*	*Dtype*	*Rage*	*Diab*	*CIT*
1	6	1384	0	63	0	44	0	25.3
2	8	1446	0	17	0	33	0	24.0
3	8	1414	0	34	0	48	0	16.7
4	5	1459	0	36	0	31	0	13.6
5	4	1385	0	63	0	58	0	30.5
6	2	1455	0	40	0	35	0	15.8
7	3	0	1	59	0	46	0	14.9
8	6	1453	0	17	0	38	0	17.4
9	8	236	1	57	1	50	0	18.7
10	8	1445	0	59	0	34	0	15.0
11	8	1428	0	53	0	63	0	13.0
12	4	1454	0	59	0	50	0	13.7
13	4	1372	0	27	1	65	0	19.3
14	4	382	1	27	1	71	0	12.2
15	3	1452	0	47	0	68	0	17.8
16	3	1436	0	29	0	37	0	12.1
17	7	1452	0	28	0	49	0	12.9
18	4	310	1	51	1	62	0	14.3
19	1	1059	1	73	1	62	0	10.6
20	1	1446	0	17	1	32	0	10.3
21	1	1397	0	17	1	51	0	19.0
22	1	1369	0	37	1	46	0	10.4
23	1	1444	0	37	1	48	0	15.1
24	8	1443	0	63	0	53	0	14.8
25	7	1395	0	32	0	60	0	19.9
26	3	1396	0	36	0	36	0	13.4
27	4	1261	0	30	0	48	0	15.1
28	5	1441	0	44	1	50	1	12.4
29	2	1439	0	54	0	27	0	11.6
30	4	1411	0	38	0	26	0	15.9

where n_j is the number of patients in the jth centre, and the expected transplant failure rate at one year can then be estimated from this survivor function. The unadjusted and adjusted one-year survival rates are shown in Table 11.4, together with the *RAFR*.

To illustrate the calculation, for Centre 1, the unadjusted and adjusted one-year survival rates are 0.9138 and 0.8920, respectively, and since overall unadjusted survival rate is 0.096, the *RAFR* is

$$\frac{1 - 0.9138}{1 - 0.8920} \times 0.096 = 0.077.$$

The corresponding risk adjusted transplant survival rate for this centre is 0.923. Across the 8 centres, the risk adjusted one-year survival rates vary between 6% and 17%.

Table 11.4 *Values of RAFR found from risk adjusted failure rates.*

Centre	Number of patients	Estimated one-year survival Unadjusted	Adjusted	*RAFR*
1	267	0.9138	0.8920	0.0768
2	166	0.8887	0.9084	0.1170
3	148	0.8986	0.9150	0.1148
4	255	0.9254	0.9061	0.0764
5	164	0.9024	0.9002	0.0941
6	160	0.9438	0.9068	0.0581
7	102	0.8922	0.8947	0.0985
8	177	0.8475	0.9128	0.1682

An alternative and more convenient way of calculating the *RAFR* in Expression (11.3) is based on an estimate of

$$\frac{\text{Observed number of failures}}{\text{Expected number of failures}} \times \text{Overall failure rate}, \tag{11.5}$$

in a given time period. To estimate the *RAFR* using this definition, we need an estimate of the expected number of failures in the time period of interest. From Section 1.3 of Chapter 1, the cumulative hazard of a failure at time t, $H(t)$, is the expected number of failures in the period to t, given that no failure has occurred before then. Therefore, for the ith individual in the jth institution who survives to time t_{ij}, $H_{ij}(t_{ij})$ is the expected number of failures during their follow-up. Using the result in Equation (1.8) of Chapter 1, the estimated number of failures in centre j is then

$$\hat{e}_j = \sum_{i=1}^{n_j} \hat{H}_{ij}(t_{ij}) = -\sum_{i=1}^{n_j} \log \hat{S}_{ij}(t_{ij}), \tag{11.6}$$

where $\hat{S}_{ij}(t_{ij})$ is defined in Equation (11.4).

Example 11.4 Comparisons between kidney transplant centres
Transplant outcomes for eight kidney transplant centres, from the data described in Example 11.3, are now used to estimate the *RAFR* using Expression (11.5). The observed number of transplant failures in the first year in each centre is first determined. Next, a Cox regression model is fitted to the data to give an estimate of the survivor function for the ith patient in the jth centre, $\hat{S}_{ij}(t)$. For patients with *Tsurv* $\leqslant 365$, their estimated survivor function is obtained at their value of *Tsurv*, while for patients with *Tsurv* > 365, their estimated survivor function at $t = 365$ is calculated. The corresponding estimate of the cumulative hazard is then obtained at the survival time for each patient, and from Equation (11.6), summing these estimates over the patients in the jth centre gives an estimate of the expected number of failures in that centre. These values are shown in Table 11.5. To illustrate the calculation, for Centre 1, we observe 23 transplant failures in the first year and the estimated

Table 11.5 *Values of RAFR found from the observed and expected numbers of transplant failures.*

Centre	Number of patients	Number of transplant failures		*RAFR*
		Observed	Expected	
1	267	23	28.96	0.0764
2	166	18	14.93	0.1160
3	148	15	12.48	0.1157
4	255	19	24.23	0.0755
5	164	16	16.68	0.0923
6	160	9	15.38	0.0563
7	102	11	10.67	0.0992
8	177	27	14.66	0.1772

expected number is 28.96. The overall failure rate is 0.096, and so the *RAFR* for this centre is

$$RAFR = \frac{23}{28.96} \times 0.096 = 0.076.$$

The *RAFR* values in this table are very similar to those given in Table 11.4.

11.4.1 Interval estimate for the RAFR*

To obtain an interval estimate for the risk adjusted failure rate, we use the definition in Expression (11.5), and assume that the expected number of failures and the overall failure rate are estimated with negligible error. This will often be the case, as these quantities will have been obtained from a large data set covering all the institutions. Now let Y_j be the random variable associated with the number of failures out of n_j in the jth institution in a given time period, and let y_j be the corresponding observed value. Also let p_j be the probability of failure in the jth institution, so that Y_j has a binomial distribution. Generally, n_j will be sufficiently large for the Poisson approximation to the binomial distribution to be valid, according to which a binomial distribution with parameters n_j, p_j tends to a Poisson distribution with mean μ_j as $n_j \to \infty$ and $p_j \to 0$, whilst $\mu_j = n_j p_j$ remains finite. Then, the random variable associated with the number of failures in the jth institution, Y_j, has a Poisson distribution with mean μ_j. Note that this result is only valid when the failure probability is small, as it will be when failures are not too frequent. Also, this result means that we do not need to dwell on the value of n_j to use in the following calculations, which is particularly useful when individuals may have censored survival times.

Approximate interval estimates for the number of deaths in the jth institution can be obtained from the result that $\log Y_j$ is approximately normally distributed with mean $\log \mu_j$ and variance given by $\text{var}\,(\log Y_j) \approx \mu_j^{-2}\,\text{var}\,(Y_j)$, using the result in Equation (2.8) of Chapter 2. Now, the variance of a Poisson random variable is equal to its mean, so that $\text{var}\,(Y_j) = \mu_j$, and the variance of $\log Y_j$ is approximately $1/\mu_j$. Since the best estimate of μ_j is simply the observed number of failures, y_j, this variance can be estimated by $1/y_j$. It then follows that a 95% interval estimate for the number of failures is the interval $\exp\{\log y_j \pm 1.96/\surd(y_j)\}$.

It is also possible to calculate 'exact' Poisson limits for the number of failures in a particular institution. Suppose that we observe a value y of a random variable Y, which has a Poisson distribution with mean μ. The lower limit of a 95% interval for μ is then y_L, which is such that $\mathrm{P}(Y \geqslant y) = 0.025$ when $\mu = y_L$. Similarly, the upper limit of the 95% interval for μ is the value y_U such that $\mathrm{P}(Y \leqslant y) = 0.025$ when $\mu = y_U$. These limits can be shown to have desirable optimality properties.

To calculate these exact limits, we can use the general result that if Y has a Poisson distribution with mean μ, and X has a gamma distribution with shape parameter $y + 1$ and unit scale parameter, that is $Y \sim P(\mu)$ and $X \sim \Gamma(y + 1, 1)$, then $P(Y \leqslant y) = 1 - P(X \leqslant \mu)$. This means that

$$\sum_{k=0}^{y} \frac{e^{-\mu}\mu^k}{k!} = 1 - \int_0^{\mu} \frac{e^{-x}x^y}{\Gamma(y+1)}\,\mathrm{d}x, \tag{11.7}$$

where $\Gamma(y + 1) = y!$ is a gamma function. The gamma distribution was introduced in Section 6.1.3 of Chapter 6, and this result can be verified using integration by parts.

The lower limit of a 95% interval for the number of events, y_L, is the expected value of a Poisson random variable, Y, which is such that $\mathrm{P}(Y \geqslant y) = 0.025$. Adapting the result in Equation (11.7),

$$\mathrm{P}(Y \geqslant y) = 1 - \mathrm{P}(Y \leqslant y-1) = 1 - \sum_{k=0}^{y-1} \frac{e^{-y_L}{y_L}^k}{k!} = \int_0^{y_L} \frac{e^{-x}x^{y-1}}{\Gamma(y)}\,\mathrm{d}x,$$

and so y_L is such that

$$\int_0^{y_L} \frac{e^{-x}x^{y-1}}{\Gamma(y)}\,\mathrm{d}x = 0.025.$$

This means that y_L is the lower 2.5% point of a gamma random variable with shape parameter y and unit scale parameter, and so can be obtained from the inverse cumulative distribution function for the gamma distribution. Similarly, the upper limit of the 95% confidence interval, y_U, is the expected value of a Poisson random variable for which $\mathrm{P}(Y \leqslant y) = 0.025$. Again using Equation (11.7),

$$\mathrm{P}(Y \leqslant y) = \sum_{k=0}^{y} \frac{e^{-y_U}{y_U}^k}{k!} = 1 - \int_0^{y_U} \frac{e^{-x}x^y}{\Gamma(y+1)}\,\mathrm{d}x,$$

so that

$$\int_0^{y_U} \frac{e^{-x}x^y}{\Gamma(y+1)}\,\mathrm{d}x = 0.975,$$

and y_U is the upper 2.5% point of a gamma distribution with shape parameter $y + 1$ and unit scale parameter.

As an illustration, suppose that the observed number of events in a particular institution is $y = 9$, as it is for Centre 6 in the data on kidney transplant failure rates in Example 11.3. The lower 2.5% point of a gamma distribution with shape parameter 9 and unit scale parameter is $y_L = 4.12$, and so $\text{P}(Y \geqslant 9) = 0.025$ when Y has a Poisson distribution with mean $\mu = 4.12$. Also, the upper 2.5% point of a gamma distribution with shape parameter 10 and unit scale parameter is $y_U = 17.08$, and so $\text{P}(Y \leqslant 9) = 0.025$ when Y has a Poisson distribution with mean 17.08. These two distributions are shown in Figure 11.7. The tail area to the right of $y = 9$ in the distribution with mean 4.12, and the tail area to the left of $y = 9$ in the distribution with mean 17.08, are both equal to 0.025. An exact 95% interval estimate for the observed number of events is then $(4.12, 17.08)$.

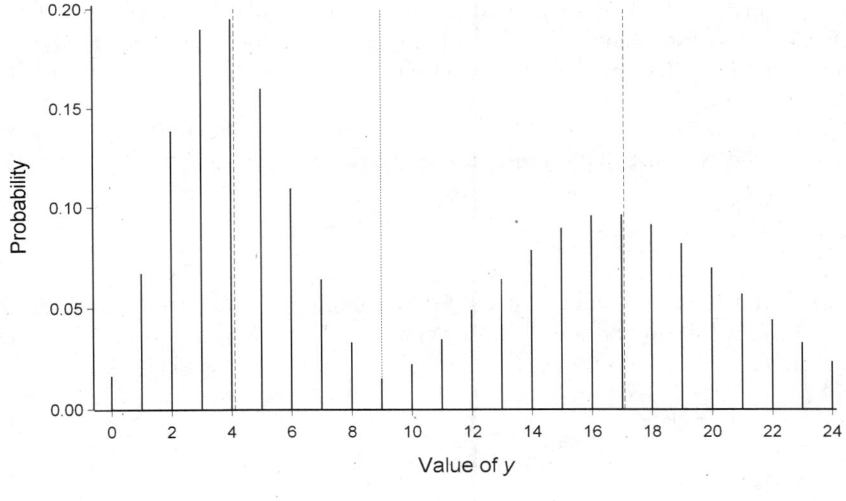

Figure 11.7 *Poisson distributions with means 4.12 and 17.09 (- - -) for deriving exact confidence limits for an observed value of 9 (·······).*

Once an interval estimate for the number of failures, (y_L, y_U), has been obtained using either the approximate or exact method, corresponding limits for the *RAFR* are

$$\frac{y_L}{e_j} \times \text{overall failure rate, and } \frac{y_U}{e_j} \times \text{overall failure rate,}$$

where here e_j is the estimated number of failures in the jth institution, obtained using Equation (11.6), but taken to have negligible error.

Example 11.5 Comparisons between kidney transplant centres

For the data on transplant outcomes in eight kidney transplant centres, given in Example 11.3, approximate and exact 95% confidence limits for the *RAFR* are shown in Table 11.6.

Table 11.6 *Approximate and exact 95% interval estimates for the RAFR.*

Centre	*RAFR*	Approximate limits		Exact limits	
		Lower	Upper	Lower	Upper
1	0.0764	0.051	0.115	0.048	0.115
2	0.1160	0.073	0.184	0.069	0.183
3	0.1157	0.070	0.192	0.065	0.191
4	0.0755	0.048	0.118	0.045	0.118
5	0.0923	0.057	0.151	0.053	0.150
6	0.0563	0.029	0.108	0.026	0.107
7	0.0992	0.055	0.179	0.050	0.178
8	0.1772	0.122	0.258	0.117	0.258

To illustrate how these interval estimates are calculated, consider the data for Centre 1, for which $y_1 = 23$ and the corresponding expected number of deaths is, from Example 11.4, estimated to be 28.96. The standard error of the logarithm of the number of transplant failures in this centre is $1/\surd(y_1) = 1/\surd(23) = 0.209$. A 95% confidence interval for y_1 is then $\exp(\log 23 \pm 1.96 \times 0.209)$, that is $(15.28, 34.61)$, and the corresponding interval for the *RAFR* is

$$\left(\frac{15.28}{28.96} \times 0.096, \quad \frac{34.61}{28.96} \times 0.096\right),$$

that is $(0.051, 0.115)$. Exact limits for the number of failures in this centre can be found from the lower 2.5% point of a $\Gamma(23, 1)$ random variable and the upper 2.5% point of a $\Gamma(24, 1)$ random variable. This leads to the interval $(14.58, 34.51)$, and corresponding limits for the *RAFR* are

$$\left(\frac{14.58}{28.96} \times 0.096, \quad \frac{34.51}{28.96} \times 0.096\right),$$

that is $(0.048, 0.115)$.

Table 11.6 shows that there is very good agreement between the approximate and exact limits, as would be expected when the observed number of failures is no smaller than 9.

11.4.2 Use of the Poisson regression model*

Approximate interval estimates for the *RAFR* can conveniently be obtained using a modelling approach. Let F_j be the risk adjusted failure rate and e_j the expected number of failures for centre j, so that

$$F_j = \frac{y_j}{e_j} \times \text{overall failure rate}.$$

Since we take the random variable associated with the number of failures in the jth institution, Y_j, to have a Poisson distribution with mean μ_j, it follows that

$$\mathrm{E}\,(F_j) = \frac{\mu_j}{e_j} \times \text{overall failure rate}. \tag{11.8}$$

To model the *RAFR* for centre j, F_j, we take $\log \mathrm{E}\,(F_j) = c_j$, where c_j is the effect due to the jth institution. Now, using Equation (11.8),

$$\log \mathrm{E}\,(F_j) = \log \mu_j - \log\{e_j/(\text{overall failure rate})\},$$

and this leads to a log-linear model for μ_j where

$$\log \mu_j = c_j + \log\{e_j/(\text{overall failure rate})\}. \tag{11.9}$$

In this model, the term $\log\{e_j/(\text{overall failure rate})\}$ is a variate with a known coefficient of unity, called an *offset*. When the log-linear model in Equation (11.9) is fitted to the observed number of failures in each institution, y_j, the model has the same number of unknown parameters as there are observations. It will therefore be a perfect fit to the data, and so the fitted values $\hat{\mu}_j$ will be equal to the observed number of failures. The parameter estimates $\hat{c}_j$ will be the fitted values of $\log \mathrm{E}\,(F_j)$, so that the *RAFR* for the jth centre is $\exp(\hat{c}_j)$. A 95% confidence interval for the *RAFR* is then $\exp\{\hat{c}_j \pm 1.96\,\mathrm{se}\,(\hat{c}_j)\}$, where $\hat{c}_j$ and its standard error can be obtained from computer output from fitting the log-linear model.

Example 11.6 Comparisons between kidney transplant centres
Interval estimates for the *RAFR*, obtained from fitting the log-linear model in Equation (11.9) to the data on the number of transplant failures in each of 8 centres, are given in Table 11.7.

Table 11.7 *The RAFR and interval estimates from fitting a log-linear model.*

Centre	$\hat{c}_j$	$\mathrm{se}\,(\hat{c}_j)$	*RAFR* ($e^{\hat{c}_j}$)	95% limits for *RAFR*	
				Lower	Upper
1	−2.571	0.209	0.0764	0.051	0.115
2	−2.154	0.236	0.1160	0.073	0.184
3	−2.157	0.258	0.1157	0.070	0.192
4	−2.584	0.229	0.0755	0.048	0.118
5	−2.382	0.250	0.0923	0.057	0.151
6	−2.877	0.333	0.0563	0.029	0.108
7	−2.310	0.302	0.0992	0.055	0.179
8	−1.730	0.192	0.1772	0.122	0.258

The *RAFR* values and their corresponding interval estimates, obtained from the fitted log-linear model, are in exact agreement with the approximate interval estimates given in Table 11.6, as they should be.

11.4.3 Random institution effects

The log-linear model for the expected number of events in Equation (11.9) provides a framework for calculating interval estimates for the $RAFR$ across institutions. In this model, the parameters associated with institution effects are fitted as fixed effects, which is entirely appropriate when the number of institutions is small, as it is in Example 11.3. This methodology can also be used when there is a much larger number of institutions, but in this situation, it would be undesirable for institution effects to be incorporated as fixed effects. Instead, random effects would be used to model the variation between institutions. Random effects were introduced in Section 10.1.1 of Chapter 10, in the context of frailty models.

Suppose that the effect due to the jth institution, c_j, is drawn from a normal distribution with mean α and variance σ_c^2, denoted $N(\alpha, \sigma_c^2)$. Since the log-linear model for the $RAFR$ in the jth centre is such that $\log \mathrm{E}\,(F_j) = c_j$, a lognormal distribution is implied for the variation in the expected $RAFR$ values, $\mathrm{E}\,(F_j)$, across the centres. Alternatively, the model in Equation (11.9) can be written as

$$\log \mu_j = \alpha + c_j + \log\{e_j/(\text{overall failure rate})\}$$

where now the c_j have a $N(0, \sigma_c^2)$ distribution, and α is the overall value of the logarithm of the $RAFR$, so that e^{α} is the overall failure rate.

Using random rather than fixed effects has two consequences. First, the estimated institution effects, $\tilde{c}_j$, are 'shrunk' towards the overall rate, $\tilde{\alpha}$, and the more extreme the $RAFR$, the greater the shrinkage. Second, interval estimates for institution effects in the random effects model will be shorter than when fixed effects are used, increasing the precision of prediction for future patients. Both these features are desirable when using centre rates to guide patient choice. The concept of shrinkage was referred to in Section 3.7 of Chapter 3, when describing the lasso method for variable selection.

Example 11.7 Comparisons between kidney transplant centres

Random centre effects are now used in modelling the observed numbers of transplant failures in the eight kidney transplant centres. The observed number of transplant failures in the jth centre, y_j, is modelled by taking y_j to be the observed value of a Poisson random variable with mean μ_j, where

$$\log \mu_j = c_j + \log\{e_j/(\text{overall failure rate})\},$$

and $c_j \sim N(\alpha, \sigma_c^2)$.

The estimate of α is $\tilde{\alpha} = -2.341$, so that $\exp(\tilde{\alpha}) = 0.096$, the same as the failure rate obtained from the Kaplan-Meier estimate of the overall survivor function. The estimated variance of the centre effects is $\tilde{\sigma}_c^2 = 0.054$ with a standard error of 0.054, and so there is no evidence of significant between centre variation. Estimates of the centre effects, $\tilde{c}_j$, lead to $RAFR$ estimates, $\exp(\tilde{c}_j)$, obtained as estimates of the modal value of the posterior distribution of the random effects (see Section 10.4 of Chapter 10), and are shown in Table 11.8.

Table 11.8 *The RAFR and interval estimates using random centre effects in a log-linear model.*

Centre	$\tilde{c}_j$	se $(\tilde{c}_j)$	$RAFR$ $(e^{\tilde{c}_j})$	95% limits for $RAFR$	
				Lower	Upper
1	−2.471	0.170	0.084	0.061	0.118
2	−2.252	0.186	0.105	0.073	0.151
3	−2.261	0.194	0.104	0.071	0.152
4	−2.468	0.179	0.085	0.060	0.120
5	−2.360	0.181	0.094	0.066	0.135
6	−2.537	0.228	0.079	0.051	0.124
7	−2.330	0.199	0.097	0.066	0.144
8	−2.000	0.232	0.135	0.086	0.214

The estimates of the $RAFR$ values on using a random effects model are similar to those found with the fixed effects model shown in Table 11.7, but closer to the overall rate of 0.096. This is particularly noticeable for Centre 8, which has the largest $RAFR$. Also, the values of se $(\tilde{c}_j)$ are generally smaller, which in turn means that the corresponding interval estimates are narrower. These two features illustrate the shrinkage effect caused by using random centre effects.

11.5 Further reading

Examples of survival analyses in situations where the proportional hazards model is not applicable have been given by Stablein, Carter and Novak (1981) and Gore, Pocock and Kerr (1984). Further details on the stratified proportional hazards model can be found in Kalbfleisch and Prentice (2002) and Lawless (2002), for example. A review of methods for dealing with non-proportional hazards in the Cox regression model is included in Schemper (1992). A discussion of strategies for dealing with non-proportional hazards is also included in Chapter 6 of Therneau and Grambsch (2000).

Royston and Parmar (2011) describe and illustrate how the restricted mean survival time can be used to summarise a treatment difference in the presence of non-proportional hazards. The use of average hazard ratios is discussed by Schemper, Wakounig and Heinze (2009). Andersen, Hansen and Klein (2004) showed how pseudo-values could be used in modelling the restricted mean, and Andersen and Perme (2010) review the applications of pseudo-values in survival analysis. Klein et al. (2008) described a SAS macro and an R package for the computation of the restricted mean.

Statistical methods for the comparison of institutional performance are described and illustrated by Thomas, Longford and Rolph (1994) and Goldstein and Spiegelhalter (1996). A detailed comparison of surgical outcomes between a number of hospitals following paediatric cardiac surgery is given by Spiegelhalter et al. (2002). Sun, Ono and Takeuchi (1996) showed how exact Poisson limits for a standardised mortality ratio can be obtained using the relationship between a Poisson distribution and a gamma or chi-squared distribution. Funnel plots, described by Spiegelhalter (2005), provide a visual comparison of institutional performance. Ohlssen, Sharples and Spiegelhalter (2007) describe techniques that can be used to identify institutions that perform differently from others, and Spiegelhalter et al. (2012) provide a comprehensive review of statistical methods used in healthcare regulation.

Chapter 12

Competing risks

In studies where the outcome is death, individuals may die from one of a number of different causes. For example, in a study to compare two or more treatments for prostatic cancer, patients may succumb to a stroke, myocardial infarction or the cancer itself. In some cases, an analysis of death from all causes may be appropriate, and standard methods for survival analysis can be used. More commonly, there will be interest in how the hazard of death from different causes depends on treatment effects and other explanatory variables. Of course, death from any one of a number of possible causes precludes its occurrence from any other cause, and this feature has implications for the analysis of data of this kind. In this chapter, we review methods for summarising data on survival times for different causes of death, and describe models for cause-specific survival data.

12.1 Introduction to competing risks

Individuals face death from a number of risks. These risks compete to become the actual cause of death, which gives rise to the situation known as *competing risks*, in which a competing risk prevents the occurrence of an event of particular interest. More generally, this term applies when an individual may experience one of a number of different end-points, where the occurrence of any one of these hinders or eliminates the potential for others to occur.

Data of this type occur in many application areas. For example, in a cancer clinical trial, we may be interested in deaths from a specific cancer, and here events such as a myocardial infarct or stroke are competing risks. A study involving the exposure of animals to a possible carcinogen may result in exposed animals dying from different cancers, where each cause of death is of interest, allowing for competing causes. In outcome studies following bone marrow transplantation in patients suffering from leukaemia, possible end-points might be discharged from hospital, relapse, the occurrence of graft versus host disease or death, with interest centering on how various factors affect the times to each event, in the presence of other risks.

There may be a number of aims when analysing data where there are multiple end-points. For example, it may be important to determine which of a number of factors are associated with a particular end-point, in the presence of competing risks. Estimates of the effect of such factors on the hazard of death from a particular cause, allowing for possible competing causes, may also be needed. In other situations, it will be of interest to compare survival times across different causes of death to identify those causes that lead to earlier or later failure times. An assessment of the consistency of estimated hazard ratios for certain factors across different end-points may also be needed. An example of a data set with multiple end-points follows.

Example 12.1 Survival of liver transplant recipients
A number of conditions lead to failure of the liver, and the only possible treatment is a liver transplant. Transplantation is generally very effective, and the median survival time for adult transplant recipients is now well over 12 years. However, following a liver transplant, the graft may fail as a result of acute or chronic organ rejection, hepatic artery thrombosis, recurrent disease or other reasons. This example is based on the times from a liver transplant to graft failure for 1761 adult patients who had a first elective transplant with an organ from a deceased donor between January 2000 and December 2010, who were followed up until the end of 2012. These data concern patients transplanted for three particular liver diseases, primary biliary cirrhosis (PBC), primary sclerosing cholangitis (PSC) and alcoholic liver disease (ALD). In addition to the graft survival time, information is given on the age and gender (1 = male, 2 = female) of the patient, their primary liver disease and the cause of graft failure (0 = functioning graft, 1 = rejection, 2 = thrombosis, 3 = recurrent disease, 4 = other). Because transplantation is so successful, these data exhibit heavy censoring, and there are only 261 (15%) patients who suffer graft failure, although an additional 211 die with a functioning graft. The failure times of this latter group have been taken to be censored at their time of death. The first 20 observations in the data set are given in Table 12.1.

12.2 Summarising competing risks data

In standard survival analysis, we have observations on a random variable T associated with the survival time. In addition, there will be an event indicator that denotes whether the end-point has actually occurred or whether the observed time has been censored. When there are competing risks, the event indicator is extended to cover the different possible end-points. The resulting data are therefore a survival time T and a cause C. The data for a given individual are then observed values of (T, C), and we will write (t_i, c_i) for the data from the ith individual, $i = 1, 2, \ldots, n$, where the possible values of c_i are $0, 1, 2, \ldots, m$, and $c_i = 0$ when no end-point has been observed.

From the data, we know that the jth of m possible causes, $j = 1, 2, \ldots, m$, has not occurred in the ith individual before time t_i. Death from a particular cause, the jth, say, may have occurred at time t_i, and all other potential causes could have occurred after t_i if cause j had not occurred. As we do not know which cause might have occurred when, difficulties in estimating a

Table 12.1 *Graft survival times for 20 liver transplant recipients and the cause of graft failure.*

Patient	Age	Gender	Primary disease	Time	Status	Cause of failure
1	55	1	ALD	2906	0	0
2	63	1	PBC	4714	0	0
3	67	1	PBC	4673	0	0
4	58	1	ALD	27	0	0
5	59	1	PBC	4720	0	0
6	35	2	PBC	4624	0	0
7	51	2	PBC	18	1	1 Rejection
8	61	2	PSC	294	1	1 Rejection
9	51	2	ALD	4673	0	0
10	59	2	ALD	51	0	0
11	53	1	PSC	8	1	2 Thrombosis
12	56	1	ALD	4592	0	0
13	55	2	ALD	4679	0	0
14	44	1	ALD	1487	0	0
15	61	2	PBC	427	1	4 Other
16	59	2	PBC	4604	0	0
17	52	2	PSC	4083	1	3 Recurrent disease
18	61	1	PSC	559	1	3 Recurrent disease
19	57	1	PSC	4708	0	0
20	49	2	ALD	957	1	4 Other

cause-specific survivor function, that is the probability of a particular end-point occurring after any time t, might be anticipated.

12.2.1 Kaplan-Meier estimate of survivor function

To summarise competing risks data, we might consider using a separate estimate of the survivor function for each cause. This would involve using the event times for each cause of interest in turn, taking the event times for all other causes as censored. This is justified on the grounds that if a specific end-point has been observed, no other causes of death could have occurred before this time. These other causes may have occurred later, had the specific end-point not occurred. Data expressed in this form is known as *cause-specific survival data.* There are, however, pitfalls to using the Kaplan-Meier estimate of the survivor function to summarise such data, as the following example shows.

Example 12.2 Survival of liver transplant recipients
Data on the times to graft failure, and the cause of failure, for eight patients from the data set used in Example 12.1 are given in Table 12.2. The data sets used to construct the survivor functions for the patients suffering

Table 12.2 *Graft survival times for eight liver transplant recipients and the cause of graft failure.*

Patient	Survival time	Cause of failure
1	18	Rejection
2	27	Thrombosis
3	63	Thrombosis
4	80	Rejection
5	143	Thrombosis
6	255	Thrombosis
7	294	Rejection
8	370	Rejection

from graft rejection and thrombosis are as follows, where an asterisk (∗) denotes a censored observation. For failure from rejection, the graft survival times are:

$$18 \quad 27^{*} \quad 63^{*} \quad 80 \quad 143^{*} \quad 255^{*} \quad 294 \quad 370$$

and for failure from thrombosis, the graft survival times are:

$$18^{*} \quad 27 \quad 63 \quad 80^{*} \quad 143 \quad 255 \quad 294^{*} \quad 370^{*}$$

The Kaplan-Meier estimate of the survivor function can be calculated from each set of cause-specific survival times, and this leads to the estimates shown in Table 12.3.

Table 12.3 *Kaplan-Meier estimates of survivor functions for two causes of graft failure in eight liver transplant recipients.*

Rejection		Thrombosis	
Time interval	$\hat{S}(t)$	Time interval	$\hat{S}(t)$
0–	1.000	0–	1.000
18–	0.875	27–	0.857
80–	0.700	63–	0.714
294–	0.350	143–	0.536
370–	0.000	255–	0.357

From the estimated survivor functions in this table, the probability of graft failure due to rejection in the period to 370 days is 1.000, and that from thrombosis is $1 - 0.357 = 0.643$. However, half of this group of 8 patients suffers graft failure from rejection in 370 days, and the other half fail from thrombosis. The survivor function should therefore be 0.5 at 370 days in each case. Also, the probability that one or other causes of graft failure occur after 370 days is zero, since all 8 patients have failed by then, rather than $1 - (1 + 0.643)$ suggested by the Kaplan-Meier estimates.

This simple example shows that the Kaplan-Meier estimate does not lead to an appropriate summary of survival data when there are competing risks. So what is the Kaplan-Meier estimate estimating? Consider the Kaplan-Meier estimate for the jth cause, where the event times from other causes are taken to be censored. The Kaplan-Meier estimate is the probability of death beyond time t, if cause j is the only cause of death, that is if all other risks were removed. Consequently, the estimate does not take proper account of the competing risks from other causes. Also, the Kaplan-Meier estimates assume that an individual will ultimately die from any given cause, and so do not allow for the possibility that a particular cause of death may never occur. In general, as in Example 12.2, the complement of the Kaplan-Meier estimator overestimates the incidence of a particular event, and so this estimate rarely has a meaningful interpretation in the context of competing risks.

12.3 Hazard and cumulative incidence functions

This section introduces two functions that are particularly useful in the context of competing risks, namely the hazard function and the cumulative incidence function for the different event types.

12.3.1 Cause-specific hazard function

The *cause-specific hazard function* for the jth cause, $h_j(t)$, for $j = 1, 2, \ldots, m$, is defined by

$$h_j(t) = \lim_{\delta t \to 0} \left\{ \frac{\mathrm{P}(t \leqslant T \leqslant t + \delta t, C = j \mid T \geqslant t)}{\delta t} \right\}. \tag{12.1}$$

This hazard function is the instantaneous failure rate from the jth cause at time t, in the presence of all other risks.

From the definition of $h_j(t)$ in Equation (12.1) and following the method used to derive Equation (1.4) in Section 1.3.2 of Chapter 1, we have that

$$\begin{aligned} h_j(t) &= \lim_{\delta t \to 0} \left\{ \frac{\mathrm{P}(t \leqslant T \leqslant t + \delta t, C = j)}{\delta t \, \mathrm{P}(T \geqslant t)} \right\}, \\ &= \frac{1}{\mathrm{P}(T \geqslant t)} \lim_{\delta t \to 0} \left\{ \frac{\mathrm{P}(t \leqslant T \leqslant t + \delta t, C = j)}{\delta t} \right\}, \end{aligned}$$

and so

$$h_j(t) = \frac{f_j(t)}{S(t)}, \tag{12.2}$$

where $f_j(t)$ is the cause-specific density function and $S(t) = \mathrm{P}(T \geqslant t)$ is the overall survivor function.

Since only one of the m possible causes can lead to an event,

$$\mathrm{P}(t \leqslant T \leqslant t + \delta t \mid T \geqslant t) = \sum_{j=1}^{m} \mathrm{P}(t \leqslant T \leqslant t + \delta t, C = j \mid T \geqslant t).$$

The overall hazard function is then $h(t) = \sum_{j=1}^{m} h_j(t)$, using the definition of the cause-specific hazard in Equation (12.1). Similarly, the overall cumulative hazard function is $H(t) = \sum_{j=1}^{m} H_j(t)$, where $H_j(t)$ is the cumulative hazard function for the jth cause. The overall survivor function is then

$$S(t) = \exp\left\{ -\sum_{j=1}^{m} H_j(t) \right\}. \tag{12.3}$$

Although $S(t)$ can also be expressed as

$$S(t) = \prod_{j=1}^{m} S_j^{\dagger}(t),$$

where $S_j^{\dagger}(t) = \exp\{-H_j(t)\}$, $S_j^{\dagger}(t)$ is not an observable survivor function. This is because we can never know the cause of a death that may occur after time t, when there is more than one possible cause.

Survival studies where there are competing risks can also be formulated in terms of m random variables, $T_1, T_2, \ldots, T_m$, that are associated with the times to the m possible causes of failure. These random variables cannot be observed directly, since only one event can occur, and so they are referred to as *latent random variables*. In practice, we observe the earliest of the m events to occur, and the random variable associated with the time to that event, T, is such that $T = \min(T_1, T_2, \ldots, T_m)$. If the different causes are independent, the hazard function in Equation (12.2) is the marginal hazard function associated with T_j, the random variable for the jth event type, which is

$$\lim_{\delta t \to 0} \left\{ \frac{\mathrm{P}(t \leqslant T_j \leqslant t + \delta t \mid T_j \geqslant t)}{\delta t} \right\}.$$

Unfortunately, the joint distribution of the random variables associated with times to the different causes, $(T_1, T_2, \ldots, T_m)$, cannot be uniquely determined, and it is not possible to use the competing risks data to test the assumption of independence of the different causes. Consequently, this formulation of competing risks will not be considered further.

12.3.2 Cause-specific cumulative incidence function

In competing risks data, no cause of death has occurred until the death of an individual from a particular cause. The *cause-specific cumulative incidence function* for a particular cause is therefore a more useful summary of the data than a survivor function. This is the probability of surviving until t and death is from cause j, in the presence of all other risks, and is given by

$$F_j(t) = \mathrm{P}(T < t, C = j),$$

for $j = 1, 2, \ldots, m$. The maximum value of the cumulative incidence function is

$$\mathrm{P}(T < \infty, C = j) = \mathrm{P}(C = j) = \pi_j,$$

where π_j is the ultimate probability of cause j occurring. Consequently, $F_j(t) \to \pi_j$ as $t \to \infty$, and since $F_j(t)$ does not tend to zero, $F_j(t)$ is not a 'proper' probability distribution function. Because of this, the cumulative incidence function is also referred to as the *subdistribution function.*

From Equation (12.2), $f_j(t) = h_j(t)S(t)$, and it then follows that $F_j(t)$ can be expressed in the form

$$F_j(t) = \int_0^t h_j(u)S(u)\,du. \tag{12.4}$$

Equation (12.4) suggests that the cause-specific cumulative incidence function can be estimated by

$$\hat{F}_j(t) = \sum_{i:t_i \leqslant t} \frac{\delta_{ij}}{n_i}\hat{S}(t_{i-1}), \tag{12.5}$$

where $\hat{S}(t_{i-1})$ is the Kaplan-Meier estimate of the overall survivor function at t_{i-1}, ignoring different causes, n_i is the number of individuals alive and uncensored just prior to t_i, and δ_{ij} is the event indicator for the cause-specific data. Thus, δ_{ij} is unity if cause j is the cause of death for the ith individual and zero otherwise, and the ratio δ_{ij}/n_i in Equation (12.5) is the Nelson-Aalen estimate of the hazard function for the jth cause; see Section 2.3.3 of Chapter 2. The summation in Equation (12.5) is over all event times up to time t, and so the estimated cumulative incidence function for a given cause uses information on the death times for all causes. This means that it is not possible to estimate the cause-specific cumulative incidence function from the corresponding cause-specific hazard function.

When there is just one event type, that is $m = 1$, we have $\delta_{i1} \equiv \delta_i$, and using Equation (2.4) of Chapter 2, we find that $\hat{F}_1(t) = 1 - \hat{S}(t)$, where $\hat{S}(t)$ is the usual Kaplan-Meier estimate of the survivor function.

The variance of the estimated cumulative incidence function at time t is given by

$$\begin{aligned}\text{var}\{\hat{F}_j(t)\} = & \sum_{i:t_i \leqslant t} \left\{\left[\hat{F}_j(t) - \hat{F}_j(t_i)\right]^2 \frac{\delta_i}{n_i(n_i - \delta_i)} + \hat{S}(t_{i-1})^2 \frac{\delta_{ij}(n_i - \delta_{ij})}{n_i^3}\right\} \\ & -2 \sum_{i:t_i \leqslant t} \left\{\hat{F}_j(t) - \hat{F}_j(t_i)\right\} \hat{S}(t_{i-1}) \frac{\delta_{ij}}{n_i^2},\end{aligned}$$

where $\delta_i = \sum_{j=1}^{m} \delta_{ij}$ and n_i is the number at risk of an event occurring at time t_i. Confidence intervals for the cumulative incidence function at any time, t, can then be found in the manner described in Section 2.2.3 of Chapter 2. When there is just one type of event, $\hat{S}(t_{i-1}) = n_i(n_i - \delta_i)^{-1}\hat{S}(t_i)$, and the square root of this variance reduces to Greenwood's formula for the standard error of the Kaplan-Meier estimate, given as Equation (2.12) of Chapter 2.

The overall cumulative incidence, $F(t)$, can be also be estimated from the m cause-specific functions, since $\hat{F}(t) = \sum_{j=1}^{m} \hat{F}_j(t)$. This in turn leads to an estimate of the overall survivor function, given by $\hat{S}(t) = 1 - \hat{F}(t)$, where in the absence of explanatory variables, $\hat{S}(t)$ is the usual Kaplan-Meier estimate, ignoring differences in death from different causes.

Example 12.3 Survival of liver transplant recipients
Example 12.2 showed that the Kaplan-Meier estimate of the survivor function cannot be used to estimate cumulative incidence. For the data shown in Table 12.2, the calculations needed to estimate the cumulative incidence function for the two causes of graft failure, rejection and thrombosis respectively, are shown in Table 12.4. The values of $\hat{S}(t_{i-1})$ are found from the Kaplan-Meier estimate of the survivor function across all event times.

Table 12.4 *Estimates of the cumulative incidence of rejection, $\hat{F}_1(t)$, and thrombosis, $\hat{F}_2(t)$, from data on the survival times of eight liver transplant recipients.*

Time interval	n_i	δ_{i1}	δ_{i2}	$\hat{S}(t_{i-1})$	$\hat{F}_1(t)$	$\hat{F}_2(t)$
0–	8	0	0	1.000	0.000	0.000
18–	8	1	0	1.000	0.125	0.000
27–	7	0	1	0.875	0.125	0.125
63–	6	0	1	0.750	0.125	0.250
80–	5	1	0	0.625	0.250	0.250
143–	4	0	1	0.500	0.250	0.375
255–	3	0	1	0.375	0.250	0.500
294–	2	1	0	0.250	0.375	0.500
370–	1	1	0	0.125	0.500	0.500

The estimate of cumulative incidence at 370 days, obtained using Equation (12.5), is now 0.5 for each cause, as required. Moreover, the overall survivor function estimate at 370 days is now $\hat{S}(370) = 1 - \sum_{j=1}^{m} \hat{F}_j(370) = 1 - (0.5 + 0.5) = 0$, as it should be.

Example 12.4 Survival of liver transplant recipients
For the data on the survival times of liver transplant recipients, the estimated cumulative incidence functions for graft failure due to rejection, hepatic artery thrombosis, recurrent disease or other reasons, are shown in Figure 12.1. This figure shows that the incidence functions vary between the four causes of graft failure, with failure due to other causes having the greatest incidence in these liver recipients. Estimates of the ultimate probability of each cause of graft failure occurring are obtained from estimates of the cumulative incidence function at 12 years, from which approximate estimates are 0.025, 0.055, 0.060 and 0.102 for rejection, hepatic artery thrombosis, recurrent disease and other reasons, respectively.

The estimated cumulative incidence function can also be used to summarise the effect of certain explanatory variables on particular end-points. As an illustration, the cumulative incidence of thrombosis for transplant recipients with each of the three indications for transplantation, PBC, PSC and

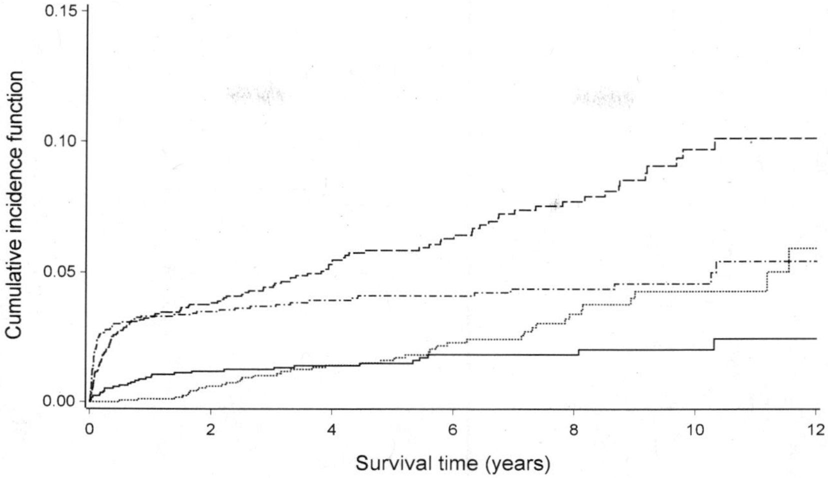

Figure 12.1 *Cumulative incidence of the four causes of graft failure, rejection (—), thrombosis (-·-), recurrent disease (······) and other reasons (- - -).*

ALD, are shown in Figure 12.2. The incidence of thrombosis is quite similar in patients with PBC and PSC, and greater than that for patients with ALD. However, a more formal analysis is needed to determine the significance of these differences.

The cumulative incidence functions provide descriptive summaries of competing risks data, but they can be supplemented by analogues of the log-rank test for comparing two or more groups, in the presence of competing risks. These tests include Gray's test (Gray, 1988) and the method due to Pepe and Mori (1993). Further details are not given here as an alternative procedure is available through a modelling approach to the analysis of competing risks data, and possible models are described in Sections 12.4 and 12.5.

12.3.3 Some other functions of interest*

The cause-specific cumulative incidence function, $F_j(t)$, leads to certain other quantities that may be of interest in a competing risks situation. For example, the probability of death before t when the cause is j is

$$\text{P}(T < t \mid C = j) = \pi_j^{-1} F_j(t),$$

where π_j is the probability of the jth cause occurring. Also, the probability of death from cause j when death has occurred before time t is

$$\text{P}(C = j \mid T < t) = \frac{F_j(t)}{F(t)},$$

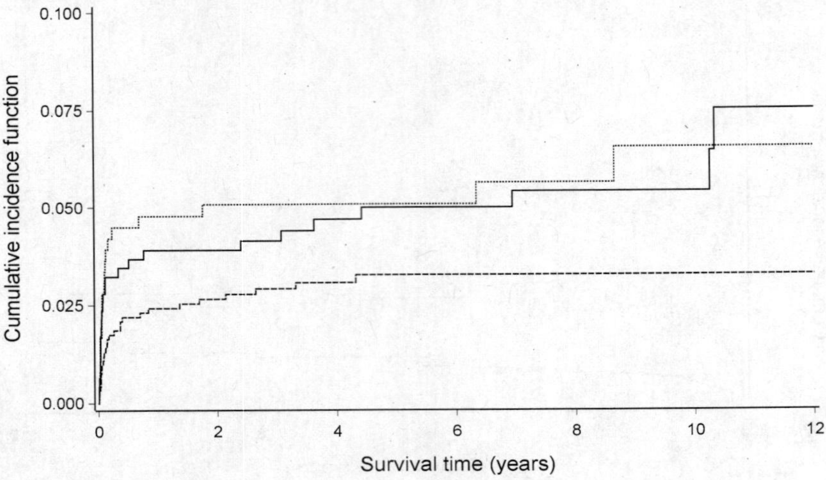

Figure 12.2 *Cumulative incidence of thrombosis for recipients with PBC (—), PSC (⋯⋯) or ALD (- - -) at the time of transplant.*

where $F(t) = 1 - S(t)$, and $S(t)$ is overall survivor function. Estimates of each of these probabilities can be readily obtained from the estimated cumulative incidence function.

12.4 Modelling cause-specific hazards

To model the dependence of the cause-specific hazard function on the values of p explanatory variables, we take the hazard of death for the ith individual, $i = 1, 2, \ldots, n$, from the jth cause, $j = 1, 2, \ldots, m$, to be

$$h_{ij}(t) = \exp(\boldsymbol{\beta}_j' \boldsymbol{x}_i) h_{0j}(t),$$

where $h_{0j}(t)$ is the baseline hazard for the jth cause, $\boldsymbol{x}_i$ is the vector of values of the explanatory variables for the ith individual, and $\boldsymbol{\beta}_j$ is the vector of their coefficients for the jth cause.

From results given in the sequel, separate models can be developed for each cause of death from the cause-specific survival data, illustrated in Example 12.2. To do this, a set of survival data is produced for each cause in turn, where death from that cause is an event and the death times for all other causes are regarded as censored. Inferences about the impact of each explanatory variable on the cause-specific hazard function can then be based on hazard ratios in the usual way, using either a Cox regression model or a parametric model.

In modelling cause-specific hazards, the event times of individuals who experience a competing risk are censored, and so are treated as if there is the possibility of the event of interest occurring in the future. Consequently, the estimated hazard ratios correspond to the situation where other causes of death are removed or assumed not to occur. This can lead to the hazard of a particular cause of failure being overestimated. Also, models for cause-specific survival data are based on the usual assumption of independent censoring. If the competing events do not occur independently of the event of interest, this assumption is not valid. Unfortunately the assumption of independent competing risks cannot be tested using the observed data. Despite these drawbacks, this approach may be warranted when interest centres on how the explanatory variables directly influence the hazard associated with a particular cause of death, ignoring deaths from other causes.

When there is just one event type, the survivor function, and hence the cumulative incidence function, can be obtained from the hazard function using Equations (1.7) and (1.6) of Chapter 1. The impact of a change in the value of an explanatory variable on the hazard function can then be interpreted in terms of the effect of this change on the cumulative incidence function. However, in the presence of competing risks, the cumulative incidence function for any cause depends on the hazard of occurrence of each potential cause of death, as indicated in Equation (12.5). This means that we cannot infer how explanatory variables affect the cumulative incidence of each cause from analysing cause-specific survival data. For this, we need to model the $F_j(t)$ directly, which we return to in Section 12.5.

12.4.1 Likelihood functions for competing risks models*

In this section, it is shown that either a Cox regression model or a fully parametric model can be used to model the dependence of the cause-specific hazard functions on the explanatory variables, by fitting separate models to the m sets of cause-specific survival data.

Models for the cause-specific hazard function, where the baseline hazard functions for each cause, $h_{0j}(t)$, $j = 1, 2, \ldots, m$, are not specified, are fitted by maximising a partial likelihood function, just as in the case of a single cause of death. Consider the probability that the ith individual, $i = 1, 2, \ldots, n$, dies from cause j at the ith ordered death time t_i, conditional on one of the individuals at risk of death at time t_i dying from cause j. Using the approach described in Section 3.3.1 of Chapter 3, this probability is

$$\frac{\exp(\boldsymbol{\beta}_j' \boldsymbol{x}_i)}{\sum_{l \in R(t_i)} \exp(\boldsymbol{\beta}_j' \boldsymbol{x}_l)}, \tag{12.6}$$

where $R(t_i)$ is the risk set at time t_i, that is the set of individuals who are alive and uncensored just prior to t_i. Setting $\delta_{ij} = 1$ if the ith individual dies from the jth cause, and zero otherwise, the partial likelihood function in

Expression (12.6) can be written as

$$\prod_{j=1}^{m}\left\{\frac{\exp(\boldsymbol{\beta}_j'\boldsymbol{x}_i)}{\sum_{l\in R(t_i)}\exp(\boldsymbol{\beta}_j'\boldsymbol{x}_l)}\right\}^{\delta_{ij}},$$

and the partial likelihood function for all n individuals is then

$$\prod_{i=1}^{n}\prod_{j=1}^{m}\left\{\frac{\exp(\boldsymbol{\beta}_j'\boldsymbol{x}_i)}{\sum_{l\in R(t_i)}\exp(\boldsymbol{\beta}_j'\boldsymbol{x}_l)}\right\}^{\delta_{ij}}.$$

This function factorises into the product of m terms of the form

$$\prod_{i=1}^{n}\left\{\frac{\exp(\boldsymbol{\beta}_j'\boldsymbol{x}_i)}{\sum_{l\in R(t_i)}\exp(\boldsymbol{\beta}_j'\boldsymbol{x}_l)}\right\}^{\delta_{ij}},$$

which is the partial likelihood function for the cause-specific survival data corresponding to the jth cause. This means that m separate Cox regression models can be fitted to the cause-specific survival data to determine how the explanatory variables affect the hazard of death from each cause.

When $h_{0j}(t)$ is fully specified, we have a parametric model that can be fitted using standard maximum likelihood methods. Again, the likelihood function factorises into a product of likelihoods for the cause-specific survival data. To show this, the contribution to the likelihood function for an individual who dies from cause c_i at t_i is $f_{c_i}(t_i)$, where $c_i = 1, 2, \ldots, m$, for the ith individual, $i = 1, 2, \ldots, n$. A censored survival time, for which the value of the cause variable c_i is zero, contains no information about the possible future cause of death, and so the corresponding contribution to the likelihood function is the overall survivor function, $S(t_i)$. Ignoring covariates for the moment, the likelihood function for data from n individuals is then

$$L = \prod_{i=1}^{n} f_{c_i}(t_i)^{\delta_i} S(t_i)^{1-\delta_i}, \tag{12.7}$$

where $\delta_i = 0$ if the ith individual has a censored survival time and unity otherwise. Using the result in Equation (12.2), and writing $h_{c_i}(t)$ for the hazard function for the ith individual who experiences cause c_i,

$$L = \prod_{i=1}^{n}\{h_{c_i}(t_i)\}^{\delta_i} S(t_i). \tag{12.8}$$

Now, from Equation (12.3), $S(t_i) = \prod_{j=1}^{m}\exp\{-H_j(t_i)\}$, where the cumulative hazard function for the jth cause at time t_i is obtained from the corresponding cause-specific hazard function, $h_j(t_i)$, and given by

$$H_j(t_i) = \int_0^{t_i} h_j(u)\,\mathrm{d}u.$$

Also, setting $\delta_{ij} = 1$ if $c_i = j$, and zero otherwise, $j = 1, 2, \ldots, m$, the likelihood in Equation (12.8) can be expressed solely in terms of the hazard functions for each of the m causes, where

$$L = \prod_{i=1}^{n} \left(\prod_{j=1}^{m} h_j(t_i)^{\delta_{ij}} \right) \prod_{j=1}^{m} \exp\{-H_j(t_i)\},$$

and this equation can be written as

$$L = \prod_{i=1}^{n} \prod_{j=1}^{m} h_j(t_i)^{\delta_{ij}} \exp\{-H_j(t_i)\}. \tag{12.9}$$

The likelihood function in Equation (12.9) is the product of m terms of the form

$$\prod_{i=1}^{n} h_j(t_i)^{\delta_{ij}} \exp\{-H_j(t_i)\},$$

and by comparing this expression with Equation (12.8), we see that this is the likelihood function for the jth cause when the event times of all other causes are taken to be censored. Consequently, the cause-specific hazard functions can be estimated by fitting separate parametric models to the cause-specific survival data. For example, if the baseline hazard function for the jth cause, $h_{0j}(t)$, is taken to have a Weibull form, so that $h_{0j}(t) = \lambda_j \gamma_j t^{\gamma_j - 1}$, the parameters λ_j and γ_j in this baseline hazard function, together with the coefficients of explanatory variables in the model, can be obtained by fitting separate Weibull models to the cause-specific survival times. Standard methods can then be used to draw inferences about the impact of the explanatory variables on the hazard of death from each cause.

Example 12.5 Survival of liver transplant recipients

To illustrate modelling cause-specific hazards, separate Cox regression models are fitted to the cause-specific data on graft failure times in liver transplant recipients. The models fitted contain the variables associated with patient age as a linear term, gender and primary disease. The corresponding hazard ratios are shown in Table 12.5, together with their 95% confidence limits.

The hazard ratios in this table can be interpreted as the effect of each variable on each of the four possible causes of graft failure, irrespective of the occurrence of the other three causes. For example, the hazard ratios for rejection apply in the hypothetical situation where a patient can only suffer graft failure from rejection. From this analysis, the risk of rejection and thrombosis is less in older patients, but the risk of graft failure from other causes increases as patients get older. There is no evidence that the hazard of graft failure is affected by gender. Patients with PBC have less risk of graft failure from recurrent disease than patients with PSC and ALD, and there is a suggestion that PBC patients have a greater incidence of graft failure from thrombosis.

Table 12.5 *Cause-specific hazard ratios and their 95% confidence intervals for the four causes of graft failure in liver transplant recipients.*

Variable		Cause of graft failure			
		Rejection	Thrombosis	Recurrent disease	Other
Age	(linear)	0.97 (0.93, 1.00)	0.98 (0.96, 1.00)	0.98 (0.95, 1.01)	1.03 (1.01, 1.05)
Gender	male	0.60 (0.26, 1.37)	1.07 (0.61, 1.90)	0.89 (0.44, 1.80)	0.92 (0.59, 1.43)
	female	1.00	1.00	1.00	1.00
Disease	PBC	0.68 (0.24, 1.91)	1.80 (0.94, 3.46)	0.34 (0.12, 1.01)	0.66 (0.38, 1.13)
	PSC	1.14 (0.46, 2.84)	1.61 (0.89, 2.92)	1.76 (0.90, 3.44)	1.34 (0.86, 2.08)
	ALD	1.00	1.00	1.00	1.00

12.4.2 Parametric models for cumulative incidence functions*

In Section 12.4.1, we saw how standard parametric models for the hazard function for the jth cause, $h_j(t)$, for $j = 1, 2, \ldots, m$, could be fitted by modelling the cause-specific survival data. However, if the hazard function for the jth cause has a Weibull form, in view of Equation (12.2), the corresponding density function, $f_j(t)$, and cumulative incidence function, $F_j(t)$, are not those of a Weibull distribution for the survival times. Indeed, since the cumulative incidence function is not a proper distribution function, we cannot model this using a standard probability distribution, and we need to account for the ultimate probability of a specific cause, $F_j(\infty)$, having a value of less than unity.

To take the simplest case, suppose that survival times are assumed to be exponential with mean θ_j^{-1} for cause j, $j = 1, 2, \ldots, m$. Then, conditional on cause j,

$$\text{P}(T < t \mid C = j) = 1 - e^{-\theta_j t},$$

so that the cumulative incidence of cause j is

$$F_j(t) = \text{P}(T < t \mid C = j)P(C = j) = \pi_j(1 - e^{-\theta_j t}),$$

where π_j is the probability of death from cause j. As $t \to \infty$, this cumulative incidence function tends to π_j, as required.

The corresponding density function is $f_j(t) = \pi_j \theta_j e^{-\theta_j t}$, and on using the result in Equation (12.2), and taking $S(t) = 1 - \sum_{j=1}^{m} F_j(t)$, the corresponding cause-specific hazard becomes

$$\lambda_j(t) = \frac{\pi_j \theta_j e^{-\theta_j t}}{\sum_j \pi_j e^{-\theta_j t}}.$$

This cause-specific hazard function is not constant, even though the conditional incidence function has an exponential form.

When a parametric model is adopted for the cumulative incidence of the jth cause, $F_j(t)$, models can be fitted by maximising the likelihood function in Equation (12.7), from which the likelihood function for the n observations (t_i, c_i) is

$$\prod_{i=1}^{n} f_{c_i}(t_i)^{\delta_i} S(t_i)^{1-\delta_i},$$

where $\delta_i = 0$ for a censored observation and unity otherwise. In this expression, $c_i = j$ if the ith individual experiences the jth event type, and $S(t_i)$ is the survivor function at t_i, obtained from $S(t_i) = 1 - \sum_{j=1}^{m} F_j(t_i)$. Even in the case of exponential cause-specific survival times, the corresponding likelihood function has a complicated form, and numerical methods are required to determine the estimates of the unknown parameters that maximise it.

12.5* Modelling cause-specific incidence

In standard survival analysis, where there is just one possible end-point, there is a direct correspondence between the cumulative incidence, survivor and hazard functions, and models for the survivor function are obtained directly from those for the hazard function. As noted in Section 12.4, this is not the case when there are competing risks. Although models for cause-specific hazards can be used to determine the impact of explanatory variables on the hazard of the competing risks, a different approach is needed to model how they affect the cumulative incidence function. In this section, a model for the dependence of cause-specific cumulative incidence functions on explanatory variables is described. This model was introduced by Fine and Gray (1999), and has become known as the *Fine and Gray model.*

12.5.1 The Fine and Gray competing risks model

The cause-specific cumulative incidence function, or subdistribution function, for the jth cause is $F_j(t) = \mathrm{P}(T < t, C = j)$. Using the relationship first given in Equation (1.5) of Chapter 1, the corresponding hazard function for the subdistribution, known as the *subdistribution hazard function* or *subhazard*, is

$$\lambda_j(t) = -\frac{\mathrm{d}}{\mathrm{d}t}\log\{1 - F_j(t)\} = \frac{1}{1 - F_j(t)}\frac{\mathrm{d}F_j(t)}{\mathrm{d}t}, \tag{12.10}$$

for the jth cause.

Now, $1 - F_j(t)$ is the probability that a person survives beyond time t or who has previously died from a cause other than the jth, and as in Section 1.3 of Chapter 1,

$$\frac{\mathrm{d}F_j(t)}{\mathrm{d}t} = \lim_{\delta t \to 0}\left\{\frac{F_j(t + \delta t) - F_j(t)}{\delta t}\right\}.$$

It then follows that the subdistribution hazard function, $\lambda_j(t)$, can be expressed as

$$\lambda_j(t) = \lim_{\delta t \to 0} \left\{ \frac{\mathrm{P}(t \leqslant T \leqslant t + \delta t, C = j \mid T \geqslant t \text{ or } \{T \leqslant t \text{ and } C \neq j\})}{\delta t} \right\}.$$

This is the instantaneous death rate at time t from cause j, given that an individual has not previously died from cause j. Since the definition of this hazard function includes those who have died from a cause other than j before time t, this subdistribution hazard function is different from the cause-specific hazard in Equation (12.1) in both definition and interpretation.

To model the cause-specific cumulative incidence function, a Cox regression model is assumed for the subhazard function for the jth cause. The hazard of cause j at time t for the ith of n individuals is then

$$\lambda_{ij}(t) = \exp(\boldsymbol{\beta}_j' \boldsymbol{x}_i)\lambda_{0j}(t), \tag{12.11}$$

where $\lambda_{0j}(t)$ is the baseline subdistribution hazard function for cause j, $\boldsymbol{x}_i$ is the vector of values of p explanatory variables for the ith individual, and the vector $\boldsymbol{\beta}_j$ contains their coefficients for the jth cause. In this model, the subdistribution hazard functions are assumed to be proportional.

The model in Equation (12.11) is fitted by adapting the usual partial likelihood in Equation (3.4) of Chapter 3 to include a weighted combination of values in the risk set. The resulting partial likelihood function for the jth of m causes is

$$\prod_{h=1}^{r_j} \frac{\exp(\boldsymbol{\beta}_j' \boldsymbol{x}_h)}{\sum_{l \in R(t_{(h)})} w_{hl} \exp(\boldsymbol{\beta}_j' \boldsymbol{x}_l)}, \tag{12.12}$$

where the product is over the r_j individuals who die from cause j at event times $t_{(1)} < t_{(2)} < \cdots < t_{(r_j)}$, and $\boldsymbol{x}_h$ is the vector of values of the explanatory variables for an individual who dies from cause j at time $t_{(h)}$, $h = 1, 2, \ldots, r_j$. The risk set $R(t_{(h)})$ is the set of all those who have not experienced an event before the hth event time $t_{(h)}$, for whom the survival time is greater than or equal to $t_{(h)}$, and those who have experienced a competing risk by $t_{(h)}$, for whom the survival time is less than or equal to $t_{(h)}$. This risk set is not straightforward to interpret, since an individual who has died from a cause other than the jth before time t is no longer at risk at t, but nevertheless they do feature in the risk set for this model. The weights in Expression (12.12) are defined as

$$w_{hl} = \frac{\hat{S}_c(t_{(h)})}{\hat{S}_c(\min\{t_{(h)}, t_l\})},$$

where $\hat{S}_c(t)$ is the Kaplan-Meier estimate of the survivor function for the censoring times. This is obtained by regarding all event times, of any type, in the data set as censored times, and likewise all censored times as event times, and calculating the Kaplan-Meier estimate from the resulting data. The weight w_{hl} will be 1.0 when $t_l \geqslant t_{(h)}$, that is for those in the risk set who have not had an event before $t_{(h)}$, and less than 1.0 otherwise. The effect of this weighting function is that individuals that die from a cause other than the jth remain in the risk set and are given a censoring time that exceeds all event times. Also, the weights become smaller with increasing time between the occurrence of a competing risk and the event time being considered, so that earlier deaths from a competing risk have a diminishing impact on the results.

The partial likelihood in Expression (12.12) is maximised to obtain estimates of the β-parameters for a given cause. Since the weights used in this partial likelihood may vary over the survival time of a particular individual, the data must first be assembled in the counting process format. This was outlined in Section 8.6 of Chapter 8. This also makes it straightforward to include time-dependent variables in this model.

The subdistribution hazard function is difficult to interpret, and the fitted model is best interpreted in terms of the effect of the explanatory variables on the cause-specific cumulative incidence function for the jth cause, which from Equation (12.10), can be estimated by

$$\hat{F}_{ij}(t) = 1 - \exp\{-\hat{\Lambda}_{ij}(t)\},$$

for the ith individual, where $\hat{\Lambda}_{ij}(t)$ is an estimate of the cumulative subdistribution hazard function, $\Lambda_{ij}(t)$. This estimate is given by

$$\hat{\Lambda}_{ij}(t) = \exp(\hat{\boldsymbol{\beta}}_j' \boldsymbol{x}_i)\hat{\Lambda}_{0j}(t),$$

where $\hat{\Lambda}_{0j}(t)$ is the baseline cumulative subdistribution hazard function for the jth event type. This function can be estimated using an adaptation of the Nelson-Aalen estimate of the baseline cumulative hazard function, given in Equation (3.28) of Chapter 3, where

$$\hat{\Lambda}_{0j}(t) = \sum_{t_{(h)} \leqslant t} \frac{d_h}{\sum_{l \in R(t_{(h)})} w_{hl} \exp(\hat{\boldsymbol{\beta}}_j' \boldsymbol{x}_l)},$$

and d_h is the number of deaths at time $t_{(h)}$.

The Fine and Gray model can also be expressed in terms of a baseline cumulative incidence function, $F_{ij}(t)$, for each cause, where

$$F_{ij}(t) = 1 - \{1 - F_{0j}(t)\}^{\exp(\boldsymbol{\beta}_j' \boldsymbol{x}_i)},$$

and $F_{0j}(t) = 1 - \exp\{-\Lambda_{0j}(t)\}$ is the baseline cumulative incidence function for the jth cause. This emphasises that a quantity of direct interest is being modelled.

Example 12.6 Survival of liver transplant recipients

In this example, the Fine and Gray model for the cumulative incidence function is used to model the data given in Example 12.1. Models for the cumulative incidence of graft rejection, thrombosis, recurrent disease and other

Table 12.6 *Subhazard ratios and their 95% confidence intervals in the Fine and Gray model for the four causes of graft failure in liver transplant recipients.*

Variable		Cause of graft failure			
		Rejection	Thrombosis	Recurrent disease	Other
Age	(linear)	0.97 (0.93, 1.00)	0.98 (0.96, 1.00)	0.98 (0.95, 1.01)	1.03 (1.01, 1.05)
Gender	male	0.60 (0.27, 1.31)	1.08 (0.67, 1.75)	0.89 (0.45, 1.74)	0.90 (0.58, 1.39)
	female	1.00	1.00	1.00	1.00
Disease	PBC	0.69 (0.25, 1.91)	1.83 (1.06, 3.17)	0.35 (0.13, 0.98)	0.67 (0.39, 1.15)
	PSC	1.10 (0.44, 2.76)	1.59 (0.87, 2.91)	1.68 (0.84, 3.39)	1.34 (0.85, 2.10)
	ALD	1.00	1.00	1.00	1.00

causes of failure are fitted in turn. Subhazard ratios and their corresponding 95% confidence intervals for these four failure types are shown in Table 12.6.

The subhazard ratios in this table summarise the direct effect of each variable on the incidence of different causes of graft failure, in the presence of competing risks. However, their values are very similar to the hazard ratios shown in Table 12.5, which suggests that there is little association between the competing causes of graft failure. In a later example, Example 12.7 in Section 12.6, this is not the case.

12.6 Model checking

Many of the model checking procedures described in Chapter 4 can be applied directly to examine the adequacy of a model for a specific cause. The methods for checking the functional form of an explanatory variable (plots of martingale and Schoenfeld residuals) and testing for proportional hazards (plot of scaled Schoenfeld residuals, tests of proportional hazards) are particularly useful. In addition, an adaptation of the method described in Section 7.3 of Chapter 7 for comparing observed survival with a model-based estimate can be used to determine the validity of an assumed parametric model for the cumulative incidence of each cause. Some of these methods are illustrated in Example 12.7.

Example 12.7 Survival of laboratory mice
In a laboratory study to compare the survival times of two groups of mice following exposure to radiation, one group was reared in a standard environment and the other group was kept in a germ-free environment. The mice were RFM strain males, a strain that is particularly susceptible to tumour development following exposure to ionising radiation. The mice were exposed to a dose of 300 rads of radiation when they were five or six weeks old, and each mouse

was followed up until death. Following an autopsy, the cause of death of each mouse was recorded as thymic lymphoma, reticulum cell sarcoma or other causes, together with the corresponding survival times in days. The data were first described by Hoel (1972), and are given in Table 12.7. These data are unusual in that there are no censored survival times.

Estimated cumulative incidence functions for deaths from the three causes are shown in Figure 12.3.

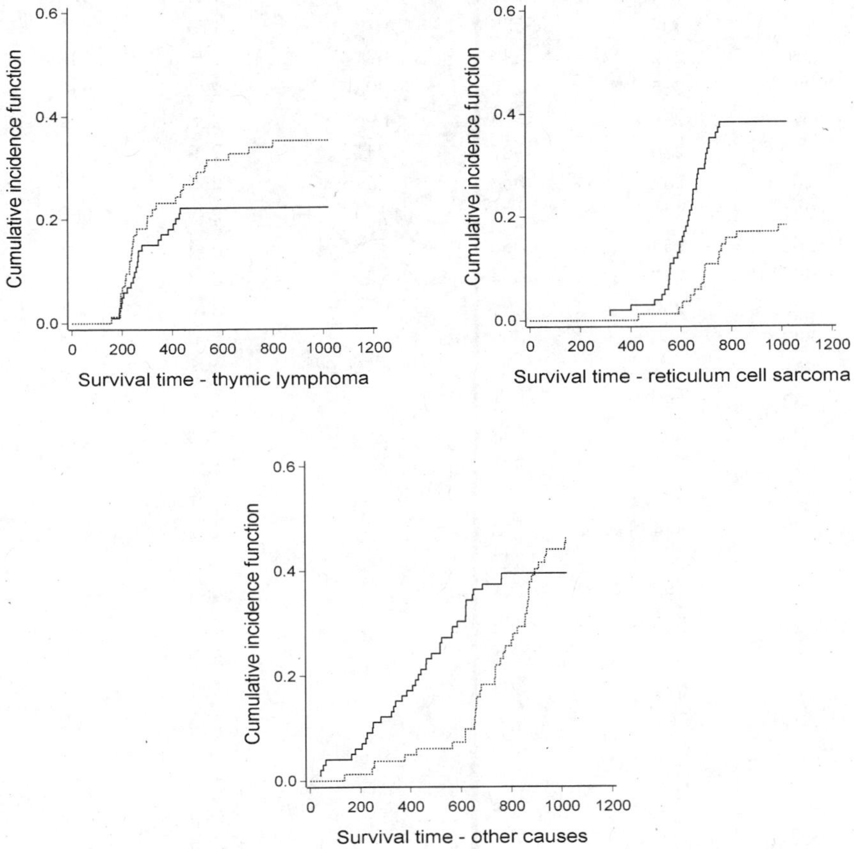

Figure 12.3 *Cumulative incidence functions for mice raised in a standard environment (—) and a germ-free environment (······) for each cause of death.*

These plots suggest that the incidence of thymic lymphoma is greater for mice raised in the germ-free environment, but that reticulum cell sarcoma has greater incidence for mice kept in the standard environment. The incidence of death from other causes also differs between the two environments.

Table 12.7 *Survival times and causes of death for two groups of irradiated mice.*

Thymic lymphoma		Reticulum cell sarcoma		Other causes	
Standard	Germ-free	Standard	Germ-free	Standard	Germ-free
159	158	317	430	40	136
189	192	318	590	42	246
191	193	399	606	51	255
198	194	495	638	62	376
200	195	525	655	163	421
207	202	536	679	179	565
220	212	549	691	206	616
235	215	552	693	222	617
245	229	554	696	228	652
250	230	557	747	249	655
256	237	558	752	252	658
261	240	571	760	282	660
265	244	586	778	324	662
266	247	594	821	333	675
280	259	596	986	341	681
343	300	605		366	734
356	301	612		385	736
383	321	621		407	737
403	337	628		420	757
414	415	631		431	769
428	434	636		441	777
432	444	643		461	800
	485	647		462	807
	496	648		482	825
	529	649		517	855
	537	661		517	857
	624	663		524	864
	707	666		564	868
	800	670		567	870
		695		586	870
		697		619	873
		700		620	882
		705		621	895
		712		622	910
		713		647	934
		738		651	942
		748		686	1015
		753		761	1019
				763	

We next fit a Cox regression model to the cause-specific survival times. For a mouse reared in the ith environment, $i = 1, 2$, the model for the jth cause-specific hazard, $j = 1, 2, 3$, is

$$h_{ij}(t) = \exp(\beta_j x_i) h_{0j}(t),$$

where $x_i = 1$ for a mouse reared in the germ-free environment and zero otherwise, so that β_j is the log-hazard ratio of death from cause j at any time for a mouse raised in the germ-free environment, relative to one from the standard environment. The estimated hazard ratio, together with the corresponding 95% confidence limits and the P-value for testing the hypothesis that the hazard ratio is 1.0, for each cause of death, are shown in Table 12.8.

Table 12.8 *Hazard ratios, confidence limits and P-value for the three causes of death in a cause-specific hazards model.*

Cause of death	Hazard ratio	95% confidence interval	P-value
Thymic lymphoma	1.36	(0.78, 2.38)	0.28
Reticulum cell sarcoma	0.13	(0.07, 0.26)	< 0.001
Other causes	0.31	(0.17, 0.55)	< 0.001

This table shows that the hazard of death from thymic lymphoma is not significantly affected by the environment in which a mouse is reared, but that mice raised in a germ-free environment have a significantly lower hazard of death from reticulum cell sarcoma or other causes.

This analysis shows how the type of environment in which the mice were raised influences the occurrence of each of the three causes of death in circumstances where the other two possible causes cannot occur. Since the cumulative incidence of any particular cause of death depends on the hazard of all possible causes, we cannot draw any conclusions about the effect of environment on the cause-specific incidence functions from modelling cause-specific hazards. For this, we fit a Fine and Gray model for the cumulative incidence of thymic lymphoma, reticulum cell sarcoma and other causes. This enables the effect of environment on each of the three causes of death to be modelled, in the presence of competing risks.

From Equation (12.11), the model for the subhazard function for a mouse reared in the ith environment that dies from the jth cause is

$$\lambda_{ij}(t) = \exp(\beta_j x_i) \lambda_{0j}(t). \tag{12.13}$$

The corresponding model for the cumulative incidence of death from cause j is

$$F_{ij}(t) = 1 - \exp\{-e^{\beta_j x_i} \Lambda_{0j}(t)\},$$

where $\Lambda_{0j}(t)$ is the baseline cumulative subhazard function and $x_i = 1$ for the germ-free environment and zero otherwise. The estimated ratio of the subhazard functions for mice raised in the germ-free environment relative to

Table 12.9 *Subhazard ratios, confidence limits and P-value for the three causes of death in the Fine and Gray model.*

Cause of death	Hazard ratio	95% confidence interval	P-value
Thymic lymphoma	1.68	(0.97, 2.92)	0.066
Reticulum cell sarcoma	0.39	(0.22, 0.70)	0.002
Other causes	1.01	(0.64, 1.57)	0.98

those in the standard environment, P-values and 95% confidence limits, are given in Table 12.9.

This table suggests that, in the presence of competing risks of death, the environment has some effect on the subhazard of death from thymic lymphoma, a highly significant effect on death from reticulum cell carcinoma, but no impact on death from other causes. The germ-free environment increases the subhazard of thymic lymphoma and reduces that for reticulum cell sarcoma.

At first sight the subhazard ratios in Table 12.9 appear quite surprising when compared to the hazard ratios in Table 12.8. Although this feature could result from the effect of competing risks on the incidence of death from thymic lymphoma or other causes, an alternative explanation is suggested by the estimates of the cumulative incidence functions, which were shown in Figure 12.3. For death from other causes, the incidence of death in the standard environment exceeds that in the germ-free environment at times when there are relatively few events. At later times, where there are more events, the incidence functions are closer together, and beyond 800 days, the incidence of death in the germ-free environment is greater. The assumption that the subhazard functions in the Fine and Gray model are proportional is therefore doubtful.

To investigate this further, techniques described in Section 4.4 of Chapter 4 are used. First a plot of the scaled Schoenfeld residuals from the model for the subhazard function for each cause is obtained, with a smoothed curve superimposed. The plot for deaths from other causes is shown in Figure 12.4. This figure shows clearly that the smoothed curve is not horizontal, and strongly suggests that the environment effect is time-dependent.

To further examine the assumption of proportional subhazards, the time-dependent variable $x_i \log t$, with a cause-dependent coefficient β_{j1}, is added to the model in Equation (12.13). The change in the value of $-2 \log \hat{L}$ on adding this term to the subhazard model is not significant for death from thymic lymphoma ($P = 0.16$), but significant for reticulum cell sarcoma ($P = 0.016$), and highly significant for death from other causes ($P < 0.001$). This demonstrates that the effect of environment on the subhazard of death from reticulum cell sarcoma and other causes is not independent of time. To illustrate this for death from other causes, where $j = 3$, Figure 12.5 shows the time-dependent subhazard ratio, $\exp\{\beta_3 + \beta_{31} \log t\}$, plotted against $\log t$, together with 95% confidence bands. The hazard ratio is significantly less than 1.0 for survival

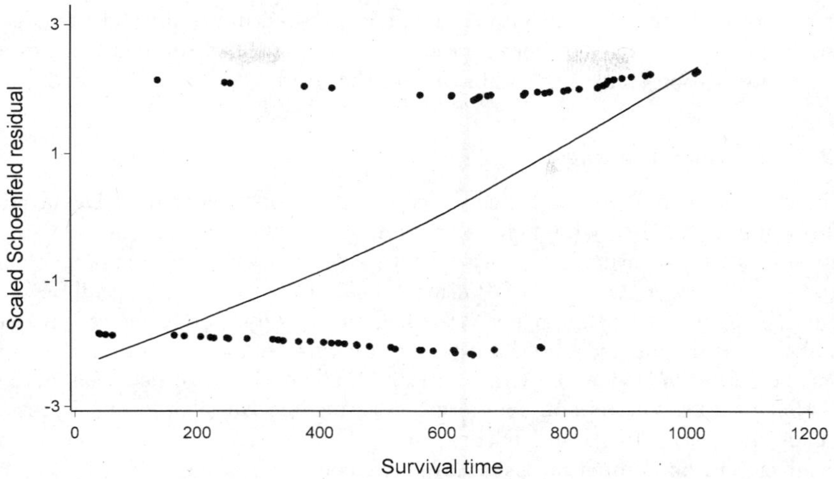

Figure 12.4 *Plot of the scaled Schoenfeld residuals against log survival time on fitting a Fine and Gray model to data on mice that die from other causes.*

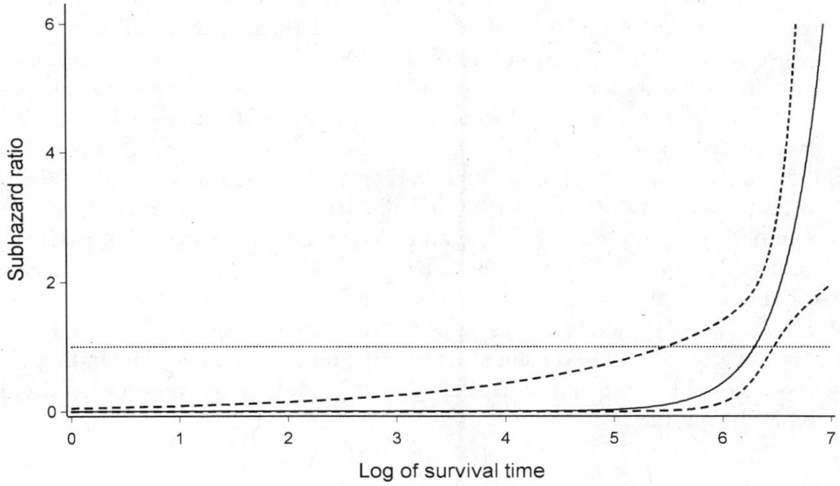

Figure 12.5 *Time-dependent subhazard ratio (—), with 95% confidence bands (- - -), for mice that die from other causes.*

times less than 240 days and significantly greater than 1.0 for survival times greater than 650 days.

Another feature of these data is that there are four unusually short times to death from other causes in mice reared in the standard environment. However, these observations have little influence on the results.

12.7 Further reading

The earliest text to be published on competing risks was that of David and Moeschberger (1978), who included a summary of the work in this area since the seventeenth century. More up to date is the paper of Moeschberger and Klein (1995), and the texts of Pintilie (2006), Crowder (2012), and Beyersmann, Allignol and Schumacher (2012). Each of these books shows how the analyses can be carried out using the R software. A more mathematical account of the area is given by Crowder (2001). General texts on survival analysis that contain chapters on competing risks include Kalbfleisch and Prentice (2002), Lawless (2002), and Kleinbaum and Klein (2012). A number of tutorial papers on competing risks have also been published, such as those of Putter, Fiocco and Geskus (2007) and Pintilie (2007a). Nomenclature is this area is notoriously inconsistent; see Wolbers and Koller (2007), and Latouche, Beyersmann and Fine (2007), for comments on that used in Pintilie (2007a), and the response in Pintilie (2007b). An illustration of the use of competing risks models in predictive modelling is given by Wolbers et al. (2009) and a comparison of four different approaches is given by Tai et al. (2001).

Expressions for the variance of the estimated cumulative incidence function are derived by Aalen (1978a), Marubini and Valsecchi (1995) and Lin (1997) amongst others. Gray (1988) and Pepe and Mori (1993) describe various models and present tests for the comparison of cumulative incidence functions for two or more groups of survival times in the presence of competing risks.

Parametric models for cause-specific hazards have been described by Kalbfleish and Prentice (2002) and Maller and Zhao (2002), while Hinchcliffe and Lambert (2013) describe and illustrate flexible parametric models for competing risks data. The Fine and Gray model for competing risks was introduced by Fine and Gray (1999). Kohl and Heinze (2012) describe a SAS macro for competing risks analysis using the Fine and Gray model, and Gray (2013) describes the `cmprsks` package for use in the R system. A number of papers have presented extensions to the Fine and Gray model, including the additive model of Sun, Sun and Zhang (2006), and the parametric model of Jeong and Fine (2007).

Chapter 13

Multiple events and event history modelling

Individuals observed over time may experience multiple events of the same type, or a number of events of different types. Studies in which there are repeated occurrences of the same type of event, such as a headache or asthmatic attack, are frequently encountered and techniques are needed to model the dependence of the rate at which such events occur on characteristics of the individuals or exposure factors. Multiple event data also arise when an individual may experience a number of outcomes of different types, with interest centering on factors affecting the time to each of these outcomes. Where the occurrence of one event precludes the occurrence of all others, we have the competing risks situation considered in Chapter 12, but in this chapter we consider situations where this is not necessarily the case.

In modelling the course of a disease, individuals may pass through a number of phases or *states* that correspond to particular stages of the disease. For example, a patient diagnosed with chronic kidney disease may be on dialysis before receiving a kidney transplant, and this may be followed by phases where chronic rejection occurs, or where the transplant fails. A patient may experience some or all of these events during the follow-up period from the time of diagnosis, and the sequence of events is termed an *event history*. *Multistate models* can be used to describe the movement of patients among the various states, and to investigate the effect of explanatory variables on the rate at which they transfer from one state to another.

Multiple event and event history data can be analysed using an extension of the Cox regression model to the situation where more than one event can occur. This extension involves the development of a probabilistic model for events that occur over time, known as a *counting process*, and so this chapter begins with an introduction to counting processes.

13.1* Introduction to counting processes

A counting process for the ith of n individuals is defined to be the sequence of values of the random variable $N_i(t), t \geqslant 0$, that counts the number of occurrences of some event over the time period $(0, t]$, for $i = 1, 2, \ldots, n$. A realisation of the counting process $N_i(t)$ is then a step-function that starts at 0 and increases in steps of one unit.

We next define $Y_i(t), t \geqslant 0$, to be a process where $Y_i(t) = 1$ when the ith individual is at risk of an event occurring at time t, and zero otherwise, so that $Y_i(t)$ is sometimes called the *at-risk process*. The value of $Y_i(t)$ must be known at a time $t-$, the time immediately before t, and when this is the case, $Y_i(t)$ is said to be a *predictable process*.

The counting process $N_i(t)$ has an associated *intensity*, which is the rate at which events occur. Formally, the intensity of a counting process is the probability that $N_i(t)$ increases by one step in unit time, conditional on the history of the process up to time t. The history or *filtration* of the process up to but not including time t is written $\mathcal{H}(t-)$, and is determined from the set of values $\{N_i(s), Y_i(s)\}$ for all values of s up to time t. If we denote the intensity process by $\lambda_i(t), t \geqslant 0$, then, in infinitesimal notation, where dt is an infinitely small interval of time, we have

$$\begin{aligned}\lambda_i(t) &= \frac{1}{\mathrm{d}t}\mathrm{P}\{N_i(t) \text{ increases by one step in an interval of length d}t \mid \mathcal{H}(t-)\},\\ &= \frac{1}{\mathrm{d}t}\mathrm{P}\{N_i(t+\mathrm{d}t) - N_i(t) = 1 \mid \mathcal{H}(t-)\}.\end{aligned}$$

If we set $\mathrm{d}N_i(t) = N_i(t+\mathrm{d}t) - N_i(t)$ to be the change in $N_i(t)$ over an infinitesimal time interval of length dt, $\lambda_i(t)$ can be expressed as

$$\lambda_i(t) = \frac{1}{\mathrm{d}t}\mathrm{P}\{\mathrm{d}N_i(t) = 1 \mid \mathcal{H}(t-)\}. \tag{13.1}$$

Since $\mathrm{d}N_i(t)$ is either 0 or 1, it follows that

$$\lambda_i(t) = \frac{1}{\mathrm{d}t}\,\mathrm{E}\,\{\mathrm{d}N_i(t) \mid \mathcal{H}(t-)\},$$

and so the intensity of the counting process is the expected number of events in unit time, conditional on the history of the process.

We can also define the cumulative intensity, or integrated intensity, $\Lambda_i(t)$, where

$$\Lambda_i(t) = \int_0^t \lambda_i(u)\,\mathrm{d}u$$

is the cumulative expected number of events in the time interval $(0, t]$, that is $\Lambda_i(t) = \mathrm{E}\,\{N_i(t)\}$.

13.1.1 Modelling the intensity function

A convenient general model for the intensity function for the ith individual is that it depends on an observable, predictable stochastic process $Y_i(t)$, and an unknown function of both time and known values of p possibly time-varying explanatory variables, $X_1(t), X_2(t), \ldots, X_p(t)$. The intensity of the counting process $N_i(t)$ is then taken to be

$$\lambda_i(t) = Y_i(t) g\{t, \boldsymbol{x}_i(t)\},$$

where $\boldsymbol{x}_i(t)$ is the vector of values of the p explanatory variables at time t. Setting $g\{t, \boldsymbol{x}_i(t)\} = \exp\{\boldsymbol{\beta}'\boldsymbol{x}_i(t)\}\lambda_0(t)$, we have

$$\lambda_i(t) = Y_i(t) \exp\{\boldsymbol{\beta}'\boldsymbol{x}_i(t)\}\lambda_0(t),$$

where $\lambda_0(t)$ is a baseline intensity function that depends on t alone.

The argument used in Section 3.3.1 of Chapter 3 to derive the partial likelihood of a sample of survival times can be adapted to obtain the likelihood of data from a realisation of a counting process. Details are omitted but in counting process notation, the partial likelihood has the form

$$\prod_{i=1}^{n} \prod_{t \geqslant 0} \left\{ \frac{Y_i(t) \exp\{\boldsymbol{\beta}'\boldsymbol{x}_i(t)\}}{\sum_{l=1}^{n} Y_l(t) \exp\{\boldsymbol{\beta}'\boldsymbol{x}_l(t)\}} \right\}^{\mathrm{d}N_i(t)}, \tag{13.2}$$

where $\mathrm{d}N_i(t) = 1$ if $N_i(t)$ increases by one unit at time t, and zero otherwise. This function is then maximised with respect to unknown parameters in the intensity function, leading to estimates of the βs.

A large body of theory has been developed for the study of counting processes, and this enables the asymptotic properties of parameter estimates to be determined. This theory is based on the properties of a type of stochastic process with zero mean known as a *martingale*. In fact, the process defined by

$$M_i(t) = N_i(t) - \Lambda_i(t) \tag{13.3}$$

is such that $\mathrm{E}\{M_i(t)\} = 0$ for all t, and is a martingale. Theoretical details will not be given here, but note that Equation (13.3) is the basis of the martingale residuals defined in Equation (4.6) of Chapter 4.

13.1.2 Survival data as a counting process

Survival data with right-censored survival times, consisting of pairs formed from a time, t_i, and an event indicator δ_i, $i = 1, 2, \ldots, n$, is a particular example of a counting process. To show this, consider a counting process in which $N_i(t) = 0$ when the ith individual is at risk of an event occurring, and $N_i(t)$ steps up to unity at the time when an event occurs. Since an individual is at risk at the time origin, $N_i(0) = 0$, and so the process $N_i(t)$ starts at 0 and increases to 1 at the event time of the ith individual, or remains at 0 for those individuals with censored survival times. The value of the at-risk process, $Y_i(t)$, is unity until the occurrence of the event, or the time is censored, and zero thereafter.

From Equation (13.1), the intensity of the counting process is such that

$$\begin{aligned}\lambda_i(t)\,\mathrm{d}t &= \mathrm{P}\{\mathrm{d}N_i(t) = 1 \mid \mathcal{H}(t-)\},\\ &= \mathrm{P}\{t \leqslant T_i \leqslant t + \mathrm{d}t \mid \mathcal{H}(t-)\},\end{aligned}$$

where T_i is the random variable associated with the time to an event for the ith individual. The intensity function can then be expressed as

$$\lambda_i(t)\,\mathrm{d}t = Y_i(t)h_i(t)\,\mathrm{d}t, \tag{13.4}$$

where

$$h_i(t)\,\mathrm{d}t = \mathrm{P}(t \leqslant T_i \leqslant t + \mathrm{d}t \mid T \geqslant t)$$

is the hazard function, $h_i(t)$, first defined in Equation (1.3) of Chapter 1. The result in Equation (13.4) follows from the fact that in survival data, the hazard of an event occurring in the interval from t to $t + \mathrm{d}t$ depends only on the individual being at risk at time $t-$, and so the relevant history at that time, $\mathcal{H}(t-)$, is that $T_i \geqslant t$. Inclusion of $Y_i(t)$ in Equation (13.4) ensures that $\lambda_i(t) = 0$ when the ith individual is not at risk.

From Equation (13.4), the intensity of the counting process is given by $\lambda_i(t) = Y_i(t)h_i(t)$, so that the intensity function is the hazard of an event occurring at time t when the ith individual is at risk of an event. Also, the intensity function of the standard Cox regression model can then be expressed as

$$Y_i(t)\exp(\boldsymbol{\beta}'\boldsymbol{x}_i)h_0(t),$$

where $h_0(t)$ is the baseline hazard function. In the sequel, this will simply be denoted $h_i(t)$, as usual.

To obtain the likelihood function for this model from the general result in Expression (13.2), we note that $\mathrm{d}N_i(t)$ is zero until the event time, when $\mathrm{d}N_i(t) = 1$. The only contributions to the partial likelihood function in Equation (13.2) are from individuals who are at risk, and so Equation (13.2) becomes

$$\prod_{i=1}^{n}\left\{\frac{\exp\{\boldsymbol{\beta}'\boldsymbol{x}_i(t)\}}{\sum_{l\in R(t_i)}\exp\{\boldsymbol{\beta}'\boldsymbol{x}_l(t)\}}\right\}^{\delta_i},$$

as given in Equation (3.5) of Chapter 8. When the explanatory variables are not time-dependent, $x_j \equiv x_j(t)$ for all values of t, $j = 1, 2, \ldots, p$, and this is Equation (3.5) in Section 3.3 of Chapter 3.

These results mean that the theory of counting processes can be used to prove many of the standard results in survival analysis, and to derive asymptotic properties of test statistics. However, the great advantage of the counting process formulation is that it can be used to extend the Cox model in many directions. These include time-varying explanatory variables, dependent censoring, recurrent events, multiple events per subject and models for correlated data. It also allows problems with more complicated censoring patterns to be managed. These include left truncation, where the follow-up process for an individual only begins some known time after the time origin, and multistate models. Some of these situations will be considered in this chapter.

13.1.3 Survival data in the counting process format

Counting process data consist of a sequence of time intervals $(t_{j-1}, t_j]$, $j = 1, 2, \ldots$, where $t_0 = 0$, over which the values of the counting process $N_i(t)$, the at-risk process $Y_i(t)$, and any time-varying explanatory variables $X_i(t)$, are constant for the ith of n individuals. Associated with each interval is the value of $N_i(t)$ at the end of the interval, $N_i(t_j)$, which marks the time when $N_i(t)$ increases by one unit, or when $Y_i(t)$ or an explanatory variable changes in value. This leads to an alternative and more flexible way of formatting survival data.

To express survival data in counting process format, suppose that t is the event time and δ is the event indicator for a particular individual. The time interval $(0, t]$ is then divided into a series of r intervals with cut points at times $t_1, t_2, \ldots, t_{r-1}$, so that $0 < t_1 < t_2 < \cdots < t_{r-1} < t$. The corresponding intervals are $(0, t_1], (t_1, t_2], \ldots, (t_{r-1}, t]$. These intervals will be such that the values of all time-varying explanatory variables are constant within each interval, and where both the at-risk process and the counting process have constant values. The event status at t_j is $N(t_j)$, so that $N(t_j) = 0$ if an individual remains at risk at t_j, and $N(t_j) = 1$ if that individual experiences an event at t_j, the end of the jth interval, $(t_{j-1}, t_j]$, for $j = 1, 2, \ldots, r$, where $t_r \equiv t$. Then, for the ith individual, the observation on a survival time and an event indicator, (t_i, δ_i), can be replaced by the sequence $\{t_{i,j-1}, t_{ij}, N_i(t_{ij})\}$, for $j = 1, 2, \ldots, r$, with $t_{i0} \equiv 0$ and $t_{ir} \equiv t_i$. This form of the survival data is often referred to as *(start, stop, status) format*, but more usually as the *counting process format*. The partial likelihood function of data expressed in this way is equivalent to that for the original data, and so the model fit is identical. Values of the $-2 \log \hat{L}$ statistic for fitted models, as well as parameter estimates and their standard errors, are then identical to those obtained when the data are analysed using the standard format.

Example 13.1 Illustration of the counting process format
Suppose that a patient in a study concerning cancer of the liver is observed from the time when they enter the study until they die 226 days later. During this time, the stage of the cancer is measured at particular time points, and the data for this individual are given in Table 13.1.

Table 13.1 *Tumour size at different times for an individual with liver cancer.*

Observation	Time	Tumour stage	Start	Stop	Status
1	0	1	0	45	0
2	45	2	45	84	0
3	84	2	84	127	0
4	127	3	127	163	0
5	163	4	163	226	1
6	226	4			

In the counting process format, a sequence of time intervals is defined, leading to the intervals $(0, 45], (45, 84], (84, 127], (127, 163], (163, 226]$. These are the start and stop times in Table 13.1. The status variable denotes whether a patient is alive (status $= 0$) or dead (status $= 1$) at the end of each interval. It is natural to use the stage of the tumour at the start of each of these intervals in the analysis, which means that the tumour stage in the period leading to a possible death at the stop time is used in the modelling process. Other possibilities include using the stage at the end of the interval, or some form of intermediate value. See Section 8.2.1 of Chapter 8 for a fuller discussion on this. Since the tumour stage is the same at 45 and 84 days, and also at 163 and 226 days, the intervals $(0, 84], (84, 127], (127, 226]$ could be used instead. Also, if the individual were still alive at 226 days, and this marked the end of follow-up for this patient, their status would be recorded as zero at that time.

13.1.4 Robust estimation of the variance-covariance matrix

When the counting process formulation of a Cox regression model is used to analyse multiple event data, the event times within an individual will not be independent. This in turn means that the standard errors of the parameter estimates in fitted models, obtained in the usual manner, may be smaller than they really should be. This overestimation of the precision of model-based estimates can be avoided by using a *robust estimate* of the variance-covariance matrix of the parameter estimates that is not so dependent on the underlying model. The most widely used robust estimate is termed the *sandwich estimate*, described in this section, and a number of studies have shown that this estimate performs well in misspecified Cox regression models.

The standard model-based estimate of the variance-covariance matrix of the parameter estimates in a Cox regression model, $\text{var}\,(\hat{\boldsymbol{\beta}})$, is the inverse of the observed information matrix. This was introduced in Section 3.3.3 of Chapter 3, and is a $p \times p$ matrix denoted $\boldsymbol{I}^{-1}(\hat{\boldsymbol{\beta}})$, where p is the number of unknown β-parameters. A robust estimate of the variance-covariance matrix due to Lin and Wei (1989) is found from $\boldsymbol{I}^{-1}(\hat{\boldsymbol{\beta}})\boldsymbol{A}(\hat{\boldsymbol{\beta}})\boldsymbol{I}^{-1}(\hat{\boldsymbol{\beta}})$, where the matrix $\boldsymbol{A}(\hat{\boldsymbol{\beta}})$ can be regarded as a correction term that allows for potential model misspecification. This correction term is sandwiched between two copies of the inverse of the information matrix, which is why it is called a sandwich estimate. The correction matrix is $\boldsymbol{A}(\hat{\boldsymbol{\beta}}) = \boldsymbol{U}'(\hat{\boldsymbol{\beta}})\boldsymbol{U}(\hat{\boldsymbol{\beta}})$, where $\boldsymbol{U}(\hat{\boldsymbol{\beta}})$ is the $n \times p$ matrix of efficient scores, evaluated at the estimates $\hat{\boldsymbol{\beta}}$, for each of the n observations.

In Section 4.3.1 of Chapter 4, the $p \times 1$ vector of efficient scores for the ith observation was written as $\boldsymbol{r}_{Ui}$ and termed the vector of score residuals for the ith observation, and so $\boldsymbol{U}(\hat{\boldsymbol{\beta}})$ is an $n \times p$ matrix whose rows are $\boldsymbol{r}'_{U1}, \boldsymbol{r}'_{U2}, \ldots, \boldsymbol{r}'_{Un}$. Now, the change in the vector of β-parameters, on omitting the ith observation, was shown in Section 4.3.1 of Chapter 4 to be approximately $\boldsymbol{r}'_{Ui}\,\text{var}\,(\hat{\boldsymbol{\beta}})$. The matrix of these values is $\boldsymbol{D}(\hat{\boldsymbol{\beta}}) = \boldsymbol{U}(\hat{\boldsymbol{\beta}})\boldsymbol{I}^{-1}(\hat{\boldsymbol{\beta}})$, in the notation of this section, and the components of the ith row of this matrix are the delta-beta statistics for assessing the effect of the ith observation on each of the p parameter estimates. It then follows that the sandwich estimate can be written as $\boldsymbol{D}'(\hat{\boldsymbol{\beta}})\boldsymbol{D}(\hat{\boldsymbol{\beta}})$, which shows how the sandwich estimate can be obtained from the delta-beta's.

In applications envisaged in this chapter, the data will consist of times to a relatively small number of events within each individual. In this situation, it is better to base the sandwich estimator on an aggregate of the event times within an individual. This is achieved by summing the efficient scores, that are the elements of the matrix $\boldsymbol{U}(\hat{\boldsymbol{\beta}})$, over the event times within each of n individuals, so that this matrix is still of dimension $n \times p$.

When the robust estimate of the variance-covariance matrix is being used, it can be helpful to compare the ratios of the robust standard errors to the usual model-based standard errors. The effect of using the robust estimator on quantities such as interval estimates for hazard ratios can then be determined.

13.2 Modelling recurrent event data

Situations where an individual experiences more than one event of the same type, known as a *recurrent event*, are common in medical research, and examples include sequences of tumour recurrences, infection episodes, adverse drug reactions, epileptic seizures, bleeding incidents, migraines and cardiothoracic events. Techniques are then needed to estimate the *rate* or *intensity* at which *recurrences* occur, and the dependence of the recurrence rate on characteristics of the individuals or exposure factors.

In an initial analysis of recurrent event data, standard methods of survival analysis can be used to model the time to the first event. Although straightforward, this approach ignores subsequent events and so is not making the most of the data available. However, more detailed analyses are complicated by two features. First, there will be variation between individuals in their susceptibility to recurrent events, and the recurrence times within an individual may not be independent. Second, following the occurrence of an event such as a heavy bleed, the treatment may mean that the individual is not at risk of a subsequent bleed for some short period of time. It will then be necessary to modify the set of individuals who are at risk of a recurrent event to take account of this.

Variations on the Cox regression model provide a convenient framework for a modelling approach to the analysis of recurrent event data. In particular, the counting process approach, described in Section 13.1, enables features such as variation in the at-risk status over time to be incorporated.

There are three models that are commonly used in recurrent event analysis. The simplest of these is due to Anderson and Gill (1982), but a rather more flexible model is due to Prentice, Williams and Peterson (1981). A third model, due to Wei, Lin and Weissfeld (1989) will also be described, but this model is more useful when there are events of different types, rather than recurrences of events of the same type, and so is introduced later in Section 13.3.1. We will follow others in referring to these as the AG, PWP and WLW models, respectively.

13.2.1 The Anderson and Gill model

In this model, the baseline intensity function is common to all recurrences and unaffected by the occurrence of previous events, and the individual recurrence times within an individual are independent. As a result, this model is particularly useful when interest centres on modelling the overall recurrence rate.

The AG model for the intensity, or hazard, of an event occurring at time t in the ith of n individuals is given by

$$h_i(t) = Y_i(t) \exp\{\boldsymbol{\beta}'\boldsymbol{x}_i(t)\} h_0(t), \tag{13.5}$$

where $Y_i(t)$ denotes whether or not the ith individual is at risk of an event at time t, $\boldsymbol{\beta}'\boldsymbol{x}_i(t)$ is a linear combination of p possibly time-dependent explanatory variables, and $h_0(t)$ is a baseline hazard function. Patients who may experience multiple events remain at risk, and so $Y_i(t)$ remains at unity unless an individual temporarily ceases to be at risk in some time period, or until the follow-up time is censored. The risk set at time t is then the set of all individuals who are still being followed up at time t, just as in the standard Cox model.

To fit this model, the recurrent event data are expressed in counting process format, where the jth time interval, $(t_{j-1}, t_j]$, is the time between the $(j-1)$th and jth recurrences, $j = 1, 2, \ldots$, where $t_0 = 0$. The status variable denotes whether or not an event occurred at the end-point of the interval, that is the jth recurrence time, and is unity if t_j was an event time and zero otherwise. An individual who experiences no events contributes a single time interval where the end-point is censored, so that the status variable is zero. Similarly, the status variable will be zero at the time marking the end of the follow-up period, unless an event is observed at that time. The format of the data that is required to fit the AG model is illustrated later in Example 13.2.

The assumption of independent recurrence times can be relaxed to some extent by including terms in the model that correspond to the number of preceding events, or the time from the origin. Since any association between recurrence times will usually result in the model-based standard errors of the estimated β-parameters being too small, the robust form of the variance-covariance matrix of the estimated β-parameters, described in Section 13.1.4, can be used.

This approach may not properly account for within-subject dependence, and so alternatively, and preferably, association between the recurrence times can be accommodated by adding a random frailty effect for the ith subject, as described in Chapter 10. The addition of a random subject effect, u_i, to the AG model leads to the model

$$h_i(t) = Y_i(t)\exp\{\boldsymbol{\beta}'\boldsymbol{x}_i(t) + u_i\}h_0(t),$$

in which u_i may be assumed to have a $N(0, \sigma_u^2)$ distribution. Fitting the AG model with and without a frailty effect allows the extent of within-subject correlation in the recurrence times to be assessed, using the methods described in Section 10.6 of Chapter 10.

Once a model has been fitted, hazard ratios and their corresponding interval estimates can be determined. In addition, the recurrence times can be summarised using the unadjusted or adjusted cumulative intensity (or hazard) function and the cumulative incidence function, estimated from the complement of the survivor function. This will be illustrated in Example 13.2.

13.2.2 The Prentice, Williams and Peterson model

A straightforward extension of the AG model in Equation (13.5) leads to a more flexible model, in which separate strata are defined for each event. This model allows the intensity to vary from one recurrence to another, so that the within-subject recurrence times are no longer independent. In the PWP model, the hazard of the jth occurrence, $j = 1, 2, \ldots$, of an event at time t in the ith of n individuals is

$$h_{ij}(t) = Y_{ij}(t)\exp\{\boldsymbol{\beta}_j'\,\boldsymbol{x}_i(t)\}h_{0j}(t), \tag{13.6}$$

where $Y_{ij}(t)$ is unity until the $(j-1)$th recurrent event and zero thereafter, $\boldsymbol{\beta}_j$ is the vector of coefficients of the p explanatory variables for the jth recurrence time, $\boldsymbol{x}_i(t)$ is the vector of values of the explanatory variables, and $h_{0j}(t)$ is the baseline hazard for the jth recurrence. In this model, the risk set for the jth recurrence is restricted to individuals who have experienced the previous $(j-1)$ recurrences. As the intensity of the jth recurrent event is conditional on the $(j-1)$th having occurred, this is termed a *conditional model*, and is widely regarded as the most satisfactory model for general use.

The PWP model, defined in Equation (13.6), can be fitted using a Cox regression model, stratified by recurrence number. The data are expressed in the same format as that used to fit the AG model, where the status indicator is unity until the jth recurrence time, and zero thereafter. In addition, a stratifying factor denotes the recurrence number. The coefficients of the explanatory variables may take different values for each recurrence, but they can be constrained to have a common value for a subset of the strata when large numbers of recurrences do not occur very often, or across all the strata. As usual, the resulting change in the value of the $-2\log\hat{L}$ statistic can be used to formally test the hypothesis of a constant hazard ratio across strata.

This model is particularly suited to situations where there is interest in the times between different recurrences of an event, and in whether hazard ratios vary with recurrence number. As for the AG model, a robust variance-covariance matrix for the parameter estimates can be used to further allow for correlated recurrence times, and the model can also be extended by using a frailty term to account for any association between recurrence times.

Example 13.2 Recurrence of mammary tumours in female rats

In animal experiments that are designed to compare an active treatment for the prevention of cancer with a control, the rate at which tumours occur is of interest. Gail, Santner and Brown (1980) describe an experiment concerning the development of mammary cancer in female rats that are allocated to one of two treatment groups. A number of rats were injected with a carcinogen and then all rats were treated with retinyl acetate, a retinoid that is a natural form of vitamin A, with the potential to inhibit tumour development. After 60 days, the 48 rats that were tumour free were randomly allocated to receive continuing prophylactic treatment with the retinoid, or to a control group with no such treatment. The rats were assessed for evidence of tumours twice weekly, and the observation period ended 122 days after randomisation to treatment. Rats with no tumour at 122 days have censored recurrence times.

The data in Table 13.2 give the times from randomisation to the development of mammary tumours for the 23 rats in the group receiving retinoid prophylaxis and 25 controls. Since the rats were not assessed on a daily basis, some rats were found to have developed more than one tumour at an assessment time. For example, one rat in the control group was found to have three tumours on day 42. To avoid the ambiguity of tied observations, these have been replaced by times of 42, 42.1 and 42.2.

A simple analysis of these data is based on modelling the time to the first event. Of the 48 rats in the experiment, just two do not develop a tumour and so contribute censored survival times. Using standard methods, the hazard of a first tumour occurring in a rat on the retinoid treatment, relative to one in the control group, is 0.50. This is significantly different from unity ($P = 0.027$), and the corresponding 95% confidence interval is (0.27, 0.93). There is strong evidence that the hazard of a first tumour in treated rats is about half that of control rats.

To illustrate how the data are organised for a recurrent event analysis, consider the data from the fifth rat in the treated group, for whom the times at which a tumour was detected are 70, 74, 85 and 92 days, and the rat was subsequently followed up until day 122 with no further tumours detected. The representation of this sequence in counting process format for the AG and PWP models is shown in Table 13.3. The treatment group is represented by an explanatory variable that is unity for a rat who receives the retinoid treatment and zero otherwise.

In the AG model, the hazard of a tumour developing at time t is given by

$$h_i(t) = Y_i(t) \exp(\beta x_i) h_0(t),$$

where $Y_i(t) = 1$ when a rat is at risk of tumour development and zero otherwise, $x_i = 1$ if the ith rat is in the treated group and zero otherwise, and β is the log-hazard ratio for a rat on the retinoid treatment, relative to one in

Table 13.2 *Recurrence times of tumours in rats on a retinoid treatment or control.*

Treatment	Times to tumour
Retinoid	122
	122*
	3, 8, 122*
	92, 122*
	70, 74, 85, 92, 122*
	38, 92, 122
	28, 35, 45, 70, 77, 107, 122*
	92, 122*
	21, 122*
	11, 24, 66, 74, 92, 122*
	56, 70, 122*
	31, 122*
	3, 8, 24, 35, 92, 122*
	45, 92, 122*
	3, 42, 92, 122*
	3, 17, 52, 80, 122*
	17, 59, 92, 101, 107, 122*
	45, 52, 85, 101, 122
	92, 122*
	21, 35, 122*
	24, 31, 42, 48, 70, 74, 122*
	122*
	31, 122*
Control	3, 42, 59, 101, 101.1, 112, 119, 122*
	28, 31, 35, 45, 52, 59, 59.1, 77, 85, 107, 112, 122*
	31, 38, 48, 52, 74, 77, 101, 101.1, 119, 122*
	11, 114, 122*
	35, 45, 74, 74.1, 77, 80, 85, 90, 90.1, 122*
	8, 8.1, 70, 77, 122*
	17, 35, 52, 77, 101, 114, 122*
	21, 24, 66, 74, 101, 101.1, 114, 122*
	8, 17, 38, 42, 42.1, 42.2, 122*
	52, 122*
	28, 28.1, 31, 38, 52, 74, 74.1, 77, 77.1, 80, 80.1, 92, 92.1, 122*
	17, 119, 122*
	52, 122*
	11, 11.1, 14, 17, 52, 56, 56.1, 80, 80.1, 107, 122*
	17, 35, 66, 90, 122*
	28, 66, 70, 70.1, 74, 122*
	3, 14, 24, 24.1, 28, 31, 35, 48, 74, 77, 119, 122*
	21, 28, 45, 56, 63, 80, 85, 92, 101, 101.1, 119, 122*
	28, 35, 52, 59, 66, 66.1, 90, 97, 119, 122*
	8, 8.1, 24, 42, 45, 59, 63, 63.1, 77, 101, 119, 122
	80, 122*
	92, 122, 122.1
	21, 122*
	3, 28, 74, 122*
	24, 74, 122

* Censored recurrence times.

Table 13.3 *Representation of the recurrence times of one rat for the AG and PWP models.*

Model	Event	Interval	Status	Stratum	Treatment
AG	1	(0, 70]	1	1	1
	2	(70, 74]	1	1	1
	3	(74, 85]	1	1	1
	4	(85, 92]	1	1	1
	5	(92, 122]	0	1	1
PWP	1	(0, 70]	1	1	1
	2	(70, 74]	1	2	1
	3	(74, 85]	1	3	1
	4	(85, 92]	1	4	1
	5	(92, 122]	0	5	1

the control group. A standard Cox regression model is then fitted to the stop times, that is the end-point of each interval, in the data arranged as illustrated in Table 13.3.

Using the robust standard error of the treatment effect, $\hat{\beta} = -0.801$ and $\text{se}(\hat{\beta}) = 0.198$. This estimate is significantly less than zero ($P < 0.001$), and the overall hazard of a tumour occurring in a rat in the retinoid group, relative to one in the control group, at any given time, is 0.45, with a 95% confidence interval of (0.30, 0.66). The tumour occurrence rate for rats in the retinoid treatment group is less than half that of rats in the control group.

The treatment difference can be summarised using the estimated cumulative intensity, or hazard, of tumour recurrences for rats in each treatment group. This is $\exp(\hat{\beta}x)\hat{H}_0(t)$, where $\hat{H}_0(t)$ is the estimated baseline cumulative intensity function, and $x = 1$ for rats exposed to the retinoid treatment and $x = 0$ for rats in the control group. This is also the cumulative expected number of tumour recurrences over time. The cumulative intensity for each treatment is shown in Figure 13.1. This shows that rats exposed to the retinoid treatment have a lower intensity of tumour occurrence than rats in the control group. At 45 days, it is estimated that one tumour would have occurred in a rat in the treated group, but two tumours would have occurred by that time in a rat in the control group.

The cumulative incidence of a recurrence can be obtained from $1 - \hat{S}_0(t)^{\exp(\hat{\beta}x)}$, for $x = 0$ or 1, where $\hat{S}_0(t) = \exp\{-\hat{H}_0(t)\}$ is the estimated baseline survivor function in the fitted AG model. The two incidence functions are shown in Figure 13.2. Again, this figure confirms that tumour incidence is substantially greater for rats in the control group. The median tumour recurrence time is 31 days for rats in the treated group and 17 days for rats in the control group.

Instead of using the robust standard error of the treatment effect, association between the recurrence times within a rat can be modelled by adding a normally distributed random effect to the AG model. This random effect

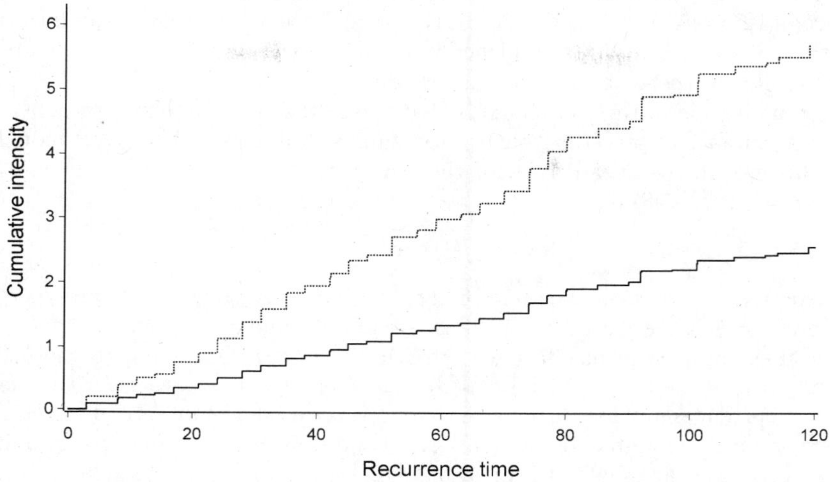

Figure 13.1 *Cumulative intensity of recurrent events for rats on the retinoid treatment (—) or a control (·······).*

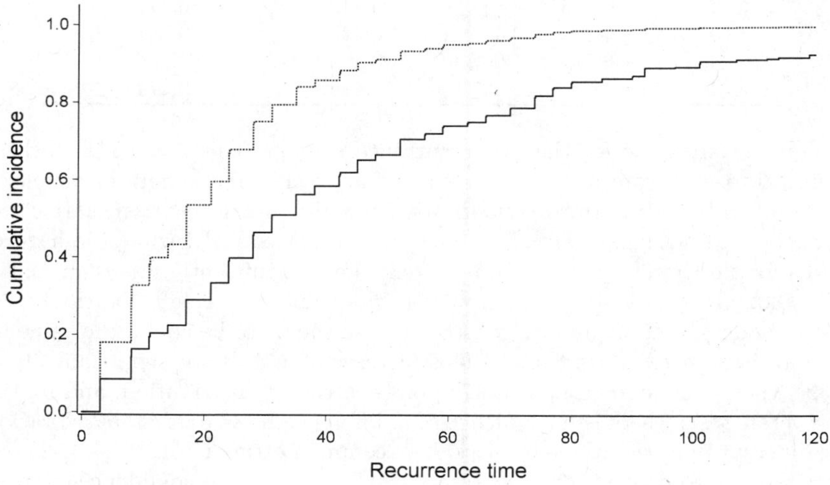

Figure 13.2 *Cumulative incidence of recurrent events for rats on the retinoid treatment (—) or a control (·······).*

differs for each rat but will be constant for the recurrence times within a rat. When this is done, the rat effect is highly significant and the estimated variance of the random effect is 0.25. In this model, the estimated overall hazard ratio is 0.46 with a 95% confidence interval of (0.31, 0.71). These estimates are similar to those obtained using the robust standard error.

A limitation of the AG model is that the recurrence rate does not depend on the number of preceding recurrences, and so we next fit the PWP model. In this model, the hazard rate for the jth recurrence, $j = 1, 2, \ldots$, in the ith rat, $i = 1, 2, \ldots, 48$, is

$$h_{ij}(t) = Y_{ij}(t) \exp(\beta_j x_i) h_{0j}(t),$$

where $Y_{ij}(t) = 1$ until the time of the $(j-1)$th recurrence and zero thereafter, $x_i = 1$ if the ith rat is in the treated group and zero otherwise, and β_j measures the treatment effect for the jth recurrence. On fitting this model, estimates $\hat{\beta}_j$, the hazard ratios $\exp(\hat{\beta}_j)$ and their standard errors, for the first four recurrences and five or more recurrences, are as shown in Table 13.4. Both the standard model-based standard errors and those obtained using the sandwich estimator are shown in this table. Unusually, those based on the robust estimator are smaller, but the sandwich estimator will be used in subsequent analyses.

Table 13.4 *Estimates on fitting a PWP model to the recurrence times.*

Recurrence	$\hat{\beta}_j$	$\exp(\hat{\beta}_j)$	se $(\hat{\beta}_j)$ [model]	se $(\hat{\beta}_j)$ [sandwich]
1	−0.686	0.503	0.312	0.283
2	−0.123	0.884	0.349	0.317
3	−0.831	0.436	0.425	0.381
4	0.060	1.062	0.482	0.296
$\geqslant 5$	−0.850	0.427	0.419	0.274

The hazard ratio for the first recurrence is $\exp(-0.686) = 0.50$, which is identical to that from just modelling the time to the first tumour occurrence, as it should be. The hazard ratio for a second and fourth recurrence are close to unity, and not significant, $P = 0.697, 0.839$, respectively, while the hazard ratios for three and five or more recurrences are significantly less than unity, $P = 0.029, 0.002$, respectively. However, the value of $-2 \log \hat{L}$ for the fitted PWP model is 812.82, and on constraining all the βs to be equal, the value of this statistic increases to 816.95. This increase of 4.13 is not significant ($P = 0.39$) when compared to percentage points of the χ^2_4 distribution, and so, on an overall basis, there is no evidence of a difference between the hazard ratios for different numbers of recurrences. The common estimate of β is -0.523, so that the hazard ratio for any recurrence is 0.59, with a 95% confidence interval of (0.46, 0.77). This is very similar to that found using the AG model, but here the recurrence times have different baseline hazards.

The hazard functions, $h_{ij}(t)$, can be constrained to be proportional by fitting an unstratified model that includes a factor associated with the recurrence number, so that

$$h_{ij}(t) = Y_{ij}(t)\exp(\beta_j x_i + \zeta_j)h_0(t),$$

where ζ_j is the effect of the jth recurrence. If the ζ_j are all zero, the model reduces to the AG model. The stratified and unstratified models are not nested, and so the two models cannot be directly compared. However, assuming proportional hazards, the overall hazard rate is 0.59, with a 95% confidence interval of (0.45, 0.77), which is very similar to that found using the stratified model.

13.3 Multiple events

Individuals suffering from chronic diseases may experience multiple events, each of which is of a different type. Any one individual may not experience all of these events, and whereas recurrent events have a natural time order, multiple events may occur in a different order in different individuals. For example, a patient diagnosed with liver disease may experience events such as histological progression of the disease, development of varices, development of ascites, an increase in serum bilirubin level, a liver transplant and death. Generally, each of these events will occur at most once in a sequence that may vary from patient to patient. Such data could be analysed by fitting separate models to the times to each event from the same time origin, but a more efficient analysis is based on the Wei, Lin and Weissfeld (WLW) model.

13.3.1 The Wei, Lin and Weissfeld model

In this model, strata are defined for each event, in such a way that the total number of strata is equal to the number of possible events. As for the PWP model, the hazard of the occurrence of the jth event at time t in the ith individual is given by

$$h_{ij}(t) = Y_{ij}(t)\exp\{\boldsymbol{\beta}_j' \boldsymbol{x}_i(t)\}h_{0j}(t),$$

but now $Y_{ij}(t)$ is unity until the jth event occurs and 0 thereafter. In this model, the risk set at time t consists of all individuals who were being followed up at time t and in whom the jth event has not occurred. This model has the same form as a Cox regression model for the jth event, except that in the WLW model, the βs are jointly estimated from the times to all events. The WLW model is termed a *marginal model* since each event time is treated as a separate event, and the time origin for each event is the start of the follow-up time for each individual. Hazard ratios may vary across the different event types, and the model also allows for differences in the underlying intensity of each event to be accommodated.

To fit this model, the total number of possible events across all the individuals in the study, r, is determined, and the time to each event is expressed as a series of intervals from the time origin, $(0, t_j]$, where t_j is the time of the jth event, $j = 1, 2, \ldots, r$. A robust variance-covariance matrix may again be used, or a frailty term can be incorporated to specifically allow for any correlation between the event times within an individual. Also, the baseline hazards could be taken to be proportional and constraints on the β-parameters may also be introduced, as for the PWP model in Section 13.2.2.

The WLW model was originally proposed as a model for recurrent events, but there is some controversy surrounding its use in this area. In particular, when the WLW model is used to model recurrent events, the definition of the risk set is such that an individual who has experienced just one recurrence is at risk of not only a second recurrence, but also a third, fourth, fifth recurrence, and so on. This makes it difficult to interpret the coefficients of the explanatory variables. Because of this inconsistency, the model is only recommended for use in situations where it is natural to consider times to separate events from the time origin.

Example 13.3 Clinical trial of tamoxifen in breast cancer patients
There is a considerable body of evidence to suggest that following breast-conserving surgery in women with breast cancer, local radiotherapy in addition to tamoxifen treatment reduces the risk of recurrence in the same breast and improves long-term survival. Breast screening is able to detect very small tumours, and there is interest in determining whether patients at low risk could avoid radiotherapy treatment. A multicentre clinical trial was begun in 1992 to determine the benefit of adjuvant treatment with radiotherapy in women aged 50 years or over, who had undergone breast-conserving surgery for an invasive adenocarcinoma with a diameter less than or equal to 5 cm. The patients were randomly assigned to receive tamoxifen treatment at the rate of 20 mg per day for five years in addition to breast irradiation, or to tamoxifen alone. Patients were seen in clinic every three months for the first three years, every six months for the next two and annually thereafter, and follow-up ended in 2002. Full details of the trial and its results were given by Fyles et al. (2004). This illustration is based on the data for one particular centre, used by Pintilie (2006), and relates to 320 women who had been randomised to tamoxifen in addition to radiotherapy, and 321 who received tamoxifen alone.

At randomisation, information was recorded on patient age, tumour size, tumour histology, hormone receptor level, haemoglobin level and whether or not axillary node dissection was performed. During the follow-up process, the time from randomisation to the first occurrence of local relapse, axillary relapse, distant relapse, second malignancy of any type and death, was recorded. For each patient, the data set contains the number of days from randomisation to the occurrence of any of these events, together with an event indicator. For women who had no events and were alive at the end of follow-up, each of the event times was censored at the last date that they were known to be alive. The variables in the data set are listed below, and the explanatory variables and survival data for 25 patients on the tamoxifen and radiotherapy treatment are shown in Table 13.5.

Table 13.5 *Data from 25 patients in a clinical trial on tamoxifen.*

Id	*Treat*	*Age*	*Size*	*Hist*	*HR*	*Hb*	*ANdis*	*Lsurv*	*Ls*	*Asurv*	*As*	*Dsurv*	*Ds*	*Msurv*	*Ms*	*Tsurv*	*Ts*
1	0	51	1.0	1	1	140	1	3019	0	3019	0	3019	0	3019	0	3019	0
2	0	74	0.5	1	1	138	1	2255	0	2255	0	493	1	2255	0	2255	0
3	0	71	1.1	1	1	157	1	2621	0	2621	0	2621	0	2621	0	2621	0
4	0	52	0.8	1	1	136	1	3471	0	3471	0	3471	0	3471	0	3471	0
5	0	62	1.5	1	1	123	1	3322	0	3322	0	3322	0	3322	0	3322	0
6	0	75	0.7	1	1	122	1	2956	0	2956	0	2956	0	2956	0	2956	1
7	0	77	2.4	1	1	139	1	265	0	265	0	220	1	265	0	265	1
8	0	78	2.0	1	1	142	1	1813	0	1813	0	1813	0	1813	0	1813	0
9	0	65	2.0	1	1	121	1	3231	0	3231	0	3231	0	3231	0	3231	0
10	0	67	1.2	1	1	132	1	1885	0	1885	0	1885	0	1885	0	1885	0
11	0	64	1.5	1	1	133	1	3228	0	3228	0	3228	0	3228	0	3228	0
12	0	58	0.5	5	1	129	1	3284	0	3284	0	3284	0	3284	0	3284	0
13	0	71	2.2	1	1	143	1	2628	0	2628	0	2628	0	2628	0	2628	0
14	0	51	1.7	1	1	140	1	3428	0	3428	0	2888	1	344	1	3428	0
15	0	57	1.3	2	1	121	1	3288	0	3288	0	3288	0	3288	0	3288	0
16	0	70	3.8	1	1	152	1	377	0	377	0	269	1	377	0	377	1
17	0	67	1.5	1	1	132	1	125	0	125	0	125	0	113	1	125	1
18	0	54	3.0	1	1	153	1	3461	0	3461	0	3461	0	959	1	3461	0
19	0	53	0.5	1	1	121	1	3485	0	3485	0	3485	0	3485	0	3485	0
20	0	72	2.0	1	1	140	0	3399	0	3399	0	3399	0	3399	0	3399	0
21	0	57	2.5	1	1	129	1	2255	1	2835	0	2835	0	2835	0	2835	0
22	0	67	1.1	1	1	126	1	3322	0	3322	0	3322	0	3322	0	3322	0
23	0	56	1.0	1	1	134	1	2620	0	2620	0	2620	0	2620	0	2620	0
24	0	86	1.5	1	1	134	0	1117	0	1117	0	1117	0	299	1	1117	1
25	0	82	1.5	2	1	114	1	2115	0	2115	0	2115	0	2115	0	2115	0

Id:	Patient identifier
Treat:	Treatment group (0 = tamoxifen + radiotherapy, 1 = tamoxifen)
Age:	Patient age (days)
Size:	Tumour size (cm)
Hist:	Tumour histology (1 = ductal, 2 = lobular, 3 = medullary; 4 = mixed, 5 = other)
HR:	Hormone receptor level (0 = negative, 1 = positive)
Hb:	Haemoglobin level (g/l)
ANdis:	Axillary node dissection (0 = no, 1 = yes)
Lsurv:	Time to local relapse or last follow-up
Ls:	Local relapse (0 = no, 1 = yes)
Asurv:	Time to axillary relapse or last follow-up
As:	Axillary relapse (0 = no, 1 = yes)
Dsurv:	Time to distant relapse or last follow-up
Ds:	Distant relapse (0 = no, 1 = yes)
Msurv:	Time to second malignancy or last follow-up
Ms:	Second malignancy (0 = no, 1 = yes)
Tsurv:	Time from randomisation to death or last follow-up
Ts:	Status at last follow-up (0 = alive, 1 = dead)

These data will be analysed using the WLW model, and the first step is to organise the data into the required format. Although no patient experienced more than three of the five possible events, the revised database will have five rows for each patient, corresponding respectively to time to local relapse, axillary relapse, distant relapse, second malignancy and death. The values of the explanatory variables are repeated in each row.

To illustrate this rearrangement, the event times and censoring indicators for four patients, one with no events, one with one event, one with two events and one with three events, are shown in Table 13.6. In this table, *Nevents* is the number of events and the explanatory variables have been omitted.

Table 13.6 *Data for four patients in the tamoxifen trial who experience 0, 1, 2 and 3 events.*

Id	*Nevents*	*Lsurv*	*Ls*	*Asurv*	*As*	*Dsurv*	*Ds*	*Msurv*	*Ms*	*Tsurv*	*Ts*
1	0	3019	0	3019	0	3019	0	3019	0	3019	0
2	1	2255	0	2255	0	493	1	2255	0	2255	0
14	2	3428	0	3428	0	2888	1	344	1	3428	0
349	3	949	1	2117	1	2775	1	3399	0	3399	0

The data for these four patients, in the required format, are given in Table 13.7. Here, the variable *Time* is the time to the event concerned and *Status* is the event status, where zero corresponds to a censored time and unity to an event. In this table, the variable *Event* is coded as 1 for local relapse, 2 for axillary relapse, 3 for distant relapse, 4 for second malignancy and 5 for death.

Table 13.7 *Rearranged data for four patients in the tamoxifen trial with 0, 1, 2 and 3 events.*

Id	*Treat*	*Age*	*Size*	*Hist*	*HR*	*Hb*	*ANdis*	*Event*	*Time*	*Status*
1	0	51	1.0	1	1	140	1	1	3019	0
1	0	51	1.0	1	1	140	1	2	3019	0
1	0	51	1.0	1	1	140	1	3	3019	0
1	0	51	1.0	1	1	140	1	4	3019	0
1	0	51	1.0	1	1	140	1	5	3019	0
2	0	74	0.5	1	1	138	1	1	2255	0
2	0	74	0.5	1	1	138	1	2	2255	0
2	0	74	0.5	1	1	138	1	3	493	1
2	0	74	0.5	1	1	138	1	4	2255	0
2	0	74	0.5	1	1	138	1	5	2255	0
14	0	51	1.7	1	1	140	1	1	3428	0
14	0	51	1.7	1	1	140	1	2	3428	0
14	0	51	1.7	1	1	140	1	3	2888	1
14	0	51	1.7	1	1	140	1	4	344	1
14	0	51	1.7	1	1	140	1	5	3428	0
349	1	74	1.3	1	1	149	1	1	949	1
349	1	74	1.3	1	1	149	1	2	2117	1
349	1	74	1.3	1	1	149	1	3	2775	1
349	1	74	1.3	1	1	149	1	4	3399	0
349	1	74	1.3	1	1	149	1	5	3399	0

A Cox regression model, stratified by *Event*, in which the coefficients of the explanatory variables are different for each event, is now fitted to the data that have been organised as shown in Table 13.7. For each event type, the hazard ratio for treatment with tamoxifen alone, relative to tamoxifen with radiotherapy, the corresponding P-value based on the Wald test, and 95% confidence limits for the hazard ratio, adjusted for the variables *Age*, *Size*, *Hist*, *HR*, *Hb* and *ANdis*, are shown in Table 13.8. A robust estimate of the variance-covariance matrix of the parameter estimates has been used.

Table 13.8 *Adjusted hazard ratio for the treatment effect for each event and 95% confidence intervals on fitting the WLW model.*

Event	Hazard ratio	P-value	95% confidence interval
1: local relapse	10.30	< 0.001	(3.68, 28.82)
2: axillary relapse	3.14	0.092	(0.83, 11.91)
3: distant relapse	0.84	0.588	(0.45, 1.57)
4: second malignancy	1.19	0.502	(0.72, 1.98)
5: death	0.79	0.416	(0.45, 1.39)

From this table, it is estimated that there is more than 10 times the risk of a local relapse if tamoxifen is used without radiotherapy, an effect that is highly significant ($P < 0.001$). There is also some evidence, significant at the 10% level, that the absence of radiotherapy increases the risk of an axillary relapse, but the estimated hazard ratios for all other events do not differ significantly from unity. Further analysis of this data set would determine the extent to which the hazards rates are proportional for different event types, and which explanatory factors were relevant to each outcome.

13.4 Event history analysis

In studies where the primary outcome is survival from the time origin to death, the occurrence of other non-fatal events during the follow-up period may help to shed further light on the underlying mortality process. The sequence of intermediate events defines an *event history*, and data of this kind can be analysed using *multistate models*.

The experience of a patient in a survival study can be thought of as a process that involves *two states*. At the point of entry to the study, the patient is in a state that corresponds to their being alive. Patients then transfer from this 'live' state to the 'dead' state at some *transition rate*, $h(t)$, which is the hazard of death at a given time t. The situation is expressed diagrammatically in Figure 13.3. The dependence of the rate of transition from one state to the other on explanatory variables is then modelled.

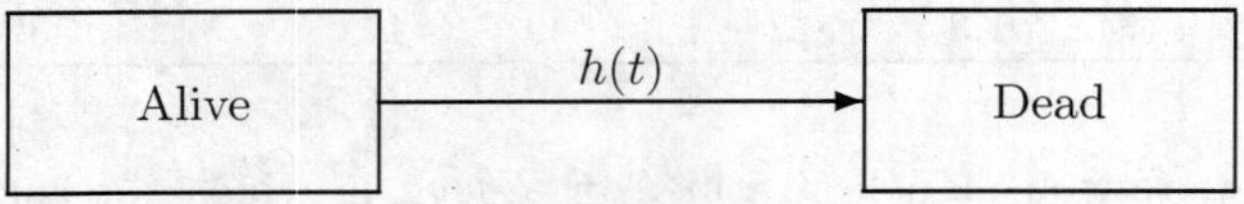

Figure 13.3 *A two-state model for survival analysis.*

As an example in which there are a number of states, consider a survival study concerning transplant patients. Following a transplant, there is the risk that the transplanted organ will fail, as well as the risk of death, and the transition rates for these two events may well be different. In addition, a patient who suffers graft failure may be retransplanted, but may also die without retransplant. The situation is shown diagrammatically in Figure 13.4.

This four-state model can be specified in terms of the transition rates from transplant to death, $h_{TD}(t)$, from transplant to graft failure, $h_{TF}(t)$, from graft failure to retransplant, $h_{FR}(t)$, from graft failure to death, $h_{FD}(t)$ and from retransplant to death, $h_{RD}(t)$. Notice that although $h_{TD}(t)$, $h_{FD}(t)$ and $h_{RD}(t)$ all denote the hazard of death at time t, the hazard rates depend on whether the patient has had graft failure or has been retransplanted, and may all be different.

It is straightforward to model the hazard of death following transplant when graft failure has not occurred, $h_{TD}(t)$. Here, the survival times of those patients who suffer graft failure are taken to be censored at the failure time. Patients who are alive and who have not experienced graft failure also contribute censored survival times. When modelling transition rates from graft

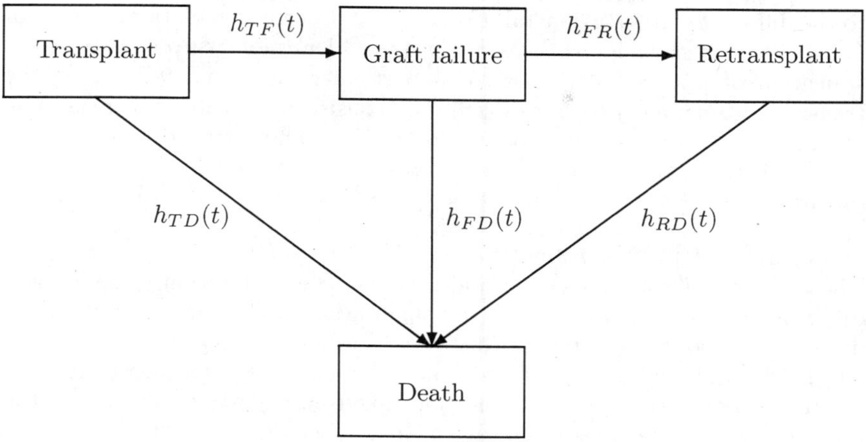

Figure 13.4 *A four-state model for recipients of a transplant.*

failure or retransplant to death, the set of patients at risk of death at any time consists of those who have had graft failure or a retransplant, respectively, and are still alive. Patients who have not yet had a graft failure or retransplant cannot be in either risk set. Fortunately, by expressing the data in counting process format, a Cox regression model can be used to model all four transitions between the states in this four-state model. Moreover, this approach can be extended to more complex multistate models.

13.4.1 Models for event history analysis

Suppose that $\boldsymbol{x}_i$ is the vector of values of p explanatory variables for the ith individual and let $\boldsymbol{\beta}_{jk}$ be the corresponding vector of their coefficients for the transition from state j to state k. Also, denote the baseline intensity function for this transition by $h_{0jk}(t)$. The transition rate of the ith individual from state j to state k at time t in a multistate model is then

$$h_{ijk}(t) = Y_{ijk}(t) \exp\{\boldsymbol{\beta}_{jk}' \boldsymbol{x}_i\} h_{0jk}(t),$$

where $Y_{ijk}(t) = 1$ if the ith of n individuals is in state j and at risk of entering state k at time t, and $Y_{ijk}(t) = 0$, otherwise. As for other models described in this chapter, the explanatory variables may also be time-dependent. Time is generally measured from the point of entry into an initial state, which marks the time origin.

When separate baseline hazards and separate regression coefficients are assumed for each transition, stratified Cox regression models can be used to model the different transition rates. Proportional hazard rates may also be assumed, and modelled by including a factor in the model that corresponds to the different states. In general, the counting process formulation of survival data will be needed for this, as the risk set definition will depend on the transition of interest. The data for a particular individual relating to the transition from state j to state k will then consist of a record giving the time of entry into state j, the time of exit from state j and a status indicator that is unity if the transition is from state j to state k and zero otherwise. The process is illustrated in Example 13.4.

Example 13.4 Patient outcome following bone marrow transplantation
The European Group for Blood and Marrow Transplantation (EBMT) was established to promote stem cell transplantation and to allow clinicians to develop collaborative studies. This is facilitated by the EBMT Registry, which contains clinical and outcome data for patients who have undergone haematopoietic stem cell transplantation. The Registry was established in the early 1970s, and transplant centres and national Registries contribute data, including annual follow-up data on their patients. As a result, the EBMT Registry is a valuable source of data for retrospective studies on the outcomes of stem cell transplantation in patients with leukaemia, lymphoma, myeloma, and other blood disorders.

This example is based on data from 2204 patients with leukaemia who received a bone marrow transplant reported to the EBMT Registry, and used in Putter, Fiocco and Geskus (2007). The transplant is designed to allow the platelet count to return to normal levels, but some individuals may relapse or die before this state has been achieved. Others may relapse or die even though their platelet count has returned to normal. A model with three states will be used to represent this event history. The time following the transplant is the initial state (state 1), and a patient may subsequently enter a state where platelet recovery has occurred (state 2) or a state corresponding to relapse or death (state 3). Transitions from state 2 to state 3 are also possible. This multistate model is shown diagrammatically in Figure 13.5. In this figure, the transition rates from state i to state j are denoted $h_{ij}(t)$, so that the three rates are $h_{12}(t)$, $h_{13}(t)$ and $h_{23}(t)$.

For each patient, data are also available on the variable *Leukaemia* that is associated with the disease type, categorised as acute myelogenous leukaemia (AML), acute lymphoblastic leukaemia (ALL) and chronic myelogenous leukaemia (CML). Their age group, *Age* ($\leqslant 20$, 21–40, > 40), was also recorded, together with the patient's donor recipient gender match, *Match* ($0 =$ no, $1 =$ yes), and whether or not there was T-cell depletion, *Tcell* ($0 =$ no, $1 =$ yes). Data for the first 20 patients are shown in Table 13.9. This table shows the times from transplantation to platelet recovery (*Ptime*) and the time to relapse or death (*RDtime*). Also shown are the event indicators at the time of platelet recovery (*Pcens*) and relapse or death (*RDcens*), which are zero for a censored observation and unity for an event.

Of the 2204 patients who had a bone marrow transplant, 1169 experienced platelet recovery and 458 relapsed or died before their platelet level

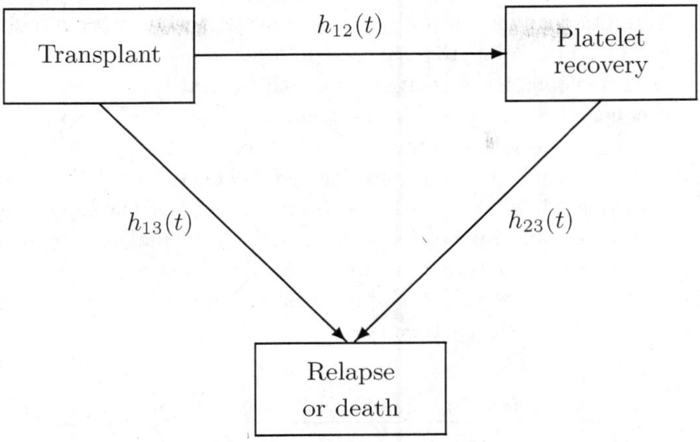

Figure 13.5 *A three-state model for recipients of a bone marrow transplant.*

Table 13.9 *Data on outcomes following bone marrow transplantation.*

Id	*Leukaemia*	*Age*	*Match*	*Tcell*	*Ptime*	*Pcens*	*RDtime*	*RDcens*
1	CML	> 40	1	0	23	1	744	0
2	CML	> 40	0	0	35	1	360	1
3	CML	> 40	0	0	26	1	135	1
4	AML	21–40	0	0	22	1	995	0
5	AML	21–40	0	0	29	1	422	1
6	ALL	> 40	0	0	38	1	119	1
7	CML	21–40	1	0	30	1	590	0
8	ALL	$\leqslant 20$	0	0	35	1	1448	0
9	AML	21–40	0	0	1264	0	1264	0
10	CML	> 40	0	0	1102	0	338	1
11	AML	21–40	1	0	50	1	84	1
12	AML	> 40	1	0	22	1	114	1
13	AML	21–40	0	0	33	1	1427	0
14	AML	> 40	0	0	29	1	775	1
15	CML	> 40	0	0	24	1	1047	1
16	AML	21–40	0	0	31	1	1618	0
17	AML	21–40	1	0	87	1	1111	0
18	AML	21–40	0	0	469	0	255	1
19	ALL	$\leqslant 20$	0	0	59	0	59	1
20	CML	21–40	0	0	1727	0	1392	1

had returned to normal. A further 383 patients relapsed or died after platelet recovery had occurred. There were also 152 patients that had experienced a relapse but remained under surveillance for platelet recovery; this includes patients 10, 18 and 20 in Table 13.9. Since the model shown in Figure 13.5 does not allow for transitions from relapse or death to platelet recovery, the times to platelet recovery are censored at the time of relapse for these patients.

To fit multistate models, the data need to be formatted in such a way that there is one row for each possible transition for each patient. There are three possible transitions, shown as 1→2, 1→3, and 2→3. For the 2→3 transition, only patients whose platelet level has returned to normal are at subsequent risk of relapse or death, so that only two possible transitions are recorded for these patients. Data for the first 10 patients in Table 13.9, expressed in this format, are shown in Table 13.10.

Table 13.10 *Reorganised data on outcomes following bone marrow transplantation.*

Id	*Leukaemia*	*Age*	*Match*	*Tcell*	*Transition*	*Start*	*Stop*	*Status*
1	CML	> 40	1	0	1→2	0	23	1
1	CML	> 40	1	0	1→3	0	23	0
1	CML	> 40	1	0	2→3	23	744	0
2	CML	> 40	0	0	1→2	0	35	1
2	CML	> 40	0	0	1→3	0	35	0
2	CML	> 40	0	0	2→3	35	360	1
3	CML	> 40	0	0	1→2	0	26	1
3	CML	> 40	0	0	1→3	0	26	0
3	CML	> 40	0	0	2→3	26	135	1
4	AML	21–40	0	0	1→2	0	22	1
4	AML	21–40	0	0	1→3	0	22	0
4	AML	21–40	0	0	2→3	22	995	0
5	AML	21–40	0	0	1→2	0	29	1
5	AML	21–40	0	0	1→3	0	29	0
5	AML	21–40	0	0	2→3	29	422	1
6	ALL	> 40	0	0	1→2	0	38	1
6	ALL	> 40	0	0	1→3	0	38	0
6	ALL	> 40	0	0	2→3	38	119	1
7	CML	21–40	1	0	1→2	0	30	1
7	CML	21–40	1	0	1→3	0	30	0
7	CML	21–40	1	0	2→3	30	590	0
8	ALL	⩽ 20	0	0	1→2	0	35	1
8	ALL	⩽ 20	0	0	1→3	0	35	0
8	ALL	⩽ 20	0	0	2→3	35	1448	0
9	AML	21–40	0	0	1→2	0	1264	0
9	AML	21–40	0	0	1→3	0	1264	0
10	CML	> 40	0	0	1→2	0	338	0
10	CML	> 40	0	0	1→3	0	338	1

The transitions between the three states are modelled by fitting a Cox regression model to the data in the format shown in Table 13.10, stratified by transition type. A stratified model that allows the parameters associated with the four explanatory factors, *Leukaemia*, *Age*, *Match* and *Tcell*, to depend on the transition type is first fitted, by including interactions between the strata and these four factors. Comparing alternative models using the $-2 \log \hat{L}$ statistic shows that there is no evidence that the factors *Tcell* and *Match* vary over the three transition types, and moreover, none of the three transitions depend on *Match*. A reduced model therefore contains the main effects of *Leukaemia*, *Age* and *Tcell*, together with interactions between *Leukaemia* and *Transition*, and *Age* and *Transition*. For this model, the hazard ratios, and their associated 95% confidence intervals, are shown in Table 13.11. In this example, a robust estimate of variance is used, but the resulting standard errors differ little from the model-based estimates.

Table 13.11 *Hazard ratios and 95% confidence intervals for each transition.*

Factor	Transition 1→2	Transition 1→3	Transition 2→3
Leukaemia			
AML	1.00	1.00	1.00
ALL	0.96 (0.83, 1.11)	1.29 (0.98, 1.69)	1.16 (0.86, 1.56)
CML	0.74 (0.65, 0.85)	1.02 (0.82, 1.26)	1.31 (1.04, 1.64)
Age			
$\leqslant 20$	1.00	1.00	1.00
21–40	0.86 (0.74, 0.99)	1.29 (0.96, 1.72)	1.02 (0.76, 1.38)
> 40	0.92 (0.78, 1.08)	1.69 (1.25, 2.29)	1.68 (1.23, 2.30)
Tcell			
No	1.00	1.00	1.00
Yes	1.42 (1.27, 1.59)	1.42 (1.27, 1.59)	1.42 (1.27, 1.59)

The effect of both type of leukaemia and age group differs for the three transitions. Patients with CML progress to platelet recovery at a slower rate than those with the other two types of disease, and are more likely to relapse after platelet recovery has occurred. Patients with ALL have a greater hazard of relapse or death before platelet recovery than those with AML or CML. Patients aged 21–40 experience platelet recovery at a slower rate than others, while those aged over 40 have an increased hazard of relapse or death, whether or not platelet recovery has occurred. T-cell depletion leads to significantly greater rates of transition to other states, with no evidence that these rates differ between transition types.

The three baseline cumulative hazard and incidence rates, that is the rates for patients in the $\leqslant 20$ age group with AML and no T-cell depletion, are shown in Figures 13.6 and 13.7. The baseline cumulative hazard plot shows that the transition to platelet recovery occurs at a much faster rate than transitions to relapse or death. The cumulative incidence functions have a very similar pattern, and from Figure 13.7, the one-year cumulative incidence of relapse or death from either of the two possible states is about one-third that of platelet recovery, for patients in the baseline group.

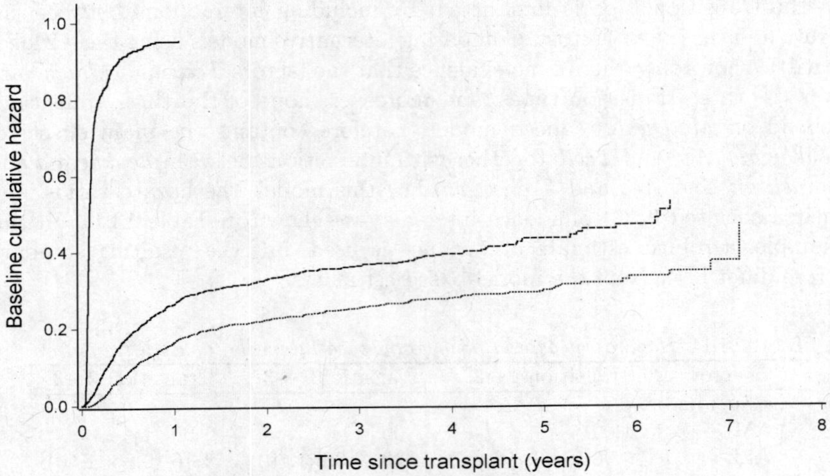

Figure 13.6 *Baseline cumulative hazard for the transitions 1→2 (—), 1→3 (- - -) and 2→3 (......).*

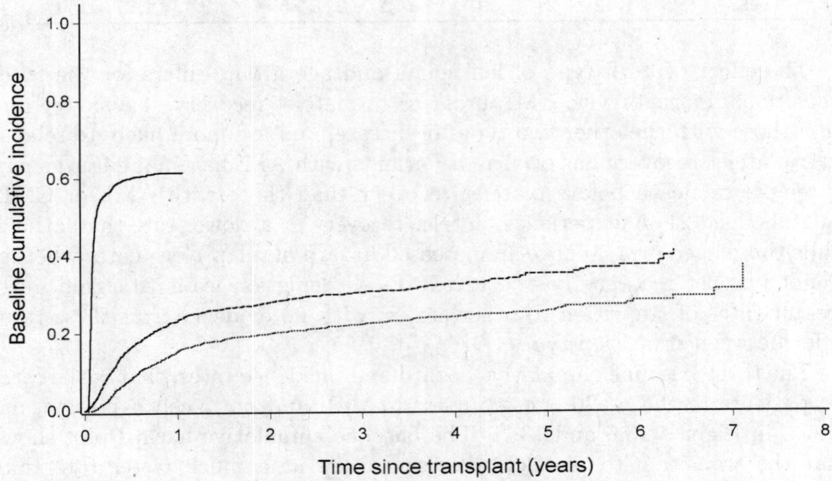

Figure 13.7 *Baseline incidence of transitions 1→2 (—), 1→3 (- - -) and 2→3 (......).*

Figure 13.6 suggests that the baseline hazard functions for the transitions to relapse or death from either of the other two states may well be proportional, although the hazard rate for the transition to a state of platelet recovery has a different shape from the other two. Some further simplification of the model is therefore possible, but this has little effect on the resulting inferences.

13.5 Further reading

A number of texts describe counting process methods in survival analysis, including Fleming and Harrington (2005), Aalen, Borgan and Gjessing (2008), and Andersen et al. (1993). A mathematical treatment of models for survival data, based on the counting process theory, is given by Andersen and Gill (1982), while a more readable summary is contained in Gill (1984). See also the comprehensive review paper of Andersen and Borgan (1985). The robust sandwich estimate of the variance-covariance matrix of parameter estimates in a Cox regression model was introduced by Lin and Wei (1989), and the link with the delta-beta's was described by Therneau and Grambsch (2000).

The three main models for recurrent and multiple events covered in this chapter are due to Andersen and Gill (1982), Prentice, Williams and Petersen (1981) and Wei, Lin and Weissfeld (1989). The text of Cook and Lawless (2007) presents a comprehensive review of methodology for recurrent events, and Therneau and Grambsch (2000) describe models for recurrent and multiple events in their text on extensions to the Cox regression model. Wei and Glidden (1997) give an overview of statistical methods for the analysis of multiple events in clinical trials. Kelly and Lim (2000) give a careful discussion of the different models for recurrent event data, concluding that the WLW model is inappropriate. Arguments for and against the WLW model for the analysis of recurrent event data are given by Metcalfe and Thompson (2007).

A thorough review of multistate models is given by Andersen and Keiding (2002), and subsequent papers, in an issue of *Statistical Methods in Medical Research* that is devoted to this topic. Other review articles include Commenges (1999), Hougaard (1999) and Meira-Machado et al. (2009). Hougaard (2000) describes and illustrates event history models in his account of multivariate survival data. The tutorial article of Putter, Fiocco and Geskus (2007) describe how the Cox regression model can be used in event history modelling, and illustrates the approach with the EBMT data that was used in Example 13.4 of Section 13.4. A number of other articles have featured multistate models for patients who have a bone marrow transplant, including Keiding, Klein and Horowitz (2001) and Klein and Shu (2002). Further examples of the use of multistate models in medical research have been given by Hougaard and Madsen (1985) and Andersen (1988).

The use of the R software for the analysis of competing risks and multistate modelling is covered in the text of Beyersmann, Allignol and Schumacher (2012), and by Putter, Fiocco and Geskus (2007). See also the special issue of the *Journal of Statistical Software*, introduced by Putter (2011).

In order to use the methods presented in this section, the recurrence times must be known. Multistate models that do not rely on the recurrence times being known have been considered by many authors in connection with animal tumourigenicity experiments. In particular, see Dinse (1991), Kodell and Nelson (1980), and McKnight and Crowley (1984). A useful review of this literature is included in Lindsey and Ryan (1993).

Chapter 14

Dependent censoring

The methods described in this book for the analysis of censored survival data are only valid if the censoring is independent or non-informative. Essentially, this means that the censoring is not associated with the actual survival time, so that individuals with censored survival times are representative of all others who are at risk at that time, and who have the same values of measured explanatory variables. For example, censoring would be considered to be independent if a censored time occurs because a patient has withdrawn from a study on relocating to a different part of the country, or when survival data are analysed at a prespecified time. On the other hand, if patients are withdrawn because they experience life-threatening side effects from a particular treatment, or if patients that do not respond to an active treatment are given rescue medication, the censoring time is no longer independent of the survival time. The censoring is then said to be *dependent* or *informative*. This chapter shows how dependent censoring can be taken account of when modelling survival data.

14.1 Identifying dependent censoring

Dependent censoring occurs when there is a dependence between the time to an event such as death and the time to the occurrence of censoring. Since both of these events cannot be observed in a given individual, it is not possible to use the observed data to determine whether a data set has dependent censoring, nor the extent of any such dependence. However, the context of a study can often give some indication of whether or not there is likely to be dependent censoring.

As an illustration, consider the double-blind clinical trial carried out by the Acquired Immunodeficiency Syndrome (AIDS) Clinical Trials Group, known as the ACTG 175 trial, and reported by Hammer et al. (1996). In this trial, 2467 patients were randomly assigned to one of four treatment regimens, and the primary end-point was the time from randomisation to at least a 50% reduction in the cluster of differentiation 4 (CD4) cell count, the development of AIDS, or death. There were 1902 censored event times, with 933 of these accounted for by the patient not having experienced any of the three events at the end of the follow-up period, and so reflect independent administrative censoring. In addition, 283 discontinued treatment because of treatment toxicity, and 380 left the study at the request of either the patient or the investigator. It might be that patients in poor health would be more likely to experience toxicity, and for these patients, their event times may be shorter. Similarly, patients may have left the study to seek alternative treatments, and again these patients may not be representative of the patient group as a whole. The possibility of dependent censoring would therefore need to be considered when analysing times to the primary end-point.

Statistical methods can be used to examine the assumption of independent censoring in a number of ways. One approach is to plot observed survival times against the values of explanatory variables, where the censored observations are distinguished from the uncensored. If a pattern is exhibited in the censoring, such as there being more censored observations at an earlier time on a particular treatment, or if there is a greater proportion of censored survival times in patients with a particular range of values of explanatory variables, dependent censoring is suggested. More formally, a model could be used to examine whether the probability of censoring is related to the explanatory variables in the model. In particular, a linear logistic model could be used in modelling a binary response variable that takes the value unity if an observed survival time is censored and zero otherwise. If the probability of censoring is found to depend on the values of certain explanatory variables, the assumption of independent censoring may have been violated.

14.2 Sensitivity to dependent censoring

Even though dependent censoring is present, this feature may not necessarily affect inferences of primary interest. It is therefore important to determine the sensitivity of such inferences to the possibility of dependent censoring, and this can be examined using two complementary analyses. In the first, we assume that individuals who contribute censored observations are actually those at high risk of an event. We therefore suppose that individuals for whom the survival time is censored would have experienced the event immediately after the censoring time, and designate all censored times as event times. In the second analysis, we assume that the censored individuals are those at low risk of an event. We then suppose that individuals with censored times experience the event only after the longest observed survival time amongst all others in the data set. The censored times are therefore replaced by the longest event time. The impact of these two assumptions on the results of the analysis can then be studied in detail. If essentially the same conclusions arise from the original analysis and the two supplementary analyses, it will be safe to assume that the results are not sensitive to the possibility of dependent censoring.

Another way to determine the potential impact of dependent censoring is to obtain bounds on the survivor function in the presence of dependent censoring. This has led to a number of proposals, but many of these lead to bounds that are too wide to be of practical value, and so this approach will not be considered further.

Since the occurrence of dependent censoring cannot be identified without additional information, it is useful to analyse the extent to which quantities such as the risk score or median survival time are sensitive to the introduction of some association between the time to failure and the time to censoring. A sensitivity analysis for dependent censoring in parametric proportional hazards models, described by Siannis, Copas and Lu (2005), will be outlined in the next section.

14.2.1 A sensitivity analysis*

Suppose that T is a random variable associated with the survival time and C is a random variable associated with time to censoring. We will assume Weibull proportional hazards models for both the hazard of death and the hazard of censoring at time t. The two hazard functions for the ith individual, $i = 1, 2, \ldots, n$, for whom $\boldsymbol{x}_i$ is a vector of values of p explanatory variables, are respectively $h_i(t)$ and $h_{ci}(t)$, where

$$h_i(t) = \exp(\boldsymbol{\beta}'\boldsymbol{x}_i)h_0(t), \qquad h_{ci}(t) = \exp(\boldsymbol{\beta}_c'\,\boldsymbol{x}_i)h_{c0}(t).$$

The baseline hazard functions for the survival and censoring times are given by

$$h_0(t) = \lambda\gamma t^{\gamma-1}, \qquad h_{c0}(t) = \lambda_c\gamma_c t^{\gamma_c-1},$$

respectively, in which λ, λ_c are scale parameters and γ, γ_c are shape parameters in underlying Weibull distributions. The models for the survival time and censoring time may contain different explanatory variables.

On fitting these models, the estimated values of $\boldsymbol{\beta}'\boldsymbol{x}_i$ and $\boldsymbol{\beta}_c'\,\boldsymbol{x}_i$ are the *risk score*, $\hat{\boldsymbol{\beta}}'\boldsymbol{x}_i$, and the *censoring score*, $\hat{\boldsymbol{\beta}}_c'\,\boldsymbol{x}_i$, respectively. A plot of the values of the risk score against the corresponding censoring score will help determine whether there is dependent censoring. In particular, if there is an association between these two scores, dependent censoring is suggested.

We now introduce a parameter ϕ that measures the extent of dependence between T and C. When $\phi = 0$, censoring is independent of the survival times, but as ϕ increases, censoring becomes more dependent on them. In fact, ϕ is an upper bound to the correlation between T and C. Now let $\hat{\eta}(\boldsymbol{x}_0)$ denote the risk score for the individual for whom $\boldsymbol{x}_0$ is the vector of values of the explanatory variables in the model, and let $\hat{\eta}_\phi(\boldsymbol{x}_0)$ be the risk score for that individual when ϕ measures the association between the survival time and time to censoring. It can then be shown that an approximation to the change in the risk score in a Weibull model that occurs when a small amount of dependence between the time to failure and time to censoring variables, ϕ, is assumed, is given by

$$B(\boldsymbol{x}_0) = \hat{\eta}_\phi(\boldsymbol{x}_0) - \hat{\eta}(\boldsymbol{x}_0) = \phi\frac{\sum_{i=1}^n \{e^{\hat{\boldsymbol{\beta}}_c'\,\boldsymbol{x}_0} t_i^{\hat{\gamma}+\hat{\gamma}_c} - (1-\delta_i)t_i^{\hat{\gamma}}\}}{\sum_{i=1}^n t_i^{\hat{\gamma}}}, \qquad (14.1)$$

where δ_i is an event indicator for the ith individual that is zero for a censored observation and unity otherwise.

The *sensitivity index*, $B(\boldsymbol{x}_0)$, only depends on the values of explanatory variables through the censoring score, $\hat{\boldsymbol{\beta}}_c' \boldsymbol{x}_0$, and Equation (14.1) shows that the risk score is most sensitive to dependent censoring when the hazard of censoring is greatest. A plot of $B(\boldsymbol{x}_0)$ against a range of values of the censoring score, $\hat{\boldsymbol{\beta}}_c' \boldsymbol{x}_0$, for a given value of ϕ, provides information about the sensitivity of the risk score to dependent censoring. Usually, ϕ is chosen to take values in the range $(-0.3, 0.3)$. This plot will indicate the values of the censoring score that may result in dependent censoring having a non-negligible impact on the risk score.

We can also examine the sensitivity of other summary statistics to dependent censoring, such as a survival rate and the median survival time. For the Weibull proportional hazards model, the estimated survivor function at time t for the ith individual is

$$\hat{S}_i(t) = \{\hat{S}_0(t)\}^{\exp(\hat{\boldsymbol{\beta}}' \boldsymbol{x}_i)},$$

where $\hat{S}_0(t) = \hat{\lambda} t^{\hat{\gamma}}$ is the estimated baseline survivor function. Using Equation (14.1), the estimated survivor function when there is dependent censoring is approximately

$$\{\hat{S}_0(t)\}^{\exp\{\hat{\boldsymbol{\beta}}' \boldsymbol{x}_i + B(\boldsymbol{x}_i)\}},$$

from which the impact of dependent censoring on survival rates can be determined, for a given value of ϕ. Similarly, the estimated median survival time of an individual with vector of explanatory variables $\boldsymbol{x}_i$ in the Weibull model is

$$\hat{t}(50) = \left\{ \frac{\log 2}{\hat{\lambda} \exp(\hat{\boldsymbol{\beta}}' \boldsymbol{x}_i)} \right\}^{1/\hat{\gamma}},$$

and again using Equation (14.1), the estimated median when there is a degree of dependence, ϕ, between the survival and censoring times is

$$\hat{t}_\phi(50) = \left\{ \frac{\log 2}{\hat{\lambda} \exp[\hat{\boldsymbol{\beta}}' \boldsymbol{x}_i + B(\boldsymbol{x}_i)]} \right\}^{1/\hat{\gamma}}.$$

An approximation to the relative reduction in the median survival time for this individual is then

$$\frac{\hat{t}(50) - \hat{t}_\phi(50)}{\hat{t}(50)} = 1 - \exp\{-\hat{\gamma}^{-1} B(\boldsymbol{x}_i)\}, \qquad (14.2)$$

for some value of ϕ. A plot of this quantity against a range of possible values of the censoring score, $\hat{\boldsymbol{\beta}}_c' \boldsymbol{x}_i$, shows how the median survival time for individuals with different censoring scores might be affected by dependent censoring. The robustness of the estimated median to different amounts of dependent censoring can also be explored by using a range of ϕ-values.

14.2.2 Impact of dependent censoring

With independent censoring, individuals who are censored are representative of the individuals at risk at the time of censoring, and estimated hazard ratios and survivor functions obtained from a standard analysis of the time to event data will be unbiased. On the other hand, if there is dependent censoring, but it is assumed to be independent, model-based estimates may be biased. The direction of this bias depends on whether there is positive or negative association between the time to event and time to censoring variables. If there is a positive association between the two variables, those with censored event times would be expected to experience a shorter event time than those who remain at risk. Similarly, if there is a negative association, individuals with censored event times may be those who would otherwise have had a longer time before the occurrence of the event of interest. Standard methods for survival analysis would then lead to an overestimate or underestimate of the survivor function, respectively, and the extent of the bias will tend to increase as the number of dependently censored observations increases.

Example 14.1 Time to death while waiting for a liver transplant
Once a patient has been judged to need a liver transplant they are added to the registration list. However, the national shortage of livers means that a patient may wait for some time for their operation, and a number die while waiting. In a study to determine the mortality rate for patients registered for a liver transplant, and the impact of certain factors on this outcome variable, data were obtained from the UK Transplant Registry on the time from registration to death on the list. The study cohort consisted of 281 adults with primary biliary cirrhosis. This condition mainly affects females, and is characterised by the progressive destruction of the small bile ducts of the liver, leading to a build-up of bile in the liver, damage to liver tissue and cirrhosis. The patients were first registered for a liver transplant in the five-year period from 1 January 2006, and the response variable of interest is the time from being registered for a liver transplant until death on the list. For patients who receive a transplant, the time from registration is censored at the time of transplant. Times at which a patient are removed from the list because their condition has deteriorated to the point where transplantation is no longer an option, are regarded as death times.

In addition to the survival time from listing, information was available on the age (years) and gender (male = 1, female = 0) of the patient, their body mass index (BMI) (kg/m^2) and the value of the UK end-stage liver disease (UKELD) score, an indicator of disease severity where higher values correspond to a disease of greater severity. The first 20 observations in this data set are given in Table 14.1, where the status variable is unity for a patient who has died while waiting for a transplant and zero when their time from listing has been censored. The data have been ordered by survival time.

Table 14.1 *Time from registration for a liver transplant until death while waiting.*

Patient	Time	Status	Age	Gender	BMI	UKELD
1	1	0	60	0	24.24	60
2	2	1	66	0	30.53	67
3	3	0	71	0	26.56	61
4	3	0	65	1	23.15	63
5	3	0	62	0	22.55	64
6	4	1	56	0	36.39	73
7	5	0	52	0	24.77	57
8	5	0	65	0	33.87	49
9	5	1	58	0	27.55	75
10	5	1	57	0	22.10	64
11	6	0	62	0	21.60	55
12	7	0	56	0	25.69	66
13	7	0	52	0	32.39	59
14	8	1	45	0	28.98	66
15	9	0	50	0	31.67	60
16	9	0	65	0	24.67	57
17	9	0	44	0	24.34	64
18	10	0	67	0	22.65	61
19	12	0	67	0	26.18	57
20	13	0	57	0	22.23	53

Livers are generally allocated on the basis of need, and so tend to be offered to those patients who are more seriously ill. As a result, patients who get a transplant tend to be those who are nearer to death. The time to censoring will then be associated with the time to death, and so the time from listing until a transplant is dependent on the time from listing until death without a transplant.

To illustrate the sensitivity analysis described in Section 14.2.1, consider a Weibull model for the hazard of death at time t that contains the explanatory variables that denote the age, gender, BMI and UKELD value of a patient on the liver registration list. From a log-cumulative hazard plot, the Weibull distribution fits well to the unadjusted survival times. The times to censoring are also well fitted by a Weibull distribution, and the same four explanatory variables will be included in this model. From these fitted models, the risk score, $\hat{\boldsymbol{\beta}}'\boldsymbol{x}_i$, and the censoring score, $\hat{\boldsymbol{\beta}}_c'\boldsymbol{x}_i$, can be obtained for each of the 281 patients, and a plot of the risk score against the censoring score for each patient is given in Figure 14.1.

This figure shows that the risk score is positively correlated with the censoring score, and so individuals that have a greater hazard of death, that is those with a higher risk score, are more likely to be censored. This indicates that there is dependent censoring in this data set.

To explore how this dependent censoring might affect the median survival time, the relative change in the median is obtained for a moderate value of

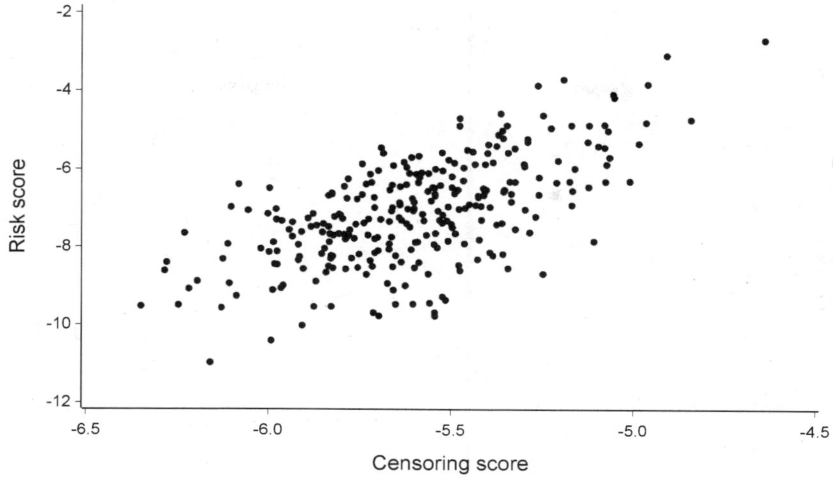

Figure 14.1 *A plot of the values of the risk score, $\hat{\boldsymbol{\beta}}'\boldsymbol{x}_i$ against the censoring score, $\hat{\boldsymbol{\beta}}_c'\boldsymbol{x}_i$, for each patient on the liver transplant waiting list.*

ϕ, using Equation (14.2). A plot of the percentage relative reduction in the median against the censoring score, $\hat{\boldsymbol{\beta}}_c'\boldsymbol{x}_i$, for values of $\hat{\boldsymbol{\beta}}_c'\boldsymbol{x}_i$ in the range $(-6.5, -4.5)$ and $\phi = 0.3$, corresponding to a moderate amount of dependent censoring, is shown in Figure 14.2.

This figure shows that the relative reduction in the median survival time is only near zero when the censoring score is around -6, corresponding to individuals with the lowest hazard of censoring, that is the lowest chance of a transplant. On the other hand, for individuals with a censoring score of -5.5, which is close to the average censoring score for the 281 patients in the data set, dependent censoring could decrease the median by about 30%. For those at greatest risk of being censored, with a censoring score of at least -5, the percentage decrease in median that might occur through dependent censoring with $\phi = 0.3$ is greater than 50%. An analysis based on the assumption of independent censoring may therefore be seriously misleading. A technique that allows account to be taken of dependent censoring in modelling survival data is described in the next section.

14.3 Modelling with dependent censoring

In the presence of dependent censoring, standard methods for the analysis of survival data must be modified. One possibility, useful when censoring does not occur too early in patient time, is to analyse survival to a time before any censoring has occurred. Alternatively, the probability of survival beyond such a time could be modelled using logistic regression modelling, although

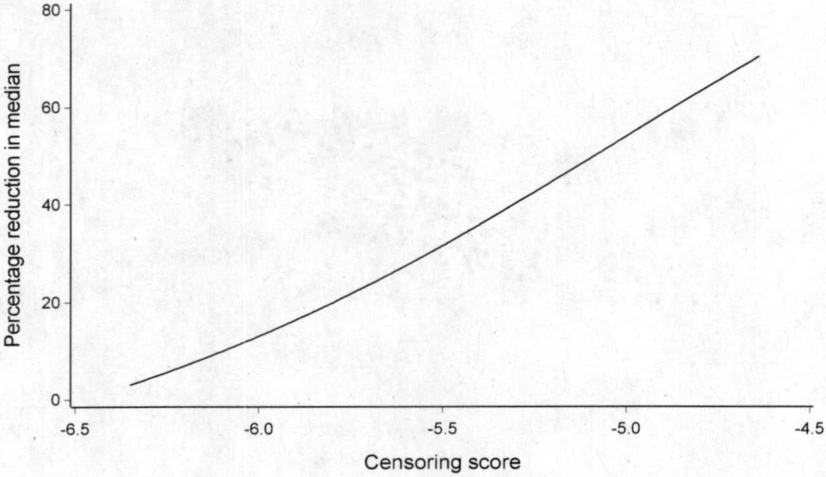

Figure 14.2 *Approximate percentage reduction in the median survival time from listing for a liver transplant, as a function of the censoring score, when* $\phi = 0.3$.

this approach is unlikely to be useful when dependent censoring occurs early in the study. A far better approach is to analyse the survival data using a Cox regression model that directly accommodates dependent censoring.

14.3.1 Cox regression model with dependent censoring

Suppose that a Cox regression model is anticipated for data on the event times of n individuals, some of which may be censored, so that the hazard of an event at time t for the ith individual is

$$h_i(t) = \exp(\boldsymbol{\beta}'\boldsymbol{x}_i)h_0(t),$$

where $\boldsymbol{x}_i$ is the vector of values of p explanatory variables, $\boldsymbol{\beta}$ is the vector of their coefficients, and $h_0(t)$ is the baseline hazard function.

To allow for dependent censoring when fitting this model, we first develop a model for the censored survival times. This is then used to weight the contribution of the observed survival times to the partial likelihood function used in the process of fitting the Cox regression model.

To summarise the basic idea of this technique, consider a particular individual, the ith say, who is at risk at an event time t. Suppose that the probability that this individual's survival time is censored at or after time t is $1/3$. This means that on average, two other individuals who are identical to the ith in terms of measured explanatory variables, will have survival times that are censored before time t. If their survival times had not been censored, these two individuals would have survived to at least t, as the ith individual has done. Had all three of these individuals survived to t without being censored, each would have made the same contribution to the partial likelihood function at time t. This can be modelled by weighting the contribution of the ith individual to the partial likelihood at an event time t by 3, the reciprocal of the censoring probability.

This process leads to *Inverse Probability of Censoring Weighted* (IPCW) estimates of the unknown parameters in the model. The effect of this weighting process is that greater weight is given to individuals that have a higher probability of censoring before t, and so this accounts for censoring that is associated with the survival time.

To calculate the weights used to adjust for dependent censoring, a model is needed for the dependence of the probability of censoring at or after time t on the values of measured explanatory variables. This is obtained from the data by modelling the time to a censored observation by taking the time of censoring as the end-point, and treating actual event times as censored observations. If the data include an event indicator, δ, that is unity for an event and zero for a censored observation, the corresponding indicator variable for censored times is $1 - \delta$. Fitting a survival model to the censored survival times leads to an estimated baseline survivor function, $\hat{S}_{c0}(t)$. From this, the probability of censoring occurring at or after time t in the ith individual, whose vector of values of the explanatory variables is $\boldsymbol{x}_i$, is

$$\hat{S}_{ci}(t) = [\hat{S}_{c0}(t)]^{\exp(\hat{\boldsymbol{\beta}}_c' \boldsymbol{x}_i)}, \tag{14.3}$$

where $\hat{\boldsymbol{\beta}}_c$ is the vector of estimated coefficients of the explanatory variables in the censoring model. The weight for the ith individual at time t is $w_i(t) = \{\hat{S}_{ci}(t)\}^{-1}$, and these weights are then used in fitting a Cox regression model for the time to an event.

The weighted partial likelihood function is found from the reformulation of the Cox regression model in terms of a counting process. From an extension of the formula given in Equation (13.2) of Chapter 13 to incorporate the weights $w_i(t)$, this likelihood function is

$$\prod_{i=1}^{n} \prod_{t \geqslant 0} \left\{ \frac{w_i(t) Y_i(t) \exp\{\boldsymbol{\beta}' \boldsymbol{x}_i\}}{\sum_{l=1}^{n} w_l(t) Y_l(t) \exp\{\boldsymbol{\beta}' \boldsymbol{x}_l\}} \right\}^{\mathrm{dN_i(t)}}, \tag{14.4}$$

where $Y_i(t) = 1$ if an individual is at risk at time t and zero otherwise, $\mathrm{d}N_i(t) = 1$ if an event occurs at time t and zero otherwise, and the inner product is taken over all event times. Time-varying explanatory variables can also be accommodated in this model.

The weights that are obtained using Equation (14.3) depend on the explanatory variables in the censoring model, have different values at each event time and change in value over the follow-up period for an individual. Because of this, it is more convenient to model the censoring times using a parametric model, as the weights are then a continuous function of t. The precise form of the chosen model is not that important and the Weibull model is suggested for general use. The hazard of censoring at time t for the ith individual is then $h_{ci}(t) = \exp(\boldsymbol{\beta}_c' \boldsymbol{x}_i)h_{c0}(t)$, where $h_{c0}(t) = \lambda_c\gamma_c t^{\gamma_c-1}$, and $\boldsymbol{x}_i$ is the vector of values of explanatory variables in the censoring model for the ith individual. The corresponding survivor function is

$$S_{ci}(t) = \exp\{-\lambda_c \exp(\boldsymbol{\beta}_c' \boldsymbol{x}_i)t^{\gamma_c}\}.$$

Note that the variables in the model for the censored survival times need not be the same as those in the model for the survival times. In terms of the log-linear formulation of Weibull model, described in Section 5.6.3 of Chapter 5,

$$S_{ci}(t) = \exp\left\{-\exp\left[\frac{\log t - \mu_c - \boldsymbol{\alpha}_c' \boldsymbol{x}_i}{\sigma_c}\right]\right\},$$

in which μ_c is the 'intercept', σ_c the 'scale', α_{cj} is the coefficient of the jth explanatory variable and $\lambda_c = \exp(-\mu_c/\sigma_c)$, $\gamma_c = 1/\sigma_c$, $\beta_{cj} = -\alpha_{cj}/\sigma_c$, for $j = 1, 2, \ldots, p$.

To handle the time dependence of the weights, the data need to be expressed in counting process format, using the (start, stop, status) notation that was described in Section 13.1.3 of Chapter 13. The stop times are taken to be the event times in the data set.

Example 14.2 Data format for dependent censoring

Suppose that the first three ordered event times in a data set are 18, 55 and 73 days. The observed survival time of 73 days in counting process format is taken to have the intervals $(0, 18], (18, 55], (55, 73]$, where the status indicator is 0 for the first two intervals and 1 for the third. If the survival time of 73 days was censored, the status would be 0 for the third interval. Suppose further that the model-based probability of censoring at or beyond times 18, 55 and 73, obtained using a model for the censored survival times, is 0.94, 0.82 and 0.75, respectively. The weights that are used in fitting Cox regression models to the data based on the counting process format are then 1.064, 1.220 and 1.333, respectively.

The weights, $w_i(t)$, calculated from Equation (14.3), can get quite large when the probability of censoring beyond t is small, and this can lead to computational problems. It can then be more efficient to use *stabilised weights*, $w_i^*(t)$, calculated using $w_i^*(t) = \hat{S}_{KM}(t)/\hat{S}_{ci}(t)$, where $\hat{S}_{KM}(t)$ is the Kaplan-Meier estimate of the probability of censoring after t. Using the term $\hat{S}_{KM}(t)$ in the numerator of the weights has no effect on parameter estimates, since $\hat{S}_{KM}(t)$ is independent of explanatory variables in the model and cancels out in the numerator and denominator of the partial likelihood function in Equation (14.4). However, it does lead to greater stability in the model fitting process.

Finally, to account for the additional uncertainty in the specification of the model, a robust estimate of the variance-covariance matrix of the parameter estimates is recommended, such as the sandwich estimate introduced in Section 13.1.4 of Chapter 13.

Example 14.3 Time to death while waiting for a liver transplant
The data from Example 14.1 on the survival times from registration for a liver transplant are now analysed using a modelling approach that makes allowance for any dependent censoring. To model the probability of censoring, a Weibull model is fitted to the time from registration until censoring, where the censoring indicator is zero when the status variable in Table 14.1 is unity, and vice-versa. Using the log-linear formulation of the Weibull model, the estimated probability of censoring at or beyond time t is

$$\hat{S}_{ci}(t) = \exp\left\{-\exp\left[\frac{\log t - \hat{\mu}_c - \hat{\alpha}_{c1}x_{1i} - \hat{\alpha}_{c2}x_{2i} - \hat{\alpha}_{c3}x_{3i} - \hat{\alpha}_{c4}x_{4i}}{\hat{\sigma}_c}\right]\right\}, \tag{14.5}$$

where x_{1i} is the age, x_{2i} the gender, x_{3i} the BMI, and x_{4i} the UKELD score at registration for the ith patient. The estimated parameters and their standard errors in this model are shown in Table 14.2. At this stage, the model could be modified by excluding variables that have no significant effect on the probability of censoring, namely age, gender and BMI, but we will continue to use a censoring model that contains all four variables.

Table 14.2 *Parameter estimates and their standard errors in a Weibull model for the censoring time.*

Variable	Parameter	Estimate	se (Estimate)
Age	$\hat{\alpha}_{c1}$	0.0070	0.0079
Sex	$\hat{\alpha}_{c2}$	−0.1839	0.1950
BMI	$\hat{\alpha}_{c3}$	0.0193	0.0141
UKELD	$\hat{\alpha}_{c4}$	−0.0535	0.0152
Intercept	$\hat{\mu}_c$	7.6261	1.0058
Scale	$\hat{\sigma}_c$	0.9813	0.0507

Next, the data in Table 14.1 are expressed in the counting process format and weights are calculated from the reciprocals of the censoring probabilities at the 'stop' times, from the inverse of the estimated censoring probability, $\hat{S}_{ci}(t)$ in Equation (14.5). Data for the first 10 patients from Table 14.1 are shown in the counting process format in Table 14.3, together with the censoring probabilities and weights that are used in fitting a Cox regression model to the survival times.

A weighted Cox regression model that contains the same four explanatory variables is then fitted, and the estimated hazard of death at time t for the ith patient is

$$\hat{h}_i(t) = \exp\{\hat{\beta}_1 x_{1i} + \hat{\beta}_2 x_{2i} + \hat{\beta}_3 x_{3i} + \hat{\beta}_4 x_{4i}\}\hat{h}_0(t),$$

where $\hat{h}_0(t)$ is the estimated baseline hazard function. The parameter estimates and their standard errors in the weighted Cox regression model that

Table 14.3 *Data from the first 10 patients in Table 14.1 in the counting process format.*

Patient	Start time	Stop time	Status	Censoring probability	Weight
1	0	1	0	0.9955	1.0045
2	0	2	1	0.9888	1.0114
3	0	2	0	0.9915	1.0085
3	2	3	0	0.9872	1.0129
4	0	2	0	0.9873	1.0128
4	2	3	0	0.9809	1.0195
5	0	2	0	0.9885	1.0116
5	2	3	0	0.9827	1.0176
6	0	2	0	0.9851	1.0151
6	2	4	1	0.9701	1.0308
7	0	2	0	0.9919	1.0081
7	2	4	0	0.9837	1.0166
7	4	5	0	0.9796	1.0208
8	0	2	0	0.9960	1.0040
8	2	4	0	0.9919	1.0081
8	4	5	0	0.9899	1.0102
9	0	2	0	0.9806	1.0198
9	2	4	0	0.9610	1.0405
9	4	5	1	0.9513	1.0511
10	0	2	0	0.9880	1.0121
10	2	4	0	0.9758	1.0248
10	4	5	1	0.9698	1.0312

takes account of dependent censoring are shown in Table 14.4. Also shown are the corresponding unweighted estimates when dependent censoring is not taken into account. The sandwich estimate of the variance-covariance matrix of the parameter estimates has been used in both cases, but this only makes a very small difference to the standard errors.

Table 14.4 *Parameter estimates and their standard errors in a weighted and unweighted Cox regression model.*

Variable	Parameter	Weighted		Unweighted	
		Estimate	se (Estimate)	Estimate	se (Estimate)
Age	$\hat{\beta}_1$	0.0118	0.0316	0.0774	0.0200
Sex	$\hat{\beta}_2$	−0.9895	0.6549	−0.1471	0.4944
BMI	$\hat{\beta}_3$	−0.0218	0.0492	0.0236	0.0210
UKELD	$\hat{\beta}_4$	0.1559	0.0427	0.2162	0.0276

The two sets of estimates are somewhat different, which shows that the adjustment for dependent censoring has affected the hazard ratios. In the unweighted analysis, both age and UKELD score are highly significant

($P < 0.001$), whereas age ceases to be significant in the weighted analysis. From the hazard ratio for UKELD after adjustment for dependent censoring, a unit increase in the UKELD leads to a 17% increase in the hazard of death.

To illustrate the effect of the adjustment for dependent censoring, Figure 14.3 shows the estimated survivor functions for a female patient aged 50 with a UKELD score of 60 and a BMI of 25, from a weighted and unweighted Cox regression model for the hazard of death.

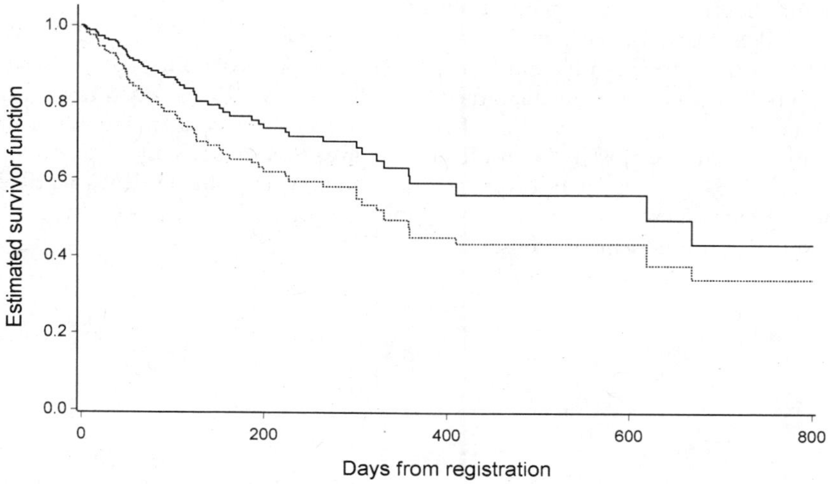

Figure 14.3 *Estimated survivor functions in a weighted (·······) and unweighted (—), Cox regression model for a 50-year-old female with a UKELD score of 60 and a BMI of 25.*

This figure shows how survival rates are overestimated if account is not taken of dependent censoring. In particular, if no allowance is made for dependent censoring, the survival rate at six months is estimated to be 77%, but after taking account of dependent censoring, the estimate is 65%. In addition, the 80% survival rate is overestimated by nearly two months. Failure to take account of the dependent censoring can therefore result in misleading estimates of the waiting list mortality for patients awaiting a liver transplant.

In an extension to this analysis, separate models could be entertained for different causes of censoring, namely transplant and removal from the registration list because of a deteriorating condition, as well as for any independent censoring. Additionally, variation in the UKELD score over time could also be incorporated so that changes in disease severity over the registration period can be accounted for.

14.4 Further reading

Bounds for the survivor function in the presence of dependent censoring have been described by a number of authors, including Peterson (1976), Slud and Rubinstein (1983) and Klein and Moeschberger (1988). Tsiatis (1975) explains why the extent of association between event times and censoring times cannot be estimated from observed data, and Siannis (2004) and Siannis, Copas and Lu (2005) have described methods for determining the sensitivity of inferences to dependent censoring in parametric models. This approach has been extended to the Cox proportional hazards model in Siannis (2011), although the method is computationally intensive.

Models for data with dependent censoring have been described by Wu and Carroll (1988) and Schlucter (1992). Inverse probability of censoring weighted estimators were introduced by Robins and Rotnitzky (1992) and Robins (1993). Robins and Finkelstein (2000) showed how these estimators could be used to adjust Kaplan-Meier estimates to take account of dependent censoring. Satten, Datta and Robins (2001) and Scharfstein and Robins (2002) showed how to estimate the survivor function for a Cox regression model in the presence of dependent censoring.

Chapter 15

Sample size requirements for a survival study

There are many aspects of the design of a medical research programme that need to be considered when the response variable of interest is a survival time. These include factors such as the inclusion and exclusion criteria for study participants, the unambiguous definition of the time origin and the end-point of the study, and the duration of patient follow-up. In a clinical trial, the specification of treatments, the method of randomisation to be employed in allocating patients to treatment group, and the use of blinding must also be specified. Consideration might also be given to whether the study should be based on a fixed number of patients, or whether a sequential design should be adopted, in which the study continues until there is a sufficient number of events to be able to distinguish between treatments. The need for interim analyses, or adaptive designs that allow planned modifications to be made to the sample size or allocated treatment as data accumulate, also needs to be discussed.

Many of these considerations are not unique to studies where survival is the outcome of interest, and are discussed in a number of texts on the design and analysis of clinical trials, such as Friedman, Furberg and DeMets (2010), Matthews (2006) and Pocock (1983). However, there is one matter in the design of fixed sample size studies that will be discussed here. This is the crucial issue of the number of patients that are required in a survival study. If too few patients are recruited, there may be insufficient information available in the data to enable a treatment difference to be pronounced significant. On the other hand, it is unethical to waste resources in studies that are unnecessarily large. Sample size calculations for survival data are presented in this chapter.

15.1 Distinguishing between two treatment groups

Many survival studies are concerned with distinguishing between two alternative treatments. For this reason, a study to compare the survival times of patients who receive a new treatment with those who receive a standard will be used as the focus for this chapter. The same formulae can of course be used in other situations and for other end-points.

Suppose that in this study, there are two groups of patients, and that the standard treatment is allocated to the patients in Group I, while the new treatment is allocated to those in Group II. Assuming a proportional hazards model for the survival times, the hazard of death at time t for a patient on the new treatment, $h_N(t)$, can be written as

$$h_N(t) = \psi h_S(t),$$

where $h_S(t)$ is the hazard function at t for a patient on the standard treatment and ψ is the unknown hazard ratio. We will also define $\theta = \log \psi$ to be the log-hazard ratio. If θ is zero, there is no treatment difference. On the other hand, negative values of θ indicate that survival is longer under the new treatment, while positive values of θ indicate that patients survive longer on the standard treatment.

In order to test the null hypothesis that $\theta = 0$, the log-rank test described in Section 2.6 can be used. As was shown in Section 3.13, this is equivalent to using the score test of the null hypothesis of equal hazards in the Cox regression model. In this chapter, sample size requirements will be based on the log-rank test statistic, but the formulae presented can also be used when an analysis based on the Cox regression model is envisaged.

In a survival study, the occurrence of censoring means that it is not usually possible to measure the actual survival times of all patients in the study. However, it is the number of actual deaths that is important in the analysis, rather than the total number of patients. Accordingly, the first step in determining the number of patients in a study is to calculate the number of deaths that must be observed. We then go on to determine the required number of patients.

15.2 Calculating the required number of deaths

To determine the sample size requirement for a study, we calculate the number of patients needed for there to be a certain chance of declaring θ to be significantly different from zero when the true, but unknown, log-hazard ratio is θ_R. Here, θ_R is the *reference value* of θ. It will be a reflection of the magnitude of the treatment difference that it is important to detect, using the test of significance. In a study to compare a new treatment with a standard, there is likely to be a minimum worthwhile improvement and a maximum envisaged improvement. The actual choice of θ_R will then lie between these two values. In practice, θ_R might be chosen on the basis of the desired hazard ratio, the change in the median survival time that is to be detected, or the difference in the probability of survival beyond a given time. This is discussed and illustrated later in Example 15.1.

More formally, the required number of deaths is taken to be such that there is a probability of $1 - \beta$ of declaring the observed log-hazard ratio to be significantly different from zero, using a hypothesis test with a specified significance level of α, when in fact $\theta = \theta_R$. The term $1 - \beta$ is the probability of rejecting the null hypothesis when it is in fact false, and is known as the *power* of the test. The quantity β is the probability of not rejecting the null hypothesis when it is false and is sometimes known as the *type II error*. Both α and β are taken to be small. Typical values will be $\alpha = 0.05$ and $\beta = 0.1$, and with these values there would be a 90% chance of declaring the observed difference between two treatments to be significant at the 5% level. The exact specification of α and β will to some extent depend on the circumstances. If it is important to detect a difference as being significant at a lower level of significance, or if there needs to be a higher chance of declaring a result to be significant, α and β will need to be modified accordingly.

The required number of deaths in a survival study, d, can be obtained from the equation

$$d = \frac{4(z_{\alpha/2} + z_\beta)^2}{\theta_R^2}, \tag{15.1}$$

where $z_{\alpha/2}$ and z_β are the upper $\alpha/2$- and upper β-points, respectively, of the standard normal distribution. It is convenient to write $c(\alpha, \beta) = (z_{\alpha/2} + z_\beta)^2$ in Equation (15.1), giving

$$d = 4c(\alpha, \beta)/\theta_R^2. \tag{15.2}$$

The values of $c(\alpha, \beta)$ for commonly chosen values of the significance level α and power $1 - \beta$ are given in Table 15.1.

Table 15.1 *Values of the function $c(\alpha, \beta)$.*

Value of α	Value of $1-\beta$			
	0.80	0.90	0.95	0.99
0.10	6.18	8.56	10.82	15.77
0.05	7.85	10.51	13.00	18.37
0.01	11.68	14.88	17.81	24.03
0.001	17.08	20.90	24.36	31.55

Calculation of the required number of deaths then requires that a value for θ_R be identified, and appropriate values of α and β chosen. Table 15.1 is then used in conjunction with Equation (15.2) to give the number of deaths required in a study.

The derivation of the result in Equation (15.2) assumes that the same number of individuals is to be assigned to each treatment group. If this is not the case, a modification has to be made. In particular, if the proportion of individuals to be allocated to Group I is π, so that a proportion $1 - \pi$ will be allocated to Group II, the required total number of deaths becomes

$$d = \frac{c(\alpha, \beta)}{\pi(1 - \pi)\theta_R^2}.$$

Notice that an imbalance in the number of individuals in the two treatment groups leads to an increase in the total number of deaths required. The derivation also includes an approximation, which means that the calculated number of deaths could be an underestimate. Some judicious rounding up of the calculated value is therefore suggested to compensate for this.

The actual derivation of the formula for the required number of deaths is important and so details are given below in Section 15.2.1. This section can be omitted without loss of continuity. It is followed by an example that illustrates the calculations.

15.2.1 Derivation of the required number of deaths*

An expression for the required number of deaths is now derived on the basis of a log-rank test to compare two treatment groups. As in Section 2.6, suppose that there are r distinct death times, $t_{(1)} < t_{(2)} < \cdots < t_{(r)}$, among the individuals in the study, and that in the ith group there are d_{ij} deaths at the jth ordered death time $t_{(j)}$, for $i = 1, 2$ and $j = 1, 2, \ldots, r$. Also suppose that the number at risk at $t_{(j)}$ in the ith group is n_{ij}, and write $n_j = n_{1j} + n_{2j}$ for the total number at risk at $t_{(j)}$ and $d_j = d_{1j} + d_{2j}$ for the number who die at $t_{(j)}$. The log-rank statistic is then

$$U = \sum_{j=1}^{r} (d_{1j} - e_{1j}),$$

where e_{1j} is the expected number of deaths in Group I at $t_{(j)}$, given by $e_{1j} = n_{1j}d_j/n_j$, and the variance of the log-rank statistic is

$$V = \sum_{j=1}^{r} \frac{n_{1j}n_{2j}d_j(n_j - d_j)}{n_j^2(n_j - 1)}. \tag{15.3}$$

When using the log-rank test, the null hypothesis that $\theta = 0$ is rejected if the absolute value of U is sufficiently large, that is, if $|U| > k$, say, where $k > 0$ is a constant. We therefore require that

$$\text{P}(|U| > k; \theta = 0) = \alpha, \tag{15.4}$$

and

$$\text{P}(|U| > k; \theta = \theta_R) = 1 - \beta,$$

for a two-sided $100\alpha\%$ significance test to have power $1 - \beta$.

We now quote without proof a result given in Sellke and Siegmund (1983), according to which the log-rank statistic, U, has an approximate normal distribution with mean θV and variance V, for small values of θ. Indeed, the result that $U \sim N(0, V)$ under the null hypothesis $\theta = 0$, is used as a basis for the log-rank test. Then, since

$$\text{P}(|U| > k; \theta = 0) = \text{P}(U > k; \theta = 0) + \text{P}(U < -k; \theta = 0),$$

and U has an $N(0, V)$ distribution when $\theta = 0$, a distribution that is symmetric about zero,

$$\mathrm{P}(U > k; \theta = 0) = \mathrm{P}(U < -k; \theta = 0).$$

It then follows from Equation (15.4) that

$$\mathrm{P}(U > k; \theta = 0) = \frac{\alpha}{2}. \tag{15.5}$$

Next, we note that

$$\mathrm{P}(|U| > k; \theta = \theta_R) = \mathrm{P}(U > k; \theta = \theta_R) + \mathrm{P}(U < -k; \theta = \theta_R).$$

For the sort of values of k that are likely to be used in the hypothesis test, either $\mathrm{P}(U < -k; \theta = \theta_R)$ or $\mathrm{P}(U > k; \theta = \theta_R)$ will be negligible. For example, if the new treatment is expected to increase survival so that θ_R is taken to be less than zero, the probability of U having a value in excess of k, $k > 0$, will be small. So without loss of generality we will take

$$\mathrm{P}(|U| > k; \theta = \theta_R) \approx \mathrm{P}(U < -k; \theta = \theta_R).$$

We now denote the upper $100p\%$ point of the standard normal distribution by z_p. Then $\Phi(z_p) = 1 - p$, where $\Phi(\cdot)$ stands for the standard normal distribution function. The quantity $\Phi(z_p)$ therefore represents the area under a standard normal density function to the left of the value z_p. Now, since $U \sim N(0, V)$ when $\theta = 0$,

$$\mathrm{P}(U > k; \theta = 0) = 1 - \mathrm{P}(U \leqslant k; \theta = 0) = 1 - \Phi\left(\frac{k}{\surd(V)}\right),$$

and using Equation (15.5) we have that

$$\Phi\left(\frac{k}{\surd(V)}\right) = 1 - (\alpha/2).$$

Therefore,

$$\frac{k}{\surd(V)} = z_{\alpha/2},$$

where $z_{\alpha/2}$ is the upper $\alpha/2$-point of the standard normal distribution, and so k can be expressed as

$$k = z_{\alpha/2}\surd(V). \tag{15.6}$$

In a similar manner, since $U \sim N(\theta_R V, V)$ when $\theta = \theta_R$,

$$\mathrm{P}(U < -k; \theta = \theta_R) = \Phi\left(\frac{-k - \theta_R V}{\surd(V)}\right) \approx 1 - \beta,$$

and so we take

$$\frac{-k - \theta_R V}{\surd(V)} = z_\beta,$$

where z_β is the upper β-point of the standard normal distribution. If we now substitute for k from Equation (15.6), we get

$$-z_{\alpha/2}\surd(V) - \theta_R V = z_\beta \surd(V),$$

and so V needs to be such that

$$V = (z_{\alpha/2} + z_\beta)^2/\theta_R^2, \tag{15.7}$$

to meet the specified requirements.

When the number of deaths is few relative to the number at risk, the expression for V in Equation (15.3) is approximately

$$\sum_{j=1}^{r} \frac{n_{1j} n_{2j} d_j}{n_j^2}. \tag{15.8}$$

Moreover, if θ is small, and recruitment to each treatment group proceeds at a similar rate, then $n_{1j} \approx n_{2j}$, for $j = 1, 2, \ldots, r$, and so

$$\frac{n_{1j} n_{2j}}{n_j^2} = \frac{n_{1j} n_{2j}}{(n_{1j} + n_{2j})^2} \approx \frac{n_{1j}^2}{(2n_{1j})^2} = \frac{1}{4}.$$

Then, V is given by

$$V \approx \sum_{j=1}^{r} d_j/4 = d/4,$$

where $d = \sum_{j=1}^{r} d_j$ is the total number of deaths among the individuals in the study.

Finally, using Equation (15.7), we now require d to be such that

$$\frac{d}{4} = \frac{(z_{\alpha/2} + z_\beta)^2}{\theta_R^2},$$

which leads to the required number of deaths being that given in Equation (15.1).

At later death times, that is, when the values of j in Expression (15.8) are close to r, the numbers of individuals at risk in the two groups will be small. This is likely to mean that n_{1j} and n_{2j} will be quite different at the later death times, and so $n_{1j} n_{2j}/n_j^2$ will be less than 0.25. This in turn means that $V < d/4$ and so the required number of deaths will tend to be underestimated.

Example 15.1 Survival from chronic active hepatitis

Patients suffering from chronic active hepatitis rapidly progress to an early death from liver failure. A new treatment has become available and so a clinical trial is planned to evaluate the effect of this new treatment on the survival times of patients suffering from the disease. As a first step, information is obtained on the survival times in years of patients in a similar age range

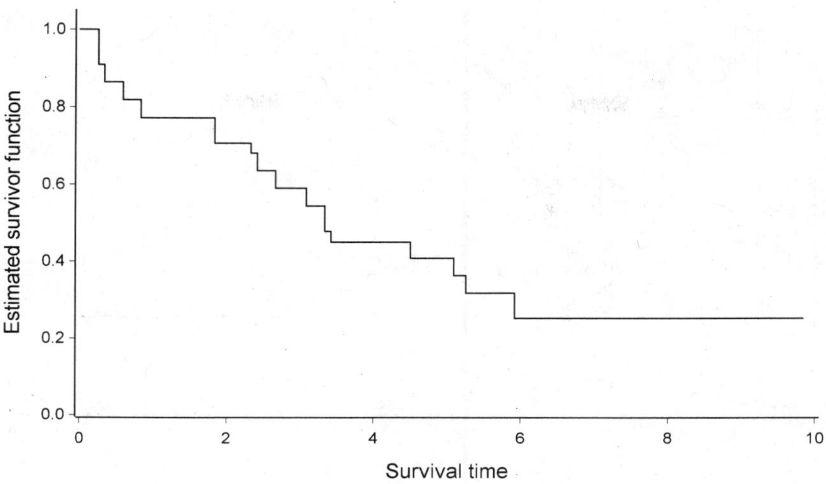

Figure 15.1 *Estimated survivor function for patients receiving a standard treatment for hepatitis.*

who have received the standard therapy. The Kaplan-Meier estimate of the survivor function derived from such data is shown in Figure 15.1.

From this estimate of the survivor function, the median survival time is 3.3 years, and the survival rates at two, four and six years can be taken to be given by $S(2) = 0.70$, $S(4) = 0.45$, and $S(6) = 0.25$.

The new treatment is expected to increase the survival rate at five years from 0.41, the value under the standard treatment, to 0.60. This information can be used to calculate a value for θ_R. To do this, we use the result that if the hazard functions are assumed to be proportional, the survivor function for an individual on the new treatment at time t is

$$S_N(t) = [S_S(t)]^{\psi}, \tag{15.9}$$

where $S_S(t)$ is the survivor function for an individual on the standard treatment at t and ψ is the hazard ratio. Therefore,

$$\psi = \frac{\log S_N(t)}{\log S_S(t)},$$

and so the value of ψ corresponding to an increase in $S(t)$ from 0.41 to 0.60 is

$$\psi_R = \frac{\log(0.60)}{\log(0.41)} = 0.57.$$

With this information, the survivor function for a patient on the new treatment is $[S_S(t)]^{\psi_R}$, and so $S_N(2) = 0.82$, $S_N(4) = 0.63$, and $S_N(6) = 0.45$. A plot of the two survivor functions is shown in Figure 15.2.

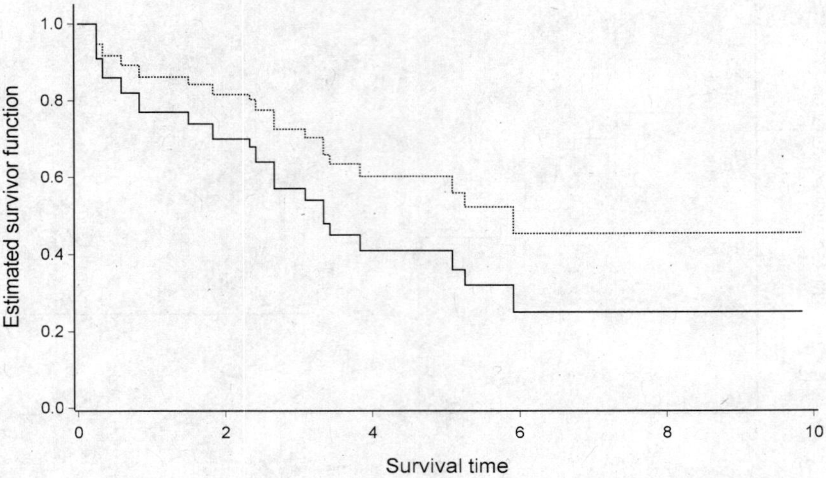

Figure 15.2 *Estimated survivor functions for individuals on the standard treatment (—) and the new treatment (·······).*

The median survival time under the new treatment can be determined from this estimate of the survivor function. Using Figure 15.2, the median survival time under the new treatment is estimated to be about six years. A hazard ratio of 0.57 therefore implies an increase in median survival time from 3.3 years on the standard treatment to 6 years on the new treatment.

To calculate the number of deaths that would be required in a study to compare the two treatments, we will take $\alpha = 0.05$ and $1 - \beta = 0.90$. With these values of α and β, the value of the function $c(\alpha, \beta)$ from Table 15.1 is 10.51. Substituting for $c(0.05, 0.1)$ in Equation (15.2) and taking $\theta_R = \log \psi_R = \log(0.57) = -0.562$, the number of deaths required to have a 90% chance of detecting a hazard ratio of 0.57 to be significant at the 5% level is given by

$$d = \frac{4 \times 10.51}{0.562^2} = 133.$$

Allowing for possible underestimation, this can be rounded up to 140 deaths in total. This means that approximately 70 deaths would need to be observed in each treatment group.

The treatment difference that it is required to detect may also be expressed in terms of the desired absolute or relative change in the median survival time. The corresponding log-hazard ratio, for use in Equation (15.1), can then be found by reversing the preceding calculation. For example, suppose that an increase in the median survival time from 3.3 years on the standard treatment to just 5 years on the new treatment is anticipated. The survivor function on the new treatment is then 0.5 when $t = 5$, and using Equation (15.9),

$S_N(5) = \{S_S(5)\}^{\psi_R} = 0.5$. Consequently, $\psi_R \log\{S_S(5)\} = \log 0.5$, and since $S_S(5) = 0.41$, $\psi_R = 0.78$. This reflects a less optimistic view of the treatment effect than when ψ_R is taken to be 0.57. The corresponding number of deaths that would need to be observed for this hazard ratio to be declared significantly different from unity at the 5% level, with 90% power, is then around 680. This is considerably greater than the number needed to identify a hazard ratio of 0.57 as significant.

The calculations described above are only going to be of direct use when a study is to be continued until a given number of those entering the study have died. Most trials will be designed on the basis of the number of patients to be recruited and so we must now examine how this number can be obtained.

15.3 Calculating the required number of patients

In order to calculate the actual number of patients that are required in a survival study, we need to consider the probability of death over the duration of a study. Typically, patients are recruited over an *accrual period* of length a. After recruitment is complete, there is an additional *follow-up period* of length f. The total duration of a study will therefore be of length $a + f$. Notice that if f is small, or even zero, there will need to be correspondingly more patients recruited in order to achieve a specific number of deaths.

Once the probability of a patient dying in the study has been evaluated, the required number of patients will be found from

$$n = \frac{d}{\mathrm{P(death)}}, \tag{15.10}$$

where d is the required number of deaths found from Equation (15.2). According to a result derived in the next section, the probability of death can be taken as

$$\mathrm{P(death)} = 1 - \frac{1}{6}\{\bar{S}(f) + 4\bar{S}(0.5a + f) + \bar{S}(a + f)\}, \tag{15.11}$$

where

$$\bar{S}(t) = \frac{S_S(t) + S_N(t)}{2},$$

and $S_S(t)$ and $S_N(t)$ are the estimated values of the survivor functions for individuals on the standard and new treatments, respectively, at time t.

The above result shows how the required number of patients can be calculated for a trial with an accrual period of a and a follow-up period of f. Of course, the duration of the accrual period and follow-up period will depend on the recruitment rate. So suppose that the recruitment rate is expected to be m patients per month and that d deaths are required. If n patients are to be entered into the study over a period of a months, this means that n/a need to be recruited in each month. In practice, information is likely to be available on the accrual rate, m, that can be expected. The number recruited in an accrual period of length a is then ma and so the expected number of deaths in the study is

$$ma \times \text{P(death)}.$$

Values of a and f which make this value close to the number of deaths required can then be found numerically, for example, by trying out different values of a and f. This algorithm could be computerised and an optimisation method used to find the value of a that makes

$$d - \{ma \times \text{P(death)}\} \tag{15.12}$$

close to zero for a range of values of f. Alternatively, the value of f that yields the result in Equation (15.12) for a range of values of a can be found. A two-way table giving the required number of patients for different combinations of values of a and f will be particularly useful in planning a study.

The following section gives details underlying the derivation of the result in Equation (15.11), and can again be omitted without loss of continuity.

15.3.1 Derivation of the required number of patients*

We begin with the general result from distribution theory that the marginal probability of a patient dying during the course of a study can be obtained from the joint probability of death and entry to the study at time t using

$$\text{P(death)} = \int_0^a \text{P(death and entry at time } t) \, \mathrm{d}t. \tag{15.13}$$

The joint probability can in turn be found from the result

$$\text{P(death and entry at time } t) = \text{P(death} \mid \text{entry at } t) \times \text{P(entry at } t), \tag{15.14}$$

which is simply a version of the result that $\text{P}(A \mid B) = \text{P}(AB)/\text{P}(B)$.

We now assume a uniform recruitment rate over the accrual period. The distribution of entry times to the study can then be taken to be uniform over the time interval $(0, a)$. Therefore, the probability of an individual being recruited to the study at time t is a^{-1}, for any value of t in the interval $(0, a)$. From Equations (15.13) and (15.14), we have

$$\text{P(death)} = \int_0^a \text{P(death} \mid \text{entry at } t) a^{-1} \, \mathrm{d}t,$$

so that

$$\text{P(death)} = 1 - \frac{1}{a} \int_0^a \text{P(survival} \mid \text{entry at } t) \, \mathrm{d}t.$$

A patient entering the study at time t who survives for the duration of the study, that is, to time $a + f$, must have been alive for a period of length

$a + f - t$ after entry. The conditional probability P(survival | entry at t) is therefore the probability of survival beyond $a + f - t$. This probability is the value of the survivor function for that individual at $a + f - t$, that is, $S(a + f - t)$. Consequently,

$$\text{P(death)} = 1 - \frac{1}{a}\int_0^a S(a + f - t)\,\mathrm{d}t,$$

and on writing $u = a + f - t$, this result becomes

$$\text{P(death)} = 1 - \frac{1}{a}\int_f^{a+f} S(u)\,\mathrm{d}u. \tag{15.15}$$

The integral of the survivor function is now approximated using numerical integration. According to Simpson's rule,

$$\int_u^v f(x)\,\mathrm{d}x \approx \frac{v-u}{6}\left\{f(u) + 4f\left(\frac{u+v}{2}\right) + f(v)\right\},$$

so that

$$\int_f^{a+f} S(u)\,\mathrm{d}u \approx \frac{a}{6}\left\{S(f) + 4S(0.5a + f) + S(a + f)\right\},$$

and hence, using Equation (15.15), the probability of death during the study is given by

$$\text{P(death)} = 1 - \frac{1}{6}\left\{S(f) + 4S(0.5a + f) + S(a + f)\right\}.$$

From this result, the approximate probability of death for an individual in Group I, for whom the survivor function is $S_S(t)$, is

$$\text{P(death; Group I)} = 1 - \frac{1}{6}\left\{S_S(f) + 4S_S(0.5a + f) + S_S(a + f)\right\},$$

and similarly that for an individual in Group II is

$$\text{P(death; Group II)} = 1 - \frac{1}{6}\left\{S_N(f) + 4S_N(0.5a + f) + S_N(a + f)\right\}.$$

On the assumption that there is an equal probability of an individual being assigned to either of the two treatment groups, the overall probability of death is the average of these two probabilities, so that

$$\text{P(death)} = \frac{\text{P(death; Group I)} + \text{P(death; Group II)}}{2}.$$

On substituting for the probabilities of death in the two treatment groups, and setting $\bar{S}(t) = \{S_S(t) + S_N(t)\}/2$, the overall probability of death can be written

$$\text{P(death)} = 1 - \frac{1}{6}\{\bar{S}(f) + 4\bar{S}(0.5a + f) + \bar{S}(a + f)\},$$

as in Equation (15.11).

If the proportion of individuals to be allocated to Group I is π, the overall probability of death becomes

$$\pi\,\text{P(death; Group I)} + (1 - \pi)\,\text{P(death; Group II)},$$

and the result for the overall probability of death given in Equation (15.11) can be modified accordingly.

Example 15.2 Survival from chronic active hepatitis
In Example 15.1, it was shown that 140 deaths needed to be observed for the study on chronic hepatitis to have sufficient power to detect a hazard ratio of 0.57 as significant, at the 5% level. Suppose that patients are to be recruited to the study over an 18-month accrual period and that there is to be a subsequent follow-up period of 24 months. From Equation (15.11), the probability of death in the 42 months of the study will then be given by

$$\text{P(death)} = 1 - \frac{1}{6}\left\{\bar{S}(24) + 4\bar{S}(33) + \bar{S}(42)\right\}.$$

Now, using the estimated survivor functions shown in Figure 15.2,

$$\bar{S}(24) = \frac{S_S(24) + S_N(24)}{2} = \frac{0.70 + 0.82}{2} = 0.76,$$

$$\bar{S}(33) = \frac{S_S(33) + S_N(33)}{2} = \frac{0.57 + 0.73}{2} = 0.65,$$

$$\bar{S}(42) = \frac{S_S(42) + S_N(42)}{2} = \frac{0.45 + 0.63}{2} = 0.54,$$

and so the probability of death is

$$1 - \frac{1}{6}\{0.76 + (4 \times 0.65) + 0.54\} = 0.350.$$

From Equation (15.10), the required number of patients is

$$n = \frac{140}{0.350} = 400,$$

and so 400 patients will need to be recruited to the study over the accrual period of 18 months. This demands a recruitment rate of about 22 patients per month.

If it is only expected that 18 patients can be found each month, the accrual period will need to be extended to ensure that there is a sufficient number of individuals to give the required number of deaths. The number of individuals that could be recruited in a period of a months would be $18a$. Various values of a can then be tried in order to make this approximately equal to the value obtained from Equation (15.10). For example, if we take $a = 24$ and continue with $f = 24$, the probability of death over the four years of the study is

$$\text{P(death)} = 1 - \frac{1}{6}\{\bar{S}(24) + 4\bar{S}(36) + \bar{S}(48)\}.$$

From Figure 15.2, the survivor functions for patients on each treatment at 24, 36 and 48 months can be estimated, and we find that $\bar{S}(24) = 0.76$, $\bar{S}(36) = 0.65$, and $\bar{S}(48) = 0.50$. The probability of death then turns out to be 0.357 and the required number of patients to give 140 deaths is now 393. This is broadly consistent with an estimated recruitment rate of 18 per month.

Now suppose that it is decided that the study will not have a follow-up period, so that the accrual period is equal to the duration of the study. If the accrual period is taken to be 20 months, so that $a = 20$ and $f = 0$, the probability of death is given by

$$\text{P(death)} = 1 - \frac{1}{6}\{\bar{S}(0) + 4\bar{S}(10) + \bar{S}(20)\}.$$

Now, $\bar{S}(0) = 1.00$, $\bar{S}(10) = 0.82$, and $\bar{S}(20) = 0.79$, and the probability of death is 0.155. The required number of patients is now $140/0.155 = 903$, and this would just about be met by a recruitment rate of 45 patients per month. This shows that the absence of a follow-up period leads to an increase in the number of patients that must be entered into the study.

15.3.2 An approximate procedure

A much simpler procedure for calculating the required number of patients in a survival study to compare two treatments is outlined in this section. The basis for this result is that $\{S_S(\tau) + S_N(\tau)\}/2$ is the average probability that a patient in the study survives beyond time τ, where $S_S(\tau)$ and $S_N(\tau)$ are the survivor functions at time τ, for patients on the standard and new treatments, respectively. The probability of death, in the period from the time origin to τ, can then be approximated by

$$1 - \frac{S_S(\tau) + S_N(\tau)}{2}.$$

Using Equation (15.10), the required number of patients becomes

$$n = \frac{2d}{2 - S_S(\tau) - S_N(\tau)},$$

where d is the required number of deaths.

A natural choice for the value of τ to use in this calculation is the average length of the follow-up period for patients in the study, $f + (a/2)$, where

a is the accrual period and f the follow-up period. This procedure is very approximate because it does not take account of patient follow-up times that extend beyond τ. As a consequence, this result will tend to overestimate the required sample size.

Example 15.3 Survival from chronic active hepatitis

The study on chronic active hepatitis is now used to illustrate the approximate procedure for determining the required number of patients. As in Example 15.2, suppose that patients are recruited over an 18-month period and that there is a further follow-up period of 24 months. The average length of the follow-up period for a patient will then be $\tau = f + (a/2) = 33$ months. From Figure 15.2, the survivor functions for patients in the two groups are given by $S_S(33) = 0.57$ and $S_N(33) = 0.73$, respectively. The approximate probability of death in the period from 0 to 33 months is therefore 0.35 and the number of patients required to give 140 deaths is $140/0.35 = 400$. In this illustration, the sample size produced by the approximate result is identical to that found using the more complicated procedure illustrated in Example 15.2, but this will not usually be the case.

15.4 Further reading

Full details on the issues to be considered when designing a clinical trial are given in Friedman, Furberg and DeMets (2010), Matthews (2006) and Pocock (1983) and the more general text of Altman (1991). Whitehead (1997) describes how a sequential clinical trial can be designed when the outcome variable of interest is a survival time, and Jennison and Turnbull (2000) describe group sequential methods.

Extensive tables of sample size requirements in studies involving different types of response variable, including survival times, are provided by Machin et al. (2009) and Julious (2010). A number of commercially available software packages for sample size calculations, including PASS (Power Analysis and Sample Size program) and nQuery Advisor, also implement methods for calculating the required number of patients in a survival study.

The formula for the required number of deaths in Equation (15.1) appears in many papers, including Bernstein and Lagakos (1978), Schoenfeld (1981), Schoenfeld and Richter (1982) and Schoenfeld (1983), although the assumptions on which the result is based are different. Bernstein and Lagakos (1978) obtain Equation (15.1) on the assumption that the survival times in each group have exponential distributions. Lachin (1981), Rubinstein, Gail and Santner (1981) and Lachin and Foulkes (1986) also discuss sample size requirements in trials where the survival times are assumed to be exponentially distributed. See also the earlier work of George and Desu (1974).

Schoenfeld (1981) obtains the same result as Bernstein and Lagakos (1978) and others when the log-rank test is used to compare treatments, without making the additional assumption of exponentiality. Schoenfeld (1983) shows that Equation (15.1) holds when information on the values of explanatory variables is allowed for.

The formulae for the required number of patients in Section 15.3 are based on Schoenfeld (1983). When the assumption of exponential survival times is made, these formulae simplify to the results of Schoenfeld and Richter (1982). Although the resulting formulae are easier to use, it is dangerous to conduct sample size calculations on the basis of restrictive assumptions about survival time distributions.

A variant on the formula for the required number of deaths is given by Freedman (1982). Freedman's result has $\{(1+\psi)/(1-\psi)\}^2$ in place of $4/(\log\psi)^2$ in Equation (15.1). However, for small values of $\log\psi$,

$$\{(1+\psi)/(1-\psi)\}^2 \approx 4/(\log\psi)^2,$$

and so the two expressions will tend to give similar results. The approximate formula for the required number of patients, given in Section 15.3.2, is also due to Freedman (1982).

Lakatos (1988) presented a method for estimating the required number of patients to compare two treatments which can accommodate matters such as staggered entry, non-compliance, loss to follow-up and non-proportional hazards. Lakatos and Lan (1992) show that the Lakatos method procedure performs well in a variety of circumstances. This approach is based on a Markov model, and requires a computer program for its implementation; a SAS macro has been given by Shih (1995).

Approximate sample size formulae for use in modelling the subdistribution hazard function in the presence of competing risks, described in Section 12.5 of Chapter 12, have been given by Latouche, Porcher and Chevret (2004).

Appendix A

Maximum likelihood estimation

This appendix gives a summary of results on maximum likelihood estimation that are relevant to survival analysis. The results presented apply equally to inferences based on a partial likelihood function, and so can be used in conjunction with the Cox regression model described in Chapter 3, and the fully parametric models introduced in Chapters 5 and 6. A full treatment of the theory of maximum likelihood estimation and likelihood ratio testing is given by Cox and Hinkley (1974).

A.1 Inference about a single unknown parameter

Suppose that the likelihood of n observed survival times, $t_1, t_2, \ldots, t_n$, is a function of a single unknown parameter β, and denoted $L(\beta)$. The *maximum likelihood estimate* of β is then the value $\hat{\beta}$ for which this function is a maximum. In almost all applications, it is more convenient to work with the natural logarithm of the likelihood function, $\log L(\beta)$. The value $\hat{\beta}$, which maximises the log-likelihood, is the same value that maximises the likelihood function itself, and is generally found using differential calculus.

Specifically, $\hat{\beta}$ is the value of β for which the derivative of $\log L(\beta)$, with respect to β, is equal to zero. In other words, $\hat{\beta}$ is such that

$$\left.\frac{\mathrm{d}\log L(\beta)}{\mathrm{d}\beta}\right|_{\hat{\beta}} = 0.$$

The first derivative of $\log L(\beta)$ with respect to β is known as the *efficient score* for β, and is denoted $u(\beta)$. Therefore,

$$u(\beta) = \frac{\mathrm{d}\log L(\beta)}{\mathrm{d}\beta},$$

and so the maximum likelihood estimate of β, $\hat{\beta}$, satisfies the equation

$$u(\hat{\beta}) = 0.$$

The asymptotic variance of the maximum likelihood estimate of β can be found from

$$\left(-\mathrm{E}\left\{\frac{\mathrm{d}^2\log L(\beta)}{\mathrm{d}\beta^2}\right\}\right)^{-1}, \tag{A.1}$$

or from the equivalent formula,

$$\left(\mathrm{E} \left\{ \frac{\mathrm{d} \log L(\beta)}{\mathrm{d}\beta} \right\}^2 \right)^{-1}.$$

The variance calculated from either of these expressions can be regarded as the approximate variance of $\hat{\beta}$, although it is usually more straightforward to use Expression (A.1). When the expected value of the derivative in Expression (A.1) is difficult to obtain, a further approximation to the variance of $\hat{\beta}$ is found by evaluating the derivative at $\hat{\beta}$. The approximate variance of $\hat{\beta}$ is then given by

$$\mathrm{var}\,(\hat{\beta}) \approx - \left(\frac{\mathrm{d}^2 \log L(\beta)}{\mathrm{d}\beta^2} \right)^{-1} \Bigg|_{\hat{\beta}}. \tag{A.2}$$

The second derivative of the log-likelihood function is sometimes known as the *Hessian*, and the quantity

$$-\,\mathrm{E} \left\{ \frac{\mathrm{d}^2 \log L(\beta)}{\mathrm{d}\beta^2} \right\}$$

is called the *information function*. Since the information function is formed from the expected value of the second derivative of $\log L(\beta)$, it is sometimes called the *expected information function*. In contrast, the negative second derivative of the log-likelihood function itself is called the *observed information function*. This latter quantity will be denoted $i(\beta)$, so that

$$i(\beta) = -\left\{ \frac{\mathrm{d}^2 \log L(\beta)}{\mathrm{d}\beta^2} \right\}.$$

The reciprocal of this function, evaluated at $\hat{\beta}$, is then the approximate variance of $\hat{\beta}$ given in Equation (A.2), that is,

$$\mathrm{var}\,(\hat{\beta}) \approx \frac{1}{i(\hat{\beta})}.$$

The standard error of $\hat{\beta}$, that is, the square root of the estimated variance of $\hat{\beta}$, is found from

$$\mathrm{se}\,(\hat{\beta}) = \frac{1}{\sqrt{\{i(\hat{\beta})\}}}.$$

This standard error can be used to construct confidence intervals for β.

In order to test the null hypothesis that $\beta = 0$, three alternative test statistics can be used. The *likelihood ratio test statistic* is the difference between the values of $-2 \log L(\hat{\beta})$ and $-2 \log L(0)$. The *Wald test* is based on the statistic

$$\hat{\beta}^2 i(\hat{\beta}),$$

and the *score test statistic* is

$$\frac{\{u(0)\}^2}{i(0)}.$$

Each of these statistics has an asymptotic chi-squared distribution on 1 d.f., under the null hypothesis that $\beta = 0$. Note that the Wald statistic is equivalent to the statistic

$$\frac{\hat{\beta}}{\text{se}\,(\hat{\beta})},$$

which has an asymptotic standard normal distribution.

A.2 Inference about a vector of unknown parameters

The results in Section A.1 can be extended to the situation where n observations are used to estimate the values of p unknown parameters, $\beta_1, \beta_2, \ldots, \beta_p$. These parameters can be assembled into a p-component vector, $\boldsymbol{\beta}$, and the corresponding likelihood function is $L(\boldsymbol{\beta})$. The maximum likelihood estimates of the p unknown parameters are the values $\hat{\beta}_1, \hat{\beta}_2, \ldots, \hat{\beta}_p$, which maximise $L(\boldsymbol{\beta})$. They are therefore found by solving the p equations

$$\left.\frac{\mathrm{d}\log L(\boldsymbol{\beta})}{\mathrm{d}\beta_j}\right|_{\hat{\boldsymbol{\beta}}} = 0,$$

for $j = 1, 2, \ldots, p$, simultaneously.

The vector formed from $\hat{\beta}_1, \hat{\beta}_2, \ldots, \hat{\beta}_p$ is denoted $\hat{\boldsymbol{\beta}}$, and so the maximised likelihood is $L(\hat{\boldsymbol{\beta}})$. The efficient score for β_j, $j = 1, 2, \ldots, p$, is

$$u(\beta_j) = \frac{\mathrm{d}\log L(\boldsymbol{\beta})}{\mathrm{d}\beta_j},$$

and these quantities can be assembled to give a p-component vector of efficient scores, denoted $\boldsymbol{u}(\boldsymbol{\beta})$. The vector of maximum likelihood estimates is therefore such that

$$\boldsymbol{u}(\hat{\boldsymbol{\beta}}) = \mathbf{0},$$

where $\mathbf{0}$ is the $p \times 1$ vector of zeroes.

Now let the matrix $\boldsymbol{H}(\boldsymbol{\beta})$ be the $p \times p$ matrix of second partial derivatives of the log-likelihood function, $\log L(\hat{\boldsymbol{\beta}})$. The (j, k)th element of $\boldsymbol{H}(\boldsymbol{\beta})$ is then

$$\frac{\partial^2 \log L(\hat{\boldsymbol{\beta}})}{\partial\beta_j\partial\beta_k},$$

for $j = 1, 2, \ldots, p$, $k = 1, 2, \ldots, p$, and $\boldsymbol{H}(\boldsymbol{\beta})$ is called the *Hessian matrix*. The matrix

$$\boldsymbol{I}(\boldsymbol{\beta}) = -\boldsymbol{H}(\boldsymbol{\beta})$$

is called the *observed information matrix*. The (j, k)th element of the corresponding *expected information matrix* is

$$-\operatorname{E}\left(\frac{\partial^2 \log L(\boldsymbol{\beta})}{\partial\beta_j \partial\beta_k}\right).$$

The variance-covariance matrix of the p maximum likelihood estimates, $\hat{\beta}_1, \hat{\beta}_2, \ldots, \hat{\beta}_p$, written $\operatorname{var}(\hat{\boldsymbol{\beta}})$, can then be approximated by the inverse of the observed information matrix, evaluated at $\hat{\boldsymbol{\beta}}$, so that

$$\operatorname{var}(\hat{\boldsymbol{\beta}}) \approx \boldsymbol{I}^{-1}(\hat{\boldsymbol{\beta}}).$$

The square root of the (j, j)th element of this matrix can be taken to be the standard error of $\hat{\beta}_j$, for $j = 1, 2, \ldots, p$.

The test statistics given in Section A.1 can be generalised to the multi-parameter situation. Consider the test of the null hypothesis that all the β-parameters in a fitted model are equal to zero. The likelihood ratio test statistic is the value of

$$2\left\{\log L(\hat{\boldsymbol{\beta}}) - \log L(\mathbf{0})\right\},$$

the Wald test is based on

$$\hat{\boldsymbol{\beta}}' \boldsymbol{I}(\hat{\boldsymbol{\beta}})\, \hat{\boldsymbol{\beta}},$$

and the score test statistic is

$$\boldsymbol{u}'(\mathbf{0}) \boldsymbol{I}^{-1}(\mathbf{0}) \boldsymbol{u}(\mathbf{0}).$$

Each of these statistics has a chi-squared distribution on p d.f. under the null hypothesis that $\boldsymbol{\beta} = \mathbf{0}$.

In comparing alternative models, interest centres on the hypothesis that some of the β-parameters in a model are equal to zero. To test this hypothesis, the likelihood ratio test is the most suitable, and so we only consider this procedure here. Suppose that a model that contains $p + q$ parameters, $\beta_1, \beta_2, \ldots, \beta_p, \beta_{p+1}, \ldots, \beta_{p+q}$, is to be compared with a model that only contains the p parameters $\beta_1, \beta_2, \ldots, \beta_p$. This amounts to testing the null hypothesis that the q parameters $\beta_{p+1}, \beta_{p+2}, \ldots, \beta_{p+q}$ in the model with $p + q$ unknown parameters are all equal to zero. Let $\hat{\boldsymbol{\beta}}_1$ denote the vector of estimates under the model with $p + q$ parameters and $\hat{\boldsymbol{\beta}}_2$ that for the model with just p parameters. The likelihood ratio test of the null hypothesis that $\beta_{p+1} = \beta_{p+2} = \cdots = \beta_{p+q} = 0$ in the model with $p + q$ parameters is then based on the statistic

$$2\left\{\log L(\hat{\boldsymbol{\beta}}_1) - \log L(\hat{\boldsymbol{\beta}}_2)\right\},$$

which has a chi-squared distribution on q d.f., under the null hypothesis. This test forms the basis for comparing alternative models, and was described in greater detail in Section 3.5 of Chapter 3.

Appendix B

Additional data sets

This appendix contains a number of data sets, together with some suggestions for analyses that could be carried out. These data sets may be downloaded from the publishers's web site, at the location given in the preface.

B.1 Chronic active hepatitis

In a clinical trial described by Kirk et al. (1980), 44 patients with chronic active hepatitis were randomised to the drug prednisolone, or an untreated control group. The survival time of the patients, in months, following admission to the trial, was the response variable of interest. The data, which were given in Pocock (1983), are shown in Table B.1.

Table B.1 *Survival times of patients suffering from chronic active hepatitis.*

Prednisolone		Control	
2	131*	2	41
6	140*	3	54
12	141*	4	61
54	143	7	63
56*	145*	10	71
68	146	22	127*
89	148*	28	140*
96	162*	29	146*
96	168	32	158*
125*	173*	37	167*
128*	181*	40	182*

* Censored survival times.

Summarise the data in terms of the estimated survivor function for each treatment group. Compare the groups using the log-rank and Wilcoxon tests. Fit Cox and Weibull proportional hazards model to determine the significance of the treatment effect. Compare the results from these different analyses in terms of the significance of the treatment effect, and, for the model-based analyses, the estimated hazard ratio and corresponding 95% confidence limits.

Obtain a log-cumulative hazard plot of the data, and comment on which method of analysis is the most appropriate.

B.2 Recurrence of bladder cancer

In a placebo-controlled trial concerning bladder cancer, conducted by the Veterans Administration Cooperative Urological Research Group, patients with superficial bladder tumours first had their tumour removed transurethrally. They were then randomised to a placebo, or to the chemotherapeutic agent, thiotepa. The initial number of tumours in each patient, and the diameter of the largest of these, was recorded at the time of randomisation. The original data set, included in Andrews and Herzberg (1985), gave the times to up to nine tumour recurrences, but the data presented in Table B.2 refer to the time to the first recurrence, in months. Patients who had not experienced a recurrence by the end of the follow-up period contribute censored observations. The variables in the data set are as follows:

Patient:	Patient number (1–86)
Time:	Survival time in months
Status:	Status of patient (0 = censored, 1 = recurrence)
Treat:	Treatment group (1 = placebo, 2 = thiotepa)
Init:	Initial number of tumours
Size:	Diameter of largest initial tumour in cm

Using a Cox proportional hazards model, determine whether the recurrence times depend on the explanatory variables *Init* and *Size*. After adjusting for relevant variables, examine the significance of the treatment effect. Check if there is any evidence of an interaction between treatment group and the two explanatory variables. Using model-checking diagnostics, comment on the suitability of the fitted model. In particular, by fitting a suitable time-dependent variable, test the assumption of proportional hazards with respect to treatment. Estimate the hazard ratio for the treatment effect and give a 95% confidence interval for the ratio. Compare this estimate with that obtained from fitting a Weibull proportional hazards model.

B.3 Survival of black ducks

In the first year of a study on the movements and overwintering survival of black ducks, *Anas rubripes*, conducted by the U.S. Fish and Wildlife Service, 50 female black ducks from two locations in New Jersey were captured and fitted with radios. The ducks were captured over a period of about four weeks from 8 November 1983 to 14 December 1983, and included 31 hatch-year birds, that is, birds born during the previous breeding season, and 19 birds of at least one year of age. The body weight and wing length were measured for each duck. The status of each duck, that is, whether it was alive, missing or dead,

Table B.2 *Time to first recurrence of a tumour in bladder cancer patients.*

Patient	*Time*	*Status*	*Treat*	*Init*	*Size*	*Patient*	*Time*	*Status*	*Treat*	*Init*	*Size*
1	0	0	1	1	1	44	3	1	1	3	1
2	1	0	1	1	3	45	59	0	1	1	1
3	4	0	1	2	1	46	2	1	1	3	2
4	7	0	1	1	1	47	5	1	1	1	3
5	10	0	1	5	1	48	2	1	1	2	3
6	6	1	1	4	1	49	1	0	2	1	3
7	14	0	1	1	1	50	1	0	2	1	1
8	18	0	1	1	1	51	5	1	2	8	1
9	5	1	1	1	3	52	9	0	2	1	2
10	12	1	1	1	1	53	10	0	2	1	1
11	23	0	1	3	3	54	13	0	2	1	1
12	10	1	1	1	3	55	3	1	2	2	6
13	3	1	1	1	1	56	1	1	2	5	3
14	3	1	1	3	1	57	18	0	2	5	1
15	7	1	1	2	3	58	17	1	2	1	3
16	3	1	1	1	1	59	2	1	2	5	1
17	26	0	1	1	2	60	17	1	2	1	1
18	1	1	1	8	1	61	22	0	2	1	1
19	2	1	1	1	4	62	25	0	2	1	3
20	25	1	1	1	2	63	25	0	2	1	5
21	29	0	1	1	4	64	25	0	2	1	1
22	29	0	1	1	2	65	6	1	2	1	1
23	29	0	1	4	1	66	6	1	2	1	1
24	28	1	1	1	6	67	2	1	2	2	1
25	2	1	1	1	5	68	26	1	2	8	3
26	3	1	1	2	1	69	38	0	2	1	1
27	12	1	1	1	3	70	22	1	2	1	1
28	32	0	1	1	2	71	4	1	2	6	1
29	34	0	1	2	1	72	24	1	2	3	1
30	36	0	1	2	1	73	41	0	2	3	2
31	29	1	1	3	1	74	41	0	2	1	1
32	37	0	1	1	2	75	1	1	2	1	1
33	9	1	1	4	1	76	44	0	2	1	1
34	16	1	1	5	1	77	2	1	2	6	1
35	41	0	1	1	2	78	45	0	2	1	2
36	3	1	1	1	1	79	2	1	2	1	4
37	6	1	1	2	6	80	46	0	2	1	4
38	3	1	1	2	1	81	49	0	2	3	3
39	9	1	1	1	1	82	50	0	2	1	1
40	18	1	1	1	1	83	4	1	2	4	1
41	49	0	1	1	3	84	54	0	2	3	4
42	35	1	1	3	1	85	38	1	2	2	1
43	17	1	1	1	7	86	59	0	2	1	3

was recorded daily from the date of release until 15 February 1984, when the study was terminated. The data set, which is included in Hand et al. (1994), contains the following variables:

Time:	Survival time in days
Status:	Status of bird (0 = alive or missing, 1 = dead)
Age:	Age group (0 = hatch-year bird, 1 = bird aged $\geqslant 1$ year)
Weight:	Weight of bird in g
Length:	Length of wing in mm

The values of each of these variables for the ducks in the study are shown in Table B.3.

Table B.3 *Survival times of 50 black ducks.*

Time	*Status*	*Age*	*Weight*	*Length*	*Time*	*Status*	*Age*	*Weight*	*Length*
2	1	1	1160	277	44	1	0	1040	255
6	0	0	1140	266	49	0	0	1130	268
6	0	1	1260	280	54	0	1	1320	285
7	1	0	1160	264	56	0	0	1180	259
13	1	1	1080	267	56	0	0	1070	267
14	0	0	1120	262	57	0	1	1260	269
16	0	1	1140	277	57	0	0	1270	276
16	1	1	1200	283	58	0	0	1080	260
17	0	1	1100	264	63	0	1	1110	270
17	1	1	1420	270	63	0	0	1150	271
20	0	1	1120	272	63	0	0	1030	265
21	1	1	1110	271	63	0	0	1160	275
22	1	0	1070	268	63	0	0	1180	263
26	1	0	940	252	63	0	0	1050	271
26	1	0	1240	271	63	0	1	1280	281
27	1	0	1120	265	63	0	0	1050	275
28	0	1	1340	275	63	0	0	1160	266
29	1	0	1010	272	63	0	0	1150	263
32	1	0	1040	270	63	0	1	1270	270
32	0	1	1250	276	63	0	1	1370	275
34	1	0	1200	276	63	0	1	1220	265
34	1	0	1280	270	63	0	0	1220	268
37	1	0	1250	272	63	0	0	1140	262
40	1	0	1090	275	63	0	0	1140	270
41	1	1	1050	275	63	0	0	1120	274

Using a proportional hazards model, examine the effect of age, weight and length on survival time. Investigate whether the coefficients of the explanatory variables, *Weight* and *Length*, differ for the ducks in each age group. Is there any evidence that non-linear functions of the variables *Weight* and *Length* are needed in the model?

B.4 Bone marrow transplantation

Following the treatment of leukaemia, patients often undergo a bone marrow transplant in order to help bring their blood cells back to a normal level. A potentially fatal side effect of this is graft-versus-host disease, in which the transplanted cells attack the host cells. In a study described by Bagot et al. (1988), 37 patients who were in complete remission from acute myeloid leukaemia (AML) or acute lymphocytic leukaemia (ALL), or in the chronic phase of chronic myeloid leukaemia (CML), received a non-depleted allogeneic bone marrow transplant. The age of the bone marrow donor, and whether or not the donor had previously been pregnant, was recorded, together with the age of the recipient, their type of leukaemia, an index of mixed epidermal lymphocyte reactions, and whether or not the recipient developed graft-versus-host disease. The variables in this data set are as follows:

Patient:	Patient number (1–37)
Time:	Survival time in days
Status:	Status of patient (0 = alive, 1 = dead)
Rage:	Age of patient in years
Dage:	Age of donor in years
Type:	Type of leukaemia (1 = AML, 2 = ALL, 3 = CML)
Preg:	Donor pregnancy (0 = no, 1 = yes)
Index:	Index of cell-lymphocyte reactions
Gvhd:	Graft-versus-host disease (0 = no, 1 = yes)

The data, which were also given in Altman (1991), are presented in Table B.4.

Using a Weibull accelerated failure time model, investigate the dependence of the survival times on the prognostic variables. Estimate and plot the baseline survivor function. Fit log-logistic and lognormal models that contain the same explanatory variables, and estimate the baseline survivor function under these models. Compare these estimates with the estimated baseline survivor function obtained from fitting a Cox proportional hazards model. Hence comment on which parametric model is the most appropriate, and further examine the adequacy of this model using model-checking diagnostics.

B.5 Chronic granulomatous disease

Chronic granulomatous disease (CGD) is a group of inherited disorders of the immune system that render patients vulnerable to recurrent infections and chronic inflammatory conditions, such as gingivitis, enlarged lymph glands, or non-malignant tumour-like masses, known as granulomas. These granulomas can obstruct the passage of food through the digestive system, and may also inhibit the flow of urine from the kidneys and bladder. The disease is generally treated with antibiotics, but a multicentre trial carried out by Genentech, Inc. compared the antiviral drug, interferon, with a placebo. Data were obtained

Table B.4 *Survival times of leukaemia patients who received a bone marrow transplant.*

Patient	*Time*	*Status*	*Rage*	*Dage*	*Type*	*Preg*	*Index*	*Gvhd*
1	95	1	27	23	2	0	0.27	0
2	1385	0	13	18	2	0	0.31	0
3	465	1	19	19	1	0	0.39	0
4	810	1	21	22	2	0	0.48	0
5	1497	0	28	38	2	0	0.49	0
6	1181	1	22	20	2	0	0.50	0
7	993	0	19	19	2	0	0.81	0
8	138	1	20	23	2	0	0.82	0
9	266	1	33	36	1	0	0.86	0
10	579	0	18	19	1	0	0.92	0
11	600	0	17	20	2	0	1.10	0
12	1182	0	31	21	3	0	1.52	0
13	841	0	23	38	2	0	1.88	0
14	1364	0	27	15	2	0	2.01	0
15	695	0	26	16	2	0	2.40	0
16	1378	0	28	25	1	0	2.45	0
17	736	0	24	21	1	1	2.60	0
18	1504	0	18	20	2	0	2.64	0
19	849	0	24	25	1	1	3.78	0
20	1266	0	20	24	3	0	4.72	0
21	186	1	23	35	1	1	1.10	1
22	41	1	21	35	2	1	1.16	1
23	667	0	21	23	3	0	1.45	1
24	112	1	33	43	3	0	1.50	1
25	572	0	29	24	3	1	1.85	1
26	45	1	42	35	2	1	2.30	1
27	1019	0	27	31	3	0	2.34	1
28	479	1	43	29	2	1	2.44	1
29	190	1	22	20	1	0	3.70	1
30	100	1	35	39	1	1	3.73	1
31	177	1	16	14	1	0	4.13	1
32	80	1	39	35	2	1	4.52	1
33	142	1	28	25	3	1	4.52	1
34	1105	0	29	32	3	0	4.71	1
35	803	0	23	19	3	0	5.07	1
36	1126	0	33	34	3	0	9.00	1
37	114	1	19	20	1	0	10.11	1

on a number of prognostic variables, and the end-point of interest was the time to the first serious infection following randomisation. The database, described in Therneau and Grambsch (2000), contains the following variables:

Patient:	Patient number (1–128)
Time:	Time to first infection in days
Status:	Status of patient (0 = censored, 1 = infection)
Centre:	Centre (1 = Harvard Medical School
	2 = Scripps Institute, California
	3 = Copenhagen
	4 = National Institutes of Health, Maryland
	5 = Los Angeles Children's Hospital
	6 = Mott Children's Hospital, Michigan
	7 = University of Utah
	8 = Children's Hospital of Philadelphia, Pennsylvania
	9 = University of Washington
	10 = University of Minnesota
	11 = University of Zurich
	12 = Texas Children's Hospital
	13 = Amsterdam
	14 = Mount Sinai Medical Center)
Treat:	Treatment group (0 = placebo, 1 = interferon)
Age:	Age in years
Sex:	Sex (1 = male, 2 = female)
Height:	Height in cm
Weight:	Weight in kg
Pattern:	Pattern of inheritance (1 = X-linked, 2 = autosomal recessive)
Cort:	Use of corticosteroids at trial entry (1 = used, 2 = not used)
Anti:	Use of antibiotics at trial entry (1 = used, 2 = not used)

Identify a suitable model for the times to first infection, and investigate the adequacy of the model. Is there any evidence that the treatment effect is not consistent across the different centres? Summarise the treatment difference in terms of a relevant point estimate and corresponding confidence interval.

Now suppose that the actual infection times are interval-censored, and that the infection status of any individual can only be recorded at 90, 180, 270 and 360 days. Construct a new observation from the survival times, that gives the interval within which an infection, or censoring, occurs. The observations from individuals who do not experience an infection, or who develop an infection after 360 days, are regarded as censored. For this constructed database, analyse the interval-censored data using the methods described in Chapter 9. Compare the estimate of the treatment effect with that found from the original data.

Fit parametric and Cox regression models with shared frailty to these data, where *Centre* is a random frailty effect. Compare and contrast the two sets of results and comment on the extent of between centre variability.

Determine the number of patients who develop a first infection in the first 180 days at each centre. By fitting a Cox regression model to the first infection times, obtain an estimate of the 180 day risk adjusted first infection rate at each centre, using the methods described in Chapter 11. By treating centres as either fixed or random, calculate corresponding interval estimates for this rate, commenting on the extent of any differences.

Investigate the impact of dependent censoring in these data. First, fit a Weibull model for the probability of censoring, and using this model, obtain weights that are inversely proportional to censoring. After expressing the infection time data in the counting process format, fit a weighted Cox regression model to allow for any dependent censoring. Compare the results with those obtained from an unweighted Cox regression analysis.

Bibliography

Aalen, O.O. (1978a) Nonparametric estimation of partial transition probabilities in multiple decrement models. *Annals of Statistics*, **6**, 534–545.

Aalen, O.O. (1978b) Nonparametric inference for a family of counting processes. *Annals of Statistics*, **6**, 701–726.

Aalen, O.O. (1994) Effects of frailty in survival analysis. *Statistical Methods in Medical Research*, **3**, 227–243.

Aalen, O.O. (1998) Frailty models. In: *Statistical Analysis of Medical Data: New Developments* (eds. B.S. Everitt and G. Dunn), Arnold, London.

Aalen, O.O. and Johansen, S. (1978) An empirical transition matrix for non-homogeneous Markov chains based on censored observations. *Scandinavian Journal of Statistics*, **5**, 141–150.

Aalen, O.O., Borgan, Ø. and Gjessing, H. (2008) *Survival and Event History Analysis: A Process Point of View*, Springer, New York.

Aitkin, M., Anderson, D.A., Francis, B. and Hinde, J.P. (1989) *Statistical Modelling in GLIM*, Clarendon Press, Oxford.

Aitkin, M., Laird, N. and Francis, B. (1983) A reanalysis of the Stanford heart transplant data (with comments). *Journal of the American Statistical Association*, **78**, 264–292.

Akaike, H. (1974) A new look at the statistical model identification. *IEEE Transactions on Automatic Control*, **19**, 716–723.

Allison, P.D. (2010) *Survival Analysis Using SAS®: A Practical Guide*, 2nd ed., SAS Institute Inc., Cary, North Carolina.

Altman, D.G. (1991) *Practical Statistics for Medical Research*, Chapman & Hall/CRC, London.

Altman, D.G. and De Stavola, B.L. (1994) Practical problems in fitting a proportional hazards model to data with updated measurements of the covariates. *Statistics in Medicine*, **13**, 301–341.

Altshuler, B. (1970) Theory for the measurement of competing risks in animal experiments. *Mathematical Biosciences*, **6**, 1–11.

Andersen, P.K. (1982) Testing goodness of fit of Cox's regression and life model. *Biometrics*, **38**, 67–77.

Andersen, P.K. (1988) Multistate models in survival analysis: A study of nephropathy and mortality in diabetes. *Statistics in Medicine*, **7**, 661–670.

Andersen, P.K. (1992) Repeated assessment of risk factors in survival analysis. *Statistical Methods in Medical Research*, **1**, 297–315.

Andersen, P.K. and Borgan, Ø. (1985) Counting process models for life history data: A review. *Scandinavian Journal of Statistics*, **12**, 97–158.

Andersen, P.K. and Gill, R.D. (1982) Cox's regression model for counting processes: A large sample study. *Annals of Statistics*, **10**, 1100–1120.

Andersen, P.K. and Keiding, N. (2002) Multi-state models for event history analysis. *Statistical Methods in Medical Research*, **11**, 91–115.

Andersen, P.K. and Perme, M.P. (2010) Pseudo-observations in survival analysis. *Statistical Methods in Medical Research*, **19**, 71–99.

Andersen, P.K., Borgan, Ø., Gill, R.D. and Keiding, N. (1993) *Statistical Methods Based on Counting Processes*, Springer, New York.

Andersen, P.K., Hansen, M.G. and Klein, J.P. (2004) Regression analysis of restricted mean survival time based on pseudo-observations. *Lifetime Data Analysis*, **10**, 335–350.

Andrews, D.F. and Herzberg, A.M. (1985) *Data*, Springer, New York.

Arjas, E. (1988) A graphical method for assessing goodness of fit in Cox's proportional hazards model. *Journal of the American Statistical Association*, **83**, 204–212.

Armitage, P., Berry, G. and Matthews, J.N.S. (2002) *Statistical Methods in Medical Research*, 4th ed., Blackwells Science Ltd, Oxford.

Atkinson, A.C. (1985) *Plots, Transformations and Regression*, Clarendon Press, Oxford.

Bagot, M., Mary, J.Y., Heslan, M., Kuentz, M., Cordonnier, C., Vernant, J.P., Dubertret, L. and Levy, J.P. (1988) The mixed epidermal cell lymphocyte-reaction is the most predictive factor of acute graft-versus-host disease in bone marrow graft recipients. *British Journal of Haematology*, **70**, 403–409.

Barlow, W.E. and Prentice, R.L. (1988) Residuals for relative risk regression. *Biometrika*, **75**, 65–74.

Barnett, V. (1999) *Comparative Statistical Inference*, 3rd ed., Wiley, Chichester.

Becker, N.G. and Melbye, M. (1991) Use of a log-linear model to compute the empirical survival curve from interval-censored data, with application to data on tests for HIV positivity. *Australian Journal of Statistics*, **33**, 125–133.

Bennett, S. (1983a) Analysis of survival data by the proportional odds model. *Statistics in Medicine*, **2**, 273–277.

Bennett, S. (1983b) Log-logistic regression models for survival data. *Applied Statistics*, **32**, 165–171.

Bernstein, D. and Lagakos, S.W. (1978) Sample size and power determination for stratified clinical trials. *Journal of Statistical Computation and Simulation*, **8**, 65–73.

Beyersmann, J., Allignol, A. and Schumacher, M. (2012) *Competing Risks and Multistate Models with R*, Springer, New York.

Box, G.E.P. and Tidwell, P.W. (1962) Transformation of the independent variables. *Technometrics*, **4**, 531–550.

Box-Steffensmeier, J.M. and Jones, B.S. (2004) *Event History Modeling: A Guide for Social Scientists*, Cambridge University Press, Cambridge.

Breslow, N.E. (1972) Contribution to the discussion of a paper by D.R. Cox. *Journal of the Royal Statistical Society, B*, **34**, 216–217.

Breslow, N.E. (1974) Covariance analysis of censored survival data. *Biometrics*, **30**, 89–100.

Breslow, N.E. and Crowley, J. (1974) A large sample study of the life table and product limit estimates under random censorship. *Annals of Statistics*, **2**, 437–453.

Breslow, N.E. and Day, N.E. (1987) *Statistical Methods in Cancer Research. 2: The Design and Analysis of Cohort Studies*, I.A.R.C., Lyon, France.

Brookmeyer, R. and Crowley, J. (1982) A confidence interval for the median survival time. *Biometrics*, **38**, 29–41.

Broström, G. (2012) *Event History Analysis with R*, Chapman & Hall/CRC, Boca Raton, Florida.

Brown, H. and Prescott, R.J. (2000) *Applied Mixed Models in Medicine*, Wiley, Chichester.

Burdette, W.J. and Gehan, E.A. (1970) *Planning and Analysis of Clinical Studies*, Charles C. Thomas, Springfield, Illinois.

Byar, D.P. (1982) Analysis of survival data: Cox and Weibull models with covariates. In: *Statistics in Medical Research* (eds. V. Mike and K.E. Stanley), Wiley, New York.

Cain, K.C. and Lange, N.T. (1984) Approximate case influence for the proportional hazards regression model with censored data. *Biometrics*, **40**, 493–499.

Chatfield, C. (1995) *Problem Solving: A Statisticians Guide*, 2nd ed., Chapman & Hall/CRC, London.

Chatfield, C. (2004) *The Analysis of Time Series*, 6th ed., Chapman & Hall/CRC, London.

Chhikara, S. and Folks, J.L. (1989) *Inverse Gaussian Distribution*, Marcel Dekker, New York.

Choodari-Oskooei, B., Royston, P. and Parmar, M.K.B. (2012) A simulation study of predictive ability measures in a survival model I: Explained variation measures. *Statistics in Medicine*, **31**, 2627–2643.

Choodari-Oskooei, B., Royston, P. and Parmar, M.K.B. (2012) A simulation study of predictive ability measures in a survival model II: Explained randomness and predictive accuracy. *Statistics in Medicine*, **31**, 2644–2659.

Christensen, E. (1987) Multivariate survival analysis using Cox's regression model. *Hepatology*, **7**, 1346–1358.

Christensen, E., Schlichting, P., Andersen, P.K., Fauerholdt, L., Schou, G., Pedersen, B.V., Juhl, E., Poulsen, H., Tygstrup, N. and Copenhagen Study Group for Liver Diseases (1986) Updating prognosis and therapeutic effect evaluation in cirrhosis with Cox's multiple regression model for time-dependent variables. *Scandinavian Journal of Gastroenterology*, **21**, 163–174.

Ciampi, A. and Etezadi-Amoli, J. (1985) A general model for testing the proportional hazards and the accelerated failure time hypotheses in the analysis of censored survival data with covariates. *Communications in Statistics, A*, **14**, 651–667.

Claeskens, G., Nguti, R. and Janssen, P. (2008) One-sided tests in shared frailty models. *Test*, **17**, 69–82.

Cleveland, W.S. (1979) Robust locally weighted regression and smoothing scatterplots. *Journal of the Americal Statistical Association*, **74**, 829–836.

Cleves, M., Gould, W., Gutierrez, R.G. and Marchenko, Y.V. (2010) *An Introduction to Survival Analysis Using Stata*, 3rd ed., Stata Press.

Cohen, A. and Barnett, O. (1995) Assessing goodness of fit of parametric regression models for lifetime data–graphical methods. *Statistics in Medicine*, **14**, 1785–1795.

Collett, D. (2003) *Modelling Binary Data*, 2nd ed., Chapman & Hall/CRC, Boca Raton, Florida.

Commenges, D. (1999) Multi-state models in epidemiology. *Lifetime Data Analysis*, **5**, 315–327.

Cook, R.D. (1986) Assessment of local influence (with discussion). *Journal of the Royal Statistical Society, B*, **48**, 133–169.

Cook, R.D. and Weisberg, S. (1982) *Residuals and Influence in Regression*, Chapman & Hall/CRC, London.

Cook, R.J. and Lawless, J.F. (2007) *The Statistical Analysis of Recurrent Events*, Springer, New York.

Copas, J.B. and Heydari, F. (1997) Estimating the risk of reoffending by using exponential mixture models. *Journal of the Royal Statistical Society, A*, **160**, 237–252.

Cox, D.R. (1972) Regression models and life tables (with discussion). *Journal of the Royal Statistical Society, B*, **74**, 187–220.

Cox, D.R. (1975) Partial likelihood. *Biometrika*, **62**, 269–276.

Cox, D.R. (1979) A note on the graphical analysis of survival data. *Biometrika*, **66**, 188–190.

Cox, D.R. and Hinkley, D. V. (1974) *Theoretical Statistics*, Chapman & Hall/CRC, London.

Cox, D.R. and Oakes, D. (1984) *Analysis of Survival Data*, Chapman & Hall/CRC, London.

Cox, D.R. and Snell, E.J. (1968) A general definition of residuals (with discussion). *Journal of the Royal Statistical Society, A*, **30**, 248–275.

Cox, D.R. and Snell, E.J. (1981) *Applied Statistics: Principles and Examples*, Chapman & Hall/CRC, London.

Cox, D.R. and Snell, E.J. (1989) *Analysis of Binary Data*, 2nd ed., Chapman & Hall/CRC, London.

Crawley, M.J. (2013) *The R Book*, 2nd ed., John Wiley & Sons Ltd, Chichester.

Crowder, M.J. (2001) *Classical Competing Risks*, Chapman & Hall/CRC, Boca Raton, Florida.

Crowder, M.J. (2012) *Multivariate Survival Analysis and Competing Risks*, Chapman & Hall/CRC, Boca Raton, Florida.

Crowder, M.J., Kimber, A.C., Smith, R.L. and Sweeting, T.J. (1991) *Statistical Analysis of Reliability Data*, Chapman & Hall/CRC, London.

Crowley, J. and Hu, M. (1977) Covariance analysis of heart transplant survival data. *Journal of the American Statistical Association*, **72**, 27–36.

Crowley, J. and Storer, B.E. (1983) Comment on a paper by M. Aitkin et al. *Journal of the American Statistical Association*, **78**, 277–281.

Dalgaard, P. (2008) *Introductory Statistics with R*, 2nd ed., Springer, New York.

David, H.A. and Moeschberger, M.L. (1978) *The Theory of Competing Risks*, Lubrecht & Cramer Ltd, New York.

Davis, H. and Feldstein, M. (1979) The generalized Pareto law as a model for progressively censored survival data. *Biometrika*, **66**, 299–306.

Day, L. (1985) Residual analysis for Cox's proportional hazards model. In: *Proceedings of STATCOM-MEDSTAT '85'*, MacQuarie University, Sydney.

Demidenko, E. (2013), *Mixed Models: Theory and Applications with R*, 2nd ed., John Wiley & Sons, Hoboken, New Jersey.

Der, G. and Everitt, B.S. (2013) *Applied Medical Statistics Using SAS*, Chapman & Hall/CRC, Boca Raton, Florida.

Dinse, G.E. (1991) Constant risk differences in the analysis of animal tumourigenicity data. *Biometrics*, **47**, 681–700.

Dobson, A.J. (2001) *An Introduction to Generalized Linear Models*, 2nd ed., Chapman & Hall/CRC, Boca Raton, Florida.

Draper, N.R. and Smith, H. (1998) *Applied Regression Analysis*, 3rd ed., Wiley, New York.

Duchateau, L. and Janssen, P. (2008) *The Frailty Model*, Springer, New York.

Durrleman, S. and Simon, R. (1989) Flexible regression models with cubic splines. *Statistics in Medicine*, **8**, 551–561.

Edmunson, J.H., Fleming, T.R., Decker, D.G., Malkasian, G.D., Jorgenson, E.O., Jeffries, J.A., Webb, M.J. and Kvols, L.K. (1979) Different chemotherapeutic sensitivities and host factors affecting prognosis in advanced ovarian carcinoma versus minimal residual disease. *Cancer Treatment Reports*, **63**, 241–247.

Efron, B. (1977) The efficiency of Cox's likelihood function for censored data. *Journal of the American Statistical Association*, **72**, 557–565.

Efron, B. (1981) Censored data and the bootstrap. *Journal of the American Statistical Association*, **76**, 312–319.

Efron, B., Hastie, T., Johnstone, I. and Tibshirani, R. (2004) Least angle regression. *Annals of Statistics*, **32**, 407–451.

Elashoff, J.D. (1983) Surviving proportional hazards. *Hepatology*, **3**, 1031–1035.

Emerson, J.D. (1982) Nonparametric confidence intervals for the median in the presence of right censoring. *Biometrics*, **38**, 17–27.

Escobar, L.A. and Meeker, W.Q. (1988) Using the SAS system to assess local influence in regression analysis with censored data. *Proceedings of the Annual SAS User's Group Conference*, 1036–1041.

Escobar, L.A. and Meeker, W.Q. (1992) Assessing influence in regression analysis with censored data. *Biometrics*, **48**, 507–528.

Everitt, B.S. (1987) *Introduction to Optimisation Methods*, Chapman & Hall/CRC, London.

Everitt, B.S. and Rabe-Hesketh, S. (2001) *Analyzing Medical Data Using S-PLUS*, Springer, New York.

Farewell V.T. (1982) The use of mixture models for the analysis of survival data with long-term survivors. *Biometrics*, **38**, 1041–1046.

Farrington, C.P. (1996) Interval censored survival data: A generalized linear modelling approach. *Statistics in Medicine*, **15**, 283–292.

Farrington, C.P. (2000) Residuals for proportional hazards models with interval-censored data. *Biometrics*, **56**, 473–482.

Fine, J.P. and Gray, R.J. (1999) A proportional hazards model for the subdistribution of a competing risk. *Journal of the American Statistical Association*, **94**, 496–509.

Finkelstein, D.M. (1986) A proportional hazards model for interval-censored failure time data. *Biometrics*, **42**, 845–854.

Finkelstein, D.M. and Wolfe, R.A. (1985) A semiparametric model for regression analysis of interval-censored failure time data. *Biometrics*, **41**, 933–945.

Fisher, L.D. (1992) Discussion of a paper by L.J. Wei. *Statistics in Medicine*, **11**, 1881–1885.

Fleming, T.R. and Harrington, D.P. (2005) *Counting Processes and Survival Analysis*, John Wiley & Sons, Hoboken, New Jersey.

Ford, I., Norrie, J. and Ahmadi, S. (1995) Model inconsistency, illustrated by the Cox proportional hazards model. *Statistics in Medicine*, **14**, 735–746.

Freedman, L.S. (1982) Tables of the number of patients required in clinical trials using the logrank test. *Statistics in Medicine*, **1**, 121–129.

Friedman, L.M., Furberg, C.D. and DeMets, D.L. (2010) *Fundamentals of Clinical Trials*, 4th ed., Springer, New York.

Fyles, A.W., McCready, D.R., Manchul, L.A., Trudeau, M.E., Merante, P., Pintilie, M., Weir, L. and Olivotto, I.A. (2004) Tamoxifen with or without breast irradiation in women 50 years of age or older with early breast cancer. *New England Journal of Medicine*, **351**, 963–970.

Gail, M.H., Santner, T.J. and Brown, C.C. (1980) An analysis of comparative carcinogenesis experiments based on multiple times to tumor. *Biometrics*, **36**, 255–266.

Gaver, D.P. and Acar, M. (1979) Analytical hazard representations for use in reliability, mortality and simulation studies. *Communications in Statistics*, **8**, 91–111.

Geerdens, C., Claeskens, G. and Janssen, P. (2013) Goodness-of-fit tests for the frailty distribution in proportional hazards models with shared frailty. *Biostatistics*, **14**, 433–446.

Gehan, E.A. (1969) Estimating survival functions from the life table. *Journal of Chronic Diseases*, **21**, 629–644.

George, S.L. and Desu, M.M. (1974) Planning the size and duration of a clinical trial studying the time to some critical event. *Journal of Chronic Diseases*, **27**, 15–24.

Gill, R.D. (1984) Understanding Cox's regression model: A martingale approach. *Journal of the American Statistical Association*, **79**, 441–447.

Gill, R.D. and Schumacher, M. (1987) A simple test of the proportional hazards assumption. *Biometrika*, **74**, 289–300.

Glidden, D.V. (1999) Checking the adequacy of the gamma frailty model for multivariate failure times. *Biometrika*, **86**, 381–393.

Goeman, J., Meijer, R. and Chaturvedi, N. (2013) L_1 (lasso and fused lasso) and L_2 (ridge) penalized estimation in GLMs and in the Cox model. R package version 0.9-42, URL http://www.msbi.nl/goeman.

Goeman, J.J. (2010) L_1 penalized estimation in the Cox proportional hazards model. *Biometrical Journal*, **52**, 70–84.

Goldstein, H. and Spiegelhalter, D.J. (1996) League tables and their limitations: statistical issues in comparisons of institutional performance, *Journal of the Royal Statistical Society, A*, **159**, 385–443.

Gönen, M. and Heller, G. (2005) Concordance probability and discriminatory power in proportional hazards regression. *Biometrika*, **92**, 965–970.

Gore, S.M., Pocock, S.J. and Kerr, G.R. (1984) Regression models and nonproportional hazards in the analysis of breast cancer survival. *Applied Statistics*, **33**, 176–195.

Grambsch, P.M. and Therneau, T.M. (1994) Proportional hazards tests and diagnostics based on weighted residuals. *Biometrika*, **81**, 515–526.

Gray, R. (1990) Some diagnostic methods for Cox regression models through hazard smoothing. *Biometrics*, **46**, 93–102.

Gray, R. (2013) Subdistribution analysis of competing risks. R package version 2.2-6, URL http://www.r-project.org.

Gray, R.J. (1988) A class of k-sample tests for comparing the cumulative incidence of a competing risk. *Annals of Statistics*, **16**, 1141–1154.

Gray, R.J. (1992) Flexible methods for analyzing survival data using splines, with applications to breast cancer prognosis. *Journal of the American Statistical Association*, **87**, 942–951.

Greenwood, M. (1926) The errors of sampling of the survivorship tables. *Reports on Public Health and Statistical Subjects*, number 33, Appendix 1, HMSO, London.

Grønnesby, J.K. and Borgan, Ø. (1996) A method for checking regression models in survival analysis based on the risk score. *Lifetime Data Analysis*, **2**, 315–328.

Hall, W.J. and Wellner, J.A. (1980) Confidence bands for a survival curve from censored data. *Biometrika*, **67**, 133–143.

Hall, W.J., Rogers, W.H. and Pregibon, D. (1982) Outliers matter in survival analysis. *Rand Corporation Technical Report P–6761*, Santa Monica, California.

Hammer, S.M., Katzenstein, D.A., Hughes, M.D., Gundacker, H., Schooley, R.T., Haubrich, R.H., Henry, W.K., Lederman, M.M., Phair, J.P., Niu, M., Hirsch, M.S. and Merigan, T.C. (1996) A trial comparing nucleoside monotherapy with combination therapy in HIV-infected adults with CD4 cell counts from 200 to 500 per cubic millimeter. *New England Journal of Medicine*, **335**, 1081–1090.

Hand, D.J., Daly, F., Lunn, A.D., McConway, K.J. and Ostrowski, E. (1994) *A Handbook of Small Data Sets*, Chapman & Hall/CRC, London.

Harrell, F.E. (2001) *Regression Modelling Strategies, with Applications to Linear Models, Logistic Regression, and Survival Analysis*, Springer-Verlag, New York.

Harrell, F.E., Lee, K.L. and Mark, D.B. (1996) Multivariable prognostic models: issues in developing models, evaluating assumptions and adequacy, and measuring and reducing errors. *Statistics in Medicine*, **15**, 361–387.

Harris, E.K. and Albert, A. (1991) *Survivorship Analysis for Clinical Studies*, Marcel Dekker, New York.

Hastie, T. and Tibshirani, R. (1990) *Generalized Additive Models*, Chapman & Hall/CRC, London.

Heinzl, H. (2000) Using SAS to calculate the Kent and O'Quigley measure of dependence for Cox proportional hazards regression model. *Computer Methods and Programs in Biomedicine*, **63**, 71–76.

Henderson, R. and Milner, A. (1991) On residual plots for relative risk regression. *Biometrika*, **78**, 631–636.

Hielscher, T., Zucknick, M., Werft, W. and Benner, A. (2010) On the prognostic value of survival models with application to gene expression signatures. *Statistics in Medicine*, **30**, 818–829.

Hinchcliffe, S.R. and Lambert, P.C. (2013) Flexible parametric modelling of cause-specific hazards to estimate cumulative incidence functions. *BioMed Central Medical Research Methodology*, **13**, 1–14.

Hinkley, D.V., Reid, N. and Snell, E.J. (1991) *Statistical Theory and Modelling*, Chapman & Hall/CRC, London.

Hjorth, U. (1980) A reliability distribution with increasing, decreasing and bathtub-shaped failure rate. *Technometrics*, **22**, 99–107.

Hoel, D.G. (1972) A representation of mortality data by competing risks. *Biometrics*, **28**, 475–488.

Hollander, M. and Proschan, F. (1979) Testing to determine the underlying distribution using randomly censored data. *Biometrics*, **35**, 393–401.

Hosmer, D.W. and Lemeshow, S. (2000) *Applied Logistic Regression*, 2nd ed., John Wiley & Sons, Hoboken, New Jersey.

Hosmer, D.W., Lemeshow, S. and May, S. (2008) *Applied Survival Analysis: Regression Modeling of Time to Event Data*, 2nd ed., John Wiley & Sons, Hoboken, New Jersey.

Hougaard, P. (1995) Frailty models for survival data. *Lifetime Data Analysis*, **1**, 255–273.

Hougaard, P. (1999) Multi-state models: A review. *Lifetime Data Analysis*, **5**, 239–264.

Hougaard, P. (2000) *Analysis of Multivariate Survival Data*, Springer, New York.

Hougaard, P. and Madsen, E.B. (1985) Dynamic evaluation of short-term prognosis of myocardial infarction. *Statistics in Medicine*, **4**, 29–38.

Jennison, C. and Turnbull, B.W. (2000) *Group Sequential Methods with Applications to Clinical Trials*, Chapman & Hall/CRC, Boca Raton, Florida.

Jeong, J.-H. and Fine, J.P. (2007) Parametric regression on cumulative incidence function, *Biostatistics*, **8**, 184–196.

Johnson, N.L. and Kotz, S. (1994) *Distributions in Statistics: Continuous Univariate Distributions*, Volume 1, John Wiley & Sons, Hoboken, New Jersey.

Johnson, N.L., Kemp, A.W. and Kotz, S. (2005) *Distributions in Statistics: Discrete Distributions*, John Wiley & Sons, Hoboken, New Jersey.

Julious, S.A. (2010) *Sample Sizes for Clinical Trials*, Chapman & Hall/CRC, Boca Raton, Florida.

Kalbfleisch, J.D. and Prentice, R.L. (1972) Contribution to the discussion of a paper by D.R. Cox. *Journal of the Royal Statistical Society, B*, **34**, 215–216.

Kalbfleisch, J.D. and Prentice, R.L. (1973) Marginal likelihoods based on Cox's regression and life model. *Biometrika*, **60**, 267–278.

Kalbfleisch, J.D. and Prentice, R.L. (2002) *The Statistical Analysis of Failure Time Data*, 2nd ed., Wiley, New York.

Kaplan, E.L. and Meier, P. (1958) Nonparametric estimation from incomplete observations. *Journal of the American Statistical Association*, **53**, 457–481.

Kay, R. (1977) Proportional hazard regression models and the analysis of censored survival data. *Applied Statistics*, **26**, 227–237.

Kay, R. (1984) Goodness of fit methods for the proportional hazards model. *Revue Epidemiologie et de Santé Publique*, **32**, 185–198.

Keiding, N., Klein, J.P. and Horowitz, M.M. (2001) Multistate models and outcome prediction in bone marrow transplantation. *Statistics in Medicine*, **20**, 1871–1885.

Kelly, P.J. and Lim, L.L.-Y. (2000) Survival analysis for recurrent event data: An application to childhood infectious diseases. *Statistics in Medicine*, **19**, 13–33.

Kent, J.T. and O'Quigley, J. (1988) Measures of dependence for censored survival data. *Biometrika*, **75**, 525–534.

Kirk, A.P., Jain, S., Pocock, S., Thomas, H.C. and Sherlock, S. (1980) Late results of the Royal Free Hospital prospective controlled trial of prednisolone therapy in hepatitis B surface antigen negative chronic active hepatitis. *Gut*, **21**, 78–83.

Klein, J.P. (1991) Small-sample moments of some estimators of the variance of the Kaplan-Meier and Nelson-Aalen estimators. *Scandinavian Journal of Statistics*, **18**, 333–340.

Klein, J.P. (1992) Semiparametric estimation of random effects using the Cox model based on the EM algorithm. *Biometrics*, **48**, 795–806.

Klein, J.P. and Moeschberger, M.L. (1988) Bounds on net survival probabilities for dependent competing risks. *Biometrics*, **44**, 529–538.

Klein, J.P. and Moeschberger, M.L. (2005) *Survival Analysis: Techniques for Censored and Truncated Data*, 2nd ed., Springer, New York.

Klein, J.P. and Shu, Y. (2002) Multi-state models for bone marrow transplantation studies. *Statistical Methods in Medical Research*, **11**, 117–139.

Klein, J.P., Gerster, M., Andersen, P.K., Tarima, S. and Perme, M.P. (2008) SAS and R functions to compute pseudo-values for censored data regression. *Computer Methods and Programs in Biomedicine*, **89**, 289–300.

Kleinbaum, D.G. and Klein, J.P. (2012) *Survival Analysis: A Self-Learning Text*, 3rd ed., Springer, New York.

Kodell, R.L. and Nelson, C.J. (1980) An illness-death model for the study of the carcinogenic process using survival/sacrifice data. *Biometrics*, **36**, 267–277.

Kohl, M. and Heinze, G. (2012) *PSHREG: A SAS macro for proportional and non proportional subdistribution hazards regression with competing risk data*, Technical Report 08/2012, Section for Clinical Biometrics, Medical University of Vienna.

Krall, J.M., Uthoff, V.A. and Harley, J.B. (1975) A step-up procedure for selecting variables associated with survival. *Biometrics*, **31**, 49–57.

Kuk, A.Y.C. and Chen, C. (1992) A mixture model combining logistic regression with proportional hazards regression. *Biometrika*, **79**, 531–541.

Lachin, J.M. (1981) Introduction to sample size determination and power analysis for clinical trials. *Controlled Clinical Trials*, **2**, 93–113.

Lachin, J.M. and Foulkes, M.A. (1986) Evaluation of sample size and power for analyses of survival with allowance for nonuniform patient entry, losses to follow-up, noncompliance, and stratification. *Biometrics*, **42**, 507–519.

Lagakos, S.W. (1981) The graphical evaluation of explanatory variables in proportional hazards models. *Biometrika*, **68**, 93–98.

Lakatos, E. (1988) Sample sizes based on the log-rank statistic in complex clinical trials. *Biometrics*, **44**, 229–241.

Lakatos, E. and Lan, K.K.G. (1992) A comparison of sample size methods for the log-rank statistic. *Statistics in Medicine*, **11**, 179–191.

Lambert, P., Collett, D., Kimber, A. and Johnson, R. (2004) Parametric accelerated failure time models with random effects and an application to kidney transplant survival. *Statistics in Medicine*, **23**, 3177–3192.

Latouche, A., Beyersmann, J. and Fine, J.P. (2007) Letter to the editor: Comments on 'Analysing and interpreting competing risk data' by M. Pintilie. *Statistics in Medicine*, **26**, 3676–3680.

Latouche, A., Porcher, R. and Chevret, S. (2004) Sample size formula for proportional hazards modelling of competing risks. *Statistics in Medicine*, **23**, 3263–3274.

Lawless, J.F. (2002) *Statistical Models and Methods for Lifetime Data*, 2nd ed., Wiley, New York.

Leathem, A.J. and Brooks, S.A. (1987) Predictive value of lectin binding on breast-cancer recurrence and survival. *The Lancet*, **329**, 1054–1056.

Lee, E.T. and Wang, J.W. (2013) *Statistical Methods for Survival Data Analysis*, 4th ed., Wiley, New York.

Lin, D.Y. (1997) Non-parametric inference for cumulative incidence functions in competing risks studies. *Statistics in Medicine*, **16**, 901–910.

Lin, D.Y. and Wei, L.J. (1989) The robust inference for the Cox proportional hazards model. *Journal of the American Statistical Association*, **84**, 1074–1078.

Lin, D.Y. and Wei, L.J. (1991) Goodness-of-fit tests for the general Cox regression model. *Statistica Sinica*, **1**, 1–17.

Lindley, D.V. and Scott, W.F. (1984) *New Cambridge Elementary Statistical Tables*, Cambridge University Press, Cambridge.

Lindsey, J.C. and Ryan, L.M. (1993) A three state multiplicative model for rodent tumourigenicity experiments. *Applied Statistics*, **42**, 283–300.

Lindsey, J.C. and Ryan, L.M. (1998) Methods for interval-censored data. *Statistics in Medicine*, **17**, 219–238.

Lindsey, J.K. (1998) A study of interval censoring in parametric regression models. *Lifetime Data Analysis*, **4**, 329–354.

Machin, D., Campbell, M.J., Tan, S.B. and Tan, S.H. (2009) *Sample Sizes for Clinical Trials*, 3rd ed., John Wiley & Sons Ltd, Chichester.

Machin, D., Cheung, Y.B. and Parmar, M.K.B. (2006) *Survival Analysis: A Practical Approach*, Wiley, New York.

Maller, R.A. and Zhao, X. (2002) Analysis of parametric models for competing risks. *Statistica Sinica*, **12**, 725–750.

Mantel, N. (1966) Evaluation of survival data and two new rank order statistics arising in its consideration. *Cancer Chemotherapy Reports*, **50**, 163–170.

Mantel, N. and Haenszel, W. (1959) Statistical aspects of the analysis of data from retrospective studies of disease. *Journal of the National Cancer Institute*, **22**, 719–748.

Marubini, E. and Valsecchi, M.G. (1995) *Analysing Survival Data from Clinical Trials and Observational Studies*, Wiley, New York.

Matthews, J.N.S. (2006) *Introduction to Randomized Controlled Clinical Trials*, 2nd ed., Chapman & Hall/CRC, Boca Raton, Florida.

May, S. and Hosmer, D.W. (1998) A simplified method of calculating an overall goodness-of-fit test for the Cox proportional hazards model. *Lifetime Data Analysis*, **4**, 109–120.

McCrink, L.M., Marshall, A.H. and Cairns, K.J. (2013) Advances in joint modelling: a review of recent developments with application to the survival of end stage renal disease patients. *International Statistical Review*, **81**, 249–269.

McCullagh, P. and Nelder, J.A. (1989) *Generalized Linear Models*, 2nd ed., Chapman & Hall/CRC, London.

McCulloch, C.E., Searle, S.R. and Neuhaus, J.M. (2008) *Generalized, Linear, and Mixed Models*, 2nd ed., John Wiley & Sons, Hoboken, New Jersey.

McGilchrist, C.A. and Aisbett, C.W. (1991) Regression with frailty in survival analysis. *Biometrics*, **47**, 461–466.

McKnight, B. and Crowley, J. (1984) Tests for differences in tumour incidence based on animal carcinogenesis experiments. *Journal of the American Statistical Association*, **79**, 639–648.

Meier, P. (1975) Estimation of a distribution function from incomplete observations. In: *Perspectives in Probability and Statistics* (ed. J. Gani), Academic Press, London, pp. 67–87.

Meira-Machado, L., de Uña-Alvarez, J., Cadarso-Suárez, C. and Andersen, P.K. (2009) Multi-state models for the analysis of time-to-event data. *Statistical Methods in Medical Research*, **18**, 195–222.

Metcalfe, C.R. and Thompson, S.G. (2007) Wei, Lin and Weissfeld's marginal analysis of multivariate failure time data: should it be applied to a recurrent events outcome? *Statistical Methods in Medical Research*, **16**, 103–122.

Miller, A.J. (2002) *Subset Selection in Regression*, 2nd ed., Chapman & Hall/CRC, Boca Raton, Florida.

Moeschberger, M.L. and Klein, J.P. (1995) Statistical methods for dependent competing risks. *Lifetime Data Analysis*, **1**, 195–204.

Montgomery, D.C., Peck, E.A. and Vining, G. (2012) *Introduction to Linear Regression Analysis*, 5th ed., Wiley, New York.

Moreau, T., O'Quigley, J. and Mesbah, M. (1985) A global goodness-of-fit statistic for the proportional hazards model. *Applied Statistics*, **34**, 212–218.

Morgan, B.J.T. (1992) *Analysis of Quantal Response Data*, Chapman & Hall/CRC, London.

Nagelkerke, N.J.D., Oosting, J. and Hart, A.A.M. (1984) A simple test for goodness of fit of Cox's proportional hazards model. *Biometrics*, **40**, 483–486.

Nair, V.N. (1984) Confidence bands for survival functions with censored data: a comparative study. *Technometrics*, **26**, 265–275.

Nardi, A. and Schemper, M. (1999) New residuals for Cox regression and their application to outlier screening. *Biometrics*, **55**, 523–529.

Nelder, J.A. (1977) A reformulation of linear models (with discussion). *Journal of the Royal Statistical Society, A*, **140**, 48–77.

Nelson, K.P., Lipsitz, S.R., Fitzmaurice, G.M., Ibrahim, J., Parzen, M. and Strawderman, R. (2006) Use of the probability integral transformation to fit nonlinear mixed-effects models with nonnormal random effects. *Journal of Computational and Graphical Statistics*, **15**, 39–57.

Nelson, W. (1972) Theory and applications of hazard plotting for censored failure data. *Technometrics*, **14**, 945–965.

Neuberger, J., Altman, D.G., Christensen, E., Tygstrup, N. and Williams, R. (1986) Use of a prognostic index in evaluation of liver transplantation for primary biliary cirrhosis. *Transplantation*, **4**, 713–716.

Nieto, F.J. and Coresh, J. (1996) Adjusting survival curves for confounders: A review and a new method. *American Journal of Epidemiology*, **143**, 1059–1068.

O'Quigley, J. and Pessione, F. (1989) Score tests for homogeneity of regression effect in the proportional hazards model. *Biometrics*, **45**, 135–144.

Ohlssen, D., Sharples, L.D. and Spiegelhalter, D.J. (2007) A hierarchical modelling framework for identifying unusual performance in health care providers. *Journal of the Royal Statistical Society, A*, **170**, 865–890.

Pan, W. (2000) A two-sample test with interval censored data via multiple imputation. *Statistics in Medicine*, **19**, 1–11.

Peng Y. and Dear K.B.G. (2000) A nonparametric mixture model for cure rate estimation. *Biometrics*, **56**, 237–243.

Pepe, M.S. and Mori, M. (1993) Kaplan-Meier, marginal or conditional probability curves in summarizing competing risks failure time data? *Statistics in Medicine*, **12**, 737–751.

Petersen, T. (1986) Fitting parametric survival models with time-dependent covariates. *Applied Statistics*, **35**, 281–288.

Peterson, A.V. (1976) Bounds for a joint distribution function with fixed subdistribution functions: application to competing risks. *Proceedings of the National Academy of Sciences*, **73**, 11–13.

Peto, R. (1972) Contribution to the discussion of a paper by D.R. Cox. *Journal of the Royal Statistical Society, B*, **34**, 205–207.

Peto, R. and Peto, J. (1972) Asymptotically efficient rank invariant procedures. *Journal of the Royal Statistical Society, A*, **135**, 185–207.

Peto, R., Pike, M.C., Armitage, P., Breslow, N.E., Cox, D.R., Howard, S.V., Mantel, N., McPherson, K., Peto, J. and Smith, P.G. (1977) Design and analysis of randomized clinical trials requiring prolonged observation of each patient. II. Analysis and examples. *British Journal of Cancer*, **35**, 1–39.

Pettitt, A.N. and Bin Daud, I. (1989) Case-weighted measures of influence for proportional hazards regression. *Applied Statistics*, **38**, 51–67.

Pettitt, A.N. and Bin Daud, I. (1990) Investigating time dependence in Cox's proportional hazards model. *Applied Statistics*, **39**, 313–329.

Pintilie, M. (2006) *Competing Risks: A Practical Perspective*, John Wiley & Sons, Chichester.

Pintilie, M. (2007a) Analysing and interpreting competing risk data. *Statistics in Medicine*, **26**, 1360–1367.

Pintilie, M. (2007b) Authors reply to letter to the editor from A. Latouche, J. Beyersmann and J.P. Fine. *Statistics in Medicine*, **26**, 3679–3680.

Pocock, S.J. (1983) *Clinical Trials: A Practical Approach*, Wiley, Chichester.

Pollard, A.H., Yusuf, F. and Pollard, G.N. (1990) *Demographic Techniques*, 3rd ed., Pergamon Press, Sydney.

Prentice, R.L. and Gloeckler, L.A. (1978) Regression analysis of grouped survival data with application to breast cancer data. *Biometrics*, **34**, 57–67.

Prentice, R.L. and Kalbfleisch, J.D. (1979) Hazard rate models with covariates. *Biometrics*, **35**, 25–39.

Prentice, R.L., Williams, B.J. and Peterson, A.V. (1981) On the regression analysis of multivariate failure time data. *Biometrika*, **68**, 373–379.

Putter, H. (2011) Special issue about competing risks and multi-state models. *Journal of Statistical Software*, **38**, 1–4.

Putter, H., Fiocco, M. and Geskus, R.B. (2007) Tutorial in biostatistics: Competing risks and multi-state models. *Statistics in Medicine*, **26**, 2389–2430.

Quantin, C., Moreau, T., Asselain, B., Maccario, J. and Lellouch, J. (1996) A regression survival model for testing the proportional hazards hypothesis. *Biometrics*, **52**, 874–885.

R Core Team. (2013) R: A language and environment for statistical computing. *R Foundation for Statistical Computing*, Vienna, Austria. URL http://www.R-project.org/.

Rabe-Hesketh, S. and Everitt, B.S. (2007) *A Handbook of Statistical Analyses Using Stata*, 4th ed., Chapman & Hall/CRC, Boca Raton, Florida.

Ramlau-Hansen, H. (1983) Smoothing counting process intensities by means of kernel functions. *Annals of Statistics*, **11**, 453–466.

Rancel, M.M.S. and Sierra, M.A.G. (2001) Regression diagnostic using local influence: A review. *Communications in Statistics–Theory and Methods*, **30**, 799–813.

Reid, N. and Crépeau, H. (1985) Influence functions for proportional hazards regression. *Biometrika*, **72**, 1–9.

Ripatti, S. and Palmgren, J. (2000) Estimation of multivariate frailty models using penalised partial likelihood. *Biometrics*, **56**, 1016–1022.

Rizopoulos, D. (2012) *Joint Models for Longitudinal and Time-to-Event Data: with Applications in R*, Chapman & Hall/CRC, Boca Raton, Florida.

Robins, J.M. (1993) Information recovery and bias adjustment in proportional hazards regression analysis of randomized trials using surrogate markers. In *Proceedings of the Biopharmaceutical Section*, American Statistical Association, Virginia, 24–33.

Robins, J.M. and Finkelstein, D.M. (2000) Correcting for non-compliance and dependent censoring in an AIDS clinical trial with inverse probability of censoring weighted (IPCW) log rank tests. *Biometrika*, **56**, 779–788.

Robins, J.M. and Rotnitzky, A. (1992) Recovery of information and adjustment for dependent censoring using surrogate markers. In *AIDS Epidemiology–Methodological Issues* (eds. N. Jewell, K. Dietz and V.T. Farewell), Birkhäuser, Boston, 297–331.

Royston, P. (2006) Explained variation for survival models. *The Stata Journal*, **6**, 83–96.

Royston, P. and Altman, D.G. (1994) Regression using fractional polynomials of continuous covariates: parsimonious parametric modelling (with discussion). *Applied Statistics*, **43**, 429–467.

Royston, P. and Lambert, P.C. (2011) *Flexible Parametric Survival Analysis Using Stata: Beyond the Cox Model*, Stata Press, Texas.

Royston, P. and Parmar, M.K.B. (2002) Flexible proportional-hazards and proportional-odds models for censored survival data, with application to prognostic modelling and estimation of treatment effects. *Statistics in Medicine*, **21**, 2175–2197.

Royston, P. and Parmar, M.K.B. (2011) The use of restricted mean survival time to estimate the treatment effect in randomized clinical trials when the proportional hazards assumption is in doubt. *Statistics in Medicine*, **30**, 2409–2421.

Royston, P. and Sauerbrei, W. (2004) A new measure of prognostic separation in survival data. *Statistics in Medicine*, **23**, 723–748.

Rubinstein, L.V., Gail, M.H. and Santner, T.J. (1981) Planning the duration of a comparative clinical trial with loss to follow-up and a period of continued observation. *Journal of Chronic Diseases*, **34**, 469–479.

Satten, G.A., Datta, S. and Robins, J.M. (2001) Estimating the marginal survival function in the presence of time dependent covariates. *Statistics and Probability Letters*, **54**, 397–403.

Sauerbrei, W. and Royston, P. (1999) Building multivariate prognostic and diagnostic models: transformations of the predictors by using fractional polynomials. *Journal of the Royal Statistical Society, A*, **162**, 71–94.

Scharfstein, D.O. and Robins, J.M. (2002). Estimation of the failure time distribution in the presence of informative censoring. *Biometrika*, **89**, 617–634.

Schemper, M. (1992) Cox analysis of survival data with non-proportional hazard functions. *The Statistician*, **41**, 455–465.

Schemper, M. and Stare, J. (1996) Explained variation in survival analysis. *Statistics in Medicine*, **15**, 1999–2012.

Schemper, M., Wakounig, S. and Heinze, G. (2009) The estimation of average hazard ratios by weighted Cox regression. *Statistics in Medicine*, **28**, 2473–2489.

Schlucter, M.D. (1992) Methods for the analysis of informatively censored longitudinal data. *Statistics in Medicine*, **11**, 1861–1870.

Schoenfeld, D.A. (1980) Chi-squared goodness of fit tests for the proportional hazards regression model. *Biometrika*, **67**, 145–153.

Schoenfeld, D.A. (1981) The asymptotic properties of comparative tests for comparing survival distributions. *Biometrika*, **68**, 316–319.

Schoenfeld, D.A. (1982) Partial residuals for the proportional hazards regression model. *Biometrika*, **69**, 239–241.

Schoenfeld, D.A. (1983) Sample-size formula for the proportional-hazards regression model. *Biometrics*, **39**, 499–503.

Schoenfeld, D.A. and Richter, J.R. (1982) Nomograms for calculating the number of patients needed for a clinical trial with survival as an endpoint. *Biometrics*, **38**, 163–170.

Schumacher, M., Bastert, G., Bojar, H., Hübner, K., Olschewski, M., Sauerbrei, W., Schmoor, C., Beyerle, C., Neumann, R.L.A. and Rauschecker, H.F. (1994) Randomized 2×2 trial evaluating hormonal treatment and the duration of chemotherapy in node-positive breast cancer patients. *Journal of Clinical Oncology*, **12**, 2086–2093.

Searle, S.R., Casella, G. and McCulloch, C.E. (2006) *Variance Components*, John Wiley & Sons, Hoboken, New Jersey.

Sellke, T. and Siegmund, D. (1983) Sequential analysis of the proportional hazards model. *Biometrika*, **70**, 315–326.

Shih, J.H. (1995) Sample size calculation for complex clinical trials with survival endpoints. *Controlled Clinical Trials*, **16**, 395–407.

Shih, J.H. (1998) A goodness-of-fit test for association in a bivariate survival model. *Biometrika*, **85**, 189–200.

Shih, J.H. and Louis, T.A. (1995) Inferences on the association parameter in copula models for bivariate survival data. *Biometrics*, **51**, 1384–1399.

Siannis, F. (2004) Applications of a parametric model for informative censoring. *Biometrics*, **60**, 704–714.

Siannis, F. (2011) Sensitivity analysis for multiple right censoring processes: Investigating mortality in psoriatic arthritis. *Statistics in Medicine*, **30**, 356–367.

Siannis, F., Copas, J. and Lu, G. (2005) Sensitivity analysis for informative censoring in parametric survival models. *Biostatistics*, **6**, 77–91.

Simon, R. (1986) Confidence intervals for reporting results of clinical trials. *Annals of Internal Medicine*, **105**, 429–435.

Simon, R. and Lee, Y.J. (1982) Nonparametric confidence limits for survival probabilities and median survival time. *Cancer Treatment Reports*, **66**, 37–42.

Slud, E.V. and Rubinstein, L.V. (1983) Dependent competing risks and summary survival curves. *Biometrika*, **70**, 643–649.

Slud, E.V., Byar, D.P. and Green, S.B. (1984) A comparison of reflected versus test-based confidence intervals for the median survival time based on censored data. *Biometrics*, **40**, 587–600.

Spiegelhalter, D.J. (2005) Funnel plots for comparing institutional performance. *Statistics in Medicine*, **24**, 1185–1202.

Spiegelhalter, D.J., Aylin, P., Best, N.G., Evans, S.J.W. and Murray, G.D. (2002) Commissioned analysis of surgical performance using routine data: lessons from the Bristol inquiry (with discussion). *Journal of the Royal Statistical Society, A*, **162**, 191–231.

Spiegelhalter, D.J., Sherlaw-Johnson, C., Bardsley, M., Blunt, I., Wood, C. and Grigg, O. (2012) Statistical methods for healthcare regulation: rating, screening and surveillance (with discussion). *Journal of the Royal Statistical Society, A*, **175**, 1–47.

Stablein, D.M. and Koutrouvelis, I.A. (1985) A two-sample test sensitive to crossing hazards in uncensored and singly censored data. *Biometrics*, **41**, 643–652.

Stablein, D.M., Carter, W.H., Jr. and Novak, J.W. (1981) Analysis of survival data with nonproportional hazard functions. *Controlled Clinical Trials*, **2**, 148–159.

Stare, J., Perme, M.P. and Henderson, R. (2011) A measure of explained variation for event history data. *Biometrics*, **67**, 750–759.

Storer, B.E. and Crowley, J. (1985) A diagnostic for Cox regression and general conditional likelihoods. *Journal of the American Statistical Association*, **80**, 139–147.

Stroup, W. (2013) *Generalized Linear Mixed Models: Modern Concepts, Methods and Applications*, Chapman & Hall/CRC, Boca Raton, Florida.

Sun, J., Ono, Y. and Takeuchi, Y. (1996) A simple method for calculating the exact confidence interval of the standardized mortality ratio with an SAS function. *Journal of Occupational Health*, **38**, 196–197.

Sun, L., Liu, J., Sun, J. and Zhang, M-J. (2006) Modeling the subdistribution of a competing risk. *Statistica Sinica*, **16**, 1367–1385.

Sy, J.P. and Taylor, J.M.G. (2000) Estimation in a Cox proportional hazards cure model. *Biometrics*, **56**, 227–236.

Tableman, M. and Kim, J.S. (2004) *Survival Analysis Using S: Analysis of Time-to-Event Data*, Chapman & Hall/CRC, Boca Raton, Florida.

Tai, B-C., Machin, D., White, I. and Gebski, V. (2001) Competing risks analysis of patients with osteosarcoma: A comparison of four different approaches. *Statistics in Medicine*, **20**, 661–684.

Taylor, J.M.G. (1995) Semi-parametric estimation in failure time mixture models. *Biometrics*, **51**, 899–907.

Therneau, T. (2014) A package for survival analysis in S. R package version 2.37-7, URL http://CRAN.R-project.org/package=survival.

Therneau, T.M. (1986) The COXREGR Procedure. In: *SAS SUGI Supplemental Library User's Guide*, version 5 ed., SAS Institute Inc., Cary, North Carolina.

Therneau, T.M. and Grambsch, P.M. (2000) *Modelling Survival Data: Extending the Cox Model*, Springer, New York.

Therneau, T.M., Grambsch, P.M. and Fleming, T.R. (1990) Martingale-based residuals for survival models. *Biometrika*, **77**, 147–160.

Therneau, T.M., Grambsch, P.M. and Pankratz, V.S. (2003) Penalized survival models and frailty. *Journal of Computational and Graphical Statistics*, **12**, 156–175.

Thisted, R.A. (1988) *Elements of Statistical Computing*, Chapman & Hall/CRC, London.

Thomas, N., Longford, N.T. and Rolph, J.E. (1994) Empirical Bayes methods for estimating hospital-specific mortality rates. *Statistics in Medicine*, **13**, 889–903.

Thompson, R. (1981) Survival data and GLIM. Letter to the editor of *Applied Statistics*, **30**, 310.

Thomsen, B.L., Keiding, N. and Altman, D.G. (1991) A note on the calculation of expected survival, illustrated by the survival of liver transplant patients. *Statistics in Medicine*, **10**, 733–738.

Tibshirani, R. (1982) A plain man's guide to the proportional hazards model. *Clinical and Investigative Medicine*, **5**, 63–68.

Tibshirani, R. (1996) Regression shrinkage and selection via the lasso. *Journal of the Royal Statistical Society, B*, **58**, 267–288.

Tibshirani, R. (1997) The lasso method for variable selection in the Cox model, *Statistics in Medicine*, **16**, 385–395.

Tseng, Y.K., Hsieh, F. and Wang J.-L. (2005). Joint modeling of accelerated failure time and longitudinal data. *Biometrika*, **92**, 587–603.

Tsiatis, A.A. (1975) A nonidentifiability aspect of the problem of competing risks. *Proceedings of the National Academy of Sciences*, **72**, 20–22.

Tsiatis, A.A. and Davidian, M. (2004) Joint modeling of longitudinal and time-to-event data: An overview. *Statistica Sinica*, **14**, 809–834.

Venables, W.N. and Ripley, B.D. (2002) *Modern Applied Statistics with S*, 4th ed., Springer, New York.

Venables, W.N. and Smith, D.M. (2009) *An Introduction to R*, 2nd ed., Network Theory Limited, Bristol.

Verweij, P.J.M., van Houwelingen, H.C. and Stijnen, T. (1998) A goodness-of-fit test for Cox's proportional hazards model based on martingale residuals. *Biometrics*, **54**, 1517–1526.

Volinsky, C.T. and Raftery, A.E. (2000) Bayesian information criterion for censored survival models, *Biometrics*, **56**, 256–262.

WHO Special Programme of Research, Development and Research Training in Human Reproduction (1987) Vaginal bleeding patterns–The problem and an example data set. *Applied Stochastic Models and Data Analysis*, **3**, 27–35.

Wei, L.J. (1992) The accelerated failure time model: a useful alternative to the Cox regression model in survival analysis. *Statistics in Medicine*, **11**, 1871–1879.

Wei, L.J. and Glidden, D.V. (1997) An overview of statistical methods for multiple failure time data in clinical trials. *Statistics in Medicine*, **16**, 833–839.

Wei, L.J., Lin, D.Y. and Weissfeld, L. (1989) Regression-analysis of multivariate incomplete failure time data by modeling marginal distributions. *Journal of the American Statistical Association*, **84**, 1065–1073.

Weissfeld, L.A. (1990) Influence diagnostics for the proportional hazards model. *Statistics and Probability Letters*, **10**, 411–417.

Weissfeld, L.A. and Schneider, H. (1990) Influence diagnostics for the Weibull model fit to censored data. *Statistics and Probability Letters*, **9**, 67–73.

Weissfeld, L.A. and Schneider, H. (1994) Residual analysis for parametric models fit to censored data. *Communications in Statistics–Theory and Methods*, **23**, 2283–2297.

West, B.T., Welch, K.B. and Galecki, A.T. (2007) *Linear Mixed Models: A Practical Guide Using Statistical Software*, Chapman & Hall/CRC, Boca Raton, Florida.

White, I.R., Royston, P. and Wood, A.M. (2011) Multiple imputation using chained equations: Issues and guidance for practice. *Statistics in Medicine*, **30**, 377–399.

Whitehead, J.R. (1989) The analysis of relapse clinical trials, with application to a comparison of two ulcer treatments. *Statistics in Medicine*, **8**, 1439–1454.

Whitehead, J.R. (1997) *The Design and Analysis of Sequential Clinical Trials*, 2nd ed., Wiley, Chichester.

Wienke, A. (2011) *Frailty Models in Survival Analysis*, Chapman & Hall/CRC, Boca Raton, Florida.

Wolbers, M. and Koller, M.T. (2007) Letter to the editor: Comments on 'Analysing and interpreting competing risk data' by M. Pintilie (original article and author's reply). *Statistics in Medicine*, **26**, 3521–3523.

Wolbers, M., Koller, M.T., Witteman, J.C.M. and Steyerberg, E.W. (2009) Prognostic models with competing risks: Methods and application to coronary risk prediction. *Epidemiology*, **20**, 555–561.

Woodward, M. (2014) *Epidemiology: Study Design and Data Analysis*, 3rd ed., Chapman & Hall/CRC, Boca Raton, Florida.

Wu, M.C. and Carroll, R.J. (1988) Estimation and comparison of changes in the presence of informative right censoring by modelling the censoring process. *Biometrics*, **44**, 175–188.

Yang, S. and Prentice, R.L. (1999) Semiparametric inference in the proportional odds regression model. *Journal of the American Statistical Association*, **94**, 124–136.

Yuan, M. and Lin, Y. (2006) Model selection and estimation in regression with grouped variables, *Journal of the Royal Statistical Society, B*, **68**, 49–67.

Zahl, P.H. (1997) Letter to the editor: Comments on 'Adjusting survival curves for confounders: A review and a new method' by F.J. Nieto and J. Coresh. *American Journal of Epidemiology*, **146**, 605.

Zhang, X., Loberiza, F.R., Klein, J.P. and Zhang, M.-J. (2007) A SAS macro for estimation of direct adjusted survival curves based on a stratified Cox regression model. *Computer Methods and Programs in Biomedicine*, **88**, 95–101.

Index of examples

For each illustrative example used in this book, the number of the example is given, followed by the page number in parentheses.

Index